Brain Disorders in Critical Illness

Mechanisms, Diagnosis, and Treatment

Brain Disorders in Critical Illness

Mechanisms, Diagnosis, and Treatment

Edited by

Robert D. Stevens
Associate Professor, Department of Anesthesiology and Critical Care Medicine; Associate Professor of Neurology,
Neurosurgery and Radiology-Radiological Sciences, Johns Hopkins University School of Medicine, Baltimore, MD, USA

Tarek Sharshar
Professor, Department of Intensive Care Medicine, Raymond Poincaré Hospital, University de Versailles Saint-Quentin-en-Yvelines, Garches, France;
Laboratory of Histopathology and Animal Models, Francois Jacob Centre, Institut Pasteur, Paris, France

E. Wesley Ely
Professor of Medicine, Division of Allergy, Pulmonary, and Critical Care Medicine, Vanderbilt University School of Medicine
and the Geriatric Research Education Clinical Center (GRECC) of Tennessee Valley Veterans Affairs Healthcare System, Nashville, TN, USA

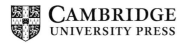

CAMBRIDGE
UNIVERSITY PRESS

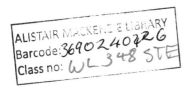
CAMBRIDGE
UNIVERSITY PRESS

University Printing House, Cambridge CB2 8BS, United Kingdom

Published in the United States of America by Cambridge University Press, New York

Cambridge University Press is part of the University of Cambridge.

It furthers the University's mission by disseminating knowledge in the pursuit of education, learning, and research at the highest international levels of excellence.

www.cambridge.org
Information on this title: www.cambridge.org/9781107029194

First published 2013

Printed in the United Kingdom by TJ International Ltd. Padstow Cornwall

A catalogue record for this publication is available from the British Library

ISBN 978-1-107-02919-4 Hardback

Contents

Section 4. Diagnosis of Brain Dysfunction

Section 5. Preventative and Therapeutic Interventions

Section 6. Clinical Encephalopathy Syndromes

Color plate section is between pp. 320 and 321.

Contributors

Ioannis P. Androulakis
Department of Biomedical Engineering, Department of Chemical and Biochemical Engineering, Rutgers University, Piscataway, and Department of Surgery, UMDNJ-Robert Wood Johnson Medical School, New Brunswick, NJ, USA

Djillali Annane
Service de reanimation, hospital Raymond Poincaré (AP-HP), University of Versailles SQY, Garches, France

Gérard Audibert
Department of Anesthesiology and Critical Care, Nancy University Hospital, Nancy, France

Lisa L. Barnes
Departments of Behavioral Sciences and Neurological Sciences, and Rush Alzheimer's Disease Center, Rush University Medical Center, Chicago, IL, USA

Paolo Bartolomeo
INSERM-U 975, Centre de Recherche de l'Institut du Cerveau et de la Moelle Epinière (CRICM) et Université Pierre et Marie Curie (UPMC), Groupe Hospitalier Pitié-Salpêtrière, Paris, France; AP-HP, Groupe Hospitalier Pitié-Salpêtrière, Fédération de Neurologie, Paris, France; Department of Psychology, Catholic University, Milan, Italy

Walter S. Bartynski
Department of Radiology and Radiological Science, Division of Neuroradiology, Medical University of South Carolina, Charleston, SC, USA

David A. Bennett
Professor of Neurological Sciences, Department of Neurological Sciences and Rush Alzheimer's Disease Center, Rush University Medical Center, Chicago, IL, USA

Nicolas Bruder
Department of Anesthesiology and Critical Care, Marseille University Hospital, Marseille, France

Nathan E. Brummel
Division of Allergy, Pulmonary and Critical Care Medicine, Vanderbilt School of Medicine, Nashville, TN, USA

Steve E. Calvano
Department of Surgery, UMDNJ-Robert Wood Johnson Medical School, New Brunswick, NJ, USA

Alain Cariou
Medical Intensive Care Unit, AP-HP, Cochin Hospital, Paris, and Paris Descartes University and Sorbonne Paris Cité Medical School, Paris, France

F. Chretien
Unité "Histopathologie Humaine et Modèles Animaux," Département Infection et Epidémiologie, Institut Pasteur, Paris, and University of Versailles Saint-Quentin-en-Yvelines, Garches, France

Jan Claassen
Division of Neurocritical Care, Neurological Institute of New York, Columbia University Medical Center, New York, NY, USA

Colm Cunningham
Trinity College Institute of Neuroscience and School of Biochemistry and Immunology, Trinity College Dublin, Republic of Ireland

Souhayl Dahmani
AP-HP, Robert Debré University Hospitals, INSERM-U 676, Paris Diderot University, Paris, France

Robert Dantzer
Department of Symptom Research, MD Anderson Cancer Center, Houston, TX, USA

Dimitry S. Davydow
Department of Psychiatry and Behavioral Sciences, University of Washington, Seattle, WA, USA

Sanjay V. Desai
Division of Pulmonary and Critical Care Medicine, The Johns Hopkins University, Baltimore, MD, USA

E. Wesley Ely
Division of Allergy, Pulmonary, and Critical Care Medicine, Vanderbilt University School of Medicine and the Geriatric Research Education Clinical Center (GRECC) of Tennessee Valley Veterans Affairs Healthcare System, Nashville, TN, USA

Frédéric Faugeras
INSERM, ICM Research Center, UMRS 975, Paris, and AP-HP, Groupe Hospitalier Pitié-Salpêtrière, Departments of Neurophysiology and Neurology, Paris, France

Karen J. Ferguson
Neuroimaging Research Fellow, School of Clinical Sciences, University of Edinburgh, UK

Brandon Foreman
Comprehensive Epilepsy Center, Neurological Institute of New York, Columbia University Medical Center, New York, NY, USA

Sadanand M. Gaikwad
Department of Neurology, Clinical Neuroscience Unit, University of Bonn, Bonn, Germany

Rebecca F. Gottesman
Department of Neurology, Johns Hopkins Bayview Medical Center, Baltimore, MD, USA

Maura A. Grega
Research Nurse Program Coordinator, The Johns Hopkins University, Baltimore, MD, USA

Richard D. Griffiths
Emeritus Professor of Medicine (Intensive Care), Whiston Hospital and Department of Musculoskeletal Biology, Institute of Ageing and Chronic Disease, Faculty of Health and Life Sciences, University of Liverpool, Liverpool, UK

Marion Griton
CNRS UMR 5536 Magnetic Resonance of Biological Systems, Victor Segalen Bordeaux 2 University, Bordeaux, France

Stefan D. Gurney
Magill Department of Anaesthesia, Intensive Care, and Pain Medicine, and Department of Anaesthetics, Intensive Care and Pain Medicine, Chelsea & Westminster Hospital, Imperial College London, UK

Hebah M. Hefzy
Department of Neurology, Henry Ford Hospital, Detroit, MI, USA

Michael T. Heneka
Department of Neurology, Clinical Neuroscience Unit, University of Bonn, Bonn, Germany

Dustin M. Hipp
Vanderbilt University School of Medicine, Nashville, TN, USA

Ramona O. Hopkins
Department of Psychology and Neuroscience Center, Brigham Young University, Provo, UT, and Department of Medicine, Pulmonary and Critical Care Division, Intermountain Medical Center, Murray, UT, USA

Christopher G. Hughes
Department of Anesthesiology, Vanderbilt University School of Medicine, Nashville, TN, USA

James C. Jackson
Division of Allergy, Pulmonary, and Critical Care Medicine, and Center for Health Services Research, Vanderbilt University School of Medicine, Nashville, TN, USA

Christina Jones
Nurse Consultant, Intensive Care Rehabilitation, Intensive Care Unit, Whiston Hospital, Prescot, Merseyside, and Honorary Reader, Institute of Ageing and Chronic Disease, Faculty of Health and Life Sciences, University of Liverpool, Liverpool, UK

Peter W. Kaplan
Department of Neurology, Johns Hopkins Bayview Medical Center, Baltimore, MD, USA

Keith W. Kelley
Department of Immunophysiology, University of Illinois at Urbana-Champaign, Urbana, IL, USA

Raymond C. Koehler
Department of Anesthesiology and Critical Care
Medicine, School of Medicine, The Johns Hopkins
University, Baltimore, MD, USA

Matthew A. Koenig
Neurocritical Care, Neuroscience
Institute, The Queen's Medical Center,
Honolulu, HI, USA

Jan Pieter Konsman
CNRS UMR 5536 Magnetic Resonance of Biological
Systems, Victor Segalen Bordeaux 2 University,
Bordeaux, France

Felix Kork
Department of Anaesthesiology and
Intensive Care Medicine, Charité –
Universitätsmedizin Berlin, Campus Virchow
Klinikum and Campus Charité Mitte, Berlin,
Germany

John P. Kress
Department of Medicine, Section of Pulmonary
and Critical Care, University of Chicago, Chicago,
IL, USA

Stephen F. Lowry
Department of Surgery, UMDNJ-Robert Wood
Johnson Medical School, New Brunswick, NJ, USA

Alawi Luetz
Department of Anaesthesiology and
Intensive Care Medicine, Charité –
Universitätsmedizin Berlin, Berlin, Germany

David Luis
Service de reanimation, hospital Raymond Poincaré
(AP-HP), University of Versailles SQY, Garches,
France

Alasdair M. J. MacLullich
Department of Geriatric Medicine, University
of Edinburgh, and Honorary Consultant in General
and Geriatric Medicine, Royal Infirmary of
Edinburgh, UK

Guy M. McKhann
Johns Hopkins University School of Medicine,
Baltimore, MD, USA

Jean Mantz
Department of Anesthesia and Critical Care,
Beaujon-Paris Val de Seine University Hospitals,
Paris, France

Panteleimon D. Mavroudis
Department of Chemical and
Biochemical Engineering, Rutgers University,
Piscataway, NJ, USA

Mervyn Maze
Department of Anesthesia & Perioperative Care,
University of California San Francisco, San
Francisco, CA, USA

Bruno Mégarbane
Medical and Toxicological Critical Care Unit,
Lariboisière Hospital, Paris Diderot University,
INSERM U705, Paris, France

Lionel Naccache
INSERM, ICM Research Center, UMRS 975,
Paris; AP-HP, Groupe Hospitalier Pitié-
Salpêtrière, Departments of
Neurophysiology and Neurology, Paris;
University Paris 6, Faculté de Médecine
Pitié-Salpêtrière, Paris, France

Dale M. Needham
Outcomes After Critical Illness and Surgery
(OACIS) Group, Division of Pulmonary
and Critical Care Medicine, and
Department of Physical Medicine and
Rehabilitation, The Johns Hopkins University,
Baltimore, MD, USA

Pratik P. Pandharipande
Vanderbilt University School of Medicine,
Anesthesia Service, VA TVHS, Nashville,
Nashville, TN, USA

Jean-Francois Payen
Department of Anesthesiology and
Critical Care, Grenoble University Hospital,
Grenoble, France

V. Hugh Perry
Experimental Neuropathology, Centre for
Biological Sciences, University of Southampton,
Southampton, UK

Margaret Pisani
Pulmonary and Critical Care Medicine,
Yale University School of Medicine, New
Haven, CT, USA

C. Rauturier
Unité "Histopathologie Humaine et
Modèles Animaux," Département
Infection et Epidémiologie, Institut
Pasteur, Paris, and University of
Versailles Saint-Quentin-en-Yvelines,
Garches, France

Benjamin Rohaut
Departments of Neurology and Intensive Care Unit,
ICM Research Center INSERM UMRS 975 and
Université Pierre et Marie Curie (Paris VI),
Pitié-Salpêtrière Hospital, Paris, France

Jennifer Ryan
Division of Mucosal Biology and Transplantation
Institute of Liver Studies, Kings College London,
Kings College Hospital, London, UK

Robert D. Sanders
Magill Department of Anaesthesia, Intensive
Care, and Pain Medicine; Department of Anaesthetics,
Intensive Care, and Pain Medicine, Chelsea &
Westminster Hospital, Imperial College London,
and Department of Leukocyte Biology, National
Heart and Lung Institute, Imperial College London,
London, UK

Jeremy D. Scheff
Department of Biomedical Engineering, Rutgers
University, Piscataway, NJ, USA

Frederic Sedel
Department of Neurology, Reference Center for
Lysosomal Diseases, Neurometabolic Function
Unit, Pitié-Salpêtrière Hospital, AP-HP, Paris, and
Université Pierre et Marie Curie (Paris VI), Paris, France

Ola A. Selnes
Department of Neurology, The Johns Hopkins
Hospital, Baltimore, MD, USA

Tarek Sharshar
Department of Intensive Care Medicine, Raymond
Poincaré Hospital, University Versailles Saint-
Quentin-en-Yvelines, Garches, France; Laboratory of
Histopathology and Animal Models, Francois Jacob
Centre, Institut Pasteur, Paris, France

Martin Siegemund
Department of Anaesthesia, Critical Care and Pre-
hospital Emergency Medicine, State Hospital AG,
Baden, Switzerland

Yoanna Skrobik
Département de soins intensifs,
Maisonneuve-Rosemont Hospital, and Critical
Care Medicine, University of Montreal, Montreal,
Quebec, Canada

Jamie W. Sleigh
Department of Anaesthesia, University of
Auckland, Waikato Hospital, Hamilton, New Zealand

Romain Sonneville
Department of Intensive Care Medicine and
Infectious Diseases, Hôpital Bichat-Claude
Bernard, Université Diderot-Paris 7, Paris;
Unité "Histopathologie Humaine et Modèles
Animaux," Département Infection et
Epidémiologie, Institut Pasteur, Paris; University
of Versailles Saint-Quentin-en-Yvelines, Garches,
France

Claudia D. Spies
Department of Anesthesiology and
Intensive Care Medicine, Charité –
Universitätsmedizin Berlin, Campus Virchow
Klinikum und Campus Charité Mitte, Berlin,
Germany

Luzius A. Steiner
Department of Anesthesia, University Hospital Center
and University of Lausanne, Lausanne, Switzerland

Robert D. Stevens
Departments of Anesthesiology and Critical Care
Medicine, and Department of Neurology,
Neurosurgery and Radiology-Radiological Sciences,
Johns Hopkins University School of Medicine,
Baltimore, MD, USA

Raoul Sutter
Departments of Anesthesiology and Critical Care
Medicine, and Department of Neurology, Johns
Hopkins University School of Medicine, Baltimore,
MD, USA

Fabio Silvio Taccone
Department of Intensive Care, Erasme Hospital,
Université Libre de Bruxelles, Bruxelles, Belgium

Richard E. Temes
Department of Neurological Sciences, Rush University
Medical Center, Chicago, IL, USA

Willem A. van Gool
Department of Neurology, Academic Medical Centre,
Amsterdam, the Netherlands

Christel C. Vanbesien
University Lille Nord de France/USTL
(Sciences & Technologies, Lille 1), and INSERM
UMR 837, Molecular events associated to early
stages of Parkinson's disease, Place de Verdun,
Lille, France

F. Verdonk
Unité "Histopathologie Humaine et
Modèles Animaux," Département
Infection et Epidémiologie, Institut
Pasteur, Paris, and University of

Versailles Saint-Quentin-en-Yvelines,
Garches, France

Odile Viltart
University Lille Nord de France/USTL (Sciences &
Technologies, Lille 1), and INSERM UMR 837,
Plasticity and Development of Postnatal Brain, Place
de Verdun, Lille, France

Julia Wendon
Division of Mucosal Biology and Transplantation,
Institute of Liver Studies, Kings College London,
Kings College Hospital, London, UK

Catherine N. Widmann
Department of Neurology, Clinical Neuroscience
Unit, University of Bonn, Bonn, Germany

Robert S. Wilson
Rush Alzheimer's Disease Center, Rush University,
Chicago, IL, USA

Foreword

Jesse Hall, MD
Professor of Medicine, Anesthesia & Critical Care,
Section Chief, Pulmonary and Critical Care Medicine,
University of Chicago,
Chicago, TL, USA

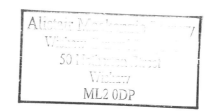

As patients emerge from the terror and abyss of early life-threatening illness, many critical care physicians have learned the wisdom of asking them – or their loved ones when the patient cannot interact and communicate – a simple but probing question: "What do you hope will be achieved by our treatments here in the intensive care unit?" Unfortunately the question is more often asked in those circumstances that lead care providers to predict that the chances for survival and recovery are becoming remote. I believe that if we asked this more routinely, of those dramatically improving and hence lifting our pride in the power of our healing, as well as those dying and bringing us to acknowledge the limitations of our interventions and engaging our commitment to provide comfort to all, the answer would be fairly straightforward and akin to: "To return to my life as I knew it" or "To be myself again."

In my experience our patients and their families show extraordinary realism and resilience. What they mean by those simple statements are not first and foremost that their hearts, and lungs, and kidneys, and limbs all return to their level of function before devastating illness or injury, although this is of course a deep wish. Yes, we discuss whether the dialysis machine or mechanical ventilator will be temporary and if it is to be eventually withdrawn what the path to liberation will entail. But their most fervent wish is to have their loved one return home. And in addition to their return to home and community and job, that they would be the same person, with the personal history, memories, ability to interact, personality and personhood that they recently left behind. In the hierarchy of all of the organs that we discuss on rounds each day when we use our organ- and problem-based approach to organize our findings and plans, they wish most to have their brains back.

Paradoxically, this pre-eminent priority embedded in their simple answers to our question is often precisely what we are least able to address, because we lack insight into what has happened to their brain in the course of critical illness, and what the arc of recovery might be. There are reasons the field of critical care medicine has found itself lacking in response to this patient-oriented outcome and priority. We are a young field of medicine, which arose in response to technology expansion and its geographic concentration in hospital units. Early means were developed and refined by pioneers of the field to halt lethal organ failure, to provide an opportunity to diagnose and treat underlying diseases and return patients to an increasingly stable state. We learned that the interplay of these disease processes and our life-support systems was complex and we wisely chose to define critical illness syndromes characterizing the state of our patients, such as the Systemic Inflammatory Response Syndrome. Careful exploration of organ function under our watch taught us that even when the patient became ill from a seemingly localized problem, such as an inflamed pancreas, coagulation, liver, renal, lung, and brain dysfunctions were more often than not present. We assumed, perhaps overly optimistically, that these organ dysfunctions seemingly acquired during critical illness would be shed if the fundamental problem was properly identified and treated, at least if our patient did not march inexorably into a dreaded state of refractory multi-system organ failure.

Because our healthcare systems lack ideal longitudinal care and follow-up – in fact far from ideal for either patients or care providers – our early hopeful supposition that conditions such as ICU delirium would be temporary and shed as the patient improved was not much tested before our own eyes. However, our increasing success in treating life-threatening illness generated large populations of survivors of critical illness, and this reality coupled with the dedication and insight of early investigators describing long-term outcomes from critical illness have challenged our early halcyon projections of recovery from presumed temporary brain dysfunction. Seminal studies of patients recovering from the acute respiratory distress syndrome (ARDS), understandably focusing upon serial lung function improvement over time, described major neurocognitive and neuropsychiatric problems persisting for years after the lung injury that so captured our attention, even when a clear and defined structural brain injury appeared absent. It was most often these deficits of the brain and psyche that precluded patients from returning to the full aspects of their premorbid lives, and which dominated their assessment of the quality of their lives.

Somewhat late to the table for the reasons stated above, a large multi-disciplinary group of investigators has arisen across the world, bringing the perspectives and tools of critical care medicine, neurology, psychology, psychiatry, pharmacology, neuroimaging, and rehabilitation medicine to this clinical problem. A handful of descriptive studies has now exploded in only a few years to become literally hundreds of publications defining, describing, and exploring the mechanisms of brain dysfunction acquired during and persisting after diverse critical illnesses. Accordingly, it is timely for the creation of a textbook to summarize where we are in this nascent field, and what the best paths to further study and treatment of our patients might be. *Brain Disorders in Critical Illness*, created by senior editors Robert Stevens, Tarek Sharshar, and Wes Ely, is a *tour de force* in the pursuit of this mission.

The assembled authors are leaders from the fields of inquiry needed to address the central questions that have arisen about brain dysfunction in critical illness. The reader will be presented with an organization of material that is logical and thorough. It begins with a section on the epidemiology and outcomes that have been increasingly described in the literature based upon longitudinal study of critically ill patients. It then moves to a series of chapters describing behavioral neurology in the ICU, a necessary preamble to

then describe biological mechanisms for dysfunction of the central nervous system with emphasis on those mechanisms most plausibly operative during the diverse insults that produce critical illness. A series of chapters then address the dilemma of diagnosis. We are still at a point of determining if there are truly unique types of injury occurring during typical treatments in the ICU, or whether we are witnessing injuries akin to those previously described during other processes (e.g., cardiopulmonary bypass, hypoxia, anesthesia), and how we may assemble tools and then definitions to identify at-risk patients during their ICU stay for special attention downstream. While we certainly are early in the course of even understanding this problem (or how many different problems the general observations will yield), the next section addresses some early studies of promising means of preventing and even treating brain dysfunction in the critically ill. Finally, the last section describes those relatively specific encephalopathies (e.g., hepatic encephalopathy, sepsis) that have been the subjects of study in their own right in the past.

Emerging fields benefit enormously from thoughtful pauses that inventory existing information, organize findings into comprehensible frameworks, offer new paradigms for understanding what has been described, and at least name the demon when there are large gaps challenging our understanding. This textbook provides those valuable contributions to the field of critical care medicine, and the authors are to be commended for their accomplishments. It is my hope the book will stimulate as much new thought and discovery as it reviews, and if so it will be poised for an even more exciting second edition in the near future.

Introduction

Tarek Sharshar, E. Wesley Ely, and Robert D. Stevens

In recent years there has been widespread acknowledgment that critical illness has a fundamental neurological dimension. A broad body of work has demonstrated that severe illnesses, possibly in conjunction with practices and interventions in the ICU, are responsible for neurological complications which have a major impact on short- and long-term outcome. This neurological burden is almost certainly an indirect product of intensive care itself, with increasing numbers of patients surviving to the recovery phase of critical illness. Scientific exploration of the relevance and impact of ICU-acquired neurological disorders has been led by an initially small, but rapidly expanding, group of dedicated researchers.

An illustration of this process is the work on delirium which started with observational studies and now includes large, multicenter randomized trials. Delirium is a complex and fascinating syndrome as its pathophysiology, expression, and severity is heavily dependent on the underlying disorder (e.g., sepsis, hepatic failure), while understanding of its biological mechanisms draws on concepts from neurology, neuropharmacology, neuroimmunology, and the cognitive neurosciences. The association between delirium and age- or disease-associated cognitive impairment is clearly reciprocal, possibly implicating subtle shifts between chronic and acute neuroinflammatory states.

Another illustration is anoxic-ischemic encephalopathy resulting from cardiac arrest, which has been the object of a major research effort mobilizing intensivists, neurologists, neurophysiologists, and neuroradiologists in order to develop prognostic models and to assess therapeutic strategies. Anoxic-ischemic encephalopathy is also a clinical paradigm for understanding the biology of consciousness and consciousness disorders.

Critical illnesses are life-threatening disturbances of homeostasis. The central nervous system is a major regulator of homeostasis, responding to physiological challenges via behavioral, neuroendocrine, autonomic, and neuroinflammatory responses. A major task for research in critical illness is to understand the fundamental differences between adaptive and maladaptive homeostatic responses, a task which will require rigorous scientific evaluation of interactions between immunological, endocrine, and autonomic systems. Knowledge of these interactions is likely to yield breakthroughs in the treatment of life-threatening diseases such as sepsis, ARDS, and their associated neurological sequelae.

Collectively, constructs elaborated in this book underscore the central relevance of neuroscience in the realm of critical care medicine, not only for clinicians in the ICU who are routinely facing acute neurological syndromes, but also for clinical and translational researchers who are evaluating novel therapeutic interventions and innovative methods to map brain perturbations via advances in neuroimaging and electrophysiology.

This book provides an overview of brain disorders in critical illness, of which delirium and anoxic-ischemic encephalopathy are emblematic. But the overarching goal is to construct a biological framework for understanding these disorders. It is our conviction that insights and methods developed in neuroscience will be the main driver of scientific progress in the neurology of critical illness. We would like to extend our deepest appreciation to each author for having enthusiastically accepted to contribute to this book. As editors of this "first-ever textbook" synthesizing *Brain Disorders in Critical Illness* we look forward to advances in care that will bring more complete healing to our patients globally as they emerge from ICUs and put the pieces of their lives back together.

Chapter 1

The epidemiology of critical illness brain dysfunction

Raoul Sutter and Robert D. Stevens

SUMMARY

Critically ill patients present with a range of alterations which relate to damage or dysfunction of the central nervous system. Acute brain dysfunction is arguably one of the most common forms of organ failure in the intensive care unit (ICU) and is linked directly to adverse short-term outcome. Mounting evidence points to a range of long-term neurological, cognitive, and behavioral changes which substantially impair quality of life following critical illness. Secular trends demonstrate that mortality following severe illnesses such as sepsis and acute respiratory distress syndrome (ARDS) has declined in the past four decades, resulting in a growing population of long-term ICU survivors with unique physical and psychological characteristics. The purpose of this chapter is to outline the epidemiological features of brain dysfunction in critical illness, distinguishing between acute and post-ICU syndromes.

Introduction

A large proportion of hospitalized adults experience acute brain dysfunction which may manifest as anxiety, agitation, delirium, seizures, focal neurological deficits, or coma. The occurrence of brain dysfunction has been linked to adverse short-term outcomes including hospital mortality and prolonged length of stay [1–3], placing significant burdens on caregivers and healthcare services [4,5]. Acute brain dysfunction may also have long-term consequences, with studies suggesting an association between delirium and an increased likelihood of post-discharge death [6], functional disability [7], institutionalization, cognitive impairment [8,9], and dementia [10]. The risk of delirium is particularly high in selected subsets of hospitalized patients such as the elderly and those with pre-existing cognitive impairments [11], subjects with terminal illnesses [12], patients undergoing major surgery [13], and those who are admitted to the ICU [14]. In this chapter we review the frequency, risk factors, and outcomes of critical illness brain dysfunction with a special emphasis on delirium, coma, and seizures.

Incidence and prevalence

Delirium

Delirium is a pathological alteration in mental status associated with inattention, a fluctuating course, and an underlying systemic illness or metabolic imbalance (Table 1.1) [15,16]. The clinical signs of delirium are protean, increasing the likelihood of under-recognition or misdiagnosis [17]. Estimates of delirium frequency are variable depending on methods of identification and populations studied. The frequency of delirium in non-ICU populations ranges from 10% to 18% on general medicine wards and up to 60% in nursing home populations. The incidence of delirium in the ICU is also variably reported, 11% in one large observational study of surgical ICU patients [18] and up to 82% in a selected medical ICU population [1]. In ICU patients older than 65 years of age, up to 70% were found to have delirium [1,14,19]. In medical ICUs nearly 50% of non-ventilated [20] and 60–82% of mechanically ventilated patients [1,21–23] are reported to have delirium. For surgical ICUs similar estimates ranging from 11% to 63% have been reported [18,24]. In a recent study involving 232 patients in 104 ICUs across 11 countries, the point prevalence of delirium was 32.3% [25].

Table 1.1 Incidence and prevalence of delirium in critical illness.

Reference	Country	Location in hospital	Examination period	Study design	No. of patients enrolled	No. (%) of patients with delirium
[17]	USA	General medical service	12 months	Prospective cohort study	229	50 (22)
[113]	Japan	Medical & surgical ICU	3 months	Prospective cohort study	238	38 (16)
[18]	Turkey	Surgical ICU	2 years	Prospective cohort study	818	90 (11)
[54]	Canada	Medical & surgical ICU	6 months	Prospective cohort study	198	38 (19)
[19]	USA	Medical ICU	8 months	Prospective cohort study	118	51 (43)
[1]; [4]	USA	Medical & cardiac ICU	1 year and 4 months	Prospective cohort study	224	183 (82)
[2]	Taiwan	Medical ICU	6 months	Prospective cohort study	102	22 (22)
[114]	USA	Medical ICU	5 months	Prospective cohort study	143	23 (16)
[20]	USA	Medical ICU	1 year	Prospective cohort study	261	125 (48)
[115]	France	Medical & surgical ICU	8 months	Prospective cohort study	182	95 (52)
[116]	USA	Medical ICU	6 months	Prospective cohort study	93	44 (47)
[117]	Australia and New Zealand	Medical & surgical ICU	6 months	Prospective cohort study	185	84 (45)
[118]	Italy	Surgical ICU	1 year and 4 months	Prospective cohort study	401	117 (29)
[21]	Canada	Medical & surgical ICU	9 months	Prospective cohort study	764	243 (32)
[119]	Canada	Medical & surgical ICU	NA	Prospective cohort study	537	189 (35)
[22]	USA	Medical ICU	2 years	Prospective cohort study	304	214 (70)
[120]	Germany	Surgical ICU	6 months	Prospective cohort study	37	17 (46)
[13]	USA	Surgical ICU	5 months	Prospective cohort study	114	34 (30)
[121]	Taiwan	Medical ICU	8 months	Prospective cohort study	143	31 (21)
[122]	Belgium	Medical & surgical ICU	4 months (Jul–Aug 2006/ Feb–Mar 2007)	Prospective cohort study	172	34 (20)
[23]	USA	Surgical & trauma ICU	3 months	Prospective cohort study	97	68 (70)
[123]	USA	Surgical ICU	4 months	Prospective cohort study	69	41 (59)
[24]	USA	2 surgical ICUs	11 months	Prospective multicenter study	134	84 (63)

Table 1.1 (cont.)

Reference	Country	Location in hospital	Examination period	Study design	No. of patients enrolled	No. (%) of patients with delirium
[124]	UK	Medical & surgical ICU	3 months	Prospective Jan 2008 Retrospective Nov-Dec 2007	71	22 (31)
[125]	the Netherlands	Medical & surgical ICU	3 months	Prospective cohort study	46	23 (50)
[52]	Belgium	Medical & surgical ICU	8 months (Jan–Apr 2007/Jan–Apr 2008)	Prospective cohort study	523	155 (30)
[126]	11 countries	104 ICUs	1 day	Prospective multicenter study	232	75 (32)
[127]	Greece	Medical & surgical ICU	1 year	Prospective cohort study	161	75 (47)
[128]	the Netherlands	Medical & surgical ICU	1 year	Prospective cohort study	1740	332 (19)
[129]	5 countries	Medical & surgical ICU	4 years and 6 months	Prospective multicenter study	354	228 (64)
[130]	Germany	Surgical ICU	8 months (Aug 2006–Nov 2006/ Feb 2007–May 2007)	Prospective cohort study	418	204 (49)
[131]	the Netherlands	Medical & surgical ICU	1 year	Prospective cohort study	1613	411 (26)

NA, not available; ICU, intensive care unit.

Coma

Coma, a state of unarousable unresponsiveness, is frequently seen in patients with severe neurological insults. However, the epidemiology of coma in non-neurological populations is less well investigated (Table 1.2). Among patients older than 65 years admitted to a medical ICU, up to one third were comatose on admission while close to 10% subsequently developed coma during their stay in the ICU [19]. Among 203 prospectively observed patients with chronic critical illness who were admitted to a respiratory care unit, 61 (30%) were found to be comatose [26]. The highest incidence of coma is reported in survivors of cardiac arrest with 80–90% being comatose acutely and 5–30% remaining unconscious at hospital discharge [27]. Coma is also observed in patients with sepsis-associated encephalopathy. In a prospective case series, 9% of patients who had sepsis were found to be comatose, and the level of consciousness was closely related to mortality [28]. In a large prospective cohort of 275 mechanically ventilated patients, 60% were comatose [1]. In another study diminished level of consciousness was related in up to one quarter of patients with failure to separate from mechanical ventilation [29].

Seizures and status epilepticus

Elucidating the true burden of seizure activity (Tables 1.3 and 1.4) in the ICU depends heavily on the method of detection. The preponderance of seizure activity in this population is non-convulsive in nature, and signs of non-convulsive seizure activity may be subtle (fluctuations in mental status, eye deviation, twitching of eyelids) and intermittent, hence overlooked by routine clinical examination or time-limited electroencephalograpy (EEG). The detection of non-convulsive seizures is increased by continuous EEG monitoring [30,31]. Non-convulsive seizure

Table 1.2 Incidence and prevalence of coma in critical illness.

Reference	Country	Location in hospital	Examination period	Study design	No. of patients enrolled	No. (%) of patients with coma
[111]	UK	NA	NA	Prospective cohort study	69 (patients with sepsis)	16 (23)
[59]	Israel	Medical ICU	22 months	Prospective cohort study	50 (patients with sepsis)	8 (16)
[132]	Denmark	Medical & cardiac ICU	8 years	NA	231 (patients with cardiopulmonary resuscitation)	116 (50); 28 (12) remained comatose
[133]	4 countries	412 Medical & surgical ICUs	1 day	Prospective multicenter study	1638 (ventilated patients)	(15)
[14]	USA	Medical & surgical ICU	6 months	Prospective cohort study	96 (patients with delirium)	15 (14)
[19]	USA	Medical ICU	8 months	Prospective cohort study	95 (of 118 patients with more than one assessment during ICU stay)	9 (9)
[1]	USA	Medical & cardiac ICU	1 year and 4 months	Prospective cohort study	275 (ventilated patients)	163 (59)
[26]	USA	Respiratory care unit	2 years and 4 months	Prospective cohort study	203	61 (30)
[109]	USA	Medical & cardiac ICU	4 years	Prospective cohort study	58 (patients with cardiopulmonary resuscitation)	58 (100)

NA, not available; ICU, intensive care unit.

Table 1.3 Incidence and prevalence of seizures in critical illness.

Reference	Country	Location in hospital	Examination period	Study design	No. of patients enrolled	No. (%) of patients with seizures
Seizures during intensive care						
[134]	USA	Medical & cardiac ICU	2 years	Prospective cohort study	1758 (without primary neurologic problem)	61 (4)
[44]	USA	Medical ICU	2, 5 years	Retrospective cohort study	201 (without primary neurologic problem)	21 (10)
Seizures following acute ischemic stroke						
[40]	Australia	Stroke unit	1 year and 5 months	Prospective cohort study	1000 (with acute stroke and TIA)	44 (4)
[32]	France	Medical ICU	NA	Prospective cohort study	1640	90 (5)
[135]	Turkey	Department of Neurology	13 years	Restrospective cohort study	1174	180 (15)
[136]	USA	NA	5 years	Prospective population-based study	904 (with first time stroke)	37 (4) early seizures of hospitalized patients

Table 1.3 (cont.)

Reference	Country	Location in hospital	Examination period	Study design	No. of patients enrolled	No. (%) of patients with seizures
[103]	USA	Neurologic ICU	5 years	Retrospective cohort study	46	3 (6)
Seizures following subarachnoid hemorrhage (SAH)						
[37]	Iceland	NA	11 years	Prospective population based study	44 (with SAH due to ruptured aneurysm and survival >6 months)	10 (23) seizures within 2 weeks after SAH
[34]	Spain	Neurosurgical ICU	7 years	Retrospective cohort study	234	38 (16)
[35]	USA	Neurologic ICU	5 years	Prospective cohort study	247	11 (4)
[33]	USA	Neurologic ICU	7 years	Prospective cohort study	116	17 (15) with non-convulsive seizures
[36]	3 countries	43 care centers	7 years and 8 months	Prospective multicenter study	2143 (with SAH due to ruptured aneurysm)	235 (11) seizures early and late after SAH
Seizures following intracerebral hemorrhage (ICH)						
[42]	China	NA	5 years	Retrospective cohort study	1402	64 (5)
[38]	4 countries	NA	2 years and 10 months	Prospective multicenter study	265	28 (11)
[41]	Italy	Neurologic & medical ICU	18 years	Prospective cohort study	761	57 (7)
[103]	USA	Neurologic ICU	5 years	Retrospective cohort study	63	18 (28)
Seizures following hypoxic-ischemic brain injury (HIE)						
[137]	USA	Medical ICU	8 years	Prospective cohort study	114	41 (36)
Seizures following traumatic brain injury (TBI)						
[138]	USA	NA	5 years	Prospective randomized trial	404	14 (3) within 24 h
[43]	USA	NA	NA	Systematic review	Patients with TBI	(12–50)
[139]	USA	Neurologic ICU	8 years	Prospective cohort study	140 (with TBI and cEEG)	32 (23)

cEEG, continuous electroencephalography; HIE, hypoxic-ischemic brain injury; ICU, intensive care unit; NA, not available; SAH, subarachnoid hemorrhage; TBI, traumatic brain injury; TIA, transient ischemic attack.

activity is described in 5% of patients with acute ischemic stroke [32], in 4–16% of patients with aneurysmal subarachnoid hemorrhage [33–37], in 10–30% of patients with intracerebral hemorrhage [38–42], and in 12–50% with head injury [43]. Seizures may occur in critically ill patients without known neurological illness at admission [44]. In comatose patients without any history of epilepsy, non-convulsive seizure activity

Table 1.4 Incidence and prevalence of status epilepticus in critical illness.

Reference	Country	Location in hospital	Examination period	Study design	No. of patients enrolled	No. (%) of patients with SE
Status epilepticus during intensive care						
[134]	USA	Medical & cardiac ICU	2 years	Prospective cohort study	1758 (without primary neurologic problem)	6 (0.3)
[68]	USA	NA	2 years	Prospective population-based study	166 (with 204 SE episodes)	41–61/100,000 per year
[45]	USA	Medical ICU	2 years	Retrospective cohort study	236 (comatose patients)	19 (8) with NCSE
[31]	Switzerland	Medical ICU	3 years	Retrospective cohort study	537 (performed EEGs)	88 (16) with NCSE
Status epilepticus following acute ischemic stroke						
[135]	Turkey	Department of Neurology	13 years	Restrospective cohort study	1174	7 (0.6)
[136]	USA	NA	5 years	Prospective population-based study	904 (with first time stroke)	10 (1)
[140]	USA	NA	9 years	Retrospective population-based study	718,531	1415 (0.2) GCSE
Status epilepticus following subarachnoid hemorrhage (SAH)						
[33]	USA	Neurologic ICU	7 years	Prospective cohort study	113	12 (11) with NCSE
Status epilepticus following intracerebral hemorrhage (ICH)						
[141]	China	NA	5 years	Retrospective cohort study	1402	11 (1)
[41]	Italy	Neurologic & medical ICU	18 years	Prospective cohort study	761	8 (1)
[140]	USA	NA	9 years	Retrospective population-based study	102,763	266 (0.3) GCSE
Status epilepticus following hypoxic-ischemic encephalopathy (HIE)						
[108]	Switzerland	Medical ICU	7 years and 8 months (retrospective), 2 years (prospective)	107 from a retrospective, 74 from a prospective cohort study	181 (with HIE and treated with therapeutic hypothermia)	6 (3)
[137]	USA	Medical ICU	8 years	Prospective cohort study	114	17 (15) with SE; 19 (17) with myoclonic SE
Status epilepticus following traumatic brain injury (TBI)						
[105]	USA	Neurologic ICU	3 years	Retrospective cohort study	20 (with moderate to severe TBI)	7 of 10 patients with seizures had SE

EEG, electroencephalography; GCSE, generalized convulsive status epilepticus; HIE, hypoxic-ischemic brain injury; ICU, intensive care unit; NA, not available; NCSE, non-convulsive status epilepticus; SAH, subarachnoid hemorrhage; SE, status epilepticus; TBI, traumatic brain injury.

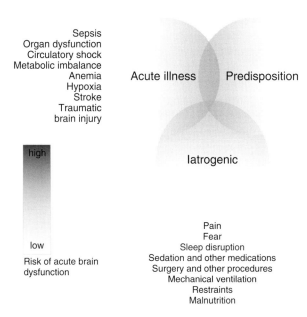

Sepsis
Organ dysfunction
Circulatory shock
Metabolic imbalance
Anemia
Hypoxia
Stroke
Traumatic
brain injury

Acute illness   Predisposition

Genetic predisposition?
Older age
Chronic organ dysfunction
Alcohol/substance use
Psychiatric disorder
Neurologic disorder
Lower educational
attainment

Figure 1.1 The interplay of risk factors for critical illness-associated brain dysfunction.

Iatrogenic

high

low

Risk of acute brain
dysfunction

Pain
Fear
Sleep disruption
Sedation and other medications
Surgery and other procedures
Mechanical ventilation
Restraints
Malnutrition

was detected in 8% of cases [45]. In one observation, over 80% of all status epilepticus was non-convulsive in nature [46].

Risk factors

Delirium

Although the biological mechanisms underlying delirium remain incompletely understood, the identification of risk factors may help develop mechanistic hypotheses. Research indicates that delirium is associated with a broad range of risk factors which may be broadly considered in terms of medical and neurological conditions preceding critical illness, physiological and metabolic alterations induced by critical illness, and iatrogenic exposures in the ICU (Figure 1.1) [47–50].

Delirium develops most commonly in susceptible patients who are exposed to precipitating factors [50]. The probability of developing delirium in the ICU increases after the age of 65 years with the odds of transitioning to delirium rising by 2% for every year above that threshold [51]. Risk factors for the development of delirium include prior cognitive impairment [19,22,52], lower educational achievement [53], malnutrition, stroke, epilepsy, depression, hypertension [21], renal insufficiency [22], smoking [54], alcohol use [21], use of illicit substances [17],

fever, and infections [17,18]. In a prospective multicenter study of 523 patients, the development of delirium was significantly associated with prior cognitive impairment (OR 2.4), smoking (OR 2.0), daily use of more than three units of alcohol (OR 3.2), and living alone (OR 1.9) [52]; environmental risk factors in the ICU were isolation (OR 2.9), the absence of family or friend visits (OR 3.7), the absence of visible daylight (OR 2.4), and the use of physical restraints (OR 33.8) [52].

Coma

Coma results from structural or metabolic alterations affecting brainstem ascending reticular arousal systems (ARAS), diencephalon, or cerebral hemispheres. Structural causes of coma impair consciousness either by directly compressing or destroying the ARAS or by distorting tissues so that they secondarily compress the ARAS or its projections [55]; this may be caused by tumors, hematomas, abscesses, and swelling caused by inflammatory processes. To be associated with coma, lesions must involve bilateral or paramedian brainstem, diencephalon, or hemispheres [55]. Non-structural processes that are associated with coma include pharmacological exposures and intoxication [56–58], sepsis [59], severe metabolic and physiological derangements [60,61], endocrine insufficiency [62,63], as well as cardiopulmonary arrest [64,65].

Different pharmacological agents in particular can interfere with neurotransmitters critically involved in maintaining arousal and awareness: these include cholinergic, glutamatergic, adrenergic, serotoninergic, and histaminergic neurons [66].

Seizures and status epilepticus

Physiologic, metabolic, inflammatory, and pharmacological exposures occurring in the setting of critical illness may decrease the threshold for seizures, possibly via disinhibition of central nervous system neurons. The development of status epilepticus during critical illness might then reflect the unmasking of an underlying, but previously unrecognized epileptic disorder. Status epilepticus has a bimodal age distribution with peaks during the first years of life and during the decades above 60 years of age [67]. Epidemiological studies have identified low subtherapeutic serum levels of antiepileptic drugs in patients with epilepsy, remote brain insults, and acute stroke as the most common risk factors for seizures in hospitalized patients [67–69]. Additional epileptogenic factors include hypoxic-ischemic encephalopathy, metabolic disorders, and history of alcohol abuse [67]. Pharmacologic agents used in critically ill patients have been associated with seizure risk; these include anesthetics [70], antiviral and antibacterial agents (i.e., cephalosporins [71–73], theophylline [74], iphosphamide [75–77]), immunomodulatory drugs (i.e., methotrexate [78]), chemotherapeutic drugs, respiratory agents (i.e., theophylline, phenylpropanolamine [74]), antiarrhythmic drugs, as well as neuroleptics, antidepressants, and lithium [79]. Sleep deprivation and hyperventilation are additional factors which may further increase the risk for seizures.

Outcomes

Delirium

The occurrence of delirium during hospitalization has been associated with adverse outcomes including prolonged hospital stay [1,14,80], institutionalization after hospital discharge [2,81], longer duration of mechanical ventilation [24], and increased risk of death both acutely [1] and in the long term [6]. In a systematic review on delirium in elderly hospitalized patients, Witlox et al. found that delirium was linked to poor outcomes independently of age, comorbid illness, or dementia [82]. The overall hazard ratio for death in this context was reported as high as 1.95 after

a mean follow-up period of 22.7 months. In a meta-analysis, these authors found a nearly two and a half fold increased odds of long-term institutionalization in studies of patients who had delirium when acutely ill. Delirium has also been linked to long-term cognitive impairment. In a recent single-center cohort study of 99 mechanically ventilated patients, severe cognitive impairment was identified in 62% at 3 months and in 36% at 12 months [83]; in this same study, the likelihood of developing cognitive impairment was linked to the duration of delirium in the acute setting. The risk of dementia following delirium has been addressed in only a few studies so far. Witlox et al. found a 12.5 (95% CI, 1.86–84.21) increased odds for the development of dementia in patients who had delirium when hospitalized [82]. In addition to the burden imposed on affected patients, delirium also has a substantial economic impact, reflected by increased costs [4]. Healthcare costs are estimated to be nearly twice as high for hospitalized patients who develop delirium when compared with those who do not [4,5].

Coma

Coma has been identified as a major predictor of death and poor outcomes in patients with ischemic strokes [84], intracerebral hemorrhage (ICH) [85], traumatic brain injury (TBI) [86,87], anoxic brain injury [84,88,89], and sepsis [28, 84]. Coma is a major factor contributing to prolongations in mechanical ventilation and ICU length of stay [90]. In a study of 558 ICU patients, the presence of coma was identified as the strongest independent predictor of death and length of stay besides cardiopulmonary resuscitation and shock [91]. In a sample of almost 16,000 patients, the admission Glasgow Coma Scale (GCS) had a strong but non-linear relationship with hospital mortality [92]; in this study, a low initial GCS in patients with sepsis was associated with a higher mortality than in patients with head trauma [92]. This result was mirrored in a more recent study of 232 patients with sepsis-associated encephalopathy whose 28-day mortality was 56% compared with 35% in septic patients without encephalopathy (p = 0.013) [93].

Seizures and status epilepticus

The case fatality rate in patients with status epilepticus is reported between 3.5% and 46% [46,67,94–96].

Distinguishing the effects of an initial brain insult from the added consequences of epileptic activity is challenging. The overall mortality of status epilepticus is reported from prospective single-center studies between 14% and 20% [97,98], excluding patients with status epilepticus following hypoxic-ischemic encephalopathy, and up to 26% including hypoxic-ischemic encephalopathy [46,67]. For generalized convulsive status epilepticus (GCSE), overall mortality was reported between 3.5% and 18% [99–101], and for non-convulsive status epilepticus (NCSE), 18% [102].

Outcome may depend not only on the type of seizures, but also on the underlying condition. For example, NCSE or seizures have been demonstrated to increase mortality in patients with TBI and with ICH [103,104]. Seizures emerging after TBI are associated with episodic or long-lasting increases of intracranial pressure [105] while seizures complicating ICH have been associated with hematoma expansion [106]. In anoxic-ischemic encephalopathy, the emergence of seizures and *malignant* EEG patterns are independent predictors for poor outcome [107–109]. Continuous EEG monitoring provides independent prognostic information in patients with poor-grade subarachnoid hemorrhage (SAH), even after controlling for clinical and neuroradiological indices of severity [33]. Seizures following ischemic stroke are related to increased resources utilization and decreasing 30-day and 1-year survival [110]. In patients with sepsis who are monitored with EEG, non-convulsive seizures and periodic epileptiform discharges are detected frequently and are also shown to be associated with poor outcome [44]. Furthermore, EEG abnormalities are linked with the severity of brain dysfunction in septic encephalopathic patients and correlate with dysfunction of other organs [111,112]. Initial diffuse slowing in the theta range (waves of 4–8 Hz) is seen in patients with mild encephalopathy, while diffuse marked slowing in the delta range (waves of less than 4 Hz), then generalized emergence of triphasic waves, and finally suppression or a generalized burst-suppression pattern are seen in more severe forms of encephalopathy.

References

1. Ely EW, Shintani A, Truman B, *et al.* Delirium as a predictor of mortality in mechanically ventilated patients in the intensive care unit. *JAMA* 2004;**291**(14):1753–62.

2. Lin S, Liu C, Wang C, *et al.* The impact of delirium on the survival of mechanically ventilated patients. *Crit Care Med* 2004;**32**(11):2254–9.

3. Pompei P, Foreman M, Rudberg MA, *et al.* Delirium in hospitalized older persons: outcomes and predictors. *J Am Geriatr Soc* 1994;**42**(8):809–15.

4. Milbrandt EB, Deppen S, Harrison PL, *et al.* Costs associated with delirium in mechanically ventilated patients. *Crit Care Med* 2004;**32**(4):955–62.

5. Leslie DL, Marcantonio ER, Zhang Y, Leo-Summers L, Inouye SK. One-year health care costs associated with delirium in the elderly population. *Arch Intern Med* 2008;**168**(1):27–32.

6. Pisani MA, Kong SY, Kasl SV, *et al.* Days of delirium are associated with 1-year mortality in an older intensive care unit population. *Am J Respir Crit Care Med* 2009;**180**(11):1092–7.

7. O'Keeffe S, Lavan J. The prognostic significance of delirium in older hospital patients. *J Am Geriatr Soc* 1997;**45**(2):174–8.

8. Girard TD, Jackson JC, Pandharipande PP, *et al.* Delirium as a predictor of long-term cognitive impairment in survivors of critical illness. *Crit Care Med* 2010;**38**(7):1513–20.

9. Saczynski JS, Marcantonio ER, Quach L, *et al.* Cognitive trajectories after postoperative delirium. *N Engl J Med* 2012;**367**(1):30–9.

10. Witlox J, Eurelings LS, de Jonghe JF, *et al.* Delirium in elderly patients and the risk of postdischarge mortality, institutionalization, and dementia: a meta-analysis. *JAMA* 2010;**304**(4):443–51.

11. Levkoff SE, Evans DA, Liptzin B, *et al.* Delirium. The occurrence and persistence of symptoms among elderly hospitalized patients. *Arch Intern Med* 1992;**152**(2):334–40.

12. Lawlor PG, Gagnon B, Mancini IL, *et al.* Occurrence, causes, and outcome of delirium in patients with advanced cancer: a prospective study. *Arch Intern Med* 2000;**160**(6):786–94.

13. Balas MC, Happ MB, Yang W, Chelluri L, Richmond T. Outcomes associated with delirium in older patients in surgical ICUs. *Chest* 2009;**135**(1):18–25.

14. Ely EW, Inouye SK, Bernard GR, *et al.* Delirium in mechanically ventilated patients: validity and reliability of the confusion assessment method for the intensive care unit (CAM-ICU). *JAMA* 2001;**286**(21):2703–10.

15. Inouye SK, Viscoli CM, Horwitz RI, Hurst LD, Tinetti ME. A predictive model for delirium in hospitalized elderly medical patients based on admission characteristics. *Ann Intern Med* 1993;**119**(6):474–81.

16. American Psychiatric Association. *Task Force on DSM-IV: Diagnostic and Statistical Manual of Mental Disorders, Fourth edition, Text Revision* (DSM–IV–TR) Washington, DC: American Psychiatric Association; 2000.

17. Francis J, Martin D, Kapoor WN. A prospective study of delirium in hospitalized elderly. *JAMA* 1990;**263**(8):1097–101.

18. Aldemir M, Ozen S, Kara IH, Sir A, Bac B. Predisposing factors for delirium in the surgical intensive care unit. *Crit Care* 2001;**5**(5):265–70.

19. McNicoll L, Pisani MA, Zhang Y, et al. Delirium in the intensive care unit: occurrence and clinical course in older patients. *J Am Geriatr Soc* 2003;**51**(5):591–8.

20. Thomason JW, Shintani A, Peterson JF, et al. Intensive care unit delirium is an independent predictor of longer hospital stay: a prospective analysis of 261 non-ventilated patients. *Crit Care* 2005;**9**(4):R375–81.

21. Ouimet S, Kavanagh BP, Gottfried SB, Skrobik Y. Incidence, risk factors and consequences of ICU delirium. *Intensive Care Med* 2007;**33**(1):66–73.

22. Pisani MA, Murphy TE, Van Ness PH, Araujo KL, Inouye SK. Characteristics associated with delirium in older patients in a medical intensive care unit. *Arch Intern Med* 2007;**167**(15):1629–34.

23. Pandharipande P, Cotton BA, Shintani A, et al. Prevalence and risk factors for development of delirium in surgical and trauma intensive care unit patients. *J Trauma* 2008;**65**(1):34–41.

24. Lat I, McMillian W, Taylor S, et al. The impact of delirium on clinical outcomes in mechanically ventilated surgical and trauma patients. *Crit Care Med* 2009;**37**(6):1898–905.

25. Salluh JI, Soares M, Teles JM, et al. Delirium epidemiology in critical care (DECCA): an international study. *Crit Care* 2010;**14**(6):R210.

26. Nelson JE, Tandon N, Mercado AF, et al. Brain dysfunction: another burden for the chronically critically ill. *Arch Intern Med* 2006;**166**(18):1993–9.

27. Puttgen HA, Geocadin R. Predicting neurological outcome following cardiac arrest. *J Neurol Sci* 2007;**261**(1–2):108–17.

28. Eidelman LA, Putterman D, Putterman C, Sprung CL. The spectrum of septic encephalopathy. *JAMA* 1996;**275**(6):470–3.

29. Kelly BJ, Matthay MA. Prevalence and severity of neurologic dysfunction in critically ill patients. Influence on need for continued mechanical ventilation. *Chest* 1993;**104**(6):1818–24.

30. Towne AR, Waterhouse EJ, Boggs JG, et al. Prevalence of nonconvulsive status epilepticus in comatose patients. *Neurology* 2000;**54**(2):340–5.

31. Sutter R, Fuhr P, Grize L, Marsch S, Rüegg S. Continuous video-EEG monitoring increases detection rate of nonconvulsive status epilepticus in the ICU. *Epilepsia* 2011;**52**(3):453–7.

32. Giroud M, Gras P, Fayolle H, et al. Early seizures after acute stroke: a study of 1,640 cases. *Epilepsia* 1994;**35**(5):959–64.

33. Claassen J, Hirsch LJ, Frontera JA, et al. Prognostic significance of continuous EEG monitoring in patients with poor-grade subarachnoid hemorrhage. *Neurocrit Care* 2006;**4**(2):103–12.

34. Martinez-Manas R, Ibanez G, Macho J, Gaston F, Ferrer E: [A study of 234 patients with subarachnoid hemorrhage of aneurysmic and cryptogenic origin]. *Neurocirugia (Astur)* 2002;**13**(3):181–93; discussion 193–5.

35. Claassen J, Peery S, Kreiter KT, et al. Predictors and clinical impact of epilepsy after subarachnoid hemorrhage. *Neurology* 2003;**60**(2):208–14.

36. Hart Y, Sneade M, Birks J, et al. Epilepsy after subarachnoid hemorrhage: the frequency of seizures after clip occlusion or coil embolization of a ruptured cerebral aneurysm. *J Neurosurg* 2011;**115**(6):1159–68.

37. Olafsson E, Gudmundsson G, Hauser WA. Risk of epilepsy in long-term survivors of surgery for aneurysmal subarachnoid hemorrhage: a population-based study in Iceland. *Epilepsia* 2000;**41**(9):1201–5.

38. Bladin CF, Alexandrov AV, Bellavance A, et al. Seizures after stroke: a prospective multicenter study. *Arch Neurol* 2000;**57**(11):1617–22.

39. Faught E, Peters D, Bartolucci A, Moore L, Miller PC. Seizures after primary intracerebral hemorrhage. *Neurology* 1989;**39**(8):1089–93.

40. Kilpatrick CJ, Davis SM, Tress BM, et al. Epileptic seizures in acute stroke. *Arch Neurol* 1990;**47**(2):157–60.

41. Passero S, Rocchi R, Rossi S, Ulivelli M, Vatti G. Seizures after spontaneous supratentorial intracerebral hemorrhage. *Epilepsia* 2002;**43**(10):1175–80.

42. Sung CY, Chu NS. Epileptic seizures in intracerebral haemorrhage. *J Neurol Neurosurg Psychiatry* 1989;**52**(11):1273–6.

43. Yablon SA. Posttraumatic seizures. *Arch Phys Med Rehabil* 1993;**74**(9):983–1001.

44. Oddo M, Carrera E, Claassen J, Mayer SA, Hirsch LJ. Continuous electroencephalography in the medical intensive care unit. *Crit Care Med* 2009;**37**(6):2051–6.

45. Towne AR, Waterhouse EJ, Boggs JG, et al. Prevalence of nonconvulsive status epilepticus in comatose patients. *Neurology* 2000;**54**(2):340–5.

46. Rudin D, Grize L, Schindler C, *et al.* High prevalence of nonconvulsive and subtle status epilepticus in an ICU of a tertiary care center: a three-year observational cohort study. *Epilepsy Res* 2011;**96**(1–2):140–50.

47. Milbrandt EB, Angus DC. Potential mechanisms and markers of critical illness-associated cognitive dysfunction. *Curr Opin Crit Care* 2005;**11**(4):355–9.

48. Pustavoitau A, Stevens RD. Mechanisms of neurologic failure in critical illness. *Crit Care Clin* 2008;**24**(1):1–24.

49. Trzepacz PT. Update on the neuropathogenesis of delirium. *Dement Geriatr Cogn Disord* 1999;**10** (5):330–4.

50. Inouye SK. Delirium in older persons. *N Engl J Med* 2006;**354**(11):1157–65.

51. Pandharipande P, Shintani A, Peterson J, *et al.* Lorazepam is an independent risk factor for transitioning to delirium in intensive care unit patients. *Anesthesiology* 2006;**104**(1):21–6.

52. Van Rompaey B, Elseviers MM, Schuurmans MJ, *et al.* Risk factors for delirium in intensive care patients: a prospective cohort study. *Crit Care* 2009;**13**(3):R77.

53. Marcantonio ER, Goldman L, Mangione CM, *et al.* A clinical prediction rule for delirium after elective noncardiac surgery. *JAMA* 1994;**271**(2):134–9.

54. Dubois MJ, Bergeron N, Dumont M, Dial S, Skrobik Y. Delirium in an intensive care unit: a study of risk factors. *Intensive Care Med* 2001;**27**(8):1297–304.

55. Posner JB, Saper CB, Schiff ND, Plum F. Examination of the comatose patient. In *Plum and Posner's Diagnosis of Stupor and Coma.* 4th edn. New York, NY: Oxford University Press; 2007:38–87.

56. Carroll WM, Mastiglia FL. Alpha and beta coma in drug intoxication. *Br Med J* 1977;**2**(6101):1518–19.

57. Goddard J, Bloom SR, Frackowiak RS, *et al.* Lithium intoxication. *Br Med J* 1991;**302**(6787):1267–9.

58. Andersen GO, Ritland S. Life threatening intoxication with sodium valproate. *J Clin Toxicol* 1995;**33**(3):279–84.

59. Eidelman LA, Putterman D, Putterman C, Sprung CL. The spectrum of septic encephalopathy. Definitions, etiologies, and mortalities. *JAMA* 1996;**275**(6):470–3.

60. Shawcross DL, Wendon JA. The neurological manifestations of acute liver failure. *Neurochem Int* 2012;**60**(7):662–71.

61. Seifter JL, Samuels MA. Uremic encephalopathy and other brain disorders associated with renal failure. *Semin Neurol* 2011;**31**(2):139–43.

62. Mahon WA, Holland J, Urowitz MB. Hyperosmolar, non-ketotic diabetic coma. *Can Med Assoc J* 1968;**99**(22):1090–2.

63. Dutta P, Bhansali A, Masoodi SR, *et al.* Predictors of outcome in myxoedema coma: a study from a tertiary care centre. *Crit Care* 2008;**12**(1):R1. doi: 10.1186/cc6211.

64. Mani R, Schmitt SE, Mazer M, Putt ME, Gaieski DF. The frequency and timing of epileptiform activity on continuous electroencephalogram in comatose post-cardiac arrest syndrome patients treated with therapeutic hypothermia. *Resuscitation* 2012;**83**(7):840–7.

65. Zandbergen EGJ. Postanoxic coma: how (long) should we treat? *Eur J Anaesthesiol Suppl* 2008;**42**:39–42.

66. Clauss RP. Neurotransmitters in disorders of consciousness and brain damage. *Medical Hypotheses* 2011;**77**(2):209–13.

67. DeLorenzo RJ, Hauser WA, Towne AR, *et al.* A prospective, population-based epidemiologic study of status epilepticus in Richmond, Virginia. *Neurology* 1996;**46**(4):1029–35.

68. DeLorenzo RJ, Pellock JM, Towne AR, Boggs JG. Epidemiology of status epilepticus. *J Clin Neurophysiol* 1995;**12**(4):316–25.

69. Knake S, Rochon J, Fleischer S, *et al.* Status epilepticus after stroke is associated with increased long-term case fatality. *Epilepsia* 2006;**47**(12):2020–6.

70. Emre M, Walser H, Baumgartner G. Non-convulsive status epilepticus after abrupt withdrawal of hypnotic-sedative drugs. *Eur Arch Psychiatry Neurol Sci* 1985;**235**(1):21–5.

71. Anzellotti F, Ricciardi L, Monaco D, *et al.* Cefixime-induced nonconvulsive status epilepticus. *Neurolog Sci* 2012;**33**(2):325–9.

72. Dixit S, Kurle P, Buyan-Dent L, Sheth RD. Status epilepticus associated with cefepime. *Neurology* 2000;**54**(11):2153–5.

73. Thabet F, Al Maghrabi M, Al Barraq A, Tabarki B. Cefepime-induced nonconvulsive status epilepticus: case report and review. *Neurocrit Care* 2009;**10**(3):347–51.

74. Krieger AC, Takeyasu M. Nonconvulsive status epilepticus in theophylline toxicity. *J Clin Toxicol* 1999;**37**(1):99–101.

75. Kilickap S, Cakar M, Onal IK, *et al.* Nonconvulsive status epilepticus due to ifosfamide. *Ann Pharmacother* 2006;**40**(2):332–5.

76. Primavera A, Audenino D, Cocito L. Ifosfamide encephalopathy and nonconvulsive status epilepticus. *Can J Neurol Sci* 2002;**29**(2):180–3.

77. Bhardwaj A, Badesha PS. Ifosfamide-induced nonconvulsive status epilepticus. *Ann Pharmacother* 1995;**29**(12):1237–9.

78. Patterson DM, Aries J, Hyare H, *et al*. Nonconvulsive status epilepticus and leucoencephalopathy after high-dose methotrexate. *J Clin Oncol* 2011;**29**(16): e459–461.

79. Ruffmann C, Bogliun G, Beghi E. Epileptogenic drugs: a systematic review. *Expert Rev Neurotherapeut* 2006;**6**(4):575–89.

80. Ely EW, Gautam S, Margolin R, *et al*. The impact of delirium in the intensive care unit on hospital length of stay. *Intensive Care Med* 2001;**27**(12):1892–900.

81. McAvay GJ, Van Ness PH, Bogardus ST, Jr., *et al*. Older adults discharged from the hospital with delirium: 1-year outcomes. *J Am Geriatr Soc* 2006;**54**(8):1245–50.

82. Witlox J, Eurelings LSM, de Jonghe JFM, *et al*. Delirium in elderly patients and the risk of postdischarge mortality, institutionalization, and dementia: a meta-analysis. *JAMA* 2010;**304**(4):443–51.

83. Girard TD, Jackson JC, Pandharipande PP, *et al*. Delirium as a predictor of long-term cognitive impairment in survivors of critical illness. *Crit Care Med* 2010;**38**(7):1513–20.

84. Sacco RL, Van Gool R, Mohr JP, Hauser WA. Nontraumatic coma. Glasgow Coma Score and coma etiology as predictors of 2-week outcome. *Arch Neurol* 1990;**47**(11):1181–4.

85. Tuhrim S, Dambrosia JM, Price TR, *et al*. Prediction of intracerebral hemorrhage survival. *Ann Neurol* 1988;**24**(2):258–63.

86. Teasdale G, Jennett B. Assessment of coma and impaired consciousness. A practical scale. *Lancet* 1974;**304**(7872):81–4.

87. Perel P, Arango M, Clayton T, *et al*. Predicting outcome after traumatic brain injury: practical prognostic models based on large cohort of international patients. *Br Med J* 2008;**336**(7641):425–9.

88. Levy DE, Caronna JJ, Singer BH, *et al*. Predicting outcome from hypoxic-ischemic coma. *JAMA* 1985;**253**(10):1420–6.

89. Booth CM, Boone RH, Tomlinson G, Detsky AS. Is this patient dead, vegetative, or severely neurologically impaired? Assessing outcome for comatose survivors of cardiac arrest. *JAMA* 2004;**291**(7):870–9.

90. Rimachi R, Vincent JL, Brimioulle S. Survival and quality of life after prolonged intensive care unit stay. *Anaesth Intensive Care* 2007;**35**(1):62–7.

91. Teres D, Brown RB, Lemeshow S. Predicting mortality of intensive care unit patients. The importance of coma. *Crit Care Med* 1982;**10**(2):86–95.

92. Bastos PG, Sun X, Wagner DP, Wu AW, Knaus WA. Glasgow Coma Scale score in the evaluation of outcome in the intensive care unit: findings from the Acute Physiology and Chronic Health Evaluation III study. *Crit Care Med* 1993;**21**(10):1459–65.

93. Zhang LN, Wang XT, Ai YH, *et al*. Epidemiological features and risk factors of sepsis-associated encephalopathy in intensive care unit patients: 2008–2011. *Chinese Med J* 2012;**125**(5):828–31.

94. DeLorenzo RJ, Kirmani B, Deshpande LS, *et al*. Comparisons of the mortality and clinical presentations of status epilepticus in private practice community and university hospital settings in Richmond, Virginia. *Seizure* 2009;**18**(6):405–11.

95. Knake S, Rosenow F, Vescovi M, *et al*. Incidence of status epilepticus in adults in Germany: a prospective, population-based study. *Epilepsia* 2001;**42**(6):714–18.

96. Shorvon SD. Prognosis and outcome of status epilepticus. In *Status Epilepticus: Its Clinical Features and Treatment in Children and Adults*. Cambridge: Cambridge University Press; 1994:293–312.

97. Novy J, Logroscino G, Rossetti AO. Refractory status epilepticus: a prospective observational study. *Epilepsia* 2010;**51**(2):251–6.

98. Alvarez V, Januel JM, Burnand B, Rossetti AO. Role of comorbidities in outcome prediction after status epilepticus. *Epilepsia* 2012;**53**(5):e89–92.

99. Waterhouse EJ, Garnett LK, Towne AR, *et al*. Prospective population-based study of intermittent and continuous convulsive status epilepticus in Richmond, Virginia. *Epilepsia* 1999;**40**(6):752–8.

100. Sagduyu A, Tarlaci S, Sirin H. Generalized tonic-clonic status epilepticus: causes, treatment, complications and predictors of case fatality. *J Neurol* 1998;**245**(10):640–6.

101. Koubeissi M, Alshekhlee A. In-hospital mortality of generalized convulsive status epilepticus: a large US sample. *Neurology* 2007;**69**(9):886–93.

102. Shneker BF, Fountain NB. Assessment of acute morbidity and mortality in nonconvulsive status epilepticus. *Neurology* 2003;**61**(8):1066–73.

103. Vespa PM, O'Phelan K, Shah M, *et al*. Acute seizures after intracerebral hemorrhage: a factor in progressive midline shift and outcome. *Neurology* 2003;**60**(9):1441–6.

104. Vespa PM, Nuwer MR, Nenov V, *et al*. Increased incidence and impact of nonconvulsive and convulsive seizures after traumatic brain injury as detected by continuous electroencephalographic monitoring. *J Neurosurg* 1999;**91**(5):750–60.

105. Vespa PM, Miller C, McArthur D, *et al*. Nonconvulsive electrographic seizures after traumatic brain injury

result in a delayed, prolonged increase in intracranial pressure and metabolic crisis. *Crit Care Med* 2007;**35**(12):2830–6.

106. Claassen J, Jette N, Chum F, *et al.* Electrographic seizures and periodic discharges after intracerebral hemorrhage. *Neurology* 2007;**69**(13):1356–65.

107. Chen R, Bolton CF, Young B. Prediction of outcome in patients with anoxic coma: a clinical and electrophysiologic study. *Crit Care Med* 1996;**24** (4):672–8.

108. Rossetti AO, Oddo M, Liaudet L, Kaplan PW. Predictors of awakening from postanoxic status epilepticus after therapeutic hypothermia. *Neurology* 2009;**72**(8):744–9.

109. Geocadin RG, Buitrago MM, Torbey MT, *et al.* Neurologic prognosis and withdrawal of life support after resuscitation from cardiac arrest. *Neurology* 2006;**67**(1):105–8.

110. Burneo JG, Fang J, Saposnik G. Impact of seizures on morbidity and mortality after stroke: a Canadian multi-centre cohort study. *Eur J Neurol* 2010;**17**(1):52–8.

111. Young GB, Bolton CF, Austin TW, *et al.* The encephalopathy associated with septic illness. *Clin Invest Med* 1990;**13**(6):297–304.

112. Young GB, Bolton CF, Archibald YM, Austin TW, Wells GA. The electroencephalogram in sepsis-associated encephalopathy. *J Clin Neurophysiol* 1992;**9**(1):145–52.

113. Kishi Y, Iwasaki Y, Takezawa K, Kurosawa H, Endo S. Delirium in critical care unit patients admitted through an emergency room. *Gen Hosp Psychiatry* 1995,**17**(5):371–9.

114. Woods JC, Mion LC, Connor JT, *et al.* Severe agitation among ventilated medical intensive care unit patients: frequency, characteristics and outcomes. *Intensive Care Med* 2004;**30**(6):1066–72.

115. Jaber S, Chanques G, Altairac C, *et al.* A prospective study of agitation in a medical-surgical ICU: incidence, risk factors, and outcomes. *Chest* 2005;**128**(4):2749–57.

116. Micek ST, Anand NJ, Laible BR, Shannon WD, Kollef MH. Delirium as detected by the CAM-ICU predicts restraint use among mechanically ventilated medical patients. *Crit Care Med* 2005;**33**(6):1260–5.

117. Roberts B, Rickard CM, Rajbhandari D, *et al.* Multicentre study of delirium in ICU patients using a simple screening tool. *Aust Crit Care: Confed Aust Crit Care Nurses J* 2005;**18**(1):6, 8–9, 11–14 passim.

118. Ranhoff AH, Rozzini R, Sabatini T, *et al.* Delirium in a sub-intensive care unit for the elderly: occurrence and risk factors. *Aging Clin Exper Res* 2006;**18**(5):440–5.

119. Marquis F, Ouimet S, Riker R, Cossette M, Skrobik Y. Individual delirium symptoms: do they matter? *Crit Care Med* 2007;**35**(11):2533–7.

120. Plaschke K, Hill H, Engelhardt R, *et al.* EEG changes and serum anticholinergic activity measured in patients with delirium in the intensive care unit. *Anaesthesia* 2007;**62**(12):1217–23.

121. Lin SM, Huang CD, Liu CY, *et al.* Risk factors for the development of early-onset delirium and the subsequent clinical outcome in mechanically ventilated patients. *J Crit Care* 2008;**23**(3):372–9.

122. Van Rompaey B, Schuurmans MJ, Shortridge-Baggett LM, *et al.* A comparison of the CAM-ICU and the NEECHAM Confusion Scale in intensive care delirium assessment: an observational study in non-intubated patients. *Crit Care* 2008;**12**(1):R16.

123. Angles EM, Robinson TN, Biffl WL, *et al.* Risk factors for delirium after major trauma. *Am J Surg* 2008;**196**(6):864–9; discussion 869–70.

124. Page VJ, Navarange S, Gama S, McAuley DF. Routine delirium monitoring in a UK critical care unit. *Crit Care* 2009;**13**(1):R16.

125. Spronk PE, Riekerk B, Hofhuis J, Rommes JH. Occurrence of delirium is severely underestimated in the ICU during daily care. *Intensive Care Med* 2009;**35**(7):1276–80.

126. Salluh JI, Soares M, Teles JM, *et al.* Delirium epidemiology in critical care (DECCA): an international study. *Crit Care* 2010;**14**(6):R210.

127. Kiekkas P, Samios A, Skartsani C, Tsotas D, Baltopoulos GI. Fever and agitation in elderly ICU patients: a descriptive study. *Intensive Crit Care Nurs* 2010;**26**(3):169–74.

128. van den Boogaard M, Peters SA, van der Hoeven JG, *et al.* The impact of delirium on the prediction of in-hospital mortality in intensive care patients. *Crit Care* 2010;**14**(4):R146.

129. Shehabi Y, Riker RR, Bokesch PM, *et al.* Delirium duration and mortality in lightly sedated, mechanically ventilated intensive care patients. *Crit Care Med* 2010;**38**(12):2311–18.

130. Heymann A, Radtke F, Schiemann A, *et al.* Delayed treatment of delirium increases mortality rate in intensive care unit patients. *J Int Med Res* 2010;**38** (5):1584–95.

131. van den Boogaard M, Pickkers P, Slooter AJ, *et al.* Development and validation of PRE-DELIRIC (PREdiction of DELIRium in ICu patients) delirium prediction model for intensive care patients: observational multicentre study. *Br Med J* 2012;**344**:e420.

132. Jorgensen EO, Holm S. The natural course of neurological recovery following

cardiopulmonary resuscitation. *Resuscitation* 1998;**36**(2):111–22.

133. Esteban A, Anzueto A, Alia I, *et al.* How is mechanical ventilation employed in the intensive care unit? An international utilization review. *Am J Respir Crit Care Med* 2000;**161**(5):1450–8.

134. Bleck TP, Smith MC, Pierre-Louis SJ, *et al.* Neurologic complications of critical medical illnesses. *Crit Care Med* 1993;**21**(1):98–103.

135. Velioglu SK, Ozmenoglu M, Boz C, Alioglu Z. Status epilepticus after stroke. *Stroke* 2001;**32**(5):1169–72.

136. Labovitz DL, Hauser WA, Sacco RL. Prevalence and predictors of early seizure and status epilepticus after first stroke. *Neurology* 2001;**57**(2):200–6.

137. Krumholz A, Stern BJ, Weiss HD. Outcome from coma after cardiopulmonary resuscitation: relation to seizures and myoclonus. *Neurology* 1988;**38**(3):401–5.

138. Temkin NR, Dikmen SS, Wilensky AJ, *et al.* A randomized, double-blind study of phenytoin for the prevention of post-traumatic seizures. *N Engl J Med* 1990;**323**(8):497–502.

139. Vespa PM, McArthur DL, Xu Y, *et al.* Nonconvulsive seizures after traumatic brain injury are associated with hippocampal atrophy. *Neurology* 2010;**75**(9):792–8.

140. Bateman BT, Claassen J, Willey JZ, *et al.* Convulsive status epilepticus after ischemic stroke and intracerebral hemorrhage: frequency, predictors, and impact on outcome in a large administrative dataset. *Neurocrit Care* 2007;**7**(3):187–93.

141. Sung CY, Chu NS. Status epilepticus in the elderly: etiology, seizure type and outcome. *Acta Neurol Scand* 1989;**80**(1):51–6.

Chapter 2

Cognitive dysfunction following critical illness

Ramona O. Hopkins and James C. Jackson

SUMMARY

Assessment of outcomes following critical illness is an important focus of intensive care unit (ICU) investigations. Historically, 28-day mortality was an outcome of predominant concern to both clinicians and researchers and interventions were considered effective if they impacted this endpoint. While short-term mortality is obviously important, the likelihood of surviving an episode of critical illness and living for an extended period of time thereafter has improved substantially, resulting in millions of ICU survivors. Survivorship brings with it potential untoward consequences including the development of post-intensive care syndrome (PICS), which refers to new or worsening physical, cognitive, or psychiatric disorders that are significant and long-lasting [1]. As a recent editorial noted, "The emerging picture of critical illness survivorship is deeply disturbing. In the year or two after discharge, patients are ravaged. They cannot walk. They cannot think clearly. They suffer from posttraumatic psychiatric syndromes. Their bodies hurt, are disfigured, and refuse to function like they did before" [2]. For these reasons, investigators are increasingly focusing on various dimensions of PICS that impact patient functioning (including and specifically, cognitive function).

Recent evidence has overwhelmingly shown that the consequences associated with serious illness, major surgery, and the like, are not merely physical in nature. On the contrary, cognitive deficits are common in diverse medical and surgical populations and are thought to result from or be worsened by the effects of the illness or its treatment [3,4]. In ICU survivors (medical and surgical, non-trauma) findings of new significant cognitive impairment are particularly striking [5]. While an emerging scientific consensus exists that ICU hospitalization is a risk factor for the acquisition of cognitive impairment, much remains to be discovered.

Prevalence of cognitive impairment

Prevalence rates of cognitive impairment after critical illness can vary widely depending on such factors as the neuropsychological test(s) employed, definitions of impairment, and assessment time points. As such, identifying prevalence of cognitive impairment with precision, as if this were a static phenomenon, is difficult. Still, studies to date provide reliable estimates of prevalence, suggesting in aggregate that cognitive impairment is very common in ICU survivors. Investigations find cognitive impairment to occur in approximately 30–70% of ICU survivors in the first year after discharge (higher impairment rates are reported immediately prior to hospital discharge), and as high as 45% at 2 years [5]. Approximately one third of general medical ICU patients have cognitive impairment at 6 months [6]. Further, the rate of moderate to severe cognitive impairment in critically ill trauma survivors (without intracranial hemorrhage) [7] and in chronically critically ill patients [8] is ~60%, and few chronically critically ill patients had a "good outcome" (defined as no cognitive impairment or functional dependency).

While trajectories of cognitive change are little studied (with many investigations relying entirely on discrete cross-sectional analyses or assessments at a single time point), ICU survivors frequently have very serious cognitive deficits in the months to years following the onset of critical illness. These deficits, particularly in some cognitive domains, may improve (and in some cases resolve) within the first year. For example, intellectual function declined from pre-ICU estimates at hospital discharge but improved to "normal levels" by 1 year with no change at 2 years.

Brain Disorders in Critical Illness, ed. Robert D. Stevens, Tarek Sharshar, and E. Wesley Ely. Published by Cambridge University Press. © Cambridge University Press 2013.

Definite – though sometimes very slight – improvement occurs beyond 1 year in other cognitive domains. However, substantial cognitive deficits remain 6 years post-ICU discharge [9]. One study found no improvement in memory comparing 2-year with 5-year outcomes in ICU survivors [10]. It is unclear if all cognitive domains improve as there are few longitudinal studies – but data from the two longitudinal studies to date suggest that while some improvements may occur between early and later follow-ups, significant cognitive impairments remain.

The fact that some improvement in cognitive function appears to be the norm – not the exception – suggests that, *in general*, the cognitive impairment observed after critical illness is not a dementia (defined as a disease of *progressive* cognitive decline), though there are likely subpopulations for whom a critical illness cognitive impairment may be the initiating event or lower the threshold for dementia presentation among predisposed individuals. While it may be the case that new post-ICU cognitive baselines are established in young ICU survivors, this is a dubious assumption among older populations who may be vulnerable or predisposed to decline or, alternatively, who may be already declining at the time of their critical illness (see sections below on dementia and acquired brain injury).

Pattern and severity of cognitive impairments

Based on current data, there appears to be no obvious "signature" pattern of cognitive deficits in ICU survivors as is the often the case in other cognitive disorders (such as Alzheimer's disease, which is primarily a disorder of memory, at least in the early to middle stages of the disease). While memory deficits are common following critical illness, it is unlikely that they are solely or primarily "amnesic" (memory deficit in which there is an inability to learn or retain new personal or factual information with sparing of other cognitive functions) in nature and are likely influenced by deficits in other domains (problems with attention are often misidentified as "memory problems" due to the role that attention mechanisms play in memory).

Existing data suggest that cognitive deficits in ICU survivors are particularly common in domains of memory, executive functioning, and attention (Table 2.1). Cognitive deficits in these domains are also common in individuals who have acquired brain injuries (e.g., traumatic and anoxic brain injury). It remains unclear whether memory, executive function, and attention are differentially affected, due to critical illness-related mechanisms that target these domains and associated brain regions, or whether these deficits are particularly notable because they have been evaluated more extensively than other cognitive domains to date. There is some evidence that mechanisms of brain injury, such as hypoxia (which differentially target brain regions, such as the hippocampus, medial temporal lobes, and frontal lobes), positively correlate with impaired memory, suggesting that some potential mechanisms of brain injury may result in specific neural injury and concomitant cognitive deficits [11]. Regardless, investigations have implicated memory, attention, and executive function as well as deficits in multiple cognitive domains in survivors of critical illness. Intellectual function, motor abilities, and many language abilities are often spared following critical illness, which is similar to impairments observed in other acquired brain injury populations (Table 2.1).

While the severity of deficits in ICU survivors varies (and may change over time), deficits are typically mild to moderate in severity, though individuals who develop anoxia during ICU treatment can demonstrate profound cognitive deficits. Though broad differences across investigations make it hard to generalize, neuropsychological test scores are often approximately 1.5 standard deviations

Table 2.1 Preserved and impaired cognitive domains following acquired brain injury.

Preserved cognitive domains	Impaired cognitive domains
Intelligence	Attention
Expressive language	Executive functioning
Receptive language	Memory
Gross motor skills	Mental processing speed
Fine motor skills	Visuospatial abilities
	Word finding difficulties

The concept of preserved and impaired abilities presumes an acquired brain injury model and depends on the degree and location (focal vs. generalized) of the brain injury. It is possible a focal lesion precisely located could result in deficits in any of the "preserved cognitive functions." For example, a lesion in Broca's area will result in expressive aphasia.

below the mean (scores worse than 95% of the overall population), and scores 2 standard deviations below the mean (worse than 98% of the overall population) are not uncommon in ICU survivors. The functional consequences of such scores, while hard to precisely determine, are likely very significant. Among individuals with relatively mild impairments, problems in higher-order activities of daily living may exist but they are likely of a magnitude that is limiting but not disabling (practical problems may include difficulties following complex instructions, remembering grocery lists, concentration in the face of distractions, multi-tasking, etc.). Among individuals with more severe impairment, functional problems may be quite pronounced and of a magnitude that may result in inability to engage in effective vocational functioning, perform effectively in academic settings, navigate complicated social situations, and drive. Current data indicate that large proportions of survivors do not return to work. For example, one study found only 49% of ICU survivors were employed at 1 year after hospital discharge [12] and a second study found that 34% were employed 2 years after hospital discharge [11]. Few studies in ICU survivors have assessed relationships between cognitive impairment and functional outcomes specifically. In the broader neuropsychological literature, the link between mild to moderate cognitive deficits and problems in "everyday functioning" is quite well established.

Factors that influence cognitive outcome

A variety of factors have the potential to influence long-term cognitive outcomes both before and during critical illness. Various factors prior to critical illness such as age, education, level of cognitive function, comorbid disease or disorders, and genetic risk factors may tip the scales towards a good or adverse cognitive outcome. For example, a patient who is young, a college graduate with no cognitive or health problems, would be less vulnerable to adverse cognitive outcomes than an older individual with 10 years of education, multiple comorbid diseases, and a genetic risk factor such as ApoE e4 (Figure 2.1). Factors during critical illness and its treatment can also impact outcome. A patient with longer ICU length of stay, high illness severity (hypotension, hypoxia, multiple organ failure, delirium, etc.) would be more vulnerable to adverse cognitive outcome (Figure 2.1).

Pre-existing vs. new cognitive impairments

Significant unresolved questions exist related to the degree to which cognitive impairment in ICU survivors is "new" as opposed to a reflection of pre-existing cognitive difficulties. In some individuals – premorbid high functioning, healthy "normal" – the presence of significant neuropsychological deficits is unquestionably new. In other cases, however, individuals may "arrive" at the ICU with unrecognized deficits – particularly those with medical comorbidities such as cardiovascular disease, diabetes, chronic obstructive pulmonary disease, and HIV-Aids that have potential neurological implications. Cognitive deficits in these medical disorders are often unknown as brain-related changes in chronic disease occur slowly over time, and cognitive function is not routinely assessed. Most studies that have tried to identify and quantify the presence and severity of pre-existing cognitive impairment and have done so with various degrees of rigor, demonstrate that when individuals with diagnosed dementia or prior cognitive impairment are excluded from studies, a relatively small number (~5–10%) of individuals screened for cognitive impairments are found to have *significant* cognitive impairment prior to the onset of acute illness. Such findings suggest that the majority of the impaired individuals identified after intensive care did not have premorbid cognitive impairment or at least not to the degree demonstrated following critical illness.

These studies do not completely answer the question of whether the cognitive impairments are newly acquired during critical illness or if some are present prior to critical illness. Two recent, large, population-based studies used their longitudinal prospective designs to assess the effect of critical illness on cognitive function [3, 4]. Cognitive function was assessed at regular time intervals in these studies which allowed assessment of cognitive function before and after critical illness. Both studies found that critical illness (critical illness hospitalization or sepsis) resulted in significant new cognitive impairments that were not present prior to the onset of critical illness. These investigations demonstrate that critical illness can and does result in significant new cognitive impairment in many ICU survivors [3, 4].

Dementia or acquired brain injury

"Dementia" is sometimes misunderstood to be a singular condition when, in fact, it refers to a broad array of

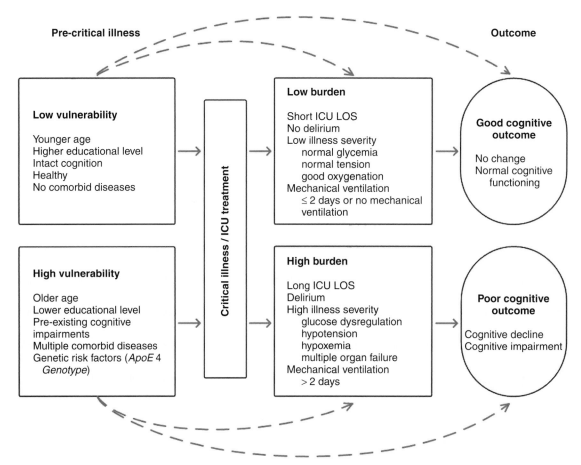

Figure 2.1 Possible explanatory model of cognitive outcomes in survivors of critical illness.

syndromes which share key features. In general, "dementia" refers to the development of cognitive deficits including impaired memory along with disturbance in at least one additional cognitive domain, and the cognitive changes often worsen over time [13]. However, the term dementia carries with it semantic baggage, is often used synonymously with Alzheimer's disease, and dementia is commonly used to refer to a progressive condition that has a gradual onset and specific pathological changes. Dementia is highlighted by predominant, though not exclusive, deficits in memory of a severity that has the ability to interfere with key aspects of daily functioning. While the role of memory is a defining feature in so called "cortical" dementias – including frontotemporal dementia (FTD), Wernicke–Korsakoff syndrome, and, importantly, Alzheimer's disease, memory is only one of several cognitive domains that may be impaired (depending on the type of dementia).

A review of existing longitudinal studies of cognition in ICU survivors suggests that relatively few individuals develop a progressive dementia; the majority of ICU survivors display a pattern of cognitive improvement and then stability as opposed to decline. Key caveats include the fact that most investigations have been carried out in middle-aged populations, while surveying cognition functioning over relatively short time periods (1–6 years). Such research "gaps" are conspicuous as aging populations, which are common in the ICU, may lower the threshold for development of dementia which may require significant time to clinically manifest. While a dementia model may not be the best fit for the cognitive impairments following critical illness, data from studies which follow large numbers of elderly ICU survivors for extended time frames are needed to see if cognitive impairment following critical illness is a risk factor for dementia.

Table 2.2 Comparison of characteristics of acquired brain injury and dementia models of brain injury.

Areas of difference	Acquired brain injury model	Dementia model
Onset	Acute	Gradual
Age at onset	Any age	Older age (generally)
Cause	An external or acute insult: Accident Anoxia Cardiac arrest drowning Electric shock Hemorrhage Serious illness Stroke Toxic exposures Trauma	Organic neurological disease or disorder: Alzheimer's disease Fronto-temporal dementia Huntington's disease Lewy body dementia Pick's disease Vascular dementia
Progression	Static or may improve over time	Progressive decline

Cognitive impairments	Attention
	Executive function
	Memory
	Mental processing speed
	Visuospatial abilities
	Word finding difficulty
		Early stage limited to one or two cognitive domains – often memory
		  (depending on dementia type)
		Middle stage – memory, executive function, language
		Late stage – most cognitive functions including sensory
		  and motor, unable to perform self-care

Associated impairments	Emotional (depression, anxiety, PTSD) Behavioral – severe brain injury Social – severe brain injury	Emotional (depression) Behavioral Social
Awareness of deficits	Often aware of deficits Severe brain injury – unaware	Early stage – aware Middle or late stage – unaware
Rehabilitation	Responds	Not respond

An alternative explanatory paradigm for post-ICU cognitive impairments is an acquired brain injury paradigm. Table 2.2 compares characteristics of dementia and acquired brain injury. In general, cognitive impairments common among ICU survivors are, by definition, "acquired" brain injuries following an acute event. To suggest this is simply to acknowledge that these cognitive deficits develop in response to one or a series of discrete external or environmental insults (e.g., they are not congenital), in this case, the effects of critical illness or its treatment. Further, the presence of cognitive impairment is thought to be a direct pathophysiological consequence of the brain injury, and the type and degree of cognitive impairment depend on the location and extent of the injury [13]. While some controversy exists regarding the definitional boundaries of certain types of brain injuries, the definition of an acquired brain injury is widely agreed upon and sufficiently broad to include not only TBI (due to external events such as a motor vehicle accidents, falls, etc. – see Table 2.2) but also those injuries occurring in the context of serious illnesses due to events such as hypoxia or cytokine-activated immune system dysregulation, or the potential neurotoxic effects of prolonged exposure to sedatives or analgesic medications.

Cognitive rehabilitation

As the number of ICU survivors increases, the need to address cognitive impairments through prevention, treatment, and rehabilitation is growing [1]. A three-step model for improving cognitive function has been proposed that includes: (1) screening for risk factors of cognitive impairments; (2) prevention of brain injury through best practices (i.e., sedation protocols, delirium screening, and early physical mobility); and (3) post-ICU physical and cognitive rehabilitation [14]. As is true with physical rehabilitation, there are potential candidates for cognitive rehabilitation who are more or less appropriate. Clearly, not all individuals with cognitive impairments can reasonably benefit from rehabilitation, even though their deficits may be severe.

This is particularly true in geriatric populations of ICU survivors who may have pre-existing deficits of a progressive nature (individuals with early or more advanced expressions of dementia). That is, these individuals may have brain injury on dementia – new cognitive impairment in addition to their pre-existing cognitive decline or dementia. Though the worsening impairment these individuals experience may have been fostered by critical illness-acquired brain injury, degenerative cognitive conditions have not been shown to respond (e.g., they neither "slow" nor improve) to rehabilitation, and as such this subpopulation of ICU survivors may not benefit from rehabilitation.

Time post-injury

Time post-injury is associated with treatment outcome as numerous studies of TBI have shown. Rehabilitation interventions may be optimal if employed within the time period in which "spontaneous or natural recovery" processes can be maximally leveraged to support full or partial recovery of cognitive function [15]. Admittedly, other perspectives abound, and some experts argue that rehabilitation interventions are most effective > 1 year post-injury, as significant time periods are required for the precise nature of cognitive and functional impairments to become clear. For example, the prominent brain injury treatment facility, the Oliver Zangwill Center, founded by leading neuropsychologist and rehabilitation researcher, Dr. Barbara Wilson, regularly treats individuals 1–10 years after their injury, predicated on the idea that such an approach is uniquely advantageous for patients. Data in stroke suggest that rehabilitation that occurs years post-stroke can improve functioning, though the rate and degree of improvement is slower and less pronounced than observed when rehabilitation occurs earlier during spontaneous recovery [16].

Effectiveness of cognitive rehabilitation

Misconceptions abound regarding the "effectiveness" of cognitive rehabilitation, as the popular conception (even among many sophisticated medical personnel) is that *cognitive rehabilitation* refers to interventions/approaches that seek to *restore* lost or degraded cognitive functions. Restoration of cognitive functioning beyond what occurs naturally during normal recovery is the "Holy Grail" of rehabilitation research and has been demonstrated only in narrowly circumscribed situations. Evidence increasingly suggests that working memory abilities can improve with the

aid of computerized training [17, 18], though similar positive findings have not been demonstrated to the same extent with regard to other aspects of memory, attention, and executive functioning. However, "restorative" approaches to rehabilitation currently represent only a small portion of rehabilitation approaches. Other approaches include pharmacological or compensatory strategies that allow individuals to "work around" their deficits.

Rehabilitation in ICU populations

While interventions have been generally ineffective in either arresting or reversing dementia, cognitive rehabilitation has been shown to improve cognitive functioning, as well as functioning more generally, in brain-injured individuals. Although various forms of rehabilitation (e.g., physical therapy) are commonly employed with ICU survivors, cognitive rehabilitation is rarely utilized (typically only in rare cases involving profound anoxic injuries). Rehabilitation following anoxic brain injury is slower and less successful than rehabilitation following TBI [19]. Despite the very limited examples in which rehabilitation is used in ICU populations, it may hold the potential to facilitate improvements in cognition, particularly among individuals with deficits in memory, attention, and executive functioning, the primary domains it has been designed to address. In the only published study of cognitive rehabilitation in ICU survivors, individuals who received a 6-week protocolized intervention (Goal Management Training) had improved executive functioning compared with their counterparts who received "usual care" (no rehabilitation-related interventions) [20]. While this study was small and obviously needs to be replicated using a much larger population, it suggests that cognitively impaired ICU survivors without pre-existing progressive dementia have the potential for significant cognitive improvement with use of focused and intensive interventions.

Although promising, the rehabilitation of cognitive deficits in ICU survivors is fraught with complexities. Among these complexities are issues such as timing of rehabilitation, selection of rehabilitation approaches, and identifying individuals who will optimally benefit from interventions (there are additional issues but a comprehensive discussion is beyond the scope of this chapter). With regard to timing, it is unclear when rehabilitation should be initiated – e.g., in the hospital, immediately after discharge, or at some later date. While the value of early interventions may seem intuitive, some rehabilitation experts believe that cognitive rehabilitation is of greatest benefit after acute issues have resolved (> 12 months post-injury), as individuals typically experience greater stability at this time point and the true nature of their deficits is more apparent [21]. Selection of rehabilitation approaches also presents a challenge, particularly in light of the fact that ICU survivors rarely present with deficits in one primary domain (unlike many survivors of TBI). In general, cognitive rehabilitation approaches target specific areas of difficulty and are not designed to be used generically. Typical rehabilitation interventions may have to be adapted to a degree to reflect the realities of diffuse cognitive impairment in individuals after critical illness. Finally, challenges exist pertaining to identifying those individuals who will benefit from cognitive rehabilitation. Certain populations with cognitive impairment may be more responsive to interventions than others. Identifying individuals likely and unlikely to respond to cognitive rehabilitation interventions is important, particularly because "supply and demand" dynamics suggest that cognitive rehabilitation – in the near future, at least – is an option that will be available to relatively small numbers of individuals due to the limited number of specialists qualified to carry this out. Rehabilitation funding is also a concern as current insurance requirements (presuming the individual has insurance) in the USA generally specify the patient must be able to tolerate at least 15 hours of rehabilitation per week; further, at least 60% of patients in acute inpatient rehabilitation must have a primary or secondary diagnosis from a list of appropriate rehabilitation diagnoses [1].

Role of ICU follow-up clinics

The use of follow-up clinics is increasingly common for patients with wide-ranging and diverse medical conditions including cardiac disease, concussion, and orthopedic issues. These clinics are staffed by specialists and focus on treating the specific problems associated with a given condition and assisting patients in adjusting to life following a significant medical event such as a hospitalization, a surgical procedure, or the receipt of a new diagnosis. Follow-up clinics are thought to contribute to improved patient outcomes and, as such, they represent an increasingly popular model of care. Experts suggest that follow-up clinics may be particularly appropriate for survivors of critical illness for a variety of reasons [22, 23]. Due to current models of service provision, patients often transition rapidly from the ICU to home (often a long geographic distance from hospital where ICU care was provided) and lack continuity of care. Additionally, the combination of cognitive, psychological, and physical comorbidities that commonly develop after critical illness is unique and not widely recognized or understood in the larger medical community and thus unlikely to be optimally addressed in any other context. In the course of our own research, we commonly encounter ICU survivors who report regularly interacting with local medical and psychological providers who fail to fully understand the details and nuances of their new conditions, thus highlighting the need for follow-up clinics. The effectiveness of these clinics is unclear, though two recent preliminary investigations suggest they do not appear to contribute to improved patient outcomes [24, 25].

Such conclusions are tentative and premature and may reflect the fact that the follow-up clinics evaluated to date have been largely nurse-led rather than specialist-led and have relied largely on psychoeducational rather than sustained psychotherapeutic interventions. Investigations regarding the role and effectiveness of ICU follow-up clinics are needed.

Conclusion

Cognitive impairment is pervasive in survivors of intensive care and contributes to meaningful and clinically significant functional decrements as well as quality of life and related difficulties. The cognitive impairments are new, improve in some patients, and appear stable over time similar to other acquired brain injuries. Despite over a decade of focused investigation, key ongoing questions pertaining to neuropsychological decrements after critical illness exist, though these are increasingly being elucidated. Presently, the precise causes of cognitive impairment remain unknown, though numerous risk factors have been identified. Treatments to prevent or reduce the severity of cognitive impairments (i.e., sedation, delirium, and early mobility protocols) need to be investigated. Similarly, recovery and remediation of cognitive impairment is a field in its infancy, though early research appears promising. Future research efforts should focus on the proactive identification of those at risk for cognitive impairment as well as on the development of methods to robustly improve and remediate deficits in ICU survivors. Furthermore, ongoing efforts should be made to educate both patients and their families regarding the impact of cognitive impairment and its practical consequences.

References

1. Needham DM, Davidson J, Cohen H, *et al.* Improving long-term outcomes after discharge from intensive care unit: report from a stakeholders' conference. *Crit Care Med* 2012;**40**(2):502–9.

2. Iwashyna TJ. Survivorship will be the defining challenge of critical care in the 21st century. *Ann Intern Med* 2010;**153**(3):204–5.

3. Ehlenbach WJ, Hough CL, Crane PK, *et al.* Association between acute care and critical illness hospitalization and cognitive function in older adults. *JAMA* 2010;**303**(8):763–70.

4. Iwashyna TJ, Ely EW, Smith DM, Langa KM. Long-term cognitive impairment and functional disability among survivors of severe sepsis. *JAMA* 2010;**304**(16):1787–94.

5. Hopkins RO, Jackson JC. Long-term neurocognitive function after critical illness. *Chest* 2006;**130**(3):869–78.

6. Jackson JC, Hart RP, Gordon SM, *et al.* Six-month neuropsychological outcome of medical intensive care unit patients. *Crit Care Med* 2003;**31**(4):1226–34.

7. Jackson JC, Obremskey W, Bauer R, *et al.* Long-term cognitive, emotional, and functional outcomes in trauma intensive care unit survivors without intracranial hemorrhage. *J Trauma* 2007;**62**(1):80–8.

8. Unroe M, Kahn JM, Carson SS, *et al.* One-year trajectories of care and resource utilization for recipients of prolonged mechanical ventilation: a cohort study. *Ann Intern Med* 2010;**153**(3):167–75.

9. Rothenhausler HB, Ehrentraut S, Stoll C, Schelling G. Kapfhammer HP. The relationship between cognitive performance and employment and health status in long-term survivors of the acute respiratory distress syndrome: results of an exploratory study. *Gen Hosp Psychiatry* 2001;**23**(2):90–6.

10. Adhikari NK, Tansey CM, McAndrews MP, *et al.* Self-reported depressive symptoms and memory complaints in survivors five years after acute respiratory distress syndrome. *Chest.* 2011; **140**(6):1484–93.

11. Hopkins RO, Weaver LK, Collingridge D, *et al.* Two-year cognitive, emotional, and quality-of-life outcomes in acute respiratory distress syndrome. *Am J Respir Crit Care Med* 2005;**171**(4):340–7.

12. Herridge MS, Cheung AM, Tansey CM, *et al.* One-year outcomes in survivors of the acute respiratory distress syndrome. *N Engl J Med* 2003;**348**(8):683–93.

13. American Psychiatric Association. *Diagnostic and Statistical Manual of Mental Disorders, Fourth edition, Text Revision* (DSM–IV–TR). Washington, DC: American Psychiatric Association; 2000.

14. Vasilevskis EE, Pandharipande PP, Girard TD, Ely EW. A screening, prevention, and restoration model for saving the injured brain in intensive care unit survivors. *Crit Care Med* 2010;**38**(10 Suppl):S683–91.

15. Stuss D, Winocur G, Robertson I. *Cognitive Neurorehabilitation: Evidence and Applications.* Cambridge: Cambridge University Press; 2006.

16. Ferrarello F, Baccini M, Rinaldi LA, *et al.* Efficacy of physiotherapy interventions late after stroke: a meta-analysis. *J Neurol Neurosurg Psychiatry* 2011;**82**(2):136–43.

17. Johansson B, Tornmalm M. Working memory training for patients with acquired brain injury: effects in daily life. *Scand J Occup Ther* 2012;**19**(2):176–83.

18. Beck SJ, Hanson CA, Puffenberger SS, Benninger KL, Benninger WB. A controlled trial of working memory training for children and adolescents with ADHD. *J Clin Child Adolesc Psychol* 2010;**39**(6):825–36.

19. Cullen NK, Crescini C, Bayley MT. Rehabilitation outcomes after anoxic brain injury: a case-controlled comparison with traumatic brain injury. *PM R* 2009;**1**(12):1069–76.

20. Jackson J, Ely EW, Morey MC, *et al.* Cognitive and physical rehabilitation of intensive care unit survivors: results of the RETURN randomized controlled pilot investigation. *Crit Care Med* 2011;**40**(4):1088–97.

21. Wilson BA, Gracey F, Evans JJ, Bateman A. *Neuropsychological Rehabilitation Theory, Models, Therapy and Outcome.* Cambridge: Cambridge University Press; 2009.

22. Williams TA, Leslie GD. Beyond the walls: a review of ICU clinics and their impact on patient outcomes after leaving hospital. *Aust Crit Care* 2008;**21**(1):6–17.

23. Modrykamien AM. The ICU follow-up clinic: a new paradigm for intensivists. *Respir Care* 2011;**57**(5):764–72.

24. Elliott D, McKinley S, Alison J, *et al.* Health-related quality of life and physical recovery after a critical illness: a multi-centre randomised controlled trial of a home-based physical rehabilitation program. *Crit Care* 2011;**15**(3):R142.

25. Cuthbertson BH, Rattray J, Campbell MK, *et al.* The PRaCTICaL study of nurse led, intensive care follow-up programmes for improving long term outcomes from critical illness: a pragmatic randomised controlled trial. *Br Med J* 2009;**339**:b3723.

Psychiatric disorders following critical illnesses

Dimitry S. Davydow

SUMMARY

As a growing number of patients survive critical illnesses, there has been increasing interest in the long-term physical and emotional outcomes of these patients.

Understanding mental health outcomes in critical illness survivors is of great public health importance due to the impact of mental health conditions on overall health outcomes such as mortality. This chapter reviews the literature on the epidemiology of, and potential interventions for, posttraumatic stress disorder (PTSD), depressive, and more general anxiety symptoms in critical illness survivors. Up to one half of all critical illness survivors may have clinically significant PTSD, depressive, or general anxiety symptoms. Patients with a prior history of anxiety or depressive disorders surviving an intensive care unit (ICU) admission for the treatment of a critical illness, as well as those who experience memories of in-ICU traumatic and/or psychotic experiences, may be at particular risk for subsequent PTSD or depression. Patients receiving a diary of their ICU experiences may have a reduced risk of PTSD following their critical illness. Additional research is needed to understand the etiology of psychiatric disorders in critical illness survivors, as well as to develop interventions to prevent and/or ameliorate these adverse outcomes in order to improve the quality of life for this growing patient population.

Patient narrative

> I remember being tied down, but I was underwater. There were fish swimming around me. I couldn't breathe, and I knew I was drowning. It was a horrible feeling.

This quotation came from a patient seen 4 months after being hospitalized in the ICU with acute respiratory distress syndrome.

Introduction

Every year, millions of people survive life-threatening critical illnesses worldwide [1]. With more individuals living through once universally fatal critical conditions such as severe sepsis and acute lung injury (ALI), there has been increasing interest in long-term outcomes following ICU admissions. Over the last decade, there has been an increasing body of research focusing on quality of life, cognitive, and mental health outcomes following critical illnesses [2–6].

Critical illnesses and their requisite ICU therapies expose patients to profound stressors, including respiratory distress, pain with endotracheal intubation and suctioning, delirium with associated psychotic experiences, hypothalamic-pituitary-adrenal axis strain, inflammation, and/or administration of exogenous catecholamines, all in the context of reduced autonomy and a limited ability to communicate. Critical illnesses are also, by definition, life-threatening, and patients who survive these conditions may face substantial physical limitations during their recovery [5]. Therefore, psychiatric disorders such as anxiety and depressive disorders are a potential concern in critical illness survivors [7].

The most commonly studied psychiatric disorders in critical illness survivors are PTSD and major depression. Posttraumatic stress disorder is a type of anxiety disorder characterized by having experienced a life-threatening (or perceived to be life-threatening), traumatic event and subsequently experiencing intrusive recollections of the event, symptoms of hyperarousal, and avoidant behavior related to the

Brain Disorders in Critical Illness, ed. Robert D. Stevens, Tarek Sharshar, and E. Wesley Ely. Published by Cambridge University Press. © Cambridge University Press 2013.

traumatic event. Major depression is characterized by at least 2 weeks of depressed mood, diminished ability/inability to experience pleasure, and neurovegetative symptoms. Importantly, inflammation is thought to play an important role in the pathophysiology of both major depression and many critical illnesses [8,9], and hypocortisolism, which has been implicated as a feature of the pathophysiology of PTSD [10], is common in critically ill patients [11]. Thus, there are plausible biological reasons to consider PTSD and major depression as potential sequelae in critical illness survivors. Greater consideration of PTSD and major depression in survivors of critical illnesses is of great public health importance. Chronic medical comorbidities are common in patients admitted to ICUs for the treatment of critical illnesses [12], and both major depression and PTSD are associated with adverse outcomes, including mortality, in patients with comorbid chronic medical illnesses [13–15]. In addition, many critical illness survivors face substantial disabilities that greatly increase the amount of caregiving they will need [4], and caregivers of critical illness survivors report substantial burdens [16,17]. There is evidence that the burden of caregiving is even greater when the patient is depressed [18], suggesting that depressed critical illness survivors may place extreme burdens on the family members that must care for them during their recovery.

The objective of the present chapter is to review the current literature on the epidemiology of PTSD, depressive, and more general anxiety symptoms in critical illness survivors. Although definitions for other common anxiety disorders have been provided in Table 3.2 for the reader, they will not be discussed in the context of critical illness survival since these conditions have not been studied in critical illness survivors. In addition to discussing potential risk factors for psychiatric morbidity following ICU admissions, current research on potential interventions that may ameliorate and/or prevent these adverse outcomes will also be described. While comprehensive, the material discussed in this chapter is not meant to be an exhaustive review of the entire known literature in this area, and the reader is advised to consult the references cited for additional information.

Epidemiology and etiology of PTSD and depressive symptoms following critical illnesses

The prevalences of PTSD, general anxiety, and depressive symptoms following critical illnesses such as severe sepsis and ALI vary in the reported literature depending upon the ascertainment methods used. The vast majority of studies have used questionnaires such as the Center for Epidemiologic Studies-Depression Scale (CES-D), the Hospital Anxiety and Depression Scale (HADS), the Impact of Events Scale (IES), and the Posttraumatic Symptom Scale-10 (PTSS-10) [1,5,6]. While questionnaires can enhance study feasibility and allow for psychiatric symptom measurements in larger sample sizes, diagnoses of psychiatric disorders cannot be made. A small minority of studies have employed clinicians using diagnostic interviews [1,5,6].

In studies using questionnaires, the point prevalence of clinically significant (i.e., reaching the appropriate questionnaire threshold of probable clinical diagnosis) PTSD symptoms in critical illness survivors has ranged from 8% [19] to 52% [20]. The point prevalence of clinically significant general anxiety symptoms in ALI survivors has ranged from 23% [21] to 48% [22]. Questionnaire-ascertained point prevalences of clinically significant depressive symptoms have ranged from 8% to 57% [5,6,23–26]. A recent study of long-term acute respiratory distress syndrome (ARDS) survivors asked about a history of physician-diagnosed psychiatric disorders following hospital discharge [27]; 51% of ARDS survivors participating in this study reported at least one episode of physician-diagnosed depression, anxiety, or both.

In studies using clinicians conducting diagnostic interviews, the point prevalence of PTSD has ranged from 10% [28] to 40% [29]. The point prevalence of depressive disorder diagnoses (including major depression, depressive disorder not otherwise specified, mood disorder due to a general medical condition, and bipolar depression) in studies using diagnostic interviews has ranged from 4% [30] to 33% [31]. To date, no studies have utilized diagnostic interviews to ascertain the point prevalences of anxiety disorders other than PTSD (e.g., generalized anxiety disorder, panic disorder, social phobia, etc.) following critical illnesses.

At least 28 studies have examined potential risk factors for psychiatric disorders following critical illnesses. Interpretation of the findings of these studies should be made with caution since the studies are primarily observational in nature, and the majority of studies did not adjust for important potential confounders in their analyses [1,5,6]. Furthermore, although numerous significant associations have been identified between various factors and increased risk of clinically significant PTSD and/or depressive symptoms following a critical illness, relatively few of these associations have been reliably reproduced across studies. Potential risk factors for psychiatric disorders following critical illnesses can be divided into three categories: pre-critical illness patient characteristics, critical illness/ICU-related factors, and post-critical illness/ICU factors.

The most consistently identified pre-critical illness patient characteristic associated with increased risk of post-critical illness, clinically significant PTSD and/or depressive symptoms is a prior history of psychiatric symptoms/disorder (variably defined using medical record review or questionnaires), with significant associations found in eight studies [23,28,31–36]. Importantly, only two of these studies utilized a standardized measure of psychiatric symptoms administered prospectively (i.e., pre-critical illness) [35,36]. Demographic factors such as age or gender have not been found to be consistent predictors of post-critical illness, clinically significant PTSD and/or depressive symptoms [1,4,6]. An interesting recent study has identified a significant unadjusted association between the presence of a homozygous allele of a glucocorticoid gene single nucleotide polymorphism (*Bcll G*) and increased risk of clinically significant PTSD symptoms 6 months following an ICU admission [37], the first genetic characteristic potentially associated with increased risk of post-critical illness psychiatric disorder.

Regarding critical illness/ICU-related characteristics, prior studies have consistently failed to find a significant association between illness severity at hospital admission (e.g., using APACHE scores) and risk of clinically significant PTSD and/or depressive symptoms [1,4,6]. Although longer durations of mechanical ventilation and ICU lengths of stay have been associated with increased risk of post-ALI PTSD and/or depressive symptoms [6], similar associations have not been identified in general ICU survivors [1,4]. Exposure to benzodiazepine sedation in the ICU has been associated with increased risk of both clinically significant PTSD and depressive symptoms in both general ICU and ALI survivors [19,23,25,38]. However, the causal pathway is unclear since prior evidence suggests that patients with premorbid histories of depression and/or anxiety disorder diagnoses may receive higher doses of benzodiazepines than those without similar histories [33]. Although one study has found a significant association between in-ICU hypoglycemia and clinically significant depressive

symptoms 3 months post-ALI [23], replication in additional studies is needed. Importantly, in the single study of critical illness survivors that adjusted for pre-illness history of psychiatric symptoms using a standardized measure administered prospectively, no clinical characteristic of a hospitalization for severe sepsis was significantly associated with post-sepsis, clinically significant depressive symptoms [36].

In the early recovery period following a critical illness, "delusional memories," or memories of in-ICU traumatic and/or psychotic experiences (e.g., hallucinations and/or delusions) have consistently been associated with increased risk of subsequent clinically significant PTSD symptoms [19,32,33,38,39], and to a lesser degree with clinically significant depressive symptoms [19,32]. Implied by the presence of in-ICU psychotic experiences, in-ICU delirium requires further study as a potential risk factor for post-critical illness PTSD, having been examined in only one study to date [38]. Cognitive impairment following a critical illness has been associated with clinically significant depressive symptoms [26,40]. Impairments in physical functioning have also been correlated with clinically significant depressive symptoms [31,36,41]. Also, early post-ICU depressive and anxiety symptoms have been found to be associated with greater risk for clinically significant PTSD and depressive symptoms later in the post-critical illness course of recovery [19].

Currently, there remains much speculation regarding the cause(s) of psychiatric disorders following critical illnesses. Since a pre-critical illness history of psychiatric disorders appears to be a potent predictor of clinically significant PTSD and/or depressive symptoms post-illness, a plausible explanation could be that the extreme stress of a critical illness could provoke exacerbations of prior conditions. Both PTSD and major depression can be recurring conditions, and extreme stress, both psychological and physiological, can precipitate both disorders in vulnerable individuals [42,43]. A contributing "neurobiological" factor in the development of PTSD and/or major depression following critical illnesses could be systemic inflammation, which is associated with conditions such as severe sepsis and ALI. Increased serum levels of inflammatory cytokines have been associated with major depression in patients with medical conditions [8]. A more "narrative" explanation of the development of psychiatric symptoms following a critical illness could be grounded in patients' feelings of loss due to cognitive and physical deficits, family life

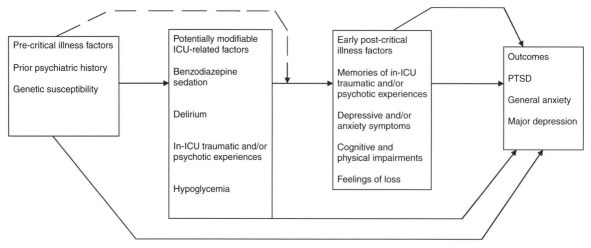

Figure 3.1 A potential causal model of psychiatric disorders following critical illnesses.

disruptions due to prolonged hospitalizations and recovery periods, and delayed return to work [6].

Figure 3.1 presents a conceptual model for the development of psychiatric disorders following critical illnesses. The model represents patient characteristics, critical illness/ICU-related factors, and early post-ICU factors as both part of a causal pathway to, and as potential individual risk factors for, the development of post-critical illness psychiatric disorders. Furthermore, the model speculates as to whether individual patient characteristics could modify the effects of critical illness/ICU-related characteristics on the development of PTSD, general anxiety, and major depression following critical illnesses. Importantly, several potential risk factors presented in the conceptual model, such as delirium, traumatic exposures, and in-ICU hypoglycemia are potentially modifiable through alterations in critical care treatment strategies, and screening of critical illness survivors with prior psychiatric histories prior to hospital discharge could lead to appropriate treatments for symptomatic patients.

Potential interventions for psychiatric disorders following critical illnesses

Recently, a small group of studies have attempted to identify interventions that could prevent post-critical illness psychiatric disorders with varying degrees of success. The types of interventions examined have included both pharmacological [29] and non-pharmacological strategies [44–46]. Although the intervention studies described are mixed in terms of yielding significantly positive findings, they represent

an initial step in attempting to ameliorate an important public health problem given the high prevalences of clinically significant PTSD and/or depressive symptoms following critical illnesses.

In one small randomized controlled trial (n = 20), patients with septic shock who received stress doses of intravenous hydrocortisone had a significantly lower risk of developing clinically significant PTSD symptoms than those who did not [29]. However, this finding is yet to be reproduced in a larger-scale randomized trial of a similar patient population. In another randomized controlled trial in critical illness survivors, patients who received a 6-week self-help rehabilitation manual had a non-significant reduction in depressive symptoms at 8 weeks post-critical illness compared with patients who did not receive the manual [44]; there was no difference in PTSD or general anxiety symptoms between groups [44]. In a large-scale randomized controlled effectiveness trial, the multisite UK PRaCTICaL trial studied a nursing-led intervention consisting of a self-help rehabilitation manual, as well as visits to nursing-led post-ICU clinics for critical illness survivors that facilitated referrals to specialty mental health providers for patients with clinically significant PTSD and/or depressive symptoms [45]. At 12 months follow-up post-ICU, the investigators failed to find any significant differences between groups in their primary outcome, quality of life, as well as in their secondary outcomes, PTSD and depressive symptoms [45]. In a multisite randomized controlled trial of a different nature, investigators found that critical illness survivors who received a diary detailing their ICU experiences (including photographs) compiled by their bedside nurse and family at 1 month post-ICU had significantly fewer PTSD symptoms at 3 months post-ICU [46]. The investigators theorized that the success of their intervention may be attributable to cognitive reframing of memories of in-ICU psychotic experiences as well as filling in gaps in memory [46]. Longer-term follow-up studies are needed to see if the apparent preventive effect of ICU diaries can be replicated and is more than a transient phenomenon.

In addition to the interventional studies described above, there are promising areas for further research into interventions that could prevent and/or treat psychiatric disorders following critical illnesses. Currently, there is a NIH-funded randomized controlled trial of empiric escitalopram, a selective serotonin reuptake inhibitor (SSRI) antidepressant, for patients undergoing mechanical ventilation (ClinicalTrials.gov identifier: NCT00872027) whose aim is to prevent post-ICU depressive and anxiety symptoms. Additional research is needed to examine if early rehabilitation in the ICU, which has been shown to improve functional outcomes at hospital discharge [21], can also prevent post-ICU psychiatric disorders through improved physical and cognitive functioning in critical illness survivors [47]. Also, if future research implicates delirium as a cause of PTSD in critical illness survivors, then it will be important to ascertain if alternative sedation strategies, some of which have been shown to minimize ICU delirium [48], may also reduce the risk of post-ICU PTSD. Finally, stepped collaborative care interventions in which care coordinators screen high-risk patients and manage psychiatric disorders in coordination with, and supervision by, primary care physicians and psychiatrists, have shown significant benefits for chronic medical conditions [49], major depression [49], and PTSD [50], and their potential benefits should be examined in critical illness survivors.

Conclusion

Psychiatric disorders such as PTSD and major depression appear to be highly prevalent in survivors of critical illnesses and represent an important public health problem. Pre-critical illness psychiatric disorders appear to be a potent predictor of PTSD and major depression following a critical illness, and future epidemiological studies of post-critical illness psychiatric disorders should adjust for this important confounder when examining whether critical illness/ ICU-related characteristics are potential risk factors for adverse mental health. Finally, additional research is needed into interventions that can prevent and/or ameliorate psychiatric disorders such as PTSD and major depression following critical illnesses.

Acknowledgment

This work was supported by grant KL2 RR025015 from the National Institutes of Health.

References

1. Davydow DS, Gifford JM, Desai SV, Needham DM, Bienvenu OJ. Posttraumatic stress disorder in general intensive care unit survivors. *Gen Hosp Psychiatry* 2008;**30**:421–34.

2. Dowdy DW, Eid MP, Sedrakyan A, *et al*. Quality of life in adult survivors of critical illnesses: a systematic review of the literature. *Intensive Care Med* 2005;**31**:611–20.

3. Hopkins RO, Jackson JC. Long-term neurocognitive function after critical illness. *Chest* 2006;**130**:869–78.

4. Iwashyna TJ, Ely EW, Smith DM, Langa KM. Long-term cognitive impairment and functional disability among survivors of severe sepsis. *JAMA* 2010;**304**:1787–94.

5. Davydow DS, Gifford JM, Desai SV, Bienvenu OJ, Needham DM. Depression in general intensive care unit survivors: a systematic review. *Intensive Care Med* 2009;**35**:796–809.

6. Davydow DS, Desai SV, Needham DM, Bienvenu OJ. Psychiatric morbidity in survivors of the acute respiratory distress syndrome: a systematic review. *Psychosom Med* 2008;**70**:512–19.

7. American Psychiatric Association. *Diagnostic and Statistical Manual of Mental Disorders, Fourth edition, Text Revision* (DSM–IV–TR). Washington, DC: American Psychiatric Association; 2000.

8. Leonard BE. Inflammation, depression, and dementia: are they connected? *Neurochem Res* 2007;**32**:1749–56.

9. Opal SM, Girard TD, Ely EW. The immunopathogenesis of sepsis in elderly patients. *Clin Infect Dis* 2005;**41**:S504–512.

10. Sherin JE, Nemeroff CB. Post-traumatic stress disorder: the neurobiological impact of psychological trauma. *Dialogues Clin Neurosci* 2011;**13**:263–78.

11. Schelling G, Roozendaal B, Krauseneck T, *et al*. Efficacy of hydrocortisone in preventing posttraumatic stress disorder following critical illness and major surgery. *Ann NY Acad Sci* 2006;**1071**:46–53.

12. Esper AM, Martin GS. The impact of comorbid conditions on critical illness. *Crit Care Med* 2011;**39**:2728–35.

13. Davydow DS, Russo JE, Ludman E, *et al.* The association of comorbid depression and intensive care unit admission in patients with diabetes: a prospective cohort study. *Psychosomatics* 2011;**52**:117–26.

14. Ahmadi N, Hajsadeghi F, Mirshkarlo HB, *et al.* Post-traumatic stress disorder, coronary atherosclerosis, and mortality. *Am J Cardiol* 2011;**108**:29–33.

15. Katon WJ, Rutter C, Simon G, *et al.* The association of comorbid depression with mortality in patients with type 2 diabetes. *Diabetes Care* 2005;**28**:2668–72.

16. Cameron JI, Herridge MS, Tansey CM, McAndrews MP, Cheung AM. Well-being in informal caregivers of survivors of acute respiratory distress syndrome. *Crit Care Med* 2006;**34**:81–86.

17. Cox CE, Docherty SL, Brandon DH, *et al.* Surviving critical illness: acute respiratory distress syndrome as experienced by patients and their caregivers. *Crit Care Med* 2009;**37**:2702–8.

18. Langa KM, Valenstein MA, Fendrick AM, Kabeto MA, Vijan S. Extent and cost of informal caregiving for older Americans with symptoms of depression. *Am J Psychiatry* 2004;**161**:857–63.

19. Samuelson KAM, Lundberg D, Fridlund B. Stressful memories and psychological distress in adult mechanically ventilated intensive care patients: a 2-month follow-up study. *Acta Anaesthesiol Scand* 2007;**51**:671–8.

20. Griffiths J, Gager M, Alder N, *et al.* A self-report based study of the incidence and associations of sexual dysfunction in survivors of intensive care treatment. *Intensive Care Med* 2006;**32**:445–51.

21. Hopkins RO, Weaver LK, Collinridge D, *et al.* Two-year cognitive, emotional, and quality-of-life outcomes in acute respiratory distress syndrome. *Am J Respir Crit Care Med* 2005;**171**:340–7.

22. Christie JD, Biester RC, Taichman DB, *et al.* Formulation and validation of a telephone battery to assess cognitive function in acute respiratory distress syndrome survivors. *J Crit Care* 2006;**21**:125–32.

23. Dowdy DW, Dinglas V, Mendez-Tellez PA, *et al.* Intensive care unit hypoglycemia predicts depression during early recovery from acute lung injury. *Crit Care Med* 2008;**36**:2726–33.

24. Adhikari NKJ, McAndrews MP, Tansey CM, *et al.* Self-reported symptoms of depression and memory dysfunction in survivors of ARDS. *Chest* 2009;**135**:678–87.

25. Dowdy DW, Bienvenu OJ, Dinglas VD, *et al.* Are intensive care factors associated with depressive symptoms 6 months after acute lung injury? *Crit Care Med* 2009;**37**:1702–7.

26. Hopkins RO, Key CW, Suchyta MR, Weaver LK, Orme JF, Jr. Risk factors for depression and anxiety in survivors of acute respiratory distress syndrome. *Gen Hosp Psychiatry* 2010;**32**:147–55.

27. Herridge MS, Tansey CM, Matté A, *et al.* Functional disability 5 years after acute respiratory distress syndrome. *N Engl J Med* 2011;**364**:1293–304.

28. Nickel M, Leiberich P, Nickel C, *et al.* The occurrence of posttraumatic stress disorder in patients following intensive care treatment: a cross-sectional study in a random sample. *J Intensive Care Med* 2004;**19**:285–290.

29. Schelling G, Briegel J, Roozendaal B, *et al.* The effect of stress doses of hydrocortisone during septic shock on posttraumatic stress disorder in survivors. *Biol Psychiatry* 2001;**50**:978–85.

30. Kapfhammer HP, Rothenhausler HB, Krauseneck T, Stoll C, Schelling G. Posttraumatic stress disorder and health-related quality of life in survivors of the acute respiratory distress syndrome. *Am J Psychiatry* 2004;**161**:45–52.

31. Weinert C, Meller W. Epidemiology of depression and antidepressant therapy after acute respiratory failure. *Psychosomatics* 2006;**47**:399–407.

32. Jones C, Griffiths RD, Humphris G, Skirrow PM. Memory, delusions, and the development of acute posttraumatic stress disorder-related symptoms after intensive care. *Crit Care Med* 2001;**29**:573–80.

33. Jones C, Backman C, Capuzzo M, *et al.* Precipitants of post-traumatic stress disorder following intensive care: a hypothesis generating study of diversity in care. *Intensive Care Med* 2007;**33**:978–85.

34. Cuthbertson BH, Hull A, Strachan M, Scott J. Post-traumatic stress disorder after critical illness requiring general intensive care. *Intensive Care Med* 2004;**30**:450–5.

35. Davydow DS, Hough CL, Russo JE, *et al.* The association between intensive care unit admission and subsequent depression in patients with diabetes. *Int J Geriatr Psychiatry* 2012;**27**(1):22–30.

36. Davydow DS, Hough CL, Langa KM, Iwashyna TJ. Symptoms of depression in survivors of severe sepsis: a prospective cohort study of older Americans. *Am J Geriatr Psychiatry* [Epub ahead of print].

37. Hauer D, Weis F, Papassotiropoulos A, *et al.* Relationship of a common polymorphism of the glucocorticoid receptor gene to traumatic memories and posttraumatic stress disorder in patients after intensive care therapy. *Crit Care Med* 2011;**39**:643–50.

38. Girard TD, Shintani AK, Jackson JC, *et al.* Risk factors for post-traumatic stress disorder symptoms following critical illness requiring mechanical ventilation: a prospective cohort study. *Crit Care* 2007;**11**:R28.

39. Rattray JE, Johnston M, Wildsmith JM. Predictors of emotional outcomes of intensive care. *Anaesthesia* 2005;**60**:1085–92.

40. Jackson JC, Hart RP, Gordon SM, *et al.* Six-month neuropsychological outcome of medical intensive care unit patients. *Crit Care Med* 2003;**31**:1226–34.

41. Sukantarat K, Greer S, Brett S, Williamson R. Physical and psychological sequelae of critical illness. *Br J Health Psychol* 2007;**12**:65–74.

42. Kendler KS, Gardner CO, Prescott CA. Toward a comprehensive developmental model for major depression in men. *Am J Psychiatry* 2006;**163**:115–24.

43. Brewin CR, Andrews B, Valentine JD. Meta-analysis of risk factors for posttraumatic stress disorder in trauma-exposed adults. *J Consult Clin Psychol* 2000;**68**:748–66.

44. Jones C, Skirrow P, Griffiths RD, *et al.* Rehabilitation after critical illness: a randomized, controlled trial. *Crit Care Med* 2003;**31**:2456–61.

45. Cuthbertson BH, Rattray J, Cambell MK, *et al.* The PRaCTICaL study of nurse led, intensive care follow-up programmes for improving long-term outcomes from critical illness: a pragmatic randomized controlled trial. *Br Med J* 2009;**339**:b3723.

46. Jones C, Bäckman C, Capuzzo M, *et al.* Intensive care diaries reduce new onset post traumatic stress disorder following critical illness: a randomized, controlled trial. *Crit Care* 2010;**14**:R168.

47. Schweickert WD, Pohlman MC, Pohlman AS, *et al.* Early physical and occupational therapy in mechanically ventilated, critically ill patients: a randomised controlled trial. *Lancet* 2009;**373**:1874–82.

48. Pandharipande PP, Pun BT, Herr DL, *et al.* Effect of sedation with dexmedetomidine versus lorazepam on acute brain dysfunction in mechanically ventilated patients: the MENDS randomized controlled trial. *JAMA* 2007;**298**:2644–53.

49. Katon WJ, Lin EHB, Von Korff M, *et al.* Collaborative care for patients with depression and chronic illnesses. *N Engl J Med* 2010;**363**: 2611–20.

50. Zatzick D, Roy-Byrne P, Russo J, *et al.* A randomized effectiveness trial of stepped collaborative care for acutely injured trauma survivors. *Arch Gen Psychiatry* 2004;**61**:498–506.

Functional status and quality of life after critical illness

Sanjay V. Desai, Nathan E. Brummel, and Dale M. Needham

SUMMARY

Neuromuscular weakness and associated impairment in physical function is a common complication experienced by survivors of critical illness. These abnormalities are generally most severe in the early months during recovery, but may be present even a few years later. Both disease- and treatment-specific risk factors and mechanisms have been implicated in neuromuscular weakness. These complications contribute to impaired quality of life in survivors of critical illness, with deficits in physical domains extending years after critical illness. Several interventions, including early physical rehabilitation programs starting within 1 or 2 days of intensive care unit (ICU) admission, may help reduce these complications.

Introduction

Demand for intensive care is expected to markedly increase in the next two decades due to the aging baby boomers [1]. When combined with improving ICU mortality, there is a large and growing number of ICU survivors [2]. These epidemiological trends mean that clinicians face an increasingly important challenge of addressing the long-term complications experienced by ICU survivors. Two of the most relevant long-term complications are impairments in physical function and quality of life (QOL), as described in this chapter.

Physical function after critical illness

Intensive care unit survivors suffer long-term impairments in physical function. These impairments have multiple mechanisms and often stem from the neuromuscular complications described in this chapter. Figure 4.1 illustrates important physical impairments after critical illness along with relevant risk factors and associations with QOL.

Neuromuscular impairments

Taxonomy

Neuromuscular weakness is common among the critically ill and may develop as the result of a specific neuropathy or myopathy. Alternatively the same patient may develop functional weakness independent of an identifiable neuropathy or myopathy, as a result of critical illness. The literature has inconsistent and overlapping nomenclature describing these disorders. While a comprehensive discussion of these disorders is beyond the scope of this chapter, a brief overview of muscle weakness and neuropathy in critically ill patients can be found in Table 4.1.

In an effort to facilitate communication and enhance research in this field, an expert group proposed a framework for understanding neuromuscular abnormalities resulting from critical illness (Figure 4.2) [3]. In this framework, "ICU-acquired weakness" (ICUAW) is used to describe diffuse, symmetric, generalized muscle weakness (detected by physical examination and meeting specific strength-related criteria) that develops after the onset of critical illness without other identifiable cause. Patients with ICUAW who have electrophysiologically documented axonal polyneuropathy have "critical illness polyneuropathy" (CIP) and those with documented myopathy have "critical illness myopathy" (CIM). Commonly, CIP and CIM occur together. When there is evidence of CIP and probable or definite CIM, this combination is designated "critical illness neuromyopathy" (CINM) [3].

Table 4.1 Muscle weakness and neuropathy in critically ill patients.

	Physical exam findings	EMG/NCS results	Muscle biopsy
Critical illness polyneuropathy (CIP)	Distal sensory deficits Distal > proximal muscle weakness Respiratory muscle weakness Normal/decreased deep tendon reflexes	Motor and sensory axonal degeneration Decreased CMAP and SNAP action potentials Preserved nerve conduction velocity	Acute degeneration with atrophy of type I and type II fibers
Critical illness myopathy (CIM)	Preserved sensation Proximal muscle weakness Respiratory muscle weakness Normal/decreased deep tendon reflexes	Decreased CMAP amplitude with prolonged duration Normal SNAP Short duration, low amplitude MUAP with early recruitment on volitional contraction	Loss of myosin (thick) filaments with varying degrees of necrosis
Combined syndromes: Critical illness neuromyopathy (CINM)	Features of both CIP and CIM	Mild: borderline decrease in CMAP duration and SNAP, normal or mildly myopathic MUAP Severe: Markedly decreased CMAP amplitude; SNAP unrecordable	Mild: usually normal Severe: generalized necrosis

CMAP, compound muscle action potential; EMG, electromyography; MUAP, motor unit action potential; NCS, nerve conduction study; SNAP, sensory nerve action potential. Modified from Fan E, Zanni JM, Dennison CR, Lepre SJ, Needham DM. Critical illness neuromyopathy and muscle weakness in patients in the intensive care unit. *AACN Adv Crit Care* 2009;**20**:243–253 [61] and Latronico N, Bolton CF. Critical illness polyneuropathy and myopathy: a major cause of muscle weakness and paralysis. *Lancet Neuro* 2011;**10**:931–41 [62].

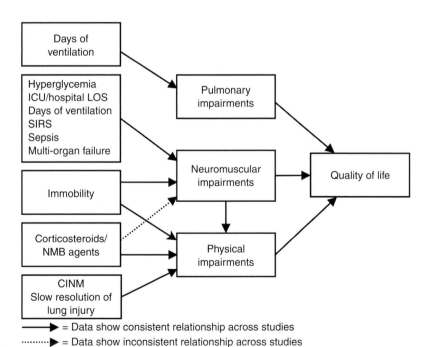

= Data show consistent relationship across studies
⋯⋯▶ = Data show inconsistent relationship across studies

Figure 4.1 Important physical impairments after critical illness along with relevant risk factors and associations with Quality of Life (QOL). CINM, critical illness neuromyopathy; ICU, intensive care unit; LOS, length of stay; NMB, neuromuscular blockade; SIRS, systemic inflammatory response syndrome.

Impairments

A systematic review demonstrated that CIP and/or CIM were observed in nearly 50% of almost 1,500 ICU patients with sepsis, multi-organ failure, or prolonged mechanical ventilation [4]. The consequences of these neuromuscular abnormalities can be dramatic. For example, in a systematic review of almost 500 ICU survivors diagnosed with CIP and/or CIM, nearly 30%

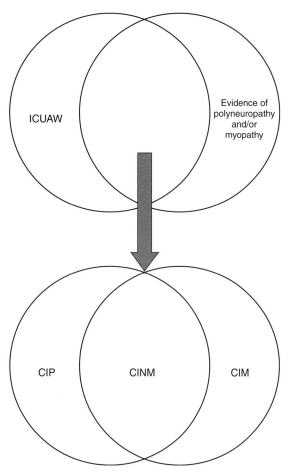

Figure 4.2 A framework for understanding neuromuscular abnormalities resulting from critical illness. CIM, critical illness myopathy; CINM, critical illness neuromyopathy; CIP, critical illness polyneuropathy; ICUAW, ICU-acquired weakness.

Mechanisms

Abnormalities with the axon, neuromuscular junction, and muscle caused by critical illness and/or critical care interventions have all been implicated in these neuromuscular impairments [11]. Relevant mechanisms include reduced nerve excitability from sodium channelopathy, bioenergetic failure, inflammatory axonal injury, and muscle breakdown [11]. Sodium channelopathy is an acquired alteration causing increased sodium inactivation and reduced nerve excitability. Bioenergetic failure is a mechanism in which the nerve cells either do not receive sufficient nourishment or cannot convert nourishment into the energy required for adequate axonal transport.

Axonal polyneuropathy, predominantly distal, occurs in both the sensory and motor nerves with evidence of fiber loss and axonal degeneration. In addition, muscle breakdown has been observed with loss of thick filaments, type II fiber atrophy, and less commonly, acute diffuse necrosis. Although less well characterized, muscle atrophy occurring, in part, from immobilization is becoming recognized as a common and likely meaningful factor in neuromuscular complications [12].

Risk factors

Commonly cited risk factors for ICUAW include hyperglycemia, systemic inflammatory response syndrome, sepsis, and multi-organ dysfunction [4]. Controlled mechanical ventilation is associated with diaphragm atrophy and proteolysis after only 18–69 hours of ventilation in a study of brain-dead organ donors [13]. Although there is some evidence that exposure to corticosteroids or neuromuscular blocking agents is associated with CINM, this has not been a consistent relationship across all studies in this area [4]. Thus, given the conflicting data regarding the harms and benefits of these treatments, particularly in ARDS, a careful balance is warranted while further studies are reported [14,15]. Similarly, tight glucose control may have a beneficial effect on the neuromuscular status of critically ill patients [16]. However, it has also been associated with increased hypoglycemia and increased mortality [17,18]. Therefore, while avoidance of hyperglycemia may be appropriate in attempts to reduce neuromuscular complications in critically ill patients, caution is warranted in aiming for tight glycemic control. Nevertheless, evidence-based strategies to reduce exposure to potentially

reported severe disability impeding independent walking or spontaneous ventilation during 3–6 month follow-up [5]. These neuromuscular abnormalities and functional impairments can be long-lasting. Nerve conduction studies were abnormal in all 13 ICU survivors studied 1–2 years after the onset of CIP [6]. Moreover, another study demonstrated clinical evidence of ICUAW in almost 60% of patients and electrophysiological evidence of CIP in 21 of 22 (95%) survivors of prolonged critical illness at a median follow-up of 3.5 (age range, 12–57) years [7]. Persistent neuromuscular abnormalities include muscle atrophy and weakness, impaired deep tendon reflexes, entrapment neuropathies, stocking and glove sensory loss, painful hyperesthesia, foot drop, and heterotopic ossification [5,8]. Some limited data suggest that recovery from CIP may be slower than from CIM [9,10].

Table 4.2 Potential risk factors and therapeutic interventions for "ICU-acquired weakness" (ICUAW).

Risk factor	Intervention to reduce risk factor exposure
Immobility	Early mobilization and rehabilitation therapy [35,36]
Prolonged mechanical ventilation	Reduce duration of mechanical ventilation with daily spontaneous awakening and breathing trials [63]
Corticosteroids	Limit use to populations where clear benefit has been demonstrated
Neuromuscular blocking agents	Limit use to populations where clear benefit has been demonstrated [15]
Hyperglycemia	Avoid high serum glucose levels [18]

modifiable risk factors may reduce the odds of a patient developing ICUAW. Selected interventions are presented in Table 4.2.

Functional limitations

Survivors of critical illness routinely report limitations in physical functioning. This outcome has been measured in several ways, including both survey- and performance-based measures. The most common survey-based measures evaluate patients' activities of daily living (ADLs) and instrumental activities of daily living (IADLs). ADLs measure daily activities of self-care, while IADLs measure higher levels of functioning, such as taking medication or shopping. The 6-minute walk distance (6MWD) is a common performance-based measure, in which a patient is instructed to walk as far as possible, on a flat surface, in 6 minutes.

Activities of daily living

Impairment in ADLs after ICU discharge is common. Within the first week after discharge, a study of 69 ICU survivors, who were mechanically ventilated for > 48 hours, reported that > 80% had moderate to severe impairments in ADLs, half of whom were completely dependent [19]. Similarly, a cohort of previously healthy ARDS survivors had a 40% mean decrement in ADLs at 28-day follow-up [20]. Although ADL function may improve with time, recovery may be incomplete in the majority of patients. Impairments have been reported in > 50% of ICU survivors in the first year after illness, and almost one third may have severe impairment at 1-year follow-up [21,22]. The presence of CIP may be related to worse ADL

functioning [23]. A large population-based study of hospitalized patients > 65 years old, who had prospective measurement of pre-ICU functional status, demonstrated that a typical patient requiring mechanical ventilation had a 30% greater impairment in ADLs at 1 year vs. those who did not require mechanical ventilation [24]. Similarly, in a prospective cohort of Medicare patients, hospitalization for severe sepsis was associated with the development of an average of 1.5 new and long-lasting functional impairments in ADLs and IADLs in patients who, prior to sepsis, had mild to moderate or no functional limitations [25]. Impairments in ADL have been correlated with physical impairments after ICU discharge, including difficulty with walking and grip strength, indicating that at least a portion of functional impairments in ICU survivors is due to physical weakness [19].

At 1-year follow-up, IADL impairments were present in > 70% of ICU survivors ventilated for > 48 hours and more than half of the survivors required caregiver support. Patients who were younger or independent at baseline were more likely to recover IADL functions at 1 year [26]. For example, of patients living at home before their critical illness, > 85% were back at home at 1-year follow-up.

Six-minute walk distance

Patients who experienced slower resolution of lung injury while critically ill had worse median 6MWD results at 5 years. However, a longitudinal study reported that, in spite of relatively normal pulmonary function, ARDS survivors' median 6MWD was 66% predicted at 1 year, 68% at 2 years, and 76% at 5 years [27,27,28]. The likelihood of persistent impairment in 6MWD at 5 years was associated with greater co-existing illnesses prior to ICU admission [27].

Early physical rehabilitation

In addition to CIP/CIM, joint contractures and other consequences of immobility may contribute to post-ICU functional limitations. The negative effects of immobility are well characterized in studies of healthy individuals [29]. Given these data, efforts to minimize deep sedation and start physical medicine and rehabilitation interventions shortly after ICU admission have been tested [30]. Early rehabilitation interventions in the ICU are safe and feasible, and have been demonstrated to improve short-term physical function and other outcomes [30–35]. The delivery and timing of rehabilitation interventions is important. For example, a two-site clinical trial demonstrated that mechanically ventilated patients randomized to early occupational and physical therapy (PT) starting within 72 hours of intubation were more likely to achieve independent functional status at hospital discharge than patients who received similar rehabilitation care starting at a median of 7 days after intubation [35]. The patients with earlier rehabilitation also had a shorter duration of delirium highlighting the likely inter-relationship of cognition and physical activity. In addition, patients randomized to routine PT plus bedside cycling exercises, for 20 minutes daily, starting at ICU day 5, had significantly improved quadriceps force, 6MWD, and physical function QOL measurements at hospital discharge vs. controls who received routine PT only [36]. Use of other technology-based rehabilitation therapies in the ICU, such as neuromuscular electrical stimulation (NMES) and a dynamic tilt-table, may also have benefits [37]. Neuromuscular electrical stimulation may help preserve muscle mass, reduce ICUAW, and hasten weaning in mechanically ventilated ICU patients [38]; modified tilt-tables can be used safely to facilitate partial weight-bearing exercises during rehabilitation in the ICU [39].

Despite these improvements observed from early ICU interventions, a randomized trial of ICU survivors receiving an individualized, home-based physical rehabilitation program showed no difference in improvement in 6MWD vs. a control group without structured post-discharge rehabilitation [40]. This finding raises many questions including how post-discharge interventions should be refined (e.g., optimal intensity and duration), whether interventions should be individually tailored for specific patient subgroups (e.g., prolonged mechanical ventilation), and whether post-discharge interventions should be focused much earlier (i.e., shortly after ICU admission). Recently published guidelines in the UK recommend initiation of an individualized, structured rehabilitation program early during ICU care, with continuation upon transfer to the ward along with education on self-guided rehabilitation [41]. A European task force also emphasized the need for structured and individualized rehabilitation in the ICU [42]. The long-term benefits of these initiatives on neuromuscular abnormalities and physical function requires greater evaluation in future studies. For further reading regarding rehabilitation following critical illness, the reader is referred to Chapter 32, this volume.

Quality of life

General ICU patients

The instruments most commonly used to measure QOL outcomes in ICU survivors include the Medical Outcomes Study 36-item Short Form General Health Survey (SF-36) and the EQ-5D. These tools measure physical and mental aspects of health-related quality of life. One important consideration in studies focusing on QOL after ICU is the lack of a baseline QOL assessment for comparison purposes. Given the unexpected nature of critical illness, QOL outcomes generally cannot be prospectively measured prior to critical illness. As a result, many studies compare ICU survivors' QOL with population norms. However, patients who become critically ill may not be at the population norm prior to illness [43,44], making it difficult to fully understand the true impact of critical illness on QOL. With this caveat, existing research indicates that QOL is commonly impaired after ICU discharge, potentially for long durations.

A systematic review of 21 studies found significantly lower QOL in > 7,000 ICU survivors, with most studies demonstrating impairments in all QOL domains except bodily pain [45]. Impairments were most commonly found in the domains related to physical QOL [21,45] and generally improve, to some degree, within 3–12 months after discharge, but generally remain below those of matched population norms [45–47]. The course of physical recovery over time may be complex. A longitudinal study of 300 ICU patients reported QOL impairment at 3 months that recovered by 1 year, but another impairment occurring between 2.5- and 5-year follow-up [43]. Throughout 5-year follow-up, the mean SF-36 physical component score of this cohort remained below population norms. However, virtually all domains of post-ICU QOL surpassed proxy-based estimates of patients' baseline QOL at 6 months after illness. This finding may be due to true recovery to baseline QOL within 6 months, a positive influence of surviving critical illness on patients' perceived QOL, or discrepancies between proxy and patient estimates of baseline QOL [43,44].

A variety of factors have been associated with QOL impairments, including ARDS, severe sepsis, age, prolonged mechanical ventilation, severe trauma, pre-existing disease, ICU severity of illness, and posttraumatic stress disorder (PTSD) and depression symptoms [48,49]. Physical QOL deficits

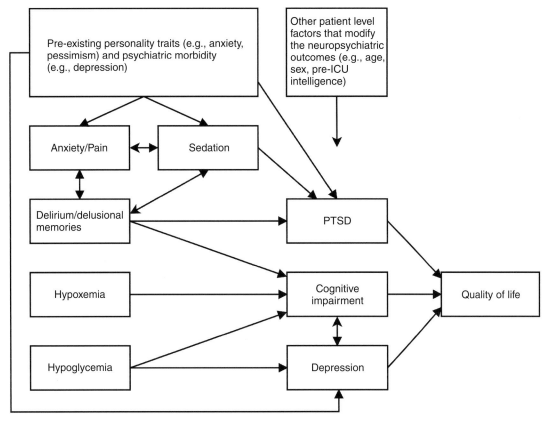

Figure 4.3 The complex associations between different physical impairments and quality of life. ICU, intensive care unit; PTSD, posttraumatic stress disorder.

have been specifically associated with CIP [21], the loss of muscle mass [50], and impaired pulmonary function [51] (Figure 4.1). A study of trauma survivors identified that delusional memories of the ICU were associated with long-lasting impairments in all QOL domains evaluated [52,53]. Figures 4.1 and 4.3 depict the complex associations between these factors and quality of life.

Acute respiratory distress syndrome

A meta-analysis of five studies of acute respiratory distress syndrome (ARDS) survivors at 1–4 years after ICU (n = 330) demonstrated significantly lower SF-36 scores vs. population norms across all eight QOL domains, with the largest decrements seen in the physical domains [54]. These decrements in QOL were profound and relatively consistent across studies. A separate systematic review evaluated psychiatric morbidity following ARDS and its effect on QOL [55]. In the 10 studies reviewed, symptoms of depression, anxiety, and PTSD were common in the months

and years after critical illness. The median prevalences for substantial symptoms of depression, PTSD, and anxiety were 28%, 28%, and 24%, respectively. Four studies explored the relationship between these psychiatric symptoms and subsequent QOL; all studies demonstrated negative associations, with the strongest decrements in QOL occurring in the domains of vitality, social functioning, role emotional, and mental health. Taken together, these analyses indicate survivors of ARDS suffer a wide range of substantial and prolonged impairments in QOL.

Sepsis

A systematic review focused on sepsis survivors found that QOL was impaired relative to population norms [56]. These QOL scores were comparable to populations of patients with chronic illnesses, such as chronic obstructive pulmonary disease and congestive heart failure. As with ARDS, these QOL decrements were observed for at least 2 years after critical illness [56]. It is unclear if sepsis is independently associated with greater declines in QOL vs. non-septic critical illnesses or ARDS [57,58]. Existing findings are mixed, and may be difficult to evaluate given considerable overlap between these ICU syndromes.

Selected interventions

Physical rehabilitation interventions have been proposed to improve survivors' post-ICU QOL. In one trial, patients randomized to cycling exercises, starting as early as ICU day 5, plus routine physical therapy (PT) had significantly improved physical QOL measurements at hospital discharge vs. controls who received only routine PT [36]. Other studies have assessed rehabilitation following hospital discharge. Intensive care unit survivors receiving a rehabilitation handbook of self-directed exercises had improved physical function-related QOL at 6 months vs. a control group without the handbook [59]. However, other randomized trials of nurse-led or home-based rehabilitation programs after hospital discharge failed to show improvements in QOL when compared with routine care [40,60]. Further investigation is needed to understand the optimal content, timing, and duration of interventions aimed at improving QOL. For further reading about interventions to improve quality of life, please refer to Chapter 32, this volume.

Conclusion

Impairments in physical function and QOL are nearly universal following critical illness. Future ICU studies should not only seek to improve mortality, but focus on long-term outcomes, such as restoring function and QOL following critical illness. Identification of factors associated with poor function and QOL after intensive care, such as neuromuscular and psychological impairments, as well as investigation of structured interventions to prevent and rehabilitate these impairments are needed.

References

1. Needham DM, Bronskill SE, Calinawan JR, et al. Projected incidence of mechanical ventilation in Ontario to 2026: preparing for the aging baby boomers. Crit Care Med 2005;33(3):574–9.

2. Spragg RG, Bernard GR, Checkley W, et al. Beyond mortality: future clinical research in acute lung injury. Am J Respir Crit Care Med 2010;181(10):1121–7.

3. Stevens RD, Marshall SA, Cornblath DR, et al. A framework for diagnosing and classifying intensive care unit-acquired weakness. Crit Care Med 2009; S299–308.

4. Stevens RD, Dowdy DW, Michaels RK, et al. Neuromuscular dysfunction acquired in critical illness: a systematic review. Intensive Care Med 2007;33(11):1876–91.

5. Latronico N, Shehu I, Seghelini E. Neuromuscular sequelae of critical illness. Curr Opin Crit Care 2005;11(4):381–90.

6. Zifko UA. Long-term outcome of critical illness polyneuropathy. Muscle Nerve Suppl 2000;9:S49–52.

7. Fletcher SN, Kennedy DD, Ghosh IR, et al. Persistent neuromuscular and neurophysiologic abnormalities in long-term survivors of prolonged critical illness. Crit Care Med 2003;31(4):1012–16.

8. Herridge MS, Cheung AM, Tansey CM, et al. One-year outcomes in survivors of the acute respiratory distress syndrome. N Engl J Med 2003;348(8):683–93.

9. Guarneri B, Bertolini G, Latronico N. Long-term outcome in patients with critical illness myopathy or neuropathy: the Italian multicentre CRIMYNE study. J Neurol Neurosurg Psychiatry 2008;79:838–41.

10. Young GB, Hammond RR. A stronger approach to weakness in the intensive care unit. Crit Care 2004;8:416–18.

11. Hough CL, Needham DM. The role of future longitudinal studies in ICU survivors: understanding determinants and pathophysiology of weakness and neuromuscular dysfunction. Curr Opin Crit Care 2007;13(5):489–96.

12. Reid CL, Campbell IT, Little RA. Muscle wasting and energy balance in critical illness. Clin Nutr 2004;23(2):273–80.

13. Levine S, Nguyen T, Taylor N, et al. Rapid disuse atrophy of diaphragm fibers in mechanically ventilated humans. N Engl J Med 2009;358(13):1327–35.

14. Hough CL, Steinberg KP, Thompson BT, Rubenfeld GD, Hudson L. Intensive care unit-acquired neuromyopathy and corticosteroids in survivors of persistent ARDS. Intensive Care Med 2009;35:63–8.

15. Papazian L, Forel JM, Gacouin A, et al. Neuromuscular blockers in early acute respiratory distress syndrome. N Engl J Med 2010;363(12):1107–16.

16. Hermans G, Wilmer A, Meersseman W, et al. Impact of intensive insulin therapy on neuromuscular complications and ventilator dependency in the medical intensive care unit. Am J Respir Crit Care Med 2007;175(5):480–9.

17. Brunkhorst FM, Engel C, Bloos F, et al. Intensive insulin therapy and pentastarch resuscitation in severe sepsis. N Engl J Med 2008;358(2):125–39.

18. NICE-SUGAR Investigators. Intensive versus conventional glucose control in critically ill patients. *N Engl J Med* 2009;**360**:1283–97.

19. van der Schaaf M, Dettling DS, Beelen A, *et al.* Poor functional status immediately after discharge from an intensive care unit. *Disabil Rehabil* 2008;**30**(23):1812–18.

20. Angus DC, Clermont G, Linde-Zwirble WT, *et al.* Healthcare costs and long-term outcomes after acute respiratory distress syndrome: a phase III trial of inhaled nitric oxide. *Crit Care Med* 2006;**34**(12):2883–90.

21. van der Schaaf M, Beelen A, Dongelmans DA, Vroom MB, Nollet F. Functional status after intensive care: a challenge for rehabilitation professionals to improve outcome. *J Rehabil Med* 2009;**41**:360–6.

22. Chaboyer W, Grace J. Following the path of ICU survivors: a quality-improvement activity. *Nursing Crit Care* 2003;**8**:149–55.

23. van der Schaaf M, Beelen A, de groot IJM. Critical illness polyneuropathy: a summary of the literature on rehabilitation outcome. *Disabil Rehabil* 2000;**22**(17):808–10.

24. Barnato AE, Albert SM, Angus DC, Lave JR, Degenholtz HB. Disability among elderly survivors of mechanical ventilation. *Am J Respir Crit Care Med* 2011;**183**(8):1037–42.

25. Iwashyna TJ, Ely EW, Smith DM, Langa KM. Long-term cognitive impairment and functional disability among survivors of severe sepsis. *JAMA* 2010;**304**(16):1787–94.

26. Chelluri L, Im K, Belle SH, *et al.* Long-term mortality and quality of life after prolonged mechanical ventilation. *Crit Care Med* 2004;**32**(1):291–3.

27. Herridge MS, Tansey CM, Matté A, *et al.* Functional disability 5 years after acute respiratory distress syndrome. *N Engl J Med* 2011;**364**(14):1293–304.

28. Cheung AM, Tansey CM, Tomlinson G, *et al.* Two-year outcomes, health care use, and costs of survivors of acute respiratory distress syndrome. *Am J Respir Crit Care Med* 2006;**174**(5):538–44.

29. Brower RG. Consequences of bed rest. *Crit Care Med* 2010;**37**(Suppl):S422–8.

30. Needham DM. Mobilizing patients in the intensive care unit: improving neuromuscular weakness and physical function. *JAMA* 2008;**300**(14):1685–90.

31. Morris PE, Goad A, Thompson C, *et al.* Early intensive care unit mobility therapy in the treatment of acute respiratory failure. *Crit Care Med* 2008;**36**(8):2238–43.

32. McWilliams DJ, Atkinson D, Carter A, *et al.* Feasibility and impact of a structured, exercise-based rehabilitation programme for intensive care survivors. *Physiother Theory Pract* 2009;**25**:566–71.

33. Needham DM, Korupolu R, Zanni JM, *et al.* Early physical medicine and rehabilitation for patients with acute respiratory failure: a quality improvement project. *Arch Phys Med Rehabil* 2010;**91**(4):536–42.

34. Morris PE, Griffin L, Berry M, *et al.* Receiving early mobility during an intensive care unit admission is a predictor of improved outcomes in acute respiratory failure. *Am J Med Sci* 2011;**341**(5):373–7.

35. Schweickert WD, Pohlman MC, Pohlman AS, *et al.* Early physical and occupational therapy in mechanically ventilated, critically ill patients: a randomised controlled trial. *Lancet* 2009;**373**(9678):1874–82.

36. Burtin C, Clerckx B, Robbeets C, *et al.* Early exercise in critically ill patients enhances short-term functional recovery. *Crit Care Med* 2009;**37**(9):2499–505.

37. Needham DM, Truong AD, Fan E. Technology to enhance physical rehabilitation of critically ill patients. *Crit Care Med* 2009;**37**(10 Suppl):S436–41.

38. Gerovasili V, Stefanidis K, Vitzilaios K, *et al.* Electrical muscle stimulation preserves the muscle mass of critically ill patients: a randomized study. *Crit Care* 2009;**13**(5):R161.

39. Trees DW, Ketelsen CA, Hobbs JA. Use of a modified tilt table for preambulation strength training as an adjunct to burn rehabilitation: a case series. *J Burn Care Rehabil* 2003;**24**:97–103.

40. Elliott D, McKinley S, Alison J, *et al.* Health-related quality of life and physical recovery after a critical illness: a multi-centre randomised controlled trial of a home-based physical rehabilitation program. *Crit Care* 2011;**15**(3):R142.

41. Tan T, Brett S, Stokes T. Rehabilitation after critical illness: summary of NICE guidance. *Br Med J* 2009;**338**:767–9.

42. Gosselink R, Bott J, Johnson M, *et al.* Physiotherapy for adult patients with critical illness: recommendations of the European Respiratory Society and European Society of Intensive Care Medicine Task Force on Physiotherapy for Critically Ill Patients. *Intensive Care Med* 2008;**34**(7):1188–99.

43. Cuthbertson BH, Roughton S, Jenkinson D, Maclennan G, Vale L. Quality of life in the five years after intensive care: a cohort study. *Crit Care* 2010;**14**(1):R6.

44. Gifford JM, Husain N, Dinglas V, Colantuoni E, Needham D. Baseline quality of life before intensive care: a comparison of patient versus proxy responses. *Crit Care Med* 2010;**38**:855–60.

45. Dowdy DW, Eid MP, Sedrakyan A, *et al.* Quality of life in adult survivors of critical illness: a systematic review of the literature. *Intensive Care Med* 2005;**31**(5):611–20.

46. Sukantarat K, Greer S, Brett S, Williamson R. Physical and psychological sequelae of critical illness. *Br J Health Psychol* 2007;**12**(Pt 1):65–74.

47. Oeyen SG, Vandijck DM, Benoit DD, Annemans L, Decruyenaere JM. Quality of life after intensive care: a systematic review of the literature. *Crit Care Med* 2011;**38**(12):2386–400.

48. Davydow DS, Gifford JM, Desai SV, Needham DM, Bienvenu OJ. Posttraumatic stress disorder in general intensive care unit survivors: a systematic review. *Gen Hosp Psychiatry* 2008;**30**(5):421–34.

49. Davydow DS, Gifford JM, Desai SV, Bienvenu OJ, Needham DM. Depression in general intensive care unit survivors: a systematic review. *Intensive Care Med* 2009;**35**(5):796–809.

50. Poulsen JB, Moller K, Kehlet H, Perner A. Long-term physical outcome in patients with septic shock. *Acta Anaesthesiol Scand* 2009;**53**:724–30.

51. Heyland DK, Groll D, Caeser M. Survivors of acute respiratory distress syndrome: relationship between pulmonary dysfunction and long-term health-related quality of life. *Crit Care Med* 2005;**33**(7):1549–56.

52. Ringdal M, Plos K, Lundberg D, Johansson L, Bergbom I. Outcome after injury: memories, health-related quality of life, anxiety, and symptoms of depression after intensive care. *J Trauma* 2009; **66**(4):1226–33.

53. Ringdal M, Plos K, Ortenwall P, Bergbom I. Memories and health-related quality of life after intensive care: a follow-up study. *Crit Care Med* 2010;**38**:38–44.

54. Dowdy DW, Eid MP, Dennison CR, *et al.* Quality of life after acute respiratory distress syndrome: a meta-analysis. *Intensive Care Med* 2006;**32**(8):1115–24.

55. Davydow DS, Desai SV, Needham DM, Bienvenu OJ. Psychiatric morbidity in survivors of the acute respiratory distress syndrome: a systematic review. *Psychosom Med* 2008;**70**(4):512–19.

56. Winters BD, Eberlein M, Leung J, *et al.* Long-term mortality and quality of life in sepsis: a systematic review. *Crit Care Med* 2010;**38**:1276–83.

57. Heyland DK, Hopman W, Coo H, Tranmer J, McColl M. Long-term health-related quality of life in survivors of sepsis. Short Form 36: a valid and reliable measure of health-related quality of life. *Crit Care Med* 2000;**28**(11):3599–605.

58. Davidson TA, Caldwell ES, Curtis JR, Hudson LD, Steinberg KP. Reduced quality of life in survivors of acute respiratory distress syndrome compared with critically ill control patients. *JAMA* 1999;**281**(4):354–60.

59. Jones C, Skirrow P, Griffiths RD, *et al.* Rehabilitation after critical illness: a randomized, controlled trial. *Crit Care Med* 2003;**31**(10):2456–61.

60. Cuthbertson BH, Rattray JE, Gager M, *et al.* The PRaCTICaL study of nurse led, intensive care follow-up programmes for improving long term outcomes from critical illness: a pragmatic randomised controlled trial. *Br Med J* 2009;**339**:1–8.

61. Fan E, Zanni JM, Dennison CR, Lepre SJ, Needham DM. Critical illness neuromyopathy and muscle weakness in patients in the intensive care unit. *AACN Adv Crit Care* 2009;**20**:243–53.

62. Latronico N, Bolton CF. Critical illness polyneuropathy and myopathy: a major cause of muscle weakness and paralysis. *Lancet Neuro* 2011;**10**:931–41.

63. Girard TD, Kress JP, Fuchs BD, *et al.* Efficacy and safety of a paired sedation and ventilator weaning protocol for mechanically ventilated patients in intensive care (Awakening and Breathing Controlled trial): a randomised controlled trial. *Lancet.* 2008;**371**(9607):126–34.

Delirium and dementia: unraveling the complex relationship

Margaret Pisani

SUMMARY

Delirium and dementia are both global disorders of cognitive impairment that occur more frequently in older patients. Both disorders have high prevalence in their respective populations with prevalence of dementia between 10.3–18.8% in older patients and delirium prevalence of 30% in hospitalized patients and up to 80% in critically ill patients. These disorders share common risk factors including age, hypertension, hearing impairment, and alcoholism among others. There are also data suggesting a common genetic predisposition to both delirium and dementia with the bulk of research focusing on apolipoprotein E e4 (ApoE e4). Systemic inflammation may be one of the pathogenic links between delirium and dementia. Infection has been demonstrated to play a role in both dementia and delirium development. Animal studies and human epidemiological data document the importance of inflammatory mediators in amyloid plaque formation and in clinical disease development and progression for Alzheimer's patients. Patients with delirium have been shown to have increased levels of inflammatory cytokines. The actual pathogenic mechanisms of how systemic inflammation impacts delirium and dementia are still being elucidated. In longitudinal studies, both delirium and dementia have been shown to lead to increased morbidity and mortality. There are multiple postulated mechanisms which can link causation of delirium and dementia, including shared risk factors, genetic susceptibility, and inflammatory mechanisms.

Introduction

Delirium and dementia are both global disorders of cognitive impairment that occur more frequently in older patients. This chapter will review the definitions of delirium and dementia, risk factors for both, and genetic and systemic inflammatory links between these two conditions. Recently there has been growing interest examining the epidemiological and pathological links between delirium and dementia, and this chapter presents the current state of the literature.

Dementia

Dementia is an acquired persistent form of cognitive impairment. It is an increasingly common and devastating problem for the aging population and is associated with increased rates of morbidity, functional disability, institutionalization, and mortality. The prevalence of dementia in community samples of older persons ranges from 10.3% to 18.8% [1]. Longitudinal studies of dementia suggest that life expectancy is increasing in patients who have Alzheimer's (AD) and multi-infarct dementia. Although severe dementia currently affects 2.2 million Americans, population projections indicate that severe dementia will affect at least 10 million Americans by 2040.

Dementia is characterized by impairment of memory and impairment in at least one other cognitive domain, including aphasia, apraxia, agnosia, or executive function. By definition, these cognitive changes must represent a decline in the patient's level of function and be severe enough to interfere with daily function and independence. Alzheimer's disease is the most common form of dementia in older patients and it is estimated to affect more than 4 million Americans. Other major dementia syndromes include dementia with Lewy bodies (DLB), frontotemporal dementia (FTD), vascular (multi-infarct) dementia, and Parkinson's disease with dementia. Each of these dementias has a different neuropathological hallmark, although there is overlap.

Brain Disorders in Critical Illness, ed. Robert D. Stevens, Tarek Sharshar, and E. Wesley Ely. Published by Cambridge University Press. © Cambridge University Press 2013.

The neuropathological hallmarks of AD are neuritic plaques and neurofibrillary tangles, although these lesions are not unique to AD and can be found in other neurodegenerative disorders and in clinically normal individuals as well. Classic neuritic plaques are spherical structures consisting of a central core of fibrous protein known as amyloid that is surrounded by degenerating or dystrophic nerve endings. Two other types of amyloid-related plaques are recognized in the brains of AD patients: diffuse plaques, which contain poorly defined amyloid but no well-circumscribed amyloid core, and "burnt-out" plaques, which consist of an isolated dense amyloid core. The amyloid protein contains a 40–42 amino acid peptide called β-amyloid (Aβ) that is derived from proteolytic processing of a larger amyloid precursor protein molecule. It is believed that abnormal processing of the amyloid precursor protein molecule results in fragments, the most toxic of which is the $A\beta_1$ peptide. Because $A\beta_1$ readily forms insoluble clumps in the brain, it has been postulated to initiate a cascade of events leading to neuronal dysfunction and death. Although increasing evidence supports the hypothesis that the accumulation of Aβ is critical to the pathogenesis of AD, some investigators believe that Aβ is not exclusively responsible for the neuronal alterations that underlie the clinical symptoms seen. Neurofibrillary tangles are the other characteristic histopathological change seen in AD. Neurofibrillary tangles are found inside neurons and are composed of paired helical filaments of hyperphosphorylated micro-tubule-associated tau protein. The intracellular deposition may cause disruption of normal cytoskeletal architecture, with subsequent neuronal cell death.

Although there are characteristic neuoropathogenic features of dementia, it remains essentially a clinical diagnosis. Readers are referred to the *Diagnostic and Statistical Manual, Fifth Edition* (DSM–5) criteria for dementia [2].

Delirium

Delirium is an acute confusional state and is increasingly being recognized as an independent predictor of adverse outcomes in medical, surgical, and critically ill patients. Delirium is a common complication in hospitalized patients, with 30% of older medical patients experiencing delirium at some point during their hospital stay. Occurrence rates of up to 50% have been documented in older postoperative patients and up to 70–80% in medically critically ill patients [3,4]. Delirium is a disorder of global cognitive function characterized by an acute onset and fluctuating course with a reduced ability to focus, sustain, or shift attention. There is a change in cognition as well as possible perceptual disturbances that are not accounted for by a pre-existing disorder. By definition, delirium is caused by a medical condition, substance intoxication, or medication side effect. Delirium can present with psychomotor disturbances such as hypoactivity or hyperactivity, as well as with sleep disturbances. Like dementia, delirium is a clinical syndrome with a wide variety of etiologies. In the *Diagnostic and Statistical Manual, Fifth Edition* (DSM–5) [2], there are some changes regarding delirium diagnosis. The first change is that the order of delirium criteria is changed with "duration of symptoms" being placed at the end of the criteria. The criteria also now include a statement that delirium symptoms can fluctuate in both duration and severity. The word "consciousness" has been changed to "awareness" as it was felt that "consciousness" was too nebulous a term to describe the symptom of delirium and that "awareness" captured the essence of delirium much better. It has been clarified that a pre-existing cognitive disorder that explains the symptoms should not be diagnosed as delirium. The DSM–5 delirium criteria mention accompanying symptoms that are not necessary or sufficient to make the diagnosis but often present in a patient with delirium. These symptoms include sleep–wake cycle disturbance, psychomotor, perceptual, and emotional disturbances, delusions, labile affect, dysarthria, and EEG abnormalities. The presence and severity of delirium is determined with standardized clinical measures and diagnostic criteria. Screening instruments for delirium are reviewed in Chapter 24, this volume.

Delirium leads to poor outcomes, including increased morbidity, mortality, a higher risk of cognitive impairment, institutionalization, longer length of ICU and hospital stays, and costlier hospitalizations [5]. Several cohort studies have demonstrated the link between delirium and increased lengths of stay. In a cohort of 238 critically ill patients admitted to the ICU through the emergency room, median ICU length of stay was three times longer in those with delirium versus those without delirium. In a cohort study of 48 mechanically ventilated medical ICU patients, delirium was the strongest predictor of hospital length of stay after controlling for severity of illness, age, gender, race, and duration of psychoactive medications [6]. The impact of delirium on length of stay was also demonstrated in non-intubated critically ill patients, suggesting that patients with delirium who are not mechanically ventilated also have increased length of stay. One study that examined the cost of delirium in the ICU found that both ICU and hospital costs were significantly higher for patients who developed delirium during their ICU stay versus those who did not [7].

Delirium pathophysiology

Delirium is the manifestation of a complex inter-relationship between a vulnerable patient, noxious insults, and precipitating risk factors. The neuropathological basis for delirium is poorly understood. Acetylcholine has been demonstrated to play a key role in the pathogenesis of delirium. Data supporting the role of acetylcholine and delirium derive from studies of healthy patients who developed delirium when given anticholinergic drugs. Other evidence comes from risk factor studies that demonstrate that conditions such as hypoxia, hypoglycemia, and thiamine deficiency which precipitate delirium also decrease acetylcholine synthesis in the central nervous system. Finally, measures of serum anticholinergic activity have been correlated with the severity of delirium. Other central nervous system neurotransmitters have been linked to delirium, including serotonin, GABA, somatostatin, norepinephrine, dopamine, among others, but the data on their roles is still being elucidated.

Pro-inflammatory cytokines such as interleukins and tumor necrosis factor alpha (TNFα) also may have a role in the pathogenesis of delirium. Experimental animal models have demonstrated central nervous system effects when cytokines or interleukins are administered. Clinical correlation studies suggest that cytokine activation may account for delirium in situations such as infection, cardiopulmonary bypass, and acute hip fracture.

The long-standing teaching has been that delirium is reversible and that all of its symptoms should resolve within days to weeks. Clinical studies have called that dogma into question. Three hypotheses that may link delirium and dementia are: (1) delirium may represent a worsening or accelerating dementia; (2) delirium and dementia may be distinct but delirium may unmask an as yet undetected dementia; (3) delirium leads to chronic cognitive impairment through irreversible central nervous system dysfunction. The remainder of the chapter will review the available evidence to support these three hypotheses. Please refer to Chapter 11, this volume, for a review of this topic.

Risk factors for delirium and dementia

There have been a multitude of studies examining risk factors for dementia and for delirium [8,9]. Many of these risk factors are common to both diseases. Age is a strong risk factor for both dementia and delirium. Other common risk factors relate to cardiovascular disease, with hypertension being a risk factor for both processes. While family history plays a role in certain forms of dementia, there are no studies examining family history and risk for delirium. Dementia is a well-recognized risk factor for delirium in a variety of patient populations including medical, surgical, and critically ill patients. Table 5.1 lists the risk factors for both delirium and dementia. The connection between delirium and dementia may lie in their shared risk factors.

Table 5.1 Risk factors for delirium and dementia.

Delirium	Dementia
Age	Age
Functional impairment	Female gender
Cognitive impairment or dementia	Mild cognitive impairment
Underlying comorbidities (e.g., heart, liver, or renal failure, diabetes, hypertension)	Delirium
	Chronic kidney disease
Neurological disease (e.g., stroke or seizure)	Gait abnormalities
Hearing or vision impairment	Alcoholism
Alcoholism	Hearing impairment
Tobacco use/nicotine withdrawal	Family history
Elevated creatinine (> 2.0 mg/dl)	Autosomal dominant forms:
Low arterial pH (< 7.35)	Amyloid precursor protein (APP) – Chromosome 21;
Severity of illness	Presenilin 1 (PS1) –
Pain	Chromosome 14; Presenilin 2 (PS2) –
Anemia	Chromosome 1
Total parenteral nutrition (TPN)	Genetic non-familial: Apolipoprotein E (ApoE)
Drug overdose or illicit drugs	Hypercholesterolemia
Opioids	Hypertension
Benzodiazepines	Diabetes mellitus
Anticholinergic medications	Tobacco use
Sleep deprivation	Metabolic syndrome
Restraint use	Low education level
Catheter use	Head trauma/loss of consciousness
Immobilization	Organophosphate and organochlorine pesticides

Genetic link

Links between delirium and dementia may also be found in studies examining genetic polymorphisms. To date, the genetic polymorphism that has been studied most frequently is apolipoprotein E e4 (ApoE e4). Apolipoprotein E is a 299 amino acid lipid binding protein. The ApoE e4 polymorphism has an allele frequency of 14% and has been identified as a major susceptibility factor for AD. The mechanism whereby ApoE e4 influences the development of AD is unknown. Apolipoprotein is involved in neuronal protection and repair, and in dementia is believed to play a role in early beta-amyloid deposition. ApoE e4 also affects plasma lipid levels and has been associated with atherosclerotic vascular disease, although it is unclear whether vascular disease is the primary mechanism by which ApoE e4 influences the development of AD. A prospective cohort study suggested that ApoE e4 was a risk factor for AD, independent from cholesterol, lipid, and lipoprotein levels. In addition, ApoE plays an immunomodulatory role in the setting of infection and acute injury and has been shown to be up-regulated in the central nervous system after injury.

ApoE e4 is a susceptibility marker for dementia in that patients who are homozygous for this allele are more likely to develop dementia and develop it at an earlier age, but are not absolutely destined to progress to disease [10]. In patients with dementia, ApoE e4 has also been associated with disease severity, including a steeper rate of cognitive decline and decreased survival than patients without the polymorphism. There are also imaging studies demonstrating associations with MRI findings of increased hippocampal atrophy and ApoE e4. Finally, there have been associations demonstrated between ApoE e4 and increased neuritic plaques and neurofibrillary tangles in patients at autopsy.

Studies have also examined the ApoE e4 polymorphism as a genetic predisposition to delirium in medical, surgical, critically ill, and hip fracture patients. In a meta-analysis of medical, cardiac, and non-cardiac surgery and hip fracture patients, the unadjusted odds ratio for delirium comparing ApoE e4 carriers with non-e4 carriers was 1.6 (95% CI, 0.9–2.7). In a study of 53 mechanically ventilated patients, ApoE e4 was associated with delirium duration in critically ill patients.

ApoE e4 may contribute to both delirium and dementia by modifying glial activation and inflammatory responses in the central nervous system. Another mechanism tying ApoE e4 to both delirium and dementia may be through promoting an anticholinergic state.

Animal models have demonstrated that ApoE-derived peptides block nicotinic acetylcholine receptors which may lead to memory loss and cognitive decline.

Systemic inflammation

The major clinical risk factors for the development of AD such as aging, obesity, diabetes, hypertension, and smoking, all comprise a significant increase in systemic inflammatory markers. While systemic inflammation is unlikely to be a major explanation for the brain pathology seen in dementia, there is good reason to believe that systemic inflammation contributes to the progression and severity of the pathology. Delirium may be the evidence that systemic inflammation contributes to the exacerbation of dementia. Dementia and age are the strongest predisposing risk factors for delirium, and one of the major precipitating risk factors for delirium is systemic inflammation often due to surgery or infection. In healthy patients, multiple precipitating factors or severe stimuli are required to cause delirium, while in older and demented patients, milder inflammatory stimuli can trigger a delirious episode.

Animal studies have demonstrated that systemic inflammation induced by pathogen-associated molecular pattern stimulators of the toll-like receptors or by pro-inflammatory cytokines and by surgery can induce changes in central nervous system function, termed "sickness behavior." These changes include decreased locomotor activity, decreased social activity and feeding, and alterations in sleep–wake cycle. There is also robust evidence that inflammatory insults have a deleterious effect on the consolidation of new memories. Systemic inflammation generated in animal models using lipopolysaccharide (LPS) demonstrated altered processing of amyloid precursor protein (APP). These animals demonstrated cognitive changes in water maze and passive avoidance tasks that were partially prevented by the anti-inflammatory medication sulindac, a COX inhibitor. Along this same vein, studies have also demonstrated that treatment of normal mice with systemic LPS can induce increased Aβ1–42 generation and deposition of amyloid plaque material. Results from mouse models show that systemic LPS or sterile systemic inflammation can induce impairments in memory consolidation in normal animals, but the deficits are accentuated in aged animals.

There are epidemiological data to suggest that infection may play a role in dementia. A review of general practitioner's databases demonstrated that two or more infections over a 4-year period increased the risk for AD by two-fold. Other similar evidence demonstrated declining Mini Mental State Examination (MMSE) scores in patients with increasing viral burden due to herpes and cytomegalovirus, and that periodontitis was a significant risk factor for AD.

Elevations in markers of systemic inflammation such as IL-1β and tumor necrosis factor alpha (TNFα) have been shown to be significantly correlated with accelerated cognitive decline in patients with dementia. Inflammation-associated exacerbations of cognitive decline were still present even when patients with delirium were excluded, raising the questions of how the pathways of inflammation, delirium, and cognitive decline in patients with dementia are occurring.

There is evidence in humans that pro-inflammatory molecules such as IL-6 and IL-8 are associated with postoperative delirium, but these associations are much weaker than the association between pre-existing cognitive impairment and the development of delirium. A prospective observational study of 516 survivors of severe sepsis also suggests biological plausibility between inflammation and cognitive impairment [11]. This study demonstrated long-term cognitive impairment in patients with severe sepsis compared with non-sepsis hospitalized patients, with deficits which persisted for at least 8 years. Figure 5.1 presents a schema for how inflammation, delirium, and dementia may be related. The exact mechanisms of how systemic inflammation affects the brain are still being elucidated, but inflammation, along with other factors, likely plays a role in the link between delirium and dementia. A recent review article discusses the role of inflammation in the pathogenesis of delirium and dementia [12]. Please refer to Chapter 18, this volume, for an in-depth review.

Clinical studies of delirium leading to dementia

There are several studies in the literature that have examined the association between the diagnosis of delirium and subsequent cognitive impairment or dementia. These studies differ widely in their design, including the choice of instruments to screen for delirium and dementia, length of follow-up, and patient populations. Most studies have small sample sizes, inadequate control for baseline cognitive impairment, and other important confounders such as severity of illness and medications. Nonetheless, taken together, these studies provide evidence of a link between delirium and cognitive impairment. The studies are summarized in Table 5.2.

Hopkins et al. reported on neuropsychological sequelae in 55 survivors of acute respiratory distress syndrome (ARDS) [13]. While they did not assess for delirium as a risk factor in this study, they documented that 100% of survivors had cognitive impairment at hospital discharge. At 1 year after ARDS hospitalization 30% of patients still had generalized cognitive decline including impaired memory, attention, and concentration or decreased mental processing speed. A study examining patients with established cognitive impairment found that delirium prevalence increased as the severity of the pre-existing cognitive impairment increased [14]. Prevalence of delirium was 50% in patients with mild cognitive impairment, increased to 82% among patients with moderate cognitive impairment, and was 86% among those with severe impairment. Delirium symptoms overall appeared to be similar, regardless of the degree of cognitive impairment. Disorganized thinking was the only

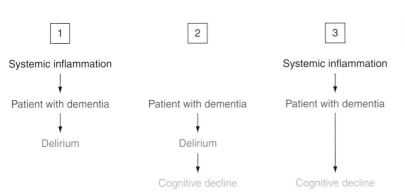

Figure 5.1 Systemic inflammation, dementia, delirium, and cognitive decline.

Table 5.2 Studies examining delirium and cognitive decline.

Reference	Patient population	Length of follow-up	Results
[19]	n = 106 Hip fracture	6 months	In patients free of dementia pre-fracture, 38% of patients who developed delirium vs. 7% (p < 0.001) of patients without delirium met criteria for dementia at 6-month follow-up
[20]	n = 263 Post-stroke	3 months	Delirium was associated with the development of dementia at 3 months post-stroke. In logistic regression the odds ratio was OR = 2.65 (95% CI, 1.17–6.02) for developing dementia after an episode of delirium
[18]	n = 77 Critically ill	12 months	Delirium duration was an independent predictor of worse cognitive performance at 3-month and 12-month follow-up after adjusting for age, education, pre-existing cognitive impairment, severity of illness, severe sepsis, and medication exposure in the intensive care unit
[21]	n = 408 Medical patients	36 months	Delirium significantly accelerated the rate of cognitive decline in patients with Alzheimer's disease as measured by the Blessed Dementia Rating Scale
[22]	n = 255 Hip surgery	8 and 38 months	Delirium was a strong independent predictor of cognitive impairment that was more marked at long-term follow-up. Cognitive impairment developed in 53.8% of the delirious group versus 4% of the non-delirious group
[23]	n = 112 Hip surgery	Average 30 months	Dementia or mild cognitive impairment diagnosed in 77.8% of patients with delirium versus 40.9% of patients without delirium (RR: 1.9, 95% CI: 1.1–1.3)
[24]	n = 103 Hip fracture	4 years	No relationship between delirium and cognitive decline. Cognitive deficit at baseline was a predictor for further cognitive decline (OR = 1.53, p = 0.024)
[25]	n = 572 Knee or hip replacement	Retrospective review	Patients with a history of postoperative delirium had a relative risk of developing dementia of 10.5 (95% CI: 3.3–33.2)
[26]	n = 102 Elective abdominal surgery	3 months	Patients with delirium had lower cognitive scores during each of three follow-up assessments
[27]	n = 34 Elective cardiac surgery	1 year	Delirium during the ICU stay was not associated with either short- or long-term cognitive deficits
[28]	n = 115 Hip surgery	6 months	Deterioration in MMSE postoperatively was greater in patients with delirium than those without (2.6 point decline versus 0.9)
[29]	n = 78 Hip fracture	5 years	Patients with delirium were 3.5 times more likely to develop dementia over the 5-year follow-up then those without delirium
[30]	n = 674 Hip fracture	1 year	Cognitive impairment first detected in the hospital persisted in over 40% of patients at 1-year follow-up
[31]	n = 34 Medical ICU patients	6 months	No significant association between delirium duration and cognitive impairment

symptom of delirium that was statistically different. It was present in 58% of patients with mild cognitive impairment compared with 92% of patients with severe cognitive impairment. There was no association between the hypoactive form of delirium and the severity of the pre-existing cognitive impairment. This study and others have demonstrated that clinical presentation of delirium is similar in patients with and without dementia.

Outcomes of delirium and dementia

There are multiple studies that indicate that both delirium and dementia lead to increased mortality

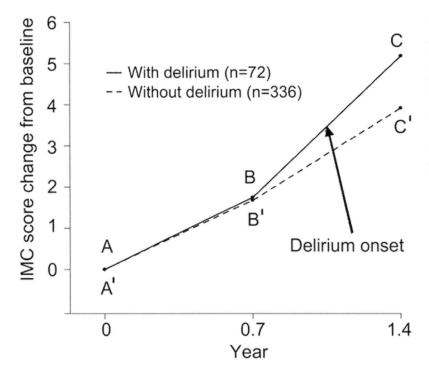

Figure 5.2 Cognitive trajectories of patients with Alzheimer's disease over time, with and without delirium [21]. The median time to delirium from point B was 0.3 years (75% interquartile range, 0.13–0.45 years). The slopes are based on the changes in the Blessed Information-Memory-Concentration (IMC) subscore over time, and the scores presented are calculated adjusting for baseline differences. These slopes are derived from linear mixed models adjusted for relevant covariables (age, sex, educational level, Massachusetts General Hospital dementia severity rating score, duration of dementia symptoms before diagnosis, family history of dementia, and number of comorbid medical diagnoses). The solid line indicates the trajectory for patients with delirium (n = 72) and the dashed line indicates the trajectory for patients without delirium (n = 336).

[15,16]. What is not clear still is the interaction between delirium and dementia and increased mortality. In a recent meta-analysis of studies examining delirium outcomes, 38% of patients had an increased risk of death compared with 27.5% of patients without delirium after a mean follow-up of 22 months [17]. This association persisted independent of pre-existing dementia. Delirium remained significantly associated with mortality when patients with delirium superimposed on dementia were compared with patients with dementia without delirium, and when patients with delirium only were compared with patients without delirium or dementia. The mechanisms by which delirium during dementia occurs are critical to understand. Alzheimer's dementia patients who experience delirium show accelerated cognitive decline, but it is unclear whether the delirium itself, or the triggers that induced the delirium, are responsible for altering the disease trajectory. Figure 5.2 illustrates the cognitive trajectories of AD patients with and without delirium and demonstrates the increased cognitive decline in patients with dementia who develop delirium compared with those who do not develop delirium. A study of critically ill patients links days of ICU delirium with 3-month and 12-month cognitive performance [18]. Duration of delirium was an independent predictor of average performance on a battery of neuropsychiatric testing after adjusting for age, education, pre-existing cognitive function, severity of illness, severe sepsis, and psychoactive medication use. Figure 5.3 presents the data from this study. Please refer to Chapter 2, this volume for an in-depth review of critical illness and cognitive impairment.

Conclusion

There are multiple postulated mechanisms which can link causation of delirium and dementia including shared risk factors, genetic susceptibility, and inflammatory mechanisms. Delirium is rarely caused by a single factor, and its development involves the complex inter-relationship between predisposing host factors and precipitating factors. Future studies are needed to clarify the pathogenesis of both delirium and dementia and to better understand the relationship between these two clinical disease states.

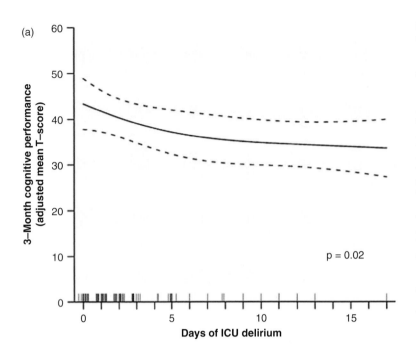

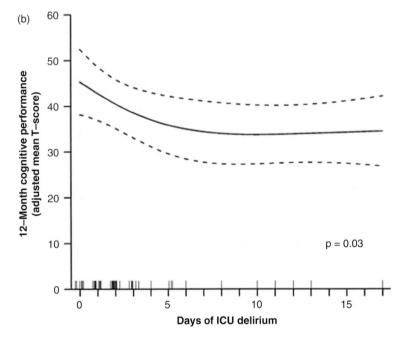

Figure 5.3 Relationship between duration of delirium and average cognitive performance measured at (a) 3-month and (b) 12-month follow-up [18]. Duration of delirium independently predicted average performance on a battery of nine neuropsychological tests after adjusting for age, education, pre-existing cognitive function, severity of illness, severe sepsis, Awakening and Breathing Controlled Trial treatment group, and total benzodiazepine, opiate, and propofol doses administered in the intensive care unit (ICU) (p = 0.02 and 0.03, respectively). A mean T-score (shown on the y-axis) of 50 indicates average performance on nine neuropsychological tests, based on age-adjusted and education-adjusted normative data. These results show that, other factors being equal, a patient with 5 days of delirium will score, on average, nearly one half of a standard deviation lower (i.e., 5 points lower) across domains of cognitive function at 3-month follow-up (and 7 points lower at 12-month follow-up) than a patient who was delirious for 1 day.

References

1. Graham JE, Rockwood K, Beattie BL, *et al.* Prevalence and severity of cognitive impairment with and without dementia in an elderly population. *Lancet* 1997;**349**(9068):1793–6.

2. American Psychiatric Association. *Diagnostic and Statistical Manual of Mental Disorders, 5th edition (DSM–5)*. Washington, DC: American Psychiatric Association; 2013.

3. McNicoll L, Pisani MA, Zhang Y, *et al.* Delirium in the intensive care unit: occurrence and clinical course in older patients. *J Am Geriatr Soc* 2003;**51**(5):591–8.

4. Ely EW, Siegel MD, Inouye SK. Delirium in the intensive care unit: an under-recognized syndrome of

organ dysfunction. *Semin Respir Crit Care Med* 2001;**22**(2):115–26.

5. Frontera JA. Delirium and sedation in the ICU. *Neurocrit Care* 2011;**14**(3):463–74.

6. Ely EW, Gautam S, Margolin R, *et al.* The impact of delirium in the intensive care unit on hospital length of stay. *Intensive Care Med* 2001;**27**(12):1892–900.

7. Milbrandt EB, Deppen S, Harrison PL, *et al.* Costs associated with delirium in mechanically ventilated patients. *Crit Care Med* 2004;**32**(4):955–62.

8. Pisani MA, Murphy TE, Van Ness PH, Araujo KL, Inouye SK. Characteristics associated with delirium in older patients in a medical intensive care unit. *Arch Intern Med* 2007;**167**(15):1629–34.

9. Ouimet S, Kavanagh BP, Gottfried SB, Skrobik Y. Incidence, risk factors and consequences of ICU delirium. *Intensive Care Med* 2007;**33**(1):66–73.

10. Myers RH, Schaefer EJ, Wilson PW, *et al.* Apolipoprotein E epsilon4 association with dementia in a population-based study: the Framingham study. *Neurology* 1996;**46**(3):673–7.

11. Iwashyna TJ, Ely EW, Smith DM, Langa KM. Long-term cognitive impairment and functional disability among survivors of severe sepsis. *JAMA* 2010;**304**(16):1787–94.

12. Simone MJ, Tan ZS. The role of inflammation in the pathogenesis of delirium and dementia in older adults: a review. *CNS Neurosci Ther* 2010;**17**(5):506–13.

13. Hopkins RO, Weaver LK, Pope D, *et al.* Neuropsychological sequelae and impaired health status in survivors of severe acute respiratory distress syndrome. *Am J Respir Crit Care Med* 1999;**160**(1):50–6.

14. Voyer P, Cole MG, McCusker J, Belzile E. Prevalence and symptoms of delirium superimposed on dementia. *Clin Nurs Res* 2006;**15**(1):46–66.

15. Ely EW, Shintani A, Truman B, *et al.* Delirium as a predictor of mortality in mechanically ventilated patients in the intensive care unit. *JAMA* 2004;**291**(14):1753–62.

16. Pisani MA, Kong SY, Kasl SV, *et al.* Days of delirium are associated with 1-year mortality in an older intensive care unit population. *Am J Respir Crit Care Med* 2009;**180**(11):1092–7.

17. Witlox J, Eurelings LS, de Jonghe JF, *et al.* Delirium in elderly patients and the risk of postdischarge mortality, institutionalization, and dementia: a meta-analysis. *JAMA* 2010;**304**(4):443–51.

18. Girard TD, Jackson JC, Pandharipande PP, *et al.* Delirium as a predictor of long-term cognitive impairment in survivors of critical illness. *Crit Care Med* 2010;**38**(7):1513–20.

19. Krogseth M, Wyller TB, Engedal K, Juliebo V. Delirium is an important predictor of incident dementia among elderly hip fracture patients. *Dement Geriatr Cogn Disord* 2011;**31**(1):63–70.

20. Melkas S, Laurila JV, Vataja R, *et al.* Post-stroke delirium in relation to dementia and long-term mortality. *Int J Geriatr Psychiatry* 2012;**27**(4): 401–8.

21. Fong TG, Jones RN, Shi P, *et al.* Delirium accelerates cognitive decline in Alzheimer disease. *Neurology* 2009;**72**(18):1570–5.

22. Bickel H, Gradinger R, Kochs E, Forstl H. High risk of cognitive and functional decline after postoperative delirium. A three-year prospective study. *Dement Geriatr Cogn Disord* 2008;**26**(1):26–31.

23. Kat MG, Vreeswijk R, de Jonghe JF, *et al.* Long-term cognitive outcome of delirium in elderly hip surgery patients. A prospective matched controlled study over two and a half years. *Dement Geriatr Cogn Disord* 2008;**26**(1):1–8.

24. Furlaneto ME, Garcez-Leme LE. Impact of delirium on mortality and cognitive and functional performance among elderly people with femoral fractures. *Clinics (Sao Paulo)* 2007;**62**(5):545–52.

25. Wacker P, Nunes PV, Cabrita H, Forlenza OV. Post-operative delirium is associated with poor cognitive outcome and dementia. *Dement Geriatr Cogn Disord* 2006;**21**(4):221–7.

26. Benoit AG, Campbell BI, Tanner JR, *et al.* Risk factors and prevalence of perioperative cognitive dysfunction in abdominal aneurysm patients. *J Vasc Surg* 2005;**42**(5):884–90.

27. Rothenhausler HB, Grieser B, Nollert G, *et al.* Psychiatric and psychosocial outcome of cardiac surgery with cardiopulmonary bypass: a prospective 12-month follow-up study. *Gen Hosp Psychiatry* 2005;**27**(1):18–28.

28. Duppils GS, Wikblad K. Cognitive function and health-related quality of life after delirium in connection with hip surgery. A six-month follow-up. *Orthop Nurs* 2004;**23**(3):195–203.

29. Lundstrom M, Edlund A, Bucht G, Karlsson S, Gustafson Y. Dementia after delirium in patients with femoral neck fractures. *J Am Geriatr Soc* 2003;**51**(7):1002–6.

30. Gruber-Baldini AL, Zimmerman S, Morrison RS, *et al.* Cognitive impairment in hip fracture patients: timing of detection and longitudinal follow-up. *J Am Geriatr Soc* 2003;**51**(9):1227–36.

31. Jackson JC, Hart RP, Gordon SM, *et al.* Six-month neuropsychological outcome of medical intensive care unit patients. *Crit Care Med* 2003;**31**(4):1226–34.

Chapter

6

Cognitive reserve

Richard E. Temes, Robert S. Wilson, Lisa L. Barnes, and David A. Bennett

SUMMARY

Cognitive reserve refers to individual differences in how tasks are processed and provide reserve against brain pathology. Measures of cognitive reserve include structural measures such as cranial capacity and synaptic density as well as more experiential measures such as occupational attainment and leisure activities (Table 6.1). Individuals who have greater cognitive reserve have less severe clinical or cognitive changes in the setting of age-related brain pathology. Cognitive reserve represents an active model that provides individuals with greater neural efficiency, capacity, and compensation in the setting of injury. Despite having its origins in dementia, cognitive reserve has been used to explain variations in disease expression in other diseases. This chapter discusses the role that neurocognitive reserve has on the disease expression of dementia, cerebrovascular disease, HIV, and critical illness encephalopathy. Specific measures of cognitive reserve such as macro- and microstructural measures, psychosocial and experiential measures, and imaging measures are reviewed.

Introduction

The concept of reserve is not a novel one and is applicable to many physiological systems outside the central nervous system. In the cardiovascular system, ventricular reserve has been used to describe the ability of the ventricles to respond to exercise or pharmacological stress. In the renal system, renal functional reserve has been used to describe the kidneys' ability to adjust glomerular filtration rates following protein loads. Similarly, reserve has been demonstrated in systems such as the pulmonary and gastrointestinal systems. Through evolutionary pressure, these organ

systems have developed compensatory mechanisms to maintain function when stressed, injured, or affected by disease. When these compensatory mechanisms fail, the manifestation of disease takes place in the forms of congestive heart failure, glomerulosclerosis, pulmonary hypertension, and liver failure. Similar to these other organ systems, the brain actively compensates for the challenges brought upon it from injury and disease through some type of cognitive reserve [1].

While threshold models of reserve take into account patho-anatomy, such as the quantity of myocytes, nephrons, neurons, and synapses, they do not take into account differences in functioning at the individual cell or cell network level in the setting of injury. Cognitive reserve represents an active model that focuses more on the mode in which tasks are processed as opposed to differences in physiology. Although two patients may have the same amount of brain reserve, the patient with more cognitive reserve may tolerate a greater injury before symptoms become clinically evident. Two types of neural mechanisms that have been implicated as underlying cognitive reserve are neural reserve and neural compensation. *Neural reserve* refers to brain networks or cognitive paradigms that are efficient and flexible, making them adaptable and less prone to disruption. This represents an important coping mechanism that brain-injured individuals utilize when faced with task demands. *Neural compensation* refers to the adoption of new neural networks due to injury or pathology interrupting pathways normally in use by healthy individuals for a given task. These neural mechanisms explain how certain individuals can sustain greater brain injury without manifesting functional deficits. Rather than the manifestation of disease solely being a function

Brain Disorders in Critical Illness, ed. Robert D. Stevens, Tarek Sharshar, and E. Wesley Ely. Published by Cambridge University Press. © Cambridge University Press 2013.

of differences in anatomy (i.e., number of synapses), it is also a function of the efficiency in the processing of information. Figures 6.1 and 6.2 demonstrate how through increased neurocognitive reserve, cognitive impairment for any given AD pathology is diminished. Neural compensation modifies this relationship between reserve and cognitive decline (Figure 6.3).

While the concept of cognitive reserve arose in large part from the observation that the severity of the neuropathological manifestations of diseases such as Alzheimer's disease (AD) did not always correlate with the severity of cognitive impairment [2], it also applies to recovery of function, for example, from traumatic brain injury or critical illness. If the interaction of neural growth, experience, and cognitive abilities is important for optimal brain function, then it is also important for how the brain responds to injury and disease. The focus of this chapter is to highlight specific measures of cognitive reserve, and to focus on the relationship that cognitive reserve has with the clinical conditions of AD, cerebrovascular disease, HIV, and critical illness encephalopathy.

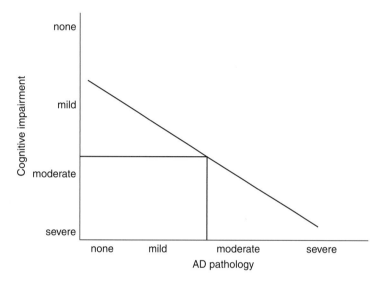

Figure 6.1 Relationship between cognitive impairment and Alzheimer's disease (AD) pathology.

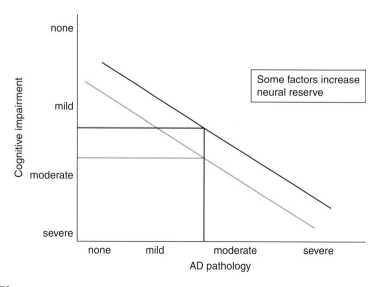

Figure 6.2 Relationship between cognitive impairment and Alzheimer's disease (AD) pathology in the setting of increased neural reserve.

Macro- and microstructural measures

Perhaps the most simplistic macrostructural measure of cognitive reserve is cranial capacity, as measured by head circumference of brain volume. The theory that individuals with more cranial capacity can afford to lose more neurons before they manifest cognitive impairment has been met with equivocal results [3–5]. While some studies found that large cranial capacity was associated with reduced age-related decline in memory, others have found no effect. Some have found brain volume to be associated with memory and intelligence [6], while others found no such association [5]. The use of cranial capacity as a surrogate measure of cognitive reserve is often insensitive and prone to variation from nutritional and metabolic exposures in utero that may be independent contributors to neural cognitive reserve. The number of neurons is directly related to cranial capacity and may be a measure of cognitive reserve. Although AD patients sustain neuronal loss that leads to atrophy, there is little direct evidence that there is an association between the number of neurons and cognitive reserve. Several microstructural measures of reserve have been identified. These generally comprise the neural elements that subserve cognition, including neuron numbers, synaptic density, dendrites, and dendritic spines [2, 7–9].

Table 6.1 Measures of cognitive reserve.

Structural measures
Cranial capacity
Neuron/dendrite count
Synaptic density
Dendritic spines
Psychosocial/experiential measures
Socioeconomic status
Educational/occupational attainment
Cognitive performance measures
Verbal/reading
Leisure activities
Personality traits
Conscientiousness
Imaging measures
Regional cerebral blood flow
Functional MRI

Psychosocial and experiential measures

A variety of psychosocial and experiential measures have been proposed and used as indicators for cognitive reserve. Measures of socioeconomic status, particularly education and occupation, have been widely used as markers of reserve because of their association with level of cognitive function. Educational and occupational attainment has also been associated with the risk of late-life dementia [10], but this may reflect, in part, their association with level of cognitive function rather than an association with rate of cognitive decline [11]. Another approach to the assessment of cognitive reserve has been to use cognitive performance measures, particularly of reading or verbal skills, to index reserve [12]. However, few studies are able to

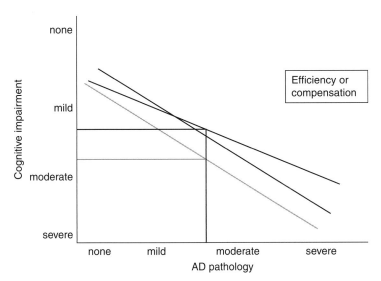

Figure 6.3 Neural compensation modifies the relationship between cognitive impairment and Alzheimer's disease (AD) pathology.

use one cognitive test, or set of tests, to explain individual differences in the effect of pathology on another set of cognitive tests [13]. This results in part because even basic lexical abilities such as reading are affected by the same neuropathological processes that impair memory and executive functioning [14]. Perhaps the most promising approach to assessing cognitive reserve has been to quantify lifestyle activities hypothesized to contribute to neural cognitive reserve. A number of self-report questionnaires have been developed to assess participation in cognitively stimulating activities such as reading a book, visiting a library, or playing chess. Those with a cognitively active lifestyle have a higher level of cognitive function than less active individuals and are less likely to experience cognitive decline or develop dementia despite equivalent levels of dementia-related pathology on postmortem examination [15]. Because personality traits refer to characteristic patterns of thought, emotion, and behavior, they may also provide some insight into cognitive reserve. Conscientiousness, which refers to impulse control and goal directedness, is associated with reduced cognitive decline but not with common neuropathological lesions associated with late-life cognitive decline and dementia [16]. Similarly, older persons who are prone to see meaning and purpose in life are at reduced risk for cognitive decline and dementia compared with those with a low sense of purpose [17], and the negative association of AD pathology with cognitive function is reduced [18]. Together, these data suggest that self-report about lifestyle and personality provides a promising means of assessing neural cognitive reserve.

Functional imaging measures

Studies of regional cerebral blood flow (rCBF) were among the first imaging techniques to assess cognitive reserve. Regional cerebral blood flow has been used as a surrogate for AD pathology based upon observations that rCBF is inversely proportional to AD pathology [19]. It has been shown that negative correlations exist between years of education and rCBF within parieto-temporal areas [20]. This suggests that patients who have achieved a greater attainment of education can withstand greater AD pathology prior to the manifestation of clinical symptoms. Similar relationships have been shown with occupational attainment [21]. Functional magnetic resonance imaging (fMRI) has been used to measure the variability in efficiency or capacity of neural networks in healthy young

subjects. It has been shown that subjects with higher IQ demonstrate greater efficiency in network expression [22], that there are individual differences in network efficiency in young healthy subjects [23], and that cognitive reserve may be associated with greater efficiency.

Dementia

There is extensive evidence for the existence of cognitive reserve in studies of age-related cognitive decline. It has been found that increased literacy is associated with slower decline in memory, executive function, and language skills [24]. Among studies of cognitive aging, slower cognitive and functional decline has been demonstrated in people with higher educational attainment [25–28]. These studies indicate that the education-related factors that seem to delay the onset of dementia also allows individuals to cope more affectively with brain changes encountered in normal aging.

While some studies show that greater reserve is associated with better outcomes in the setting of cognitive aging, others also indicate that once AD emerges, those with higher reserve have poorer outcomes. Prospective studies of AD have shown that individuals with a premorbid history of frequent cognitive activity experience more rapid cognitive decline than individuals with a premorbid history of infrequent cognitive activity [29,30]. Furthermore, patients with greater educational or occupational attainment die sooner than those with lower attainment [31]. Higher educational attainment has also been shown to be associated with more rapid cognitive decline in patients with both prevalent [31] and incident [32] AD.

The finding that a more rapid cognitive decline is found in individuals with greater cognitive reserve suggests that individuals with higher reserve can tolerate more AD pathology allowing the clinical manifestation of disease to occur later in life, after more pathology has accumulated. If it is assumed that at some point AD pathology becomes too severe to support the processes that mediate neural cognitive reserve and/or memory function and that the timing of this endpoint is the same regardless of the level of reserve, it follows that the time between the clinical manifestations of disease and complete loss of function will be shorter in patients with greater cognitive reserve [33]. This model explains how dementia in individuals with greater reserve is diagnosed later in life and how there is a more rapid time to death in those with greater reserve due to the presence of more advanced AD pathology.

These assumptions have been supported by findings from both clinical and neuroimaging studies. Higher education was found to be associated with clinical manifestations of AD occurring later in life and a more rapid decline in memory following diagnosis [34–36]. Similar findings have been reported with cognitive activity [37]. As discussed previously, rCBF with PET imaging has been used as a surrogate for AD pathology and has correlated with psychosocial measures such as education, occupational attainment, and leisure activities [19–21]. These radiographic findings have been confirmed with a prospective clinical study demonstrating that education was found to modify the association between AD pathology-assessed postmortem and level of cognitive function prior to death. Better cognitive function was seen for each year of education for the same degree of brain pathology [38–40]. Similar findings were seen with amyloid load measured pathologically or by positron emission tomography [41,42]. This suggests that education is not related to global Alzheimer's pathology but, rather, modifies the relationship between the effects of AD pathology on cognition. However, a recent study found that early and midlife cognitive activity was related to amyloid load on PET [43].

Cerebrovascular disease

There is growing interest in how cognitive reserve mediates the relationship between cerebrovascular disease and cognition. The concept of cognitive reserve also has been proposed to account for the discrepancy seen between stroke volume and its clinical manifestations (i.e., cognition). There is evidence that small, subcortical infarcts, for instance, are associated with deficits in executive functioning and activities of daily living. Importantly, several population-based studies reported that subcortical infarcts are related to not only cognitive impairment but also to cognitive decline [44,45]. However, at the individual level, large inter-individual variability on the clinical presentation of patients with subcortical infarcts exists. The association between subcortical infarct volume and cognitive function is imperfect. If cognitive neural reserve contributes to the association of cerebral vascular disease with clinical signs, it would follow that patients with a high amount of cognitive reserve would tolerate a greater infarct burden through compensatory mechanisms than patients with low levels of reserve.

Support for this concept is derived from neuroimaging where an MRI-defined infarct resulted in a greater decline in cognitive function among individuals with a low level of educational attainment compared with those with a high level of education. Education also modified the change in cognitive function before and after acute cerebral infarction [46]. It is interesting to note that the majority of MRI-defined infarcts in this study were small, subcortical, and did not lead to a clinical diagnosis of stroke. Brickman and colleagues provided additional support by demonstrating that patients who had more cognitively stimulating activities across the lifespan, such as years of education, exhibited more severe white matter pathology for any given level of cognitive function [47]. Saczynski and colleagues found that the presence of white matter lesions was significantly associated with lower speed of processing and that this effect was modified by high leisure activity [48]. These studies suggest that those with greater amounts of cognitive reserve are able to tolerate more cerebrovascular pathology and that cognitive reserve mitigates the impact of cerebrovascular disease on cognitive function. It is through neural cognitive reserve as measured by developmental experiences and exposures that provide the compensatory mechanisms to protect against the expression of pathology once it emerges in later life.

A "multiple hit" hypothesis, whereby different diseases and patterns of mixed pathology work synergistically to contribute to an overall decline in cognitive function, may occur in the setting of cerebrovascular disease. These events may exceed compensatory mechanisms provided by neural cognitive reserve and contribute to the phenotypic expression of disease in individuals already at risk for cognitive decline. For instance, patients with pre-existing cerebrovascular disease are prone to cognitive impairment when exposed to factors such as sedation or in-hospital events such as surgery. Several studies have found that premorbid cerebral infarction increased the risk of postoperative cognitive impairment and delirium [49–51]. Preoperative ischemic brain lesions on MRI have been shown to increase risk of postoperative cognitive dysfunction [52] and postoperative delirium [53]. It has also been shown that patients with decreased verbal memory prior to surgery predict postoperative delirium [54]. Vascular risk factors such as hyperlipidemia [55,56] and diabetes [57] have also been associated with an accelerated cognitive decline. Vascular risk factors may increase oxidative stress or activate a neuroinflammatory response, triggering amyloid production. Thus it has been shown that Alzheimer's pathology and cerebrovascular disease may work synergistically to cause cognitive decline [58–62]. Diabetes may influence AD progression via an inflammatory mechanism, or by contributing to amyloid plaque and neurofibrillary tangle formation, or simply by contributing to cerebrovascular disease [63].

Human immunodeficiency virus

Human immunodeficiency virus (HIV) penetrates the blood–brain barrier early in the disease and can be found within the cerebrospinal fluid prior to the manifestations of clinical disease [64]. Although both cortical and subcortical areas are affected in HIV-associated neurocognitive disturbance (HAND), subcortical structures appear to be at particular risk [65,66]. What results is a pattern of impairment that is commonly observed in subcortical dementias, such as Parkinson's disease and Hungtingtons's disease – that is, slowing in reaction time and processing speed, difficulties with executive functioning, and memory impairment. However, not all patients with HIV develop symptoms of neurocognitive impairment. Many studies looking at the role of potential cofactors such as traumatic brain injury, depression, and substance abuse have yielded negative or equivocal results, leaving the question of why some individuals with early HIV are more likely to exhibit signs of neurocognitive impairment than others [67]. Evidence that cognitive reserve modifies the relationship between HIV and cognitive impairment stems from early studies demonstrating that neuropsychological impairment was more prevalent among HIV-seropositive individuals with fewer years of education than those with more education [68]. By contrast, there was no relationship between educational attainment and neuropsychological function in seronegative controls. These findings have been extended in further studies with other measures of cognitive reserve (e.g., occupational attainment, premorbid intelligence), and associations between a lower reserve capacity and seropositive status appear to be independent of age, ethnicity, CD4 count, or substance abuse [69,70]. Studies [70,71] have shown that HIV-positive patients with low neural cognitive reserve perform more poorly on neurocognitive testing than both HIV-positive patients with high neural cognitive reserve and HIV-negative controls with low neural cognitive reserve. In addition, HIV patients with high neural cognitive reserve perform as well as HIV-negative patients with high and low cognitive reserve, irrespective of disease stage [72]. Among older patients with HIV, it has been shown that clinical outcomes are worse relative to younger patients, and there is a shorter latency between the diagnosis of HIV and the onset of dementia [73]. Although studies have provided evidence that older individuals with HIV are at higher risk for the development of neurocognitive decline, some aging HIV patients fail to demonstrate the expected declines in cognition. It has been shown that older HIV-positive patients with greater cognitive reserve (i.e., level of education, estimated premorbid intelligence) have preserved cognitive function despite the double jeopardy of older age and HIV infection, even after controlling for other psychiatric, immunological, and psychosocial protective factors [74]. While the role of cognitive reserve on cognition appears to diminish as the degree of neuropathology worsens in conditions such as AD, with a more rapid cognitive decline noted after reserve depletion, we are not aware of any studies that have examined the relationship between cognitive reserve and rate of cognitive decline with increasing HIV severity (e.g., low CD4 count, elevated viral load, or AIDS).

Critical illness encephalopathy

Cognitive changes following critical illness have been described for many years. The cause of this cognitive dysfunction, which may manifest itself as subtle impairments of memory, concentration, and information processing, is likely multifactorial and has been seen following treatment for conditions such as adult respiratory distress syndrome (ARDS), sepsis, and delirium [75,76]. It has been estimated that up to one third of patients will develop chronic neurocognitive impairment following critical illness [77]. It has been estimated that among survivors of ARDS, about a quarter of patients continue to suffer neurocognitive impairment 6 years after their treatment [78]. The consequences of this chronic neurocognitive impairment are far reaching and contribute to a decreased ability to perform activities of daily living, decreased quality of life, increased medical costs, and the inability to return to work.

There is mounting evidence that a complex interaction takes place between a susceptible individual with potentially noxious exposures in the intensive care unit (ICU), such as certain sedative medications, that together promote the development of cognitive impairment, or critical illness encephalopathy. For example, the use of anticholinergic and central nervous system (CNS)-active medications has been associated with low cognitive performance in older adults [79] and delirium and cognitive decline in individuals with dementia [80]. In a controlled clinical trial, it has been shown that a non-pharmacological sleep protocol was the most effective intervention in the prevention of delirium among hospitalized patients with dementia [81]. Just as patients who are discharged from the ICU may exhibit chronic organ failure such as heart, kidney, or lung disease from their critical illness, so too may they manifest brain failure as indicated by irreversible cognitive impairment. If cognitive reserve provides protection from cognitive impairment following exposures to conditions such as dementia, stroke, and HIV, it may afford the same protection from critical illness encephalopathy.

Among survivors of ARDS, it has been shown that estimated premorbid intelligence scores are inversely related to the magnitude of cognitive sequelae, suggesting greater neural cognitive reserve in patients with fewer cognitive decrements [82]. In large prospective studies of elderly patients over the age of 70 years and free from delirium on admission, educational attainment was found to be an important predictor of delirium [83,84]. A 5-year difference in educational attainment was associated with a 1.6-fold decrease in the odds of delirium. It has also been shown that regular physical exercise significantly predicted a lower risk of delirium while controlling for sociodemographic factors. Similarly, leisure activity participation before hospitalization predicted lower risk for delirium and mediated the relationship between education and risk for delirium [85].

Conclusion

There is strong epidemiological evidence from different disease states to support the idea that cognitive reserve mediates or modifies the relationship between brain pathology and neurological signs. Cognitive reserve relies on the idea that there are individual differences in how tasks are processed that allow some people to cope with injury and pathology better than others. Cognitive reserve is believed to be an active process where brain pathology is met with greater efficiency in pre-existing cognitive processes (neural reserve) or the recruitment of alternative

processes (neural compensation) to achieve cognitive tasks. Several measures of cognitive reserve have been examined including anatomic measures such as synaptic density, psychosocial measures such as cognitive activity and purpose in life, and measures of socioeconomic status such as educational and occupational attainment. Neuroimaging represents a promising technology to both measure reserve and ascertain the efficiency of neural networks in the setting of existing pathology.

Although the concept of cognitive reserve originated in Alzheimer's dementia, interest in its involvement in acute conditions without a long prodromal phase, such as critical illness, is on the rise. Future clinical research should focus on how cognitive reserve mediates or modifies acute insults differently from chronic ones and the impact that socioeconomic factors and cognitive activity level have on the risk of developing delirium. The impact that pharmacological treatments such as sedation and opiate use have on cognitive reserve and network efficiency should also be investigated.

Acknowledgments

Supported by NIH grants P30AG10161, R0AG15819, R01AG17917, R01AG22018, and P20MD6886.

References

1. Stern Y. What is cognitive reserve? Theory and research application of the reserve concept. *J Int Neuropsycholog Soc* 2002;**8**:448–60.

2. Katzman R, Terry R, DeTeresa R, *et al.* Clinical, pathological, and neurochemical changes in dementia: a subgroup with preserved mental status and numerous neocortical plaques. *Annals Neurol* 1988;**23**(2):138–44.

3. Borenstein Graves, A., Mortimer, J.A., Bowen, J.D., *et al.* Head circumference and incident Alzheimer's disease: modification by apolipoprotein E. *Neurology* 2001;**57**(8):1453–60.

4. Drachman DA. Hat size, brain size, intelligence, and dementia: what morphometry can tell us about brain function and disease. *Neurology* 2002;**59**(2):156–7.

5. Edland SD, Xu Y, Plevak M, *et al.* Total intracranial volume: normative values and lack of association with Alzheimer's disease. *Neurology* 2002;**59**(2), 272–4.

6. MacLullich AM, Ferguson KJ, Deary IJ, *et al.* Intracranial capacity and brain volumes are associated with cognition in healthy elderly men. *Neurology* 2002;**59**(2):169–74.

7. Honer WG, Barr AM, Sawada K, *et al.* Cognitive reserve, presynaptic proteins and dementia in the elderly. *Transl Psychiatry* 2012;**2**:e114.

8. Arnold SE, Louneva N, Cao K, *et al.* Neuropathological, cellular and molecular features of pathological Alzheimer's disease with normal cognition. *Neurobiol Aging* 2012; [Epub].

9. Soetanto A, Wilson RS, Talbot K, *et al.* Association of anxiety and depression with microtubule-associated protein 2- and synaptopodin-immunolabeled dendrite and spine densities in hippocampal CA3 of older humans. *Arch Gen Psychiatry* 2010;**67**:448–57.

10. Stern Y, Gurland B, Tatemichi TK, *et al.* Influence of education and occupation on the incidence of Alzheimer's disease. *JAMA* 1994;**271**(13):1004–10.

11. Wilson RS, Bennett DA, Bienias JL, *et al.* Cognitive activity and incident AD in a population-based sample of older persons. *Neurology* 2002;**59**(12):1910–14.

12. Jefferson AL, Gibbons LE, Rentz DM, *et al.* A life course of cognitive abilities, socioeconomic status, education, reading ability, and cognition. *J Am Geriatr Soc* 2011;**59**(8):1403–11.

13. Boyle PA, Wilson RS, Schneider JA, Bienias JL, Bennett DA. Processing resources reduce the effect of AD pathology on other cognitive systems. *Neurology* 2008;**70**:1534–42.

14. Wilson RS, Leurgans SE, Boyle PA, Bennett DA. Cognitive decline in prodromal Alzheimer disease and mild cognitive impairment. *Arch Neurol* 2011;**68**(3):351–6.

15. Wilson, R.S., Schenider, J.A., Boyle, P.A., *et al.* Relation of cognitive activity to risk of developing Alzheimer's disease. *Neurology* 2007;**69**(20):1911–20.

16. Wilson RS, Schneider JA, Arnold SE, Bienias JL, Bennett DA. Conscientiousness and the incidence of Alzheimer disease and mild cognitive impairment. *Arch Gen Psychiatry* 2007;**64**(10):1204–12.

17. Boyle PA, Buchman AS, Barnes LL, Bennett DA. Purpose in life is associated with a reduced risk of incident Alzheimer's disease among community-dwelling older persons. *Arch Gen Psychiatry* 2010;**67**:304–10.

18. Boyle PA, Buchman AS, Wilson RS, *et al.* Effect of purpose in life on the relation between Alzheimer disease pathologic changes on cognitive function in advanced age. *Arch Gen Psychiatry* 2012;**69**(5):499–504.

19. DeCarli C, Atack JR, Ball MJ, *et al.* Post-mortem neurofibrillary tangle densities but not senile plaque densities are related to regional cerebral metabolic rates for glucose during life in Alzheimer's disease patients. *Neurodegeneration* 1992;**1**:113–21.

20. Stern Y, Alexander GE, Prohovnik I, Mayeux R. Inverse relationship between eduation and parietotemporal perfusion deficit in Alzheimer's disease. *Ann Neurol* 1992;**32**:371–5.

21. Stern Y, Alexander GE, Prohovnik I, *et al.* Relationship between lifetime occupation and parietal flow: implications for a reserve against Alzheimer's disease pathology. *Neurology*, 1995;**45**:55–60.

22. Grober E, Sliwinski M. Development and validation of a model for estimating premorbid verbal intelligence in the elderly. *J Clin Exp Neuropsychol* 1991;**13**:933–49.

23. Habeck C, Hilton HJ, Zarahn E, *et al.* Relation of cognitive reserve and task performance to expression of regional covariance networks in an event-related fMRI study of non-verbal memory. *Neuroimage* 2003;**20**:1723–33.

24. Manly JJ, Touradji P, Tang MX, Stern Y. Literacy and memory decline among ethnically diverse elders. *J Clin Exp Neuropsychol* 2004;**25**(5):680–90.

25. Albert MS. How does education affect cognitive function? *Ann Epidemiol* 1995;**5**(1):76–8.

26. Butler SM, Ashford JW, Snowdon DA. Age, education, and changes in the Mini-Mental State Exam scores of older women: findings from the Nun Study. *Am Geriatr Soc* 1996;**44**(6):675–81.

27. Colsher PL, Wallace RB. Longitudinal application of cognitive function measures in a defined population of community-dwelling elders. *Ann Epidemiol* 1991;**1**(3):215–30.

28. Snowdon DA, Ostwald SK, Kane RL. Education, survival, and independence in elderly Catholic sisters, 1936–1988. *Am J Epidemiol* 1989;**130**(5):999–1012.

29. Wilson RS, Bennett DA, Gilley DW, *et al.* Premorbid reading activity and patterns of cognitive decline in Alzheimer disease. *Arch Neurol* 2000;**57**:1718–23.

30. Wilson RS, Barnes LL, Aggarwal NT, *et al.* Cognitive activity and the cognitive morbidity of Alzheimer disease. *Neurology* 2010;**75**:990–6.

31. Stern Y, Tang MX, Deanaro J, Mayeaux R. Increased risk of mortality in Alzheimer's disease patients with more advanced educational and occupational attainment. *Ann Neurology* 1995;**37**:590–5.

32. Stern Y, Albert S, Tang MX, Tsai WY. Rate of memory decline in AD is related to education and occupation: cognitive reserve? *Neurology* 1999;**53**(9):1942–7

33. Scarmeas N, Albert SM, Manly JJ, Stern Y. Education and rates of cognitive decline in incident Alzheimer's disease. *J Neurol Neurosurg Psychiatry* 2006;**77**(3):308–16.

34. Tucker AM, Stern Y. Cognitive reserve in aging. *Curr Alzheimer Res* 2011;**8**(4):354–60.

35. Hall CB, Derby C, LeValley A, *et al.* Education delays accelerated decline on a memory test in persons who develop dementia. *Neurology* 2007;**69**(17):1657–64.

36. Yu L, Boyle PA, Wilson RS, *et al.* A random change point model for cognitive decline in Alzheimer's disease and mild cognitive impairment. *Neuroepidemiology* 2012;**39**(2):73–83.

37. Hall CB, Lipton RB, Sliwinski M, *et al.* Cognitive activities delay onset of memory decline in persons who develop dementia. *Neurology* 2009;**73**(5):356–61.

38. Bennett DA, Wilson RS, Schneider JA, *et al.* Education modifies the relation of AD pathology to level of cognitive function in older persons. *Neurology* 2003;**60**(12):1909–15.

39. Roe CM, Xiong C, Miller JP, Morris JC. Education and Alzheimer disease without dementia: support for the cognitive reserve hypothesis. *Neurology* 2007;**68**(3):223–8.

40. Koepsell TD, Kurland BF, Harel O, *et al.* Education, cognitive function, and severity of neuropathology in Alzheimer disease. *Neurology* 2008;**70**(19 Pt 2):1732–9.

41. Bennett DA, Schneider JA, Wilson RS, Bienias JL, Arnold SE. Education modifies the association of amyloid, but not tangles, with cognitive function. *Neurology* 2005;**65**:953–5.

42. Rentz DM, Locascio JJ, Becker JA, *et al.* Cognition, reserve, and amyloid deposition in normal aging. *Ann Neurol* 2010;**67**(3):353–64.

43. Landau SM, Marks SM, Mormino EC, *et al.* Association of lifetime cognitive engagement and low β-amyloid deposition. *Arch Neurol* 2012;**69**(5):623–9.

44. Prins ND, van Dijk EJ, den Heijer T, *et al.* Cerebral small-vessel disease and decline in information processing speed, executive function and memory. *Brain* 2005;**128**:2034–41.

45. Schmidt R, Ropele S, Enzinger C, *et al.* White matter lesion progression, brain atrophy, and cognitive decline: the Austrian stroke prevention study. *Ann Neurol* 2005;**58**:610–16.

46. Elkins JS, Longstreth WT Jr., Manolio TA, *et al.* Education and the cognitive decline associated with MRI-defined brain infarct. *Neurology* 2006;**67**:435–40.

47. Brickman AM, Siedlecki KL, Muraskin J, *et al.* White matter hyperintensities and cognition: testing the reserve hypothesis. *Neurobiol Aging* 2011;**32**:1588–98.

48. Saczynski JS, Jonsdottir MK, Sigurdsson S, *et al.* White matter lesions and cognitive performance: the role of cognitively complex leisure activity. *J Gerontol A Biol Sci Med Sci* 2008;**63**(8):848–54.

49. Monk TG, Weldon BC, Garvan CW, *et al.* Predictors of cognitive dysfunction after non-cardiac surgery. *Anesthesiology* 2008;**108**:18–30.

50. Greene NH, Attix DK, Weldon BC, *et al.* Measures of executive function and depression identify patients at risk for post-operative delirium. *Anesthesiology* 2009;**110**:788–95.

51. Smith PJ, Attix DK, Weldon BC, *et al.* Executive function and depression as independent risk factors for post-operative delirium. *Anesthesiology* 2009;**110**:781–7.

52. Maekawa K, Goto T, Baba T, *et al.* Impaired cognition preceding cardiac surgery is related to cerebral ischemic lesions. *J Anesth* 2011;**25**(3):330–6.

53. Shiori A, Kurumaji A, Takeuchi T, *et al.* White matter abnormalities as a risk factor for postoperative delirium revealed by diffusion tensor imaging. *Am J Geriatr Psychiatry* 2010;**18**:743–53.

54. Jankowski CJ, Trenerry MR, Cook DJ, *et al.* Cognitive and functional predictors and sequelae of postoperative delirium in elderly patients undergoing elective joint arthroplasty. *Anesth Analg* 2011;**112**:1186–93.

55. Evans RM, Hui S, Perkins A, *et al.* Cholesterol and APOE genotype interact to influence Alzheimer disease progression. *Neurology* 2004;**62**(10):1869–71.

56. Helzner EP, Luchsinger JA, Scarmeas N, *et al.* Contribution of vascular risk factors to the progression in Alzheimer disease. *Arch Neurol* 2009;**66**(3):343–8.

57. Lesort M, Johnson GVW. Insulin-like growth factor-1 and insulin mediate transient site-selective increases in tau phosphorylation in primary cortical neurons. *Neuroscience* 2000;**99**(2):305–16.

58. Petrovitch H, Ross GW, Steinhorn SC, *et al.* AD lesions and infarcts in demented and non-demented Japanese-American men. *Ann Neurol* 2005;**57**(1):98–103.

59. Sonnen JA, Larson EB, Crane PK, *et al.* Pathological correlates of dementia in a longitudinal, population-based sample of aging. *Ann Neurol* 2007;**62**:406–13.

60. Troncoso JC, Zonderman AB, Resnick SM, *et al.* Effect of infarcts on dementia in the Baltimore longitudinal study of aging. *Ann Neurol* 2008;**64**(2):168–76.

61. Schneider JA, Arvanitakis Z, Leurgans SE, Bennett DA. Neuropathology of probable AD and amnestic and non-amnestic MCI. *Ann Neurol* 2009;**66**:200–8.

62. James BD, Bennett DA, Boyle PA, Leurgans S, Schneider JA. Dementia in the old versus oldest old: the role of Alzheimer's and mixed pathologies. *J Am Med Assoc* 2012;**307**:1798–800.

63. Arvanitakis Z, Schneider JA, Wilson RS, *et al.* Diabetes mellitus is related to cerebral infarction but not Alzheimer's disease pathology in older persons. *Neurology* 2006;**67**:1960–5.

64. McArthur J. Neurologic manifestations of AIDS. *Medicine* 1987;**66**:407–37.

65. Navia BA, Cho E-S, Petito CK, Price RW. The AIDS dementia complex: II. Neuropathology. *Ann Neurol* 1986;**19**:525–35.

66. Van Gorp WG, Mandelkern M, Gee M, *et al.* Cerebral metabolic dysfunction in AIDS: findings in a sample with and without dementia. *J Neuropsychiatry Clin Neurosci* 1987;**4**:280–7.

67. Satz P. Brain reserve capacity on symptom onset after brain injury: a formulation and review of evidence for threshold theory. *Neuropsychology* 1993;**7**:273–95.

68. Satz P, Morgenstern H, Miller EN, *et al.* Low education as a possible risk factor for cognitive abnormalities in HIV-1: findings from the Multicenter AIDS Cohort Study (MACS). *J Acquir Immune Defic Syndr* 1993;**6**(5):503–11.

69. Stern RA, Silva SG, Chaisson N, Evans DL. Influence of cognitive reserve on neuropsychological functioning in asymptomatic human immunodeficiency virus-1 infection. *Arch Neurol* 1996;**53**(2):148–53.

70. Pereda M, Ayuso-Mateos JL, Gomez del Barrio A, *et al.* Factors associated with neuropsychological performance in HIV-seropositive subjects. *Psychol Med* 2000;**30**(1):205–17.

71. Basso MR, Bornstein RA. Estimated premorbid intelligence mediates neurobehavioral change in individuals infected with HIV across 12 months. *J Clin Exp Neuropsychol* 2000;**22**(2):208–18.

72. Morgan EE, Woods SP, Smith C, *et al.*; The HIV Neurobehavioral Research Program (HNRP) Group. Lower cognitive reserve among individuals with syndromic HIV-associated neurocognitive disorders (HAND). *AIDS Behav* 2012;**16**(8):2279–85.

73. Butt AA, Dascomb KK, DeSalvo KB, *et al.* Human immunodeficiency virus infection in elderly patients. *Southern Med J* 2001;**94**, 397–400.

74. Foley JM, Ettenhofer ML, Kim MS, *et al.* Cognitive reserve as a protective factor in older HIV-positive patients at risk for cognitive decline. *Appl Neuropsychol Adult* 2012;**19**(1):16–25.

75. Angus DC, Musthafa AA, Clermont G, *et al.* Quality-adjusted survival in the first year after the acute respiratory distress syndrome. *Am J Respir Crit Care Med* 2001;**163**:1389–94.

76. Herridge MS, Cheung AM, Tansey CM, *et al.* One year outcomes in survivors of the acute respiratory distress syndrome. *N Engl J Med* 2003;**31**:1226–34.

77. Jackson JC, Hart RP, Gordon SM, *et al.* Six-month neuropsychological outcome of medical intensive care unit patients. *Crit Care Med* 2003;**167**:690–4.

78. Rothenhausler HB, Ehrentraut S, Stoll C, *et al.* The relationship between cognitive performance and employment and health status in long-term survivors of the acute respiratory distress syndrome: results of an exploratory study. *Gen Hosp Psychiatry* 2001;**23**:90–6.

79. Mintzer MZ, Griffiths RR. Differential effects of scopolamine and lorazepam in working memory maintenance versus manipulation processes. *Cogn Affect Behav Neurosci* 2007;**7**:120–9.

80. Fick DM, Mion LC. How to try this: delirium superimposed on dementia. *Am J Nurs* 2008;**108**(1):52–60.

81. Innouye SK, Bogardus ST, Charpentier PA, *et al.* A multicomponent intervention to prevent delirium in hospitalized elderly patients. *N Engl J Med* 1999;**340**:669–76.

82. Larson MJ, Weaver LK, Hopkins RO. Cognitive sequelae in acute respiratory distress syndrome patients with and without recall of the intensive care unit. *Int Neuropsychol Soc* 2007;**13**(4):595–605.

83. Jones C, Griffiths SD, Slater T, *et al.* Significant cognitive dysfunction in non-delirious patients identified during and persisting following critical illness. *Intensive Care Med*; 2006;**32**:923–6.

84. Inouye SK, van Dyck CH, Alessi CA, *et al.* (1990). Clarifying confusion: the confusion assessment method. A new method for detection of delirium. *Ann Intern Med* 1990;**113**:941–8.

85. Yang FM, Inouye SK, Fearing M, *et al.* Participation in activity and risk for incident delirium. *J Am Geriatr Soc* 2008;**56**:1479–84.

Neurology of consciousness impairments

Benjamin Rohaut, Frédéric Faugeras, and Lionel Naccache

SUMMARY

Probing consciousness in non-communicating patients at bedside can be very challenging. In this chapter, we describe some of the key goals, caveats, and pitfalls of the evaluation of consciousness in non-communicating patients. First, we will address the importance of neurological and behavioral examination, and then briefly outline the current developments of functional brain-imaging tools able to provide important additional evidence. Current approaches include: (i) active paradigms in which a patient is asked to perform a specific cognitive task; (ii) "resting state" conditions in which the spontaneous patterns of brain activity can be instructive of patients conscious state; and (iii) passive paradigms in which cortical functional connectivity can be explored by recording, for instance, EEG in response to focal transmagnetic stimulation (TMS) pulses.

Introduction

In this chapter, we intend to summarize the key goals, caveats, and pitfalls of the evaluation of consciousness in non-communicating patients, and in particular in awake patients in whom this issue is the most difficult to solve. Distinguishing minimally conscious (MCS) and conscious states from vegetative (VS) and comatose states can be extremely challenging at bedside. We will first address the importance of neurological and behavioral examination, and then briefly outline the current developments of functional brain-imaging tools able to provide important additional evidence. Far from being systematically categorical, we will also try to provide the reader with the current weights of (un)certainty associated with each clinical sign or neurophysiological measure mentioned in this chapter.

Caveats and pitfalls of consciousness examination

Examining an awake, eyes open, and yet non-interactive patient with no clear evidence of consciousness can be a very awkward situation. For instance, both MCS and VS patients can perform behaviors such as laughing, crying, grimacing, and they can demonstrate withdrawal movements to nociceptive stimulation. All these rich behavioral, and sometimes emotional, manifestations are difficult to interpret in relation to the conscious status of the patient, and the observers can easily overestimate them as univocal evidence of a voluntary conscious state. This problem is frequent in clinical practice, and can be the source of contradictory interpretations within a team of caregivers, and with patients' relatives. Assessing consciousness and/or residual cognitive abilities of a disorders of consciousness (DOC) patient obviously requires neurological expertise. We will adopt here the classical definition of consciousness as a "state of full awareness of the self and one's relationship to the environment" [1].

Do not overestimate consciousness

Visual fixation

Visual fixation is defined by at least two consecutive ocular saccades to a target followed by a fixation longer than 2 seconds [2] (see for instance the revised version of the Coma Recovery Scale (CRS-R) [3] (see Table 7.1). It is admitted that visual fixation does not require conscious access to the visual target, given that it can be observed for instance in some patients with cortical blindness ("blindsight" phenomenon), but it is still not clear whether visual fixation needs primary

Brain Disorders in Critical Illness, ed. Robert D. Stevens, Tarek Sharshar, and E. Wesley Ely. Published by Cambridge University Press. © Cambridge University Press 2013.

Table 7.1 Coma Recovery Scale – Revised

- **AUDITORY FUNCTION SCALE**
  - 4 – Consistent movement to command*
  - 3 – Reproducible movement to command*
  - 2 – Localization to sound
  - 1 – Auditory startle
  - 0 – None

- **VISUAL FUNCTION SCALE**
  - 5 – Object recognition*
  - 4 – Object localization: reaching*
  - 3 – Visual pursuit*
  - 2 – Fixation*
  - 1 – Visual startle
  - 0 – None

- **MOTOR FUNCTION SCALE**
  - 6 – Functional object use**
  - 5 – Automatic motor response*
  - 4 – Object manipulation*
  - 3 – Localization to noxious stimulation*
  - 2 – Flexion withdrawal
  - 1 – Abnormal posturing
  - 0 – None/flaccid

- **OROMOTOR/VERBAL FUNCTION SCALE**
  - 3 – Intelligible verbalization*
  - 2 – Vocalization/oral movement
  - 1 – Oral reflexive movement
  - 0 – None

- **COMMUNICATION SCALE**
  - 2 – Functional: accurate**
  - 1 – Non-functional: intentional*
  - 0 – None

- **AROUSAL SCALE**
  - 3 – Attention
  - 2 – Eye opening without stimulation
  - 1 – Eye opening with stimulation
  - 0 – Unarousable

*Denotes MCS.
**Denotes emergence from minimally conscious state (MCS).

visual cortex, or may be mediated through the superior colliculus pathway [4]. In the CRS-R the presence of this behavior rules out the diagnosis of VS, while it is not the case according to the Multi-Society Task Force on the persistent vegetative state (PVS) [5], and to the Royal College of Physicians' report [6]. Accordingly, a recent PET study did not report any difference in brain metabolism between VS patients with preservation of visual fixation and VS lacking this behavior. Similarly, both groups shared the same 1-year outcome [7]. From a theoretical point of view, a long-lasting intentional behavior is a gold standard criterion of consciousness [8]. As a consequence, one

may consider that a fixation sustained over several seconds belongs to this category of conscious behaviors. However it is highly notable that fixation is dependent on the continuous presence of the visual target, and may therefore correspond to a continuously stimulated visuomotor reflex, rather than to a long-lasting internally generated behavior. A patient able to fixate on a target, and to maintain fixation on instructions even after the disappearance of the stimulus, and even if presented with competing stimuli, would demonstrate a much stronger evidence of conscious processing.

Blink to threat

In contrast with auditory startle – or maybe also of visual fixation – blink to visual threat (BVT) probably requires cortical processing [9–11]. Functional integrity of primary visual cortex is a mandatory stage, but note that patients with cortical lesions located away from cortical pathways (e.g., frontal or parietal) can lose BVT [10]. The Multi-Society Task Force stated that the diagnosis of persistent VS (PVS) should be extremely cautious in the presence of BVT [5]. However, BVT is not a criterion taken into account to distinguish VS from MCS [12]. In terms of consciousness recovery, BVT does not seem to be a predictor of a better outcome [11]. Therefore, while BVT requires richer cortical processing than visual fixation, it does not guarantee a patient to be conscious, or even minimally conscious. However, presence of a BVT requires the examiner to be even more cautious to look for additional signs of cortical integrity, and for the presence of more reliable signs of consciousness. To close with that sign, note that it is highly important not to confound it with corneal reflex elicited by an air puff caused by target motion.

Oro-facial behaviors

Oral reflexes such as chewing, teeth grinding, or swallowing are not problematic but other behaviors such as facial movements (smiles or grimaces), tears, grunting, or groaning sounds could be easily considered as conscious behavior. In this case, a possible adapted emotional behavior should be carefully searched for, and for example if a patient cries only in the presence of one of his or her relatives, one has to look for the presence of more univocal signs of MCS or of conscious state. Clearly, current knowledge is insufficient to provide any strong claim about these complex and sometimes specific emotional responses.

Additional signs

Noxious or noisy stimuli can elicit arousal responses, with autonomous reaction (e.g., increases of respiration and heart rates), grimaces or limb movements, and cause the extensor or flexor withdrawal of a limb. None of these signs should be confounded with a conscious behavior. Similarly, gaze or head orientation toward a loud sound is considered as reflex, and does not exclude VS [6,12]. In the same vein, grasping reflex and triple withdrawal should not be confounded with intentional movements.

Do not miss consciousness

While it is crucial not to overestimate consciousness (the "false positive" issue), it is even more dramatic to miss conscious patients. However, many factors can lead to such an error. Consider a conscious but non-communicating patient. On the basis of clinical observation and testing, consciousness is never probed as a "pure" and isolated process but rather in relation to many distinct cognitive abilities, to sensorimotor processes, and to mental contents [13]. Therefore, trivial or subtle impairments in any of those abilities, processes, or contents may lead to the absence of clinical evidence of conscious processing in a conscious but severely disabled patient. Illustrations of "trivial" impairments correspond to deaf, blind, or paralyzed conscious patients. Note that even these "trivial" or "easy" cases are not that easy to deal with. An astonishing study on locked-in syndrome (LIS) patients reported that the mean time of LIS diagnosis since the initial event was around 2.5 months [14]. One has to take into account that at the initial stage of a massive brainstem stroke, patients are usually in a genuine comatose state during a variable period. Recovery of consciousness from this initial comatose state may be missed if clinical evaluations are not repeated very regularly. Therefore, this long diagnostic delay emphasizes the need of repeating these evaluations, and of varying the ways of assessing consciousness.

Visual pursuit

When looking for visual pursuit, the use of the patient's own eyes (and even own face) as a visual target seems to be the most powerful stimulus, probably due to self-referencing (e.g., the "cocktail party effect" which corresponds to the powerful ability to react to one's own name when heard in a complex auditory scene) [15]. Indeed, the utilization of a mirror to detect visual pursuit has been shown to be more sensitive than any other visual stimuli (other faces, contrasted, or colored targets) [16]. As mentioned below, visual pursuit is one of the most informative signs to classify a patient as MCS or conscious.

Cognitive impairments

Less trivial situations are encountered in DOC patients suffering from aphasia, or from massive anterograde amnesia, or severe dysexecutive syndrome impacting attentional, working memory, and strategic abilities. In many of the clinical tests used with DOC patients, one may miss some form of conscious processing. Obviously, there is no easy solution to this point. However, a rigorous examination using both verbal and non-verbal instructions and stimulations (e.g., imitation or automatic behavior) may help to overcome some of these limitations. Additionally, systematic assessment of any possible movement (hands, feet, eyes, blinks, mouth, and tongue movements) will maximize the probability to detect an intentional response. Repetition of clinical evaluations is particularly important in the "acute" stage (first days and weeks), given the presence of frequent and major fluctuations in arousal and also possibly in consciousness, in particular in MCS patients.

Neglect

Attentional disorders such as spatial hemi-neglect – observed in patients with a non-dominant hemispheric lesion – could explain both perceptual difficulties (culminating in the neglect of instructions delivered in the neglected hemispace) and behavioral response impairments (motor neglect) in the absence of any central or peripheral motor neuron dysfunction. Patients have to be stimulated and observed from both sides (right and left).

Aphasia

Patients with dominant hemispheric lesions could be expected to have language impairments. In this case intentional and voluntary behaviors should be tested using non-verbal communication and instructions. This consideration is not yet implemented in standard behavioral scales, but most verbal commands could be delivered by gestural description. For example, the examiner can show the movement of a handshake to the patient with one hand, while testing the patient's response with the other hand [17].

Taken together, these elements contribute to explain that up to 40% of patients considered as VS demonstrate univocal evidence of MCS when examined by expert teams used to current detailed scales [18].

Finally, one has to be aware of the possible persistence of sedative agent effects. Electroencephalography and, most importantly, pharmacological measurements and pharmacological antagonistic tests (e.g., for benzodiazepines and morphinic agents) are sometimes extremely valuable here, in particular in comatose patients. Similarly one has to systematically check body temperature and hemodynamic constants when examining a DOC patient, and in particular when examining a comatose patient and a suspicion of brain death.

Overview of clinical and behavioral assessment of consciousness

Consciousness first requires a minimal level of arousal, the absence of which is observed in comatose states.

Arousal and basic neurological assessment

Arousal depends on the ascending reticular arousal system distributed within the tegmentum of the upper pons and midbrain, and in paramedian diencephalic structures along with the basal forebrain. These structures widely project onto the cortex including the thalamo-fronto-parietal network which plays a major role in consciousness, as theorized for instance in the conscious "global workspace" model [19]. Therefore coma can result from diffuse bihemispheric lesions (e.g., anoxia, trauma) or dysfunction (e.g., status epilepticus), or from focal brainstem lesions affecting in particular the ponto-mesencephalic tegmentum, or paramedian diencephalic structures bilaterally.

In front of a comatose patient, neurological examination aims at three major goals: (1) to confirm the diagnosis of comatose, and therefore to discard differential diagnoses such as locked-in syndrome, for instance; (2) to estimate the functional depth of the comatose state from profound and poorly reversible comatose to "diencephalic" comatose associated with a better prognosis of consciousness recovery; and (3) to provide potential cues to the etiological diagnosis (e.g., presence of discrete palpebral myoclonus in a status epilepticus; fever and meningitis syndrome in an acute meningo-encephalitis). Here, we will only underline the "functional depth" issue: basically, comatose is probably the clinical condition in which Hughlings Jackson's seminal concept of the central nervous system (CNS) described as a "hierarchical vertical axis" is the most relevant [20]. According to Jackson's theory, the higher a CNS region is, the more it controls and inhibits the CNS regions located below it, and the weaker it is to CNS "aggressions." This famous conception was the first to provide a satisfactory account of the positive signs secondary to a CNS lesion (e.g., disinhibition of medulla reflexes associated to primary motor cortex lesion). As a consequence, examination of brainstem reflexes in relation to the vertical location of their neural substrates within this hierarchical axis plays a major role: the lower reflexes are usually the most resistant, and one can frequently observe a gradient of reflex preservation. This "neo-jacksonian" view inspired for instance the scoring of the famous Glasgow Coma Scale and its variants, including brainstem reflex scoring (such as the Glasgow–Liège scale) or the more recent FOUR-score (see Tables 7.2 and 23.2): the upper reflexes are more weighted than the inferior ones, and the scoring of motor reactivity to stimulation also follows this supero-inferior gradient: a decortication response is scored better than a decerebration response. As a matter of fact it is extremely rare to observe the presence of oculocephalic reflexes in a comatose patient in whom oculocardiac reflex would be abolished. Combining all these observations with the inspection of pupil diameter, reactivity, and symmetry, and with the spontaneous breathing pattern (e.g., from Cheynes–Stokes dyspnea to apneustic or ataxic respiration) usually allows definition of the "functional depth" of comatose, and to monitor it

Table 7.2 Glasgow Coma Scale

- Eye response
    - 4 – eyes open spontaneously
    - 3 – eyes opening to verbal command
    - 2 – eyes opening to pain
    - 1 – no eyes opening

- Motor response
    - 6 – obeys commands
    - 5 – localizing pain
    - 4 – withdrawal from pain
    - 3 – flexion response to pain
    - 2 – extension response to pain
    - 1 – no response to pain

- Verbal response
    - 5 – oriented
    - 4 – confused
    - 3 – inappropriate words
    - 2 – incomprehensible sounds
    - 1 – no verbal response

across time in a given patient. When this detailed clinical examination does not fit with this functional gradient view, one has to look for focal lesions within the brainstem, or for additional factors which may interfere (e.g., drugs, metabolic dysfunctions).

Consciousness assessment

A more subtle alteration of consciousness is the vegetative state, which is characterized by preserved wakefulness [21] – even if circadian rhythms may not be strictly normal [22] – in the absence of any purposeful behavior and of any sign of intentional reactions to the external environment. Note that VS is, by definition, a clinical syndrome and not a specific condition. For this reason, and in order to avoid too radical interpretations of a patient's cognitive state only based on behavioral observations, a group of experts recently proposed the 'Unresponsive Wakefulness Syndrome' expression to describe VS [23]. The mere existence of VS demonstrates that wakefulness and consciousness can be dissociated, and therefore that they cannot be identified one with another.

Consequently, several scales have been created in order to distinguish VS patients from MCS patients. All these scales enable the clinician to administer various language, auditory, visual, somatosensory, and noxious stimuli and judge whether a patient's responses are indicative of conscious processing. Stimulations have to be repeated within the same examination session, in particular when spontaneous behavioral fluctuations are frequent. It is also important to gather all sources of observational evidence, including various caregivers and relatives who deserve a special consideration: while not being experts of behavioral assessment and being frequently the most motivated to interpret the behavior of their companion as conscious, they are also the most meaningful, or as Damasio phrases it: the most "emotionally competent" to the patient. It means that they are sometimes the most active stimuli to elicit a patient's richest behaviors. It is therefore sometimes useful to include the relatives in some stages of consciousness assessment. Furthermore, confounding variables (sedation, noisy environment, physical limitations) must be reduced to a minimum.

All these scales share a common design, combining: (1) items which appreciate coma exit [e.g., item 2 of the Wessex Head Injury Matrix (WHIM); arousal scale of the Coma Recovery Scale Revised (CRS-R)], with (2) items (see Table 7.1) probing purely reflexive behaviors integrated at a brainstem level and

indicative of a vegetative state if isolated despite repeated assessment (e.g., item 3 of the WHIM, or item 2 of the auditory function scale of the CRS-R which imply integrity of the colliculi and the tectospinal tracts), and with (3) items exploring behaviors requiring cortical integration and sustained activity, properties which are considered as specific to conscious processing (item 18 of the WHIM or items 2 and 3 of the vision function scale of the CRS-R which imply integrity of parietal and frontal eye fields area).

Note that a recent study explored a clinical sign previously described and emphasized by Plum and Posner as a marker of preserved cortical integration. The authors assessed the fast nystagmic return to mid-position of the eyes after ipsilateral tonic deviation towards the cold water-irrigated ear during testing of the oculovestibular reflexes [24]. This saccadic return – probably mediated by a long-range fronto-parietal cortical network – predicted consciousness recovery in a group of 26 clinically defined VS patients. Thirteen out of these 26 patients ultimately recovered consciousness. All patients who recovered consciousness presented a fast-component of nystagmus compared with only one of 11 patients who remained unconscious.

Using cognitive neuroscience to look for consciousness in patients

A complementary approach to clinical neurology originates from cognitive neurosciences of consciousness. Although the issue remains debated, two decades of experimental and theoretical work have led to the characterization of psychological and neurophysiological attributes that may be unique to conscious processing. Many cognitive processes may occur unconsciously either in conscious subjects, in visual neglect patients or related patients, and in non-conscious patients [25–27], reaching such complex levels as abstract semantics, phonological or emotional processing. Still, three properties seem to be exclusively associated with conscious processing of reportable mental contents [19]: (1) active maintenance of mental representations in working memory; (2) strategic processing; and (3) spontaneous intentional behavior. Similarly, while unconscious processing may engage multiple isolated cortical areas, neural signatures of conscious processing are defined by late and long-lasting brain activations that mobilize long-distance coherent thalamo-cortical networks, particularly involving bilateral prefrontal, cingulate, and parietal areas [25,28].

On the basis of these studies, original experimental "active" paradigms can therefore be designed in order to improve our ability to diagnose consciousness in non-communicating patients, beyond clinical evaluations. For instance, at the behavioral level, Bekinschtein and colleagues [29] capitalized on the working memory property mentioned above, and used an eye blink conditioning paradigm in which a tone stimulus can be paired with an air puff delivered on the cornea. Delayed conditioning – where the conditioned stimulus and the unconditioned air puff overlap in time – does not require conscious processing of the stimuli. In contrast, trace conditioning where a

temporal gap is inserted between the two stimuli seems to require conscious processing in working memory [30]. Interestingly, they showed that some clinically defined VS patients were able to demonstrate trace conditioning. Functional brain-imaging approaches are also emerging [31]. For instance, Owen and colleagues (32) probed with functional magnetic resonance imaging (fMRI) the active maintenance of task-instructed cognitive tasks, such as the ability to perform motor or spatial imagery tasks for an extended duration of 30 seconds (see Figure 7.1). Using this approach on 54 patients, they could identify five patients able to willfully modulate their

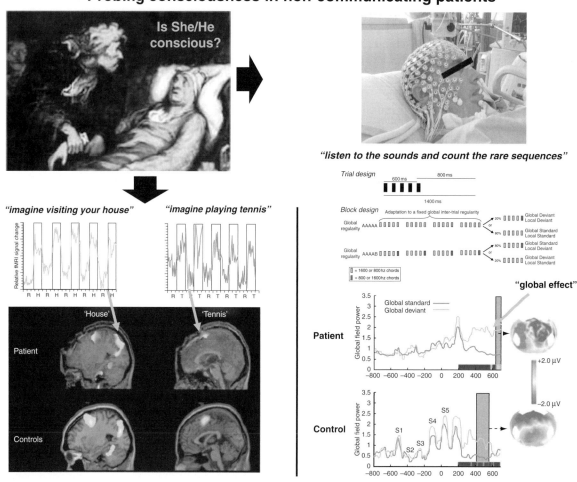

Figure 7.1 Two recent illustrations of active paradigms using functional brain imaging (EEG and fMRI) to probe consciousness in non-communicating patients. The mental navigation and mental motor imagery tasks designed by the group of Owen (left) allow the detection of sustained fMRI BOLD activations in cortical networks specific to each of these two mental imagery tasks [32]. The global regularity auditory task designed by the group of Naccache [42] allows the detection of late and sustained P3-like EEG responses when patients detect the occurrence of global regularity violations. In these two paradigms, the presence of a significant effect is highly suggestive of conscious processing. This figure is presented in color in the color plate section.

brain activity [33]. Among these five patients, two were clinically classified as VS. In one clinically MCS patient, fMRI could be used to define an arbitrary code and communicate a single piece of information (a yes/no answer), while such a communication was not possible behaviorally.

In parallel to such fMRI experiments, EEG paradigms may constitute a highly promising research direction for at least two reasons. First, EEG is a time-resolved tool able to sample brain activity at the millisecond scale. This offers a unique opportunity to monitor the flow of consciousness and eventually to interact with the patient in real time. Second, given that EEG is a non-invasive technique, has a relatively low cost, and can be recorded at bedside, one may ultimately design dedicated systems for recurrent and even continuous daily recording of brain activity in patients. In that respect, EEG monitoring seems more likely to truthfully reflect VS and MCS patients' complex fluctuating states than a single fMRI scan lasting a few tens of minutes. Schnakers and colleagues showed the utility of using active EEG paradigms to probe voluntary brain responses to stimuli. They could confirm the presence of conscious processing in a locked-in syndrome patient and in clinically defined MCS patients [34].

Active paradigms are important because they provide a way to probe various cognitive processes by looking for their specific neural signatures. However, this very same property confers a severe limitation: if for any reason the patient does not engage in the cognitive performance requested by the experimenter, then the test will fail to identify this patient as conscious even if she or he is conscious. If the patient is not awake during the task (e.g., confusional states, sleep cycles), or is conscious but cognitively impaired (aphasia, amnesia, poor working memory, dysexecutive syndrome), or refuses to obey the instructions, active paradigms will fail to diagnose this conscious patient as conscious.

For all these reasons, it is therefore useful to develop additional neurophysiological measures which could escape some of the limits of active paradigms. One promising path of research consists in recording brain activity in the absence of external stimulation. This approach, grounded on the seminal work of Raichle's group on the "resting state" or "default mode" (DM) networks, aims at exploring the spontaneous patterns of brain activity [35]. One of these DM networks include mesial cortical areas, including the precuneus and the posterior cingulate cortex, and seems to be related to self-consciousness and to introspective processes. Some key regions of this network may contribute to a general "projective system" enabling the individual to escape from immediate contingencies, e.g., projection in time (past and future), in space (mental navigation), and in mind (theory of mind) [36]. Functional MRI recordings of these DM networks seem to be informative about the level of consciousness in non-communicating patients [37]. It is important to note that while recording of resting state activity is not complex as compared with active paradigms, the selection of the most relevant analyses to be done on these raw data still remain a subject of research. Resting state measurements were initiated with fMRI but recent electrophysiological works pave the way to explore more finely these dynamics [38].

Lastly, a very elegant method combining EEG and TMS offers an easy way to probe the functionality of long-distance cortico-cortical networks at bedside without relying on a specific cognitive process. The principle consists in recording EEG with a fairly good spatial sampling over the whole cortex (from 32 up to 256 electrodes) immediately after the delivery of a single pulse of TMS over a local region of the cortex. By observing both early local, but most importantly late and sustained global responses, in particular over fronto-parietal regions, one may probe the existence of a functional "global workspace" network. First applications of this method during sleep [39], under midazolam anesthesia [40], and in DOC patients [41] strengthen its ability to isolate neural correlates of long-distance coherent cortical activities related to conscious states.

The "local global" test of consciousness

We will now focus on one "active" paradigm which provides a very specific (but not a very sensitive) way to probe consciousness in patients. We recently designed an auditory paradigm that evaluates the cerebral responses to violations of temporal regularities [42]. Local violations due to the unexpected occurrence of a single deviant sound amongst a repeated train of standard sounds led to an early response in auditory cortex, the mismatch negativity (MMN) ERP component, independent of attention and of the presence of a concurrent visual task. On the other hand, global violations, defined as the presentation of a rare and unexpected series of five sounds, led to a late and spatially distributed response that was only present when subjects were attentive and aware of the violations (P3b ERP component). We could detect the global effect in individual subjects using fMRI and both scalp and intracerebral event-related potentials. Since the original publication [42], we reported the results obtained in 65 recordings of non-communicating patients (28 recordings in MCS, 24 VS, and 13 in conscious patients) and confirmed that only conscious individuals (MCS or CS) presented a global effect (see Figure 7.1). When focusing on the group of VS patients, we confirmed the absence of global effect in the vast majority of patients, but identified two patients showing this neural signature of consciousness [43,44]. Interestingly, these two patients showed unequivocal clinical signs of consciousness within the 3–4 days following ERP recording, strongly suggesting they were misclassified as VS due to limitations of clinical examination. Taken together, these observations were highly suggestive that the global effect might be a signature of conscious processing, although it can be absent in conscious subjects who are not aware of the global auditory regularities.

Conclusion

In this non-exhaustive overview, we tried to emphasize the crucial importance of expert and informed clinical examination. Currently, up to 40% of patients may be misdiagnosed, most often considered as VS while they show univocal behavioral evidence of conscious or minimally conscious states (e.g., sustained visual pursuit in the mirror test of the CRS-R). It is probably the case that such a high error rate also reflects a prevailing opinion that being able to distinguish VS from MCS does not impact so much on the way we manage these patients. While this opinion highlights our weak therapeutic efficacy in these patients, in particular in chronic situations, we think it is important to remember that recognizing an MCS from VS is crucial for the patient, and for the relatives and caregivers. Note also that MCS patients seem to have a better functional prognosis outcome than VS patients [45]. Several new and valuable clinical scales and procedures are now increasing the power and standardization of consciousness probing in these patients. In parallel to this emphasis on clinical observation, we also tried to briefly show some of the very promising functional brain-imaging tools (in particular EEG, fMRI), taking advantage of the psychological properties of conscious processing to directly look for them in brain activity rather than in behavior. We think such tools will be integrated with the clinical assessment in these difficult situations. Finally, in identified conscious but non-communicating patients, current developments of EEG-based brain–computer interfaces may constitute a major therapeutic improvement by restoring to these patients the ability to "action their mind."

References

1. Posner JB, Plum F, Saper CB. *Plum and Posner's Diagnosis of Stupor and Coma.* New York, NY: Oxford University Press; 2007.

2. Wijdicks EFM, Bamlet WR, Maramattom BV, Manno EM, McClelland RL. Validation of a new coma scale: the FOUR score. *Ann Neurol* 2005;**58**(4):585–93.

3. Kalmar K, Giacino JT. The JFK Coma Recovery Scale – Revised. *Neuropsychol Rehabil* 2005;**15**(3–4):454–60.

4. Ro T, Shelton D, Lee OL, Chang E. Extrageniculate mediation of unconscious vision in transcranial magnetic stimulation-induced blindsight. *Proc Natl Acad Sci USA* 2004;**101**(26):9933–5.

5. The Multi-Society Task Force on PVS. Medical aspects of the persistent vegetative state (1). *N Engl J Med* 1994;**330**(21):1499–508.

6. Royal College of Physicians. *The Vegetative State: Guidance on Diagnosis and Management.* London: Royal College of Physicians; 2003.

7. Bruno MA, Vanhaudenhuyse A, Schnakers C, *et al.* Visual fixation in the vegetative state: an observational case series PET study. *BMC Neurol* 2010;**10**:35.

8. Naccache L. Psychology. Is she conscious? *Science* 2006;**313**(5792):1395–6.

9. Wade DT, Johnston C. The permanent vegetative state: practical guidance on diagnosis and management. *Br Med J* 1999;**319**(7213):841–4.

10. Liu GT, Ronthal M. Reflex blink to visual threat. *J Clin Neuroophthalmol* 1992;**12**(1):47–56.

11. Vanhaudenhuyse A, Giacino J, Schnakers C, *et al.* Blink to visual threat does not herald consciousness in the vegetative state. *Neurology* 2008;**71**(17):1374–5.

12. Giacino JT, Ashwal S, Childs N, *et al.* The minimally conscious state: definition and diagnostic criteria. *Neurology* 2002;**58**(3):349–53.

13. Cohen MA, Dennett DC. Consciousness cannot be separated from function. *Trends Cogn Sci* 2011;**15**(8):358–64.

14. Leon-Carrion J, van Eeckhout P, Dominguez-Morales Mdel R, Perez-Santamaria FJ. The locked-in syndrome: a syndrome looking for a therapy. *Brain Inj* 2002;**16**(7):571–82.

15. Cherry EC. Some experiments on the recognition of speech, with one and with two ears. *J Acoust Soc Am* 1953;**25**(5):975–9.

16. Vanhaudenhuyse A, Schnakers C, Bredart S, Laureys S. Assessment of visual pursuit in post-comatose states: use a mirror. *J Neurol Neurosurg Psychiatry* 2008;**79**(2):223.

17. Majerus S, Bruno MA, Schnakers C, Giacino JT, Laureys S. The problem of aphasia in the assessment of consciousness in brain-damaged patients. *Prog Brain Res* 2009;**177**:49–61.

18. Schnakers C, Vanhaudenhuyse A, Giacino J, *et al*. Diagnostic accuracy of the vegetative and minimally conscious state: clinical consensus versus standardized neurobehavioral assessment. *BMC Neurol* 2009;**9**:35.

19. Dehaene S, Naccache L. Towards a cognitive neuroscience of consciousness: basic evidence and a workspace framework. *Cognition* 2001;**79**(1–2):1–37.

20. Jackson JH. The Croonian Lectures on evolution and nervous system. *Br Med J* 1884;**1**:591–3;660–3;703–7.

21. Jennett B, Plum F. Persistent vegetative state after brain damage. A syndrome in search of a name. *Lancet* 1972;**1**(7753):734–7.

22. Bekinschtein TA, Golombek DA, Simonetta SH, Coleman MR, Manes FF. Circadian rhythms in the vegetative state. *Brain Inj* 2009;**23**(11):915–19.

23. Laureys S, Celesia GG, Cohadon F, *et al*. Unresponsive wakefulness syndrome: a new name for the vegetative state or apallic syndrome. *BMC Med* 2010;**8**:68.

24. Weiss N, Tadie JM, Faugeras F, *et al*. Can fast-component of nystagmus on caloric vestibulo-ocular responses predict emergence from vegetative state in ICU? *J Neurol* 2012;**259**(1):70–6.

25. Dehaene S, Changeux JP, Naccache L, Sackur J, Sergent C. Conscious, preconscious, and subliminal processing: a testable taxonomy. *Trends Cogn Sci* 2006;**10**(5):204–11.

26. Laureys S. The neural correlate of (un)awareness: lessons from the vegetative state. *Trends Cogn Sci* 2005;**9**(12):556–9.

27. Owen AM, Coleman MR, Menon DK, *et al*. Residual auditory function in persistent vegetative state: a combined PET and fMRI study. *Neuropsychol Rehabil* 2005;**15**(3–4):290–306.

28. Gaillard R, Dehaene S, Adam C, *et al*. Converging intracranial markers of conscious access. *PLoS Biol* 2009;**7**(3):e61.

29. Bekinschtein TA, Shalom DE, Forcato C, *et al*. Classical conditioning in the vegetative and minimally conscious state. *Nat Neurosci* 2009;**12**(10):1343–9.

30. Clark RE, Squire LR. Classical conditioning and brain systems: the role of awareness. *Science* 1998;**280**(5360):77–81.

31. Coleman MR, Davis MH, Rodd JM, *et al*. Towards the routine use of brain imaging to aid the clinical diagnosis of disorders of consciousness. *Brain* 2009;**132**(Pt 9):2541–52.

32. Owen AM, Coleman MR, Boly M, *et al*. Detecting awareness in the vegetative state. *Science* 2006;**313**(5792):1402.

33. Monti MM, Vanhaudenhuyse A, Coleman MR, *et al*. Willful modulation of brain activity in disorders of consciousness. *N Engl J Med* 2010;**362**(7):579–89.

34. Schnakers C, Perrin F, Schabus M, *et al*. Detecting consciousness in a total locked-in syndrome: an active event-related paradigm. *Neurocase* 2009;**15**(4):271–7.

35. Raichle ME, MacLeod AM, Snyder AZ, *et al*. A default mode of brain function. *Proc Natl Acad Sci USA* 2001;**98**(2):676–82.

36. Buckner RL, Carroll DC. Self-projection and the brain. *Trends Cogn Sci* 2007;**11**(2):49–57.

37. Vanhaudenhuyse A, Noirhomme Q, Tshibanda LJ-F, *et al*. Default network connectivity reflects the level of consciousness in non-communicative brain-damaged patients. *Brain* 2010;**133**(1):161–71.

38. He BJ, Snyder AZ, Zempel JM, Smyth MD, Raichle ME. Electrophysiological correlates of the brain's intrinsic large-scale functional architecture. *Proc Natl Acad Sci USA* 2008;**105**(41):16039–44.

39. Massimini M, Ferrarelli F, Murphy M, *et al*. Cortical reactivity and effective connectivity during REM sleep in humans. *Cogn Neurosci* 2010;**1**(3):176–83.

40. Ferrarelli F, Massimini M, Sarasso S, *et al*. Breakdown in cortical effective connectivity during midazolam-induced loss of consciousness. *Proc Natl Acad Sci USA* 2010;**107**(6):2681–6.

41. Rosanova M, Gosseries O, Casarotto S, *et al*. Recovery of cortical effective connectivity and recovery of consciousness in vegetative patients. *Brain* 2012;**135**(4):1308–20.

42. Bekinschtein TA, Dehaene S, Rohaut B, *et al*. Neural signature of the conscious processing of auditory regularities. *Proc Natl Acad Sci USA* 2009;**106**(5):1672–7.

43. Faugeras F, Rohaut B, Weiss N, *et al*. Probing consciousness with event-related potentials in the vegetative state. *Neurology* 2011;**77**(3):264–8.

44. Faugeras F, Rohaut B, Weiss N, *et al*. Event related potentials elicited by violations of auditory regularities in patients with impaired consciousness. *Neuropsychologia* 2012;**50**(3):403–18.

45. Luauté J, Maucort-Boulch D, Tell L, *et al*. Long-term outcomes of chronic minimally conscious and vegetative states. *Neurology* 75(3):246–52.

Chapter 8

Mechanisms of attention and attentional impairment

Paolo Bartolomeo

SUMMARY

Attention refers to a family of neurocognitive mechanisms which enable organisms to select stimuli appropriate to their goals while ignoring other, less important objects. Attentional mechanisms allow us to actively explore the external world and to achieve a conscious experience of it. A popular taxonomy of attention distinguishes between (1) *selection*, that is, mechanisms determining more extensive processing of some input rather than another; (2) *vigilance*, the capacity of sustaining attention over time; (3) *control*, the ability of planning and coordinating different activities. Patients in intensive care units (ICUs) can suffer from neurological impairments of each of these attentional processes. In particular, deficits of sustained attention (also referred to as vigilance or intrinsic alertness) are definitory characteristics of delirium, a frequent occurrence in these patients. Brain damage, especially if it implicates the right hemisphere, may determine a complex syndrome known as spatial neglect, whereby patients behave as if a part of the world (usually the left hemispace) did not exist anymore. Neglect is a severe disabling condition for patients, but can easily pass undetected. Diagnosis can be made by using simple, paper-and-pencil bedside tests. Attentional processes are not strictly localized in the human brain. Their functioning requires the coordinated activity of fronto-parietal networks, with a peculiar, although not yet completely elucidated role for the right hemisphere. Our knowledge of these systems is still too limited to enable us to offer specific interventions for the whole range of attentional impairments, but it is expanding at a fast pace, raising hopes for the development of effective strategies to improve the functioning of the attentional networks in brain-damaged patients.

Introduction

Biological organisms live in an environment cluttered with a multitude of objects. To behave in a coherent and goal-driven way, organisms need to select stimuli appropriate to their goals. On the other hand, because of capacity limitations, they must be capable of ignoring other, less important objects. Thus, objects in the world compete for recruiting the organism's attention in order to be the focus of the organism's subsequent behavior. Neural mechanisms of attention resolve this competition by taking into account both the goals of the organisms and the salience of the sensorial stimuli. In fact, attention and its neural correlates are not a unitary phenomenon, but they can better be understood as a heterogeneous set of processes. For example, Parasuraman [1] identified at least three independent but interacting components of attention: (1) *selection*, that is, mechanisms determining more extensive processing of some input rather than another; (2) *vigilance*, the capacity of sustaining attention over time; (3) *control*, the ability of planning and coordinating different activities.

Inattention in delirium

Patients in ICUs often show signs of delirium. Inattention is one main diagnostic criterion of delirium [2]. Attention deficits in delirium can affect each of the main components of attention. In particular, patients with delirium typically suffer from a diminished capacity of sustaining attention over time [3]. This can be an important criterion of differential diagnosis from dementia without delirium, where sustained attention can be relatively spared. Brain networks important for sustained attention, such as prefrontal and parietal cortex primarily in the right hemisphere [4], with additional contribution from thalamic and brainstem nuclei [5] (Figure 8.1), may

Brain Disorders in Critical Illness, ed. Robert D. Stevens, Tarek Sharshar, and E. Wesley Ely. Published by Cambridge University Press. © Cambridge University Press 2013.

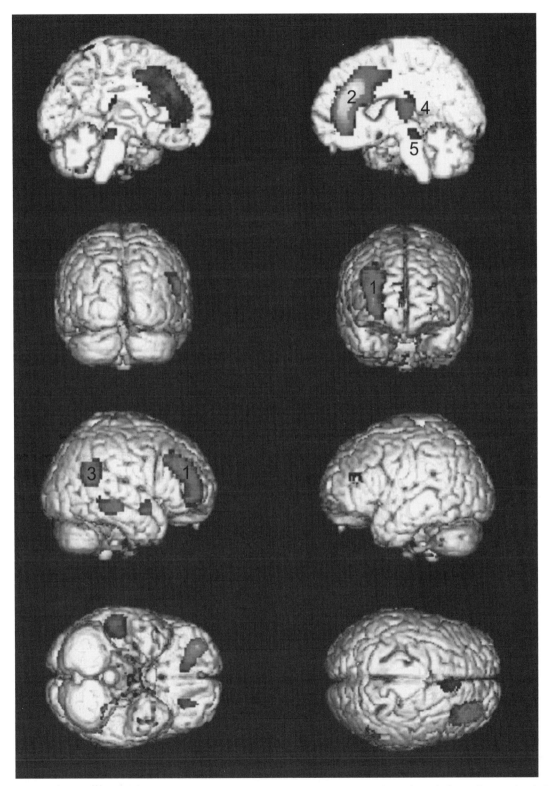

Figure 8.1 Positron emission tomography activations for a task of sustained attention with visual stimuli. The predominantly right hemisphere network encompasses the dorsolateral prefrontal cortex (1), the anterior cingulate gyrus (2), the inferior parietal cortex (3), the thalamus (4) and the ponto-mesencephalic tegmentum, possibly involving the locus coeruleus (5). From Sturm, W. (2009). Aufmerksamkeitsstörungen. In Sturm W, Herrmann M, Münte TF. (Hrsg.): *Lehrbuch der Klinischen Neuropsychologie*. 2. Aufl. (421–443). Heidelberg: Spektrum. Reprinted with the authors' permission. This figure is presented in color in the color plate section.

therefore be dysfunctional in patients with delirium. The substantial overlapping, both conceptual and anatomical, between sustained attention and general arousal/consciousness (see Chapters 7 and 9, this volume) makes it difficult or impossible to separate their respective contribution to inattention in delirium patients.

Selective attention

The concept of spatial selective attention, which will be the main object of the remaining sections of this chapter, refers operationally to the advantage in speed and accuracy of processing for objects lying in attended regions of space as compared with objects located in non-attended regions [6].

When several events compete for limited processing capacity and control of behavior, attentional selection may resolve the competition. In their influential neurocognitive model of selective attention, Desimone and Duncan [7] proposed that competition is biased toward some stimuli over others. Two types of processes determine this bias. Bottom-up processes are related to the sensory salience of stimuli; top-down processes result from the current behavioral goals. Thus, neural attentional processes resolve the competition [8], on the basis of the organisms' goals and of the sensory properties of the objects, by giving priority to some objects over others. A subset of selective attention processes deals with objects in space. In ecological settings, agents usually orient toward important stimuli by turning their gaze, head, and trunk toward their spatial location. This is done in order to align the stimulus with the part of the sensory surface with highest resolution (e.g., the retinal fovea) [9]. This allows further perceptual processing of the detected stimulus, for example its classification as a useful or as a dangerous object. Even very simple artificial organisms display orienting behavior when their processing resources are insufficient to process the whole visual scene in parallel [9]. However,

attention can also be oriented in space without eye movements (so-called "covert" orienting) [6].

The exogenous/endogenous dichotomy

To successfully cope with a continuously changing environment, an organism needs mechanisms that (1) allow for the processing of novel, unexpected events, that could be either advantageous or dangerous, in order to respond appropriately with either approaching or avoidance behavior; (2) allow for the maintenance of finalized behavior in spite of distracting events [9]. It is thereby plausible that different attentional processes serve these two partially conflicting goals. Attention can be directed to an object in space either in a relatively reflexive way (e.g., when a honking car attracts the attention of a pedestrian) or in a more controlled mode (e.g., when the pedestrian monitors the traffic light waiting for the 'go' signal to appear). Exogenous orienting processes are good candidates for being involved in drawing attention to novel events [10]. Endogenous orienting processes, on the other hand, would be responsible for directing the organism's attention towards its target despite the presence of distractors in the environment [11].

Covert orienting of spatial attention

Posner and his co-workers (see [6], for review) developed a manual response time (RT) paradigm to study the covert orienting of attention. Subjects are presented with three horizontally arranged boxes (Figure 8.2).

They fixate the central box and respond by pressing a key to a target (an asterisk) appearing in one of two lateral boxes. The target is preceded by a cue indicating one of the two lateral boxes. Cues can be either central (an arrow or another symbol presented in the central box), or peripheral (a brief brightening of one peripheral box). Valid cues correctly predict the box in which the target will appear, whereas invalid cues indicate the

Figure 8.2 Example of a trial from the Posner response time paradigm. A peripheral invalid cue precedes a left-sided target, to which a manual response (keypress) is to be made.

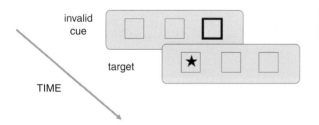

wrong box. Normal subjects usually show an advantage of valid cue-target trials as compared with invalid trials (cue validity effect). This suggests that the cue prompts an attentional orienting toward the cued location, which speeds up the processing of targets appearing in that region and slows down responses to targets appearing in other locations.

In this paradigm, it is often the case that a large majority (e.g., 80%) of cues are valid; in this case, cues are said to be informative of the future emplacement of the target. Alternatively, cues may be non-informative, when targets can appear with equal probabilities in the cued or in the uncued location. Peripheral, non-informative cues attract attention automatically, or exogenously. This exogenous attentional shift (revealed by a cue validity effect) is typically observed only for short stimulus onset asynchronies (SOAs) between cue and target. For SOAs longer than ~300 ms, uncued targets evoke faster responses than cued targets [12–14], as if attention was inhibited from returning to previously explored objects. This phenomenon is known as inhibition of return (IOR) [15,16], and is often interpreted as reflecting a mechanism which promotes the exploration of the visual scene by inhibiting repeated orientations towards the same locations [13,17]. Exogenous, or stimulus-dependent, and endogenous, or strategy-driven, mechanisms of attentional orienting are thus qualitatively different, though highly interactive, processes.

Fronto-parietal networks of spatial attention

Today, we know a fair amount of detailed information on the anatomy, functions, dynamics, and pathology of the brain networks that subserve the orienting of gaze and attention in the human brain. Important components of these networks include the dorsolateral prefrontal cortex (PFC) and the posterior parietal cortex (PPC). Physiological studies indicate that these two structures show interdependence of neural activity. In the monkey, analogous PPC and PFC areas show coordinated activity when the animal selects a visual stimulus as a saccade target [18]. Importantly, PFC and PPC show distinctive dynamics and seem to use two different languages when attention is selected by the stimulus (bottom-up or exogenous orienting) or when it is directed by more top-down (or endogenous) goals. Bottom-up signals appear first in the parietal cortex and are characterized by an increase of fronto-parietal coherence in the gamma band, whereas top-down signals emerge first in the frontal cortex and tend to synchronize in the beta band [18]. Not surprisingly, PFC and PPC are directly and extensively interconnected. Several distinct fronto-parietal, long-range pathways have been identified (see [19] for a recent review). These pathways include the arcuate fasciculus (AF) and the superior longitudinal fasciculus (SLF). The AF links the caudal portions of the temporal lobe, at the junction with the parietal lobe, with the dorsal portions of the areas 8, 46, and 6 in the frontal lobe. Within the SLF, three distinct branches can be identified in the monkey on the basis of cortical terminations and course [20]. The SLF I links the superior parietal region and the adjacent medial parietal cortex with the supplementary and premotor areas in the frontal lobe. The SLF II originates in the caudal inferior parietal lobe (corresponding to the human angular gyrus) and the occipito-parietal area and projects to the dorsolateral prefrontal cortex. The SLF III (which corresponds to the anterior segment of the AF, asAF) connects the rostral portion of the inferior parietal lobe (homologous to the human supramarginal gyrus) with the ventral premotor area 6, the adjacent area 44, the frontal operculum, and area 46. A similar architecture seems to exist in the human brain [21] (Figure 8.3).

The asAF/SLF III connects a ventral attentional network (VAN), which shows increased BOLD responses in fMRI when participants have to respond to invalidly cued targets [22]. According to Corbetta and Shulman, the VAN is thus responsible for reorienting of attention, whereas a more dorsal fronto-parietal pathway, the dorsal attentional network (DAN), connected by the human homolog of SLF I [23], would orient spatial attention during valid cueing. Importantly, the VAN seems only present in the right hemisphere, whereas the DAN is symmetrically represented in both hemispheres. The SLF II connects the parietal component of the VAN to the prefrontal component of the DAN, thus allowing direct communication between ventral and dorsal attentional networks [23]. Importantly, there is substantial anatomical overlap between these right hemisphere networks and the neural substrates of sustained attention [5,24] (see Figure 8.1). Not surprisingly, neglect patients do show impairments of sustained attention [25]. This deficit can in part be compensated by engaging patients' phasic alertness (e.g., by giving short auditory tones) [26,27].

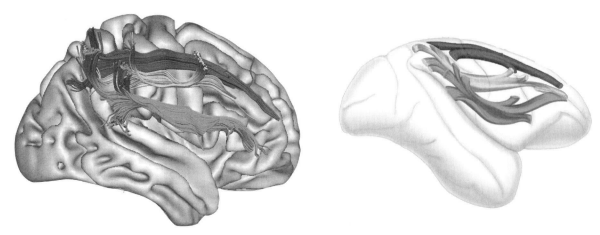

Figure 8.3 The three branches of the superior longitudinal fasciculus in a human brain (left) and a monkey brain (right). Modified from [25] with the author's permission. This figure is presented in color in the color plate section.

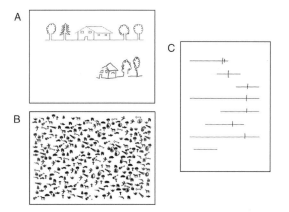

Figure 8.4 Performance of a patient with left spatial neglect on paper-and-pencil tests. A, copy of a linear drawing with omission of left-sided elements; B, target cancellation task, with omission of left-sided targets (bells); C, bisection of horizontal lines, with rightward deviation of the bisection mark and complete omission of one left-sided line.

Dysfunctions of attentional networks

Temporary inactivation of the SLF in the human right hemisphere impairs the symmetrical distribution of visual attention [21]. Vascular, traumatic, or degenerative damage to SLF networks in the right hemisphere is frequently associated to a disabling condition known as left visual neglect [28,29]. About half of the patients with a lesion in the right hemisphere suffer from neglect for the left side of space [30]. They are unaware of the left half of their environment. Neglect patients do not eat from the left part of their dish, they bump their wheelchair into obstacles situated on their left, and have a tendency to look to right-sided details as

soon as a visual scene deploys, as if their attention were "magnetically" attracted by these details [31]. They are usually unaware of their deficits (anosognosia), and often obstinately deny being hemiplegic. Patients with left brain damage may also show signs of contralesional, right-sided neglect, albeit more rarely and usually in a less severe form [32,33]. Neglect is a substantial source of handicap and disability for patients, and entails a poor functional outcome. Diagnosis is important, because effective rehabilitation strategies are available, and there are promising possibilities for pharmacological treatments [34]. Furthermore, in many cases the nature of neglect deficits (impaired active exploration of a part of space) renders the diagnosis difficult or impossible if signs of neglect are not searched for. Diagnosis is easily made by asking the patient to perform a few paper-and-pencil tests, such as target cancellation (omission of a variable amount of left-sided targets), line bisection (deviation of the subjective midpoint towards the right side), and copy of a drawing (omission of left-sided details), which can usually be done at bedside (Figure 8.4).

Since neglect is especially evident in the acute stages of brain dysfunction, patients in ICUs are particularly concerned. In addition to its clinical importance, neglect also raises important issues concerning the brain mechanisms of consciousness, perception, and attention.

Neglect is characterized, among other symptoms, by severe problems in orienting attention towards left-sided objects [35]. Indeed, an association of attentional deficits seems typical of unilateral neglect [35], including deficits of spatial orienting and impaired sustained attention/vigilance [26,27]. This is not surprising, given the substantial overlapping between orienting and sustained attention networks in the right hemisphere [5]. Some of the attentional deficits operate in a specific temporal sequence in neglect patients; an early attraction of attention toward the right is followed by an impairment in redirecting attention toward the left [31,36,37]. Importantly, these deficits seem mainly to concern exogenous, or stimulus-related, orienting of attention, with relative sparing of endogenous, or voluntary, orienting [31,32]. Thus, the simple presence of right-sided distractors can disrupt patients' performance by capturing their attention [38]. In neglect patients, damage to right-hemisphere VAN could cause a functional imbalance between the left and right DANs, with a hyperactivity of the left dorsal fronto-parietal network, which would provoke an attentional bias towards right-sided objects and neglect of left-sided items [39]. Consistent with this hypothesis, suppressive TMS on the left parieto-motor pathway correlated with an improvement of patients' performance on cancellation tests [40].

How attention shapes our experience of the world

Neglect patients may have a perfectly functioning primary visual cortex, and yet they behave as if they were blind to a part of the visual world. Thus, conscious perception does not simply depend on activity in the primary visual cortices, but needs the integrated functioning of higher-level brain areas [41]. Activity in ventral areas of the lateral temporal cortex has been related to conscious perception [42]; however, localized temporal activity does not seem sufficient to elicit a conscious state [36,38]. Several lines of evidence indicate that additional activity in parietal and pre-frontal regions is important to achieve a conscious, reportable visual experience [21,43]. Thus, there seems to be at least a certain degree of anatomical overlap between some of the putative cerebral correlates of conscious perception and the fronto-parietal networks of spatial attention [44].

Indeed, cognitive neuroscientists have often considered attentional processes as "the mechanisms of consciousness" [45]. Introspection does suggest that we need to attend to an object in order to be conscious of it, and that the objects of our attention are necessarily part of our conscious experience. More recently, however, the relationship between attention and consciousness has

become a matter of debate. In particular, the commonly accepted notion that attention is necessary and sufficient for consciousness has been challenged. For example, Koch and Tsuchiya [46] reviewed psychophysical evidence on normal participants and concluded that "top-down attention and consciousness are distinct phenomena that need not occur together."

No one disputes that attention and consciousness describe different processes, which to some extent belong to distinct conceptual categories. Attention has observable behavioral correlates in terms of response times/accuracy and perceptual discrimination. Consciousness, on the other hand, refers to subjective experience, not necessarily reflected in verbal reportability [47]. Despite this conceptual distinction, however, evidence from both normal participants and brain-damaged patients seems to confirm the introspective intuition of a tight relationship between attention and consciousness. In particular, evidence suggests that some attentional processes can be a crucial antecedent to consciousness.

With reference to the exogenous/endogenous dichotomy outlined above, accumulating evidence supports the hypothesis that exogenous attention is a necessary, although not sufficient, step for the emergence of conscious visual perception. Endogenous attention, on the other hand, seems to be less relevant for conscious perception, consistent with claims for double dissociations between attention and consciousness [46,48]. Systematic behavioral data on the importance of exogenous and endogenous attention for conscious perception were obtained by Chica et al. [49], by using Posner-like response time paradigms in which a near-threshold target was preceded by either exogenous or endogenous cues. Only exogenous (peripheral) cues improved conscious perception of the targets. In an ERP study [50] using similar paradigms, cue-locked potentials revealed a systematic relationship between the amplitude of a P100 component elicited by exogenous cues and the conscious perception of the targets. Valid cues led to the conscious perception of the subsequent targets when they captured attention to their location, as indexed by the P100 component distributed over occipito-parietal areas. On the other hand, invalid cues led to the conscious perception of the subsequent targets only when they failed to capture attention at their location (opposite to the target location). Finally, functional connectivity analyses in fMRI [51] further stressed the importance of fronto-parietal networks in the orienting of attention and its influence on conscious perception. During the cue epoch, a fronto-parietal network largely lateralized to the right hemisphere supports the significant interaction between spatial orienting and its modulation of conscious perception. These results demonstrating the importance of spatial orienting networks for consciousness in normal participants are consistent with the severe signs of spatial unawareness demonstrated by brain-damaged patients with dysfunction of right hemisphere attentional networks and visual neglect.

In conclusion, attentional processes in the brain, mainly subserved by fronto-parietal networks, with a peculiar although not yet completely elucidated role for the right hemisphere, are at the basis of our capacity to actively explore the external world. Their impairment as a result of brain damage can hamper the conscious perception of objects in space, and is a source of significant disability for patients. Our knowledge of these systems is still too limited to enable us to offer specific interventions for the whole range of attentional impairments, but it is expanding at a fast pace, raising hopes for the development of effective strategies to improve the functioning of the attentional networks in brain-damaged patients.

Acknowledgments

The author acknowledges with thanks the help of Alexia Bourgeois, Michel Thiebaut de Schotten, and Walter Sturm for the figures, and of the book editors for comments on a previous version of this chapter.

References

1. Parasuraman R. The attentive brain: issues and prospects. In Parasuraman R, editor. Cambridge, MA: MIT Press; 1998:3–15.

2. American Psychiatric Association. *Diagnostic and Statistical Manual of Mental Disorders, Fourth edition.* Washington, DC: American Psychiatric Association; 1994.

3. Brown LJ, Fordyce C, Zaghdani H, Starr JM, MacLullich AM. Detecting deficits of sustained visual attention in delirium. *J Neurol Neurosurg Psychiatry* 2011;**82**(12):1334–40.

4. Pardo JV, Fox PT, Raichle ME. Localization of a human system for sustained attention by positron emission tomography. *Nature* 1991;**349**:61–4.

5. Sturm W, de Simone A, Krause BJ, *et al.* Functional anatomy of intrinsic alertness: evidence for a fronto-parietal-thalamic-brainstem network in the right hemisphere. *Neuropsychologia* 1999;**37**(7):797–805.

6. Posner MI. Orienting of attention. *Q J Exp Psychol* 1980;**32**:3–25.

7. Desimone R, Duncan J. Neural mechanisms of selective visual attention. *Annu Rev Neurosci* 1995;**18**:193–222.

8. Di Ferdinando A, Parisi D, Bartolomeo P. Modeling orienting behavior and its disorders with "ecological" neural networks. *J Cogn Neurosci* 2007;**19**(6):1033–49.

9. Allport DA. Visual attention. In Posner MI, editor. *Foundations of Cognitive Science.* Cambridge, MA: MIT Press; 1989:631–87.

10. Yantis S. Attentional capture in vision. In Kramer AF, Coles GH, Logan GD, editors. *Converging Operations in the Study of Visual Selective Attention.* Washington, DC: American Psychological Association; 1995:45–76.

11. LaBerge D, Auclair L, Siéroff E. Preparatory attention: experiment and theory. *Conscious Cogn* 2000;**9**:396–434.

12. Maylor EA, Hockey R. Inhibitory component of externally controlled covert orienting in visual space. *J Exp Psychol Hum Percept Perform* 1985;**11**:777–87.

13. Posner MI, Cohen Y. Components of visual orienting. In Bouma H, Bouwhuis D, editors. *Attention and Performance X.* London: Lawrence Erlbaum; 1984:531–56.

14. Rafal RD, Henik A. The neurology of inhibition: integrating controlled and automatic processes. In Dagenbach D, Carr TH, editors. *Inhibitory Processes in Attention, Memory and Language.* San Diego, CA: Academic Press; 1994:1–51.

15. Posner MI, Rafal RD, Choate LS, Vaughan J. Inhibition of return: neural basis and function. *Cogn Neuropsychol* 1985;**2**:211–28.

16. Bartolomeo P, Lupiáñez J, editors. *Inhibitory After-effects in Spatial Processing: Experimental and Theoretical Issues on Inhibition of Return.* Hove: Psychology Press; 2006.

17. Klein RM. Inhibition of return. *Trends Cogn Sci* 2000;**4**(4):138–47.

18. Buschman TJ, Miller EK. Top-down versus bottom-up control of attention in the prefrontal and posterior parietal cortices. *Science* 2007;**315**(5820):1860–2.

19. Urbanski M, Thiebaut de Schotten M, Rodrigo S, *et al.* DTI-MR tractography of white matter damage in stroke patients with neglect. *Exp Brain Res* 2011;**208**(4):491–505.

20. Schmahmann JD, Pandya DN. *Fiber Pathways of the Brain.* New York, NY: Oxford University Press; 2006.

21. Thiebaut de Schotten M, Urbanski M, Duffau H, *et al.* Direct evidence for a parietal-frontal pathway subserving spatial awareness in humans. *Science* 2005;**309**(5744):2226–8.

22. Corbetta M, Shulman GL. Control of goal-directed and stimulus-driven attention in the brain. *Nat Rev Neurosci* 2002;**3**(3):201–15.

23. Thiebaut de Schotten M, Dell'Acqua F, Forkel S, *et al.* A lateralized brain network for spatial attention. *Nat Neurosci* 2911;**14**(10):1245–6.

24. Sturm W, Willmes K. On the functional neuroanatomy of intrinsic and phasic alertness. *Neuroimage* 2001;**14**(1 Pt 2):S76–84.

25. Robertson IH. Do we need the "lateral" in unilateral neglect? Spatially nonselective attention deficits in unilateral neglect and their implications for rehabilitation. *NeuroImage* 2001;**14**(1):S85–90.

26. Robertson IH, Mattingley JB, Rorden C, Driver J. Phasic alerting of neglect patients overcomes their spatial deficit in visual awareness. *Nature* 1998;**395**(6698):169–72.

27. Chica AB, Thiebaut de Shotten M, Toba MN, *et al.* Attention networks and their interactions after right-hemisphere damage.*Cortex* 2012;**48**(6):654–63.

28. Bartolomeo P. A parieto-frontal network for spatial awareness in the right hemisphere of the human brain. *Arch Neurol* 2006;**63**:1238–41.

29. Bartolomeo P, Thiebaut de Schotten M, Doricchi F. Left unilateral neglect as a disconnection syndrome. *Cereb Cortex* 2007;**45**(14):3127–48.

30. Azouvi P, Bartolomeo P, Beis J-M, *et al.* A battery of tests for the quantitative assessment of unilateral neglect. *Restorative Neurology Neurosci* 2006;**24**(4–6):273–85.

31. Gainotti G, D'Erme P, Bartolomeo P. Early orientation of attention toward the half space ipsilateral to the lesion in patients with unilateral brain damage. *J Neurol Neurosurg Psychiatry* 1991;**54**:1082–9.

32. Beis JM, Keller C, Morin N, *et al.* Right spatial neglect after left hemisphere stroke: qualitative and quantitative study. *Neurology* 2004;**63**(9):1600–5.

33. Bartolomeo P, Chokron S, Gainotti G. Laterally directed arm movements and right unilateral neglect after left hemisphere damage. *Neuropsychologia* 2001;**39**(10):1013–21.

34. Bartolomeo P. Visual neglect. *Curr Opin Neurol* 2007;**20**(4):381–6.

35. Bartolomeo P, Chokron S. Orienting of attention in left unilateral neglect. *Neurosci Biobehav Rev* 2002;**26**(2):217–34.

36. D'Erme P, Robertson I, Bartolomeo P, Daniele A, Gainotti G. Early rightwards orienting of attention on simple reaction time performance in patients with left-sided neglect. *Neuropsychologia* 1992;**30**(11):989–1000.

37. Rastelli F, Funes MJ, Lupiáñez J, Duret C, Bartolomeo P. Left neglect: is the disengage deficit space- or object-based? *Exp Brain Res* 2008;**187**(3):439–46.

38. Bartolomeo P, Urbanski M, Chokron S, *et al.* Neglected attention in apparent spatial compression. *Neuropsychologia* 2004;**42**(1):49–61.

39. Corbetta M, Kincade MJ, Lewis C, Snyder AZ, Sapir A. Neural basis and recovery of spatial attention deficits in spatial neglect. *Nat Neurosci* 2005;**8**(11):1603–10.

40. Koch G, Oliveri M, Cheeran B, *et al.* Hyperexcitability of parietal-motor functional connections in the intact left-hemisphere of patients with neglect. *Brain* 2008;**131**(12):3147–55.

41. Rees G, Kreiman G, Koch C. Neural correlates of consciousness in humans. *Nat Rev Neurosci* 2002;**3**(4):261–70.

42. Zeki S. The Ferrier Lecture 1995 behind the seen: the functional specialization of the brain in space and time. *Philos Trans R Soc Lond B Biol Sci* 2005;**360**(1458):1145–83.

43. Beck DM, Rees G, Frith CD, Lavie N. Neural correlates of change detection and change blindness. *Nat Neurosci* 2001;**4**(6):645–50.

44. Bartolomeo P. Varieties of attention and of consciousness: evidence from neuropsychology. *Psyche* 2008;**14**(1).

45. Posner MI. Attention: the mechanisms of consciousness. *Proc Natl Acad Sci USA* 1994;**91**(16): 7398–403.

46. Koch C, Tsuchiya N. Attention and consciousness: two distinct brain processes. *Trends Cogn Sci* 2007;**11**(1):16–22.

47. Dalla Barba G. *Memory, Consciousness and Temporality.* Boston, MA: Kluwer Academic Publishers; 2002.

48. Wyart V, Tallon-Baudry C. Neural dissociation between visual awareness and spatial attention. *J Neurosci* 2008;**28**(10):2667–79.

49. Chica AB, Lasaponara S, Chanes L, *et al.* Spatial attention and conscious perception: the role of endogenous and exogenous orienting. *Attent Percept Psychophys* 2011;**73**:1065–81.

50. Chica AB, Lasaponara S, Lupiáñez J, Doricchi F, Bartolomeo P. Exogenous attention can capture perceptual consciousness: ERP and behavioural evidence. *NeuroImage* 2010;**51**(3):1205–12.

51. Chica AB, Paz-Alonso PM, Valero-Cabré A, Bartolomeo P. Neural bases of the interactions between spatial attention and conscious perception. *Cerebral Cortex* 2013;**23**(6):1269–79.

75

Neurology of sleep and sleep disorders

Robert D. Sanders, Stefan D. Gurney, Jamie W. Sleigh, and Mervyn Maze

SUMMARY

Sleep is a fundamental biological process involved in multiple homeostatic processes. Yet in critically ill patients, perhaps those in most need of a good night's rest, sleep is fragmented and of poor quality. This sleep deprivation likely contributes to the significant burden of delirium and immune dysfunction that is evident in the critically ill. While most sedatives appear to produce a state akin to "pharmacologically induced sleep," there are important differences to natural sleep. One exception appears to be alpha-2 agonists that produce a state of sedation that is closer to natural sleep than drugs that target the GABA$_A$ receptor (that includes the benzodiazepines and propofol). Here we review the function and neurobiology of natural sleep, comparing and contrasting it with different types of sedation, and discuss the potential consequences thereof. We also cover a major impediment to the research into sleep in the intensive care unit (ICU): the difficulty in identifying it. Finally we cover the implications of sleep-disordered breathing (encompassing obstructive sleep apnea and obesity hypoventilation syndrome) in the ICU.

Introduction

Brain dysfunction, epitomized by the acute confusional state of delirium, is common in critically ill patients and is associated with significant morbidity and mortality (see Chapter 1, this volume). Sleep disruption is emerging as an important risk factor for developing critical care delirium. Most sedatives appear to produce a state akin to "pharmacologically induced sleep;" but in fact produce a state with important differences to natural sleep. An important exception are alpha-2 agonist drugs that produce a state of sedation that appears closer to natural sleep.

Function and stages of sleep

Sleep has anabolic, restorative properties that improves both neurocognitive and immune function [1]. The circadian rhythm determines the appropriate timing of sleep while homeostatic processes regulate sleep debt and depth depending on wakeful activity [2]. It follows that a subject can regulate the type of sleep (e.g., duration of slow wave activity) that is required based on need, and that sleep is not a homogeneous state. There are four stages to NREM sleep (with stages 3 and 4 comprising slow wave sleep depending on the extent of slow wave activity) and REM sleep (Table 9.1). As yet we do not have complete understanding of the function of the different stages of sleep but some interesting observations have been made. For example, during NREM sleep slow wave activity performs a homeostatic function to reduce the strength of synapses that has been acquired during wakeful activity [2]. This synaptic homeostasis improves subsequent cognitive function by allowing new changes in synaptic strength. Furthermore, both NREM and REM sleep are necessary for the consolidation of learning and memory and sleep deprivation results in cognitive dysfunction [3].

It has been hypothesized that sleep deprivation-induced cognitive dysfunction shares similarities with delirium, particularly hypoactive delirium [4]. Indeed both delirium and sleep deprivation are characterized by inattention, fluctuating mental status, mood disturbance, and cognitive impairment. Furthermore the underlying cognitive changes may be driven by a shared mechanism of an up-regulation of inhibitory GABA signaling in the brain [5]. This change in inhibitory tone is suggested to break down network connectivity in the brain leading to various neural symptoms including those described above [5]. Currently there are insufficient data to confirm a definite link between delirium and sleep deprivation

Brain Disorders in Critical Illness, ed. Robert D. Stevens, Tarek Sharshar, and E. Wesley Ely. Published by Cambridge University Press. © Cambridge University Press 2013.

Table 9.1 The different stages of sleep.

	Awake	Stage 1 NREM sleep	Stage 2 NREM sleep	Stage 3/4 NREM sleep	REM sleep
Arousal state	Wakeful	Hypnosis	Hypnosis	Hypnosis	Hypnosis
Predominant EEG pattern	Alpha	Theta	Theta and spindles	Delta	Theta
Cholinergic	↓	↓	↓	↓	↑
Noradrenergic	↓	↓	↓	↓	↓
Histaminergic	↓	↓	↓	↓	↓
Orexinergic	↓	↓	↓	↓	↓

partly due to the difficulties in assessing sleep in the ICU. However one small study defined a link between greater sleep deprivation and adverse cognitive performance in critically ill patients [6]. Further work focusing on the impact of sleep deprivation on the risk of delirium, and subtypes of delirium, is required.

Lack of sleep probably has a significant impact on mortality. Animal models of sleep deprivation typically result in the animal dying from a curious multi-organ failure associated with immune suppression, hypothermia, weight loss, hepatic derangement, and bacterial invasion [7]. Less extreme sleep deprivation has been shown to reduce viral clearance in mice after influenza challenge, and immunized, sleep-deprived mice responded to viral challenge similar to unimmunized mice. In addition, thermoregulation, metabolism, and hormonal dysregulation occur following sleep deprivation. While both total and REM sleep deprivation result in weight loss and temperature dysregulation in rats [7], REM sleep appears to play a unique role in temperature regulation, and given the tight temperature band in which humans function, it is unsurprising that REM sleep deprivation results in significant physiological dysfunction.

Most clinical studies examining the effects of sleep deprivation on immune function in humans have utilized healthy volunteers. It seems logical to assume that any immune dysfunction observed in sleep-deprived healthy subjects is likely to be more pronounced in patients with acute or chronic illnesses. However, a direct relationship between severity of illness and the degree of immune dysfunction resulting from sleep deprivation remains to be established. Early studies of healthy men demonstrated that sleep deprivation and disruption altered the immunological functions of peripheral blood lymphocytes, polymorphonucleocytes,

and natural killer cells in vitro. Later studies have shown that sleep deprivation impairs critical immune responses such as the production of antibodies post-immunization [8].

It is likely that disruption of baseline circadian rhythms, caused by sleep deprivation, induces changes in cortisol and other hormones. Growth hormone secretion is increased during sleep and growth hormone-releasing hormone has been found to potentiate sleep in sleep-deprived subjects. Reduced growth hormone has been associated with increased mortality in critically ill patients; we hypothesize that this may be a biomarker of sleep deprivation in these patients. Long-term complications of prolonged critical illness, which include continued sleep disruption, are being more readily recognized. Loss of sleep in the critical care setting has been associated with a decrease in subjective quality of life measures [9].

Because essential homeostatic functions occur during sleep, it seems logical that sleep disruption and/or deprivation occurring in critically ill patients will impair their ability to recover. From the end of the bed it is not possible to distinguish between a patient that is "asleep" versus a patient that is chemically immobilized with a sedative; evidence is emerging that there are important differences between sleep and sedation. Next we discuss the difficulties in identifying sleep in critically ill patients before reviewing the neurobiology of sedation and sleep, highlighting some crucial differences and their clinical significance.

Identifying sleep in critically ill patients

The issue of disturbance of the sleep pattern in ICU patients has recently received increased research interest, and is the subject of some excellent reviews [10]. However evaluation of insomnia in the ICU is beset with problems. Few ICU patients show the classical sleep architecture [11]. Clinical assessment of sleep by both the carer and the patient is inaccurate. Actigraphy is a simple and robust method of assessing sleep in the normal population, but has also been shown to overestimate the amount of sleep – because ICU patients tend not to move much even when they are awake. Of the processed EEG methods, only the bispectral index (BIS) has been investigated as a relatively clinically robust way of assessing sleep in the ICU; but the results are equivocal. Although full polysomnography is considered the gold standard in sleep assessment, it is unclear if the traditional formulaic sleep staging system, that is used in healthy subjects, has any functional validity in the extreme disturbances of physiology that occur in ICU patients. The causes of the insomnia are likewise poorly understood. Traditionally ICU patients' poor sleep is attributed to the obvious ICU environmental disturbances; however quantitative studies of arousals suggest that the noisy, painful environment only explains less than 30% of the wakefulness. It is likely that the influences of pathological and pharmacological disruption of normal neurophysiology are very important factors. In particular, ICU patients often have extreme systemic and central nervous system aminergic activation – both as the result of their critical illness and also through opioid and benzodiazepine withdrawal. The usual ICU sedative regimens tend to rely on the administration of GABAergic drugs. These drugs are a potent cause of delirium, likely resulting from suppression of a range of neurotransmitters but not noradrenaline. As we will review next, it would be rational to include alpha-2 agonists as part of the ICU sedation regimen, to reduce the aminergic activation and potentiate a more natural sleep state. There are data indicating the use of alpha-2 agonists results in less delirium and improved patient survival – possibly through reduced sleep disruption and thereby preservation of both cognitive and immune function [12].

Overlapping neural mechanisms of sleep and sedation/anesthesia

Sleeps results from a shift in the balance between the ascending reticular arousal and sleep promoting systems. These circuits are probably arranged in a manner analogous to a flip-flop or bi-stable switch of mutual inhibition to provide stability – so that once in a particular state (awake or asleep), each side of the switch inhibits the activity of the other side (i.e., the wake cells inhibit the sleep cells and vice versa). This arrangement ensures that the person does not frequently transition between states of sleep and wakefulness.

A pivotal role for inhibitory hypothalamic nuclei, the venterolateral preoptic (VLPO) and median preoptic nucleus have been demonstrated in numerous studies of sleep [13]. During sleep these inhibitory nuclei are active (i.e., they are inactive in the awake state; Figure 9.1a) releasing inhibitory neurotransmitters to suppress excitatory nuclei (that release arousal promoting, amine-based neurotransmitters). The majority of the sleep-active neurons of the median preoptic nucleus release GABA into the arousal promoting nuclei of the lateral hypothalamus including the orexinergic perifornical nucleus (PeF). The VLPO contains both inhibitory γ-aminobutyric acid type (GABAergic) and galanin type neurons. When activated, during sleep, the VLPO inhibits the histaminergic tuberomamillary nucleus (TMN), the orexinergic perifornical nucleus (PeF), and the noradrenergic locus coeruleus (LC), reducing the excitatory drive produced by histamine, orexin, and noradrenergic neurotransmission [13]. Conversely, during wakefulness the VLPO is itself inhibited by excitatory activity in the TMN and LC. Excitatory orexinergic neurons act to stabilize this sleep–wake switch, as they do not innervate the VLPO and thus reinforce activity in arousal systems when activated.

Another bi-stable switch that is proposed to control state transitions between NREM and REM sleep is located in the mesopontine tegmentum. The REM-off neurons (that are activated by orexin neurons) are GABAergic and the REM-on neurons include both GABAergic and excitatory glutamate type (glutamatergic) neurons. The GABAergic connections inhibit REM-off neurons when activated and the glutamatergic neurons project upward to the cortex to produce the active EEG, and project distally to produce atonia. It is important to note that reduced aminergic transmission is present during both NREM and REM sleep, the activated EEG evident during REM sleep being driven by active cholinergic neurotransmission.

Sedatives and anesthetics target the sleep pathway to produce some of their sedative-hypnotic effects [14,15]. The majority of sedatives, such as the

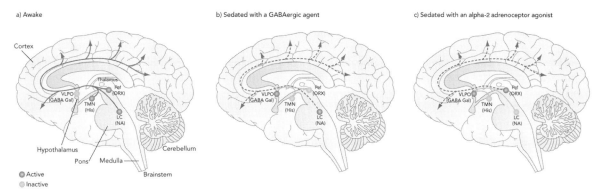

Figure 9.1 Brainstem and hypothalamic nuclei mediate the hypnotic effects of GABAergic anesthetics but do not affect noradrenergic signaling. Active nuclei are depicted in red and inactive nuclei are depicted in blue. (a) In the awake state, certain "awake-active" neural nuclei, including the noradrenergic (NA) locus coeruleus (LC), the orexinergic (ORX) perifornical nucleus (Pef) and the histaminergic (His) tuberomamillary nucleus (TMN) provide excitatory input to the corticothalamic network. When awake a "sleep-active" nucleus, the venterolateral preoptic nucleus (VLPO) is silent. During sleep the VLPO is active and the LC, Pef, and TMN are inactive. (b) During GABAergic hypnosis, potentiated inhibitory actions of the VLPO reduce neural activity in both the Pef and TMN but allow activity to proceed unimpeded in the LC (resulting in intact noradrenergic signaling; active signaling shown with a dotted red line). Reproduced with permission from *Intensetimes*. This figure is presented in color in the color plate section.

benzodiazepines and propofol, act by activating GABA$_A$ receptors [15]. GABAergic anesthetics increase activity in the VLPO (though to a lesser degree than in NREM sleep [16]) and inhibit activity in critical arousal-promoting nuclei such as the histaminergic TMN [14,17] and the orexinergic PeF [18] similar to sleep (Figure 9.1b). Unlike natural sleep, however, they exert little effect on noradrenergic activity in the LC (Figure 9.1b) [14,19]. Sedatives also act in a less discrete fashion (than sleep), targeting the cortex at lower doses, and at higher doses targeting the spinal cord to inhibit motor reflexes.

In contrast, alpha-2 agonists reduce noradrenergic activity in the LC and thus activate the VLPO, so their mechanism of action overlaps more closely with sleep (Figure 9.1c). However alpha-2 agonists do not blunt orexinergic signaling – this may explain the relative rousability of patients from dexmedetomidine sedation [3]. In turn this may allow better neurological examination of the patient and weaning from mechanical ventilation.

In addition to disrupted sleep architecture and quality, critically ill patients also show profound disruption of circadian rhythm correlating with perturbed melatonin secretion. Melatonin is released by the pineal gland and helps synchronize sleep–wake cycles. Reduced melatonin levels have been associated with altered sleep–wake patterns in the ICU, leading to interest in exogenous melatonin as an adjunct to improve sleep in critically ill patients.

Overlapping neuroimaging and electroencephalographic signatures of sleep and sedative-hypnosis

Many of the restorative properties of sleep occur during the slow wave activity phase of NREM sleep; here delta waves predominate. In lighter stages of sleep, waxing and waning alpha frequency oscillations (so-called "sleep spindles" characteristic of stage II NREM sleep) occur as the thalamus becomes hyperpolarized and enters a bursting mode. In contrast, the EEG during REM sleep shows asynchronous high frequency activity and hippocampal theta rhythm (Table 9.1).

The EEG patterns under sedative-hypnosis are typically poorly defined versions of the patterns seen during NREM sleep (e.g., spindles are typically slower). While GABAergic drugs may induce sleep-like patterns of activity (likely via modulating hypothalamic activity), they also distort the EEG by direct effects on corticothalamic networks. Notably, alpha-2 agonists produce a state that shares remarkable similarities with NREM sleep: showing both spindles and delta waves. Spindles are a late phenomenon during GABAergic sedation as the thalamus is only deactivated at higher drug doses. We attribute this to unperturbed noradrenergic signaling from the LC during GABAergic sedation maintaining thalamic activation.

In contrast, alpha-2 agonists suppress noradrenergic signaling and thus reduce thalamic activity earlier during sedation. We have recently proposed that curtailing noradrenergic signaling during sedation is important to reduce connectedness to the environment (akin to lack of awareness of our surroundings in sleep where noradrenergic signaling is also blunted; Table 9.1) [20]. GABAergic drugs primarily suppress consciousness, but not necessarily connectedness, and thus patients are in danger of interacting with their environment at reduced levels of consciousness. This produces an acute confusional state (delirium) similar to sleep inertia. Sleep inertia is rare on arousal from REM sleep as the patients are conscious (dreaming) before they become connected to the external world. However in contrast to abundant evidence for NREM patterns of neural activity, evidence for REM-like activity during sedation is rare. In the critically ill, REM-like rhythms are apparent [11], but the physiological mechanisms underlying these states remain unclear since REM activity is not noted in volunteer studies of sedation. Therefore, it is unknown whether the physiological roles of REM sleep (a high cholinergic and low aminergic state) are fulfilled by sedation (typically a low cholinergic and high aminergic state). The high aminergic state is probably not a conducive neuromodulatory environment for the synaptic downscaling that seems to be an important part of the restorative function of sleep.

An aim of sedation should be to reduce connectedness to the environment, limiting the unpleasant experience of critical illness and the ability to interact with the environment [20]. The latter is important at reduced levels of consciousness where interaction with the environment may lead to the inadvertent removal of lines or endotracheal tubes as occurs in delirium.

Can sedation fulfill the physiological role of sleep?

In humans, EEG data support the concept that alpha-2 agonists produce a state more akin to NREM sleep than GABAergic agents. This is supported by the drugs' mechanisms of action and further indirect evidence such as the release of growth hormone. Growth hormone is released during slow wave sleep and is higher in patients sedated with dexmedetomidine than propofol [21]. Patients sedated with dexmedetomidine are also less susceptible to infections than counterparts on GABAergic medication [12]; it is unclear if this is a direct immune stimulatory effect of dexmedetomidine, or secondary to the induction of a more natural sleep pattern, or due to a deleterious effect of the GABAergic drug [3]. Nonetheless we stress that definitive outcome studies showing patients sedated with dexmedetomidine have "better" sleep than patients on GABAergic drugs are still lacking.

It is unclear whether hypnotic anesthetic drugs can effectively restore sleep deficit. In animal studies propofol was shown to induce recovery of sleep deficit for both NREM and REM sleep [22]. To our knowledge, comparable studies using dexmedetomidine have not been performed. Volatile anesthetics may compensate for NREM sleep deprivation but not REM sleep deprivation [23]. Understanding of how sedatives can compensate for different sleep stages is important. Sedation may need to be correctly titrated to the state that we wish to achieve: if we want to compensate for deep NREM sleep we may need to produce slow wave activity; if we wish to compensate for REM sleep we need to produce "paradoxical" activity. This is clearly logical, though it questions the findings of the original propofol studies, as EEG during the anesthetic phase was not reported and it is unclear whether NREM–REM state cycling occurs during propofol sedation to a similar degree to natural sleep. Nonetheless, we have observed "paradoxical" activity (also termed beta arousals) during anesthesia and sedation in the ICU [11], so further studies aiming to identify REM-like activity are urgently required. It is clear we have many avenues to explore to potentially improve sedation practice.

Recommendations: sedative practice

Sedation and analgesia in the ICU, to provide patient comfort and permit mechanical ventilation, provide a vital function. However, sedation itself can cause iatrogenic harm through effects on hemodynamics, neural connectivity, and immune dysfunction [5,24]. Adequate evidence shows that choice of sedative and sedation holds can improve patient outcomes [12,25,26]. The next step will be to identify which drugs (or combinations of drugs), if any, can mimic the restorative state of sleep and tailor sedative regimens to this goal (see Chapter 29, this volume).

Based on mechanisms of action, neuroimaging, and EEG data, and accumulating clinical outcomes data [12], we recommend sedative practices in which alpha-2 agonists are included where possible – either as replacement, or as an adjunct, to the traditional GABAergic drugs. Indeed the noradrenergic suppression that is achieved with alpha-2 agonists likely has profound effects on the quality of "restorative sedation;" secondary advantages include reduced sympathetic drive and improved immune responses. Nonetheless, further studies are required to confirm these advantages.

Preliminary data also suggests that melatonin may increase sleep duration and depth in the ICU (measured by BIS) in patients with a tracheostomy who are weaning from a ventilator [27]. While this needs to be confirmed in larger studies, further data are also required to clarify whether melatonin could be added during sedation to improve circadian rhythm.

Sleep-disordered breathing in the ICU

Sleep-disordered breathing (SDB) encompasses two main syndromes of relevance in the ICU: obstructive sleep apnea (OSA) and obesity hypoventilation syndrome (OHS) (Pickwickian syndrome). Obstructive sleep apnea is defined as repetitive episodes of partial or complete upper airway obstruction during sleep leading to hypoxemia, hypercarbia, and repeated arousal from sleep due to the need to restore upper airway patency. This leads to daytime hypersomnolence and is implicated in cardio-respiratory dysfunction. The prevalence of overt OSA is estimated at approximately 2% in females and 4% in males. Obesity hypoventilation syndrome is diagnosed by criteria in Table 9.2. It occurs in the morbidly obese (BMI > 30) and unlike eucapnic OSA, is associated with daytime hypoventilation and is more likely to lead to daytime symptoms of dyspnea and severe

sequelae such as cor pulmonale. There are multiple long-term sequelae of SDB (Table 9.3) and several implications for ICU management of postoperative patients, the use of analgesics and sedatives, and airways, respiratory failure, and weaning.

Airway management is higher risk in patients with OSA and obesity. Additionally, prior to intubation, maintaining the airway may be more difficult due to the tendency to upper airway obstruction, and oxygen consumption is higher, causing a reduction in safe apneic time. Obstructive sleep apnea predisposes to esophageal reflux, resulting in an increased aspiration risk. Extubation requires special attention in patients with OSA. Tracheostomy on the ICU is associated with more complications in obese patients. Impairment of conscious level due to underlying disease or sedative drugs will increase the risk of post-extubation airway obstruction. Non-invasive positive pressure ventilation immediately post-extubation has demonstrated a reduction in the incidence of post-extubation respiratory failure in these patients and may be used as an aid to weaning.

Undiagnosed SDB may present as acute respiratory failure. Prompt diagnosis and appropriate initiation of continuous positive airway pressure (CPAP) may prevent the need for invasive ventilation in this subgroup of patients. Sleep-disordered breathing may also co-exist with diseases such as COPD, exacerbating the existing ventilatory problems. If this remains undiagnosed on the ICU, it may lead to difficulties in weaning the patient from invasive ventilation, especially as daytime

Table 9.2 Diagnosis of obesity hypoventilation syndrome.

Required condition	Description
Obesity	Body Mass Index > 30
Chronic hypoventilation	$PaCO_2 > 45$ mmHg and $PaO_2 < 70$ mmHg
Sleep-disordered breathing	Obstructive sleep apnea with apnea–hypopnea index (AHI) > 5 events/hour Non-obstructive sleep hypoventilation AHI < 5 events/hour
Exclusion of other causes of hypercapnia	

Table 9.3 Long-term sequelae of sleep-disordered breathing.

Organ system	Sequelae
Cardiac	Hypertension Cerebrovascular accidents Ischemic heart disease Right heart failure Atrial flutter/fibrillation
Respiratory	Pulmonary hypertension Cor pulmonale Secondary polycythemia
Neurological	Neurocognitive dysfunction Depression
Metabolic	Diabetes Endothelial dysfunction Dyslipidemia
Various	Road accidents

respiratory function may seem adequate. Once SDB has been diagnosed then appropriate treatment consists of titration of nocturnal positive airway pressure (PAP) to improve the patency of the upper airway. Positive airway pressure significantly reduced apneas and hypopneas, REM duration, arousal indexes, and nocturnal oxygen desaturation. The PAP is usually titrated over one night to reduce the occurrence of hypoxic events. If there is a significant central component to the SDB, such as in OHS, then it may be necessary to institute bi-level PAP, also known as non-invasive ventilation (NIV). There are no recognized guidelines on which to base the selection of the mode of PAP, rather it should be individualized to each patient.

Clearly in these high-risk patients, sedatives must be used judiciously. Alpha-2 agonists and melatonin may have a unique role due to their reduced levels of respiratory depression and the relative rousability they induce. Opioids and GABAergic drugs must be used with caution but should not necessarily be withheld if indicated.

Conclusions

While our understanding of the mechanisms of sleep and sedation expand we will increasingly understand how the two overlap and their important differences. This will drive improvements in patient comfort and outcomes. Both are important aims and both are achievable through continued efforts at the bench and rigorous clinical trials conducted at the bedside.

References

1. Takahashi Y, Kipnis DM, Daughaday WH. Growth hormone secretion during sleep. *J Clin Invest* 1968;**47**(9):2079–90.

2. Tononi G, Cirelli C. Sleep function and synaptic homeostasis. *Sleep Med Rev* 2006;**10**(1):49–62.

3. Sanders RD, Maze M. Contribution of sedative-hypnotic agents to delirium via modulation of the sleep pathway. *Can J Anaesth* 2011;**58**(2):149–56.

4. Weinhouse GL, Schwab RJ, Watson PL, *et al.* Bench-to-bedside review: delirium in ICU patients – importance of sleep deprivation. *Crit Care* 2009;**13**(6):234.

5. Sanders RD. Hypothesis for the pathophysiology of delirium: role of baseline brain network connectivity and changes in inhibitory tone. *Med Hypotheses* 2011;**77**(1):140–3.

6. Helton MC, Gordon SH, Nunnery SL. The correlation between sleep deprivation and the intensive care unit syndrome. *Heart Lung* 1980;**9**(3):464–8.

7. Rechtschaffen A, Bergmann BM, Everson CA, Kushida CA, Gilliland MA. Sleep deprivation in the rat: X. Integration and discussion of the findings. 1989. *Sleep* 2002;**25**(1):68–87.

8. Spiegel K, Sheridan JF, Van Cauter E. Effect of sleep deprivation on response to immunization. *JAMA* 2002;**288**(12):1471–2.

9. Jones C, Griffiths RD, Humphris G. Disturbed memory and amnesia related to intensive care. *Memory* 2000;**8**(2):79–94.

10. Kamdar BB, Needham DM, Collop NA. Sleep deprivation in critical illness: its role in physical and psychological recovery. *J Intensive Care Med* 2011;**27**(2):97–111.

11. Nicholson T, Patel J, Sleigh JW. Sleep patterns in intensive care unit patients: a study using the bispectral index. *Crit Care Resusc* 2001;**3**(2):86–91.

12. Pandharipande PP, Sanders RD, Girard TD, *et al.* Effect of dexmedetomidine versus lorazepam on outcome in patients with sepsis: an a priori-designed analysis of the MENDS randomized controlled trial. *Crit Care* 2010;**14**(2):R38.

13. Saper CB, Scammell TE, Lu J. Hypothalamic regulation of sleep and circadian rhythms. *Nature* 2005;**437**(7063):1257–63.

14. Nelson LE, Guo TZ, Lu J, *et al.* The sedative component of anesthesia is mediated by GABA(A) receptors in an endogenous sleep pathway. *Nat Neurosci* 2002;**5**(10):979–84.

15. Franks NP. General anaesthesia: from molecular targets to neuronal pathways of sleep and arousal. *Nat Rev Neurosci* 2008;**9**(5):370–86.

16. Lu J, Greco MA. Sleep circuitry and the hypnotic mechanism of GABAA drugs. *J Clin Sleep Med* 2006;**2**(2):S19–26.

17. Nelson LE, Lu J, Guo T, *et al.* The alpha2-adrenoceptor agonist dexmedetomidine converges on an endogenous sleep-promoting pathway to exert its sedative effects. *Anesthesiology* 2003;**98**(2):428–36.

18. Zecharia AY, Nelson LE, Gent TC, *et al.* The involvement of hypothalamic sleep pathways in general anesthesia: testing the hypothesis using the GABAA receptor beta3N265M knock-in mouse. *J Neurosci* 2009;**29**(7):2177–87.

19. Lu J, Nelson LE, Franks N, *et al.* Role of endogenous sleep-wake and analgesic systems in anesthesia. *J Comp Neurol* 2008;**508**(4):648–62.

20. Sanders RD, Tononi G, Laureys S, Sleigh JW. Unresponsiveness ≠ Unconsciousness. *Anesthesiology* 2012;**116**(4):946–59.

21. Venn RM, Bryant A, Hall GM, Grounds RM. Effects of dexmedetomidine on adrenocortical function, and the cardiovascular, endocrine and inflammatory responses in post-operative patients needing sedation in the intensive care unit. *Br J Anaesth* 2001;**86**(5):650–6.

22. Tung A, Bergmann BM, Herrera S, Cao D, Mendelson WB. Recovery from sleep deprivation occurs during propofol anesthesia. *Anesthesiology* 2004;**100**(6):1419–26.

23. Pal D, Lipinski WJ, Walker AJ, Turner AM, Mashour GA. State-specific effects of sevoflurane anesthesia on sleep homeostasis: selective recovery of slow wave but not rapid eye movement sleep. *Anesthesiology* 2011;**114**(2):302–10.

24. Sanders RD, Hussell T, Maze M. Sedation and immunomodulation. *Crit Care Clin* 2009;**25**(3):551–70.

25. Girard TD, Kress JP, Fuchs BD, *et al.* Efficacy and safety of a paired sedation and ventilator weaning protocol for mechanically ventilated patients in intensive care (Awakening and Breathing Controlled trial): a randomised controlled trial. *Lancet* 2008;**371**(9607):126–34.

26. Pandharipande PP, Pun BT, Herr DL, *et al.* Effect of sedation with dexmedetomidine vs lorazepam on acute brain dysfunction in mechanically ventilated patients: the MENDS randomized controlled trial. *JAMA* 2007;**298**(22):2644–53.

27. Bourne RS, Mills GH, Minelli C. Melatonin therapy to improve nocturnal sleep in critically ill patients: encouraging results from a small randomised controlled trial. *Critical Care* 2008;**12**(2):R52.

Chapter 10

Neural basis of fear and anxiety

Odile Viltart and Christel C. Vanbesien

SUMMARY

Fear and acute stress induce a plasma release of catecholamines and corticosteroids, respectively through the sequential activation of the sympathetic nervous system (SNS) and the hypothalamic-pituitary-adrenal (HPA) axis. These hormones act both at central and peripheral levels to adapt the organism to external and/or internal challenges. They also act upon the immune system to promote an efficient and adapted array of responses. These activations of the SNS and HPA axis prepare the organisms to deal with a threat. Additionally, by mounting inflammatory and analgesic responses they adjust internal parameters to deal with potential subsequent infections and resulting pain, and to appropriately remove invading pathogens. However, when the situation is not resolved despite such adjustments of internal parameters, the stress can become chronic and might then generate stress-induced disorders ranging from anxiety to major depression. In such situations, important alterations of immune and stress responses are observed. Indeed, clinical depression is characterized by a chronic activation of the SNS and the HPA axis, which is paralleled by a state of chronic low-grade inflammation concomitantly maintaining the depressive state. In fact, recent data support the hypothesis according to which pro-inflammatory cytokines promote depressive symptoms via an inappropriate activation of the kynurenine pathway, thus maintaining individuals in a vicious circle of inflammation/depression. Through the examination of neural bases of fear and anxiety and their impact on the immune reactivity, this chapter attempts to understand the higher mortality risk of depressive patients hospitalized for sepsis/septic shock in the intensive care unit (ICU) as compared with patients without psychiatric comorbidity.

Introduction

The survival of living organisms has always depended on their ability to cope with environmental vicissitudes. In this view, evolution has selected an array of defense mechanisms including fear and stress reactivity aimed at enabling the individual to face the many challenges of daily life and to promote its survival. Fear is an emotion usually described as an adaptive state of apprehension that rapidly begins and quickly dissipates once the threat is removed, commonly named phasic fear. On the contrary, anxiety appears as a sustained fear elicited by threats whose causes cannot be determined. Both mechanisms are known to activate stress responses and mobilize underlying neuroendocrine axes. Indeed, the survival of an individual is conditioned by a well-balanced response to internal and environmental pressures, whether physical, physiological, or psychological. As initially suggested by Claude Bernard, the organism has to mobilize its energy to maintain an adequate internal integrity to face various stressors. The physiologist Hans Selye defined the physiological responses to stressors and adapted the word *stress* from physics and engineering to its current use in the medical vocabulary; he was the first to use the terms *stress* and *stress response* in this context [1]. The response to stressors, whatever their nature, consists of a process defined by Selye as the general adaptation syndrome, which is composed of three phases: alarm, adaptation, and exhaustion. The organism has to *fight* or *flight* to survive or it may eventually *freeze* as well, which reflects the inhibition of action described by Laborit [2]. The physiological adaptations to overcome the stressful situation mainly result in higher blood pressure, faster cardiac rhythm, suppression of digestive and sexual processes, as well as re-distribution of blood to muscles (Figure 10.1). All these changes enable the organism to cope with the

Brain Disorders in Critical Illness, ed. Robert D. Stevens, Tarek Sharshar, and E. Wesley Ely. Published by Cambridge University Press. © Cambridge University Press 2013.

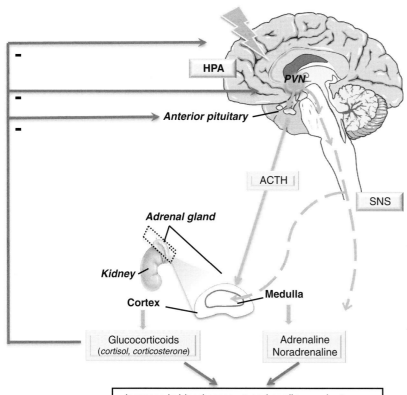

Figure 10.1 Functional anatomy of the hypothalamic-pituitary-adrenal axis (HPA) and sympathetic nervous system (SNS). Stressful situations activate various brain structures which results in the stimulation of the hypothalamic paraventricular nucleus (PVN). PVN neurons release corticotropin-releasing hormone (CRH) that induce the secretion of the adrenocorticotropin hormone (ACTH) from the anterior pituitary. In turn, ACTH acts on the adrenal cortex and triggers the release of glucocorticoids. These steroid hormones target various organs to mobilize energy and control the brain via a negative feedback. In parallel, sympathetic brain areas located in hypothalamic PVN and brainstem nuclei (including nucleus tractus solitarius) control the release of catecholamines from chromaffin cells of the adrenal medulla via the activation of the SNS. Adrenaline and noradrenaline target various organs to induce an adapted physiological response to acute stress. Adapted from Viltart and Vanbesien-Mailliot [57].

potential danger and provide enough energy to survive. Overall, the response to stressors might result either in a fast and reversible response essential for survival, or in maladaptation due to the establishment, after a long-lasting and/or very intense stress, of an inappropriate biological balance detrimental for the organism. Such stressors can weaken the organism and alter its resistance to infections and thus to systemic inflammation and/or to development of mood disorders due to its ineffectiveness to cope with the stressful event.

The systemic inflammatory response syndrome (SIRS) has been described by the American College of Chest Physicians and the Society of Critical Care Medicine as the host response to a critical illness of infectious or non-infectious origins, such as burns, trauma, or pancreatitis [3]. Sepsis, severe sepsis, septic shock, and refractory septic shock are the major clinical outcomes of this syndrome. In SIRS, the production of stress hormones during the inflammatory reaction when the organism is invaded by pathogens is highly similar to the stress response. Both responses are closely related and have been preserved among species [4,5]. Therefore, the SIRS can be considered as an inescapable stress leading to chronic alterations of the stress response which might ultimately lead to mood disorders. In fact, comorbidity with psychiatric conditions such as depression, anxiety, or posttraumatic stress disorders is commonly observed among patients admitted into the ICU (see Chapter 3, this volume) [6–9]. The impact of pre-existing comorbid conditions on hospital outcomes is however not clear. The main source of discrepancy between clinical studies is the variation in the methods used to collect data on comorbid psychiatric conditions [8]. A better understanding of the impact of such comorbidity before an ICU admission on the response to inflammation might be of importance to better adjust care procedures (sedative/analgesic administration, wakefulness, treatment of organ dysfunction) and to decrease the risk of mortality for the patients.

Although the link between physiological stress response, SIRS, and psychiatric diseases is obvious, the interaction between stress hormones and the response to inflammation in the case of sepsis is currently not well understood. The objective of this chapter is to analyze the neuronal bases of fear and anxiety and their link with psychiatric disorders, to assess the effects of existing psychiatric conditions before ICU admissions on the outcomes of patients, with a particular focus on the impact of alterations in stress responses on immune reactivity. For this purpose, we will review data from both human and animal studies to outline potential underlying mechanisms that could lead to improved therapeutic approaches.

Neural basis of stress reactivity

The word stress usually has a negative connotation. However, it is a familiar and ubiquitous aspect of life, being a stimulant for some people and enhancing natural fundamental survival mechanisms, but a burden for many others. These different perceptions reflect various coping abilities between individuals and depend on the duration of stress. Whether acute or repetitive and chronic, stress begins with an external (environmental) or internal (psychological or physiological) challenge perceived by the organism as a stimulus or a disturbance [10–12] that threatens the homeostasis. The stress response is initiated by a cerebral cortical integration of the stimulus via the activation of sensory systems or with the recall of a previous stressful experience (see below, the role of stress hormones in memory; Figures 10.1 and 10.2). In the case of a psychological stress, impulses arising from high cortical centers are relayed through various limbic structures, such as the hippocampus, the amygdala, and the medial prefrontal cortex, directly or indirectly resulting in the release of neurotransmitters such as glutamate, noradrenaline (NA), serotonin, or acetylcholine.

Whatever the stressful event, it sequentially activates the SNS and the HPA axis resulting in adapted physiological changes enabling the organism to deal with the threat (Figures 10.1 and 10.2) [13,14]. In fact, an organism confronted with a dangerous situation potentially menacing its integrity first elicits an immediate and short-lasting response, measured in seconds.

This *emergency reaction* aims at initiating adequate coping responses (fight, flight, or immobility) and involves the SNS with a plasma release of NA and adrenaline (A) from the varicose sympathetic nerve terminals and the adrenal medulla [1]. In fact, brainstem and hypothalamic nuclei control sympathetic preganglionic neurons located in thoracolumbar spinal segments whose efferent fibres innervate paravertebral ganglia or chromaffin cells of the adrenal medulla [15]. From these ganglia, postganglionic sympathetic fibers innervate different organs, such as the heart, lungs, intestines, blood vessels, sweat glands, and lymphoid organs. Importantly, the activation of the SNS wanes quickly, owing to a reflex parasympathetic activation that results in short-lived responses. When the potential threat lasts longer, this initial emergency reaction is followed by a complex reaction to stress triggered by the HPA axis called the *alarm response* (Figure 10.2) [1]. The mobilization of the HPA axis starts with the activation of the hypothalamic paraventricular nucleus, leading to the secretion of the corticotroph secretagogues, namely corticotropin-releasing hormone (CRH) and arginine vasopressin (AVP), that rapidly respond to the stressor. Both CRH and AVP are released from the hypothalamic median eminence into the portal venous system reaching the corticotroph cells of the anterior pituitary to stimulate the production of pro-opiomelanocortin, a precursor polypeptide which is subsequently cleaved into adrenocorticotropic hormone (ACTH), beta-endorphin, and alphamelanocyte stimulating hormone. Arginine vasopressin acts synergistically with CRH upon ACTH release into the peripheral blood. Adrenocorticotropic hormone then targets the adrenal cortex to trigger the release of glucocorticoid (GC) hormones, namely cortisol in humans and corticosterone in the rat. As a result, a peak in plasma GC levels occurs within 10 minutes after the initiation of the stress reaction. In addition to its action on peripheral targets enabling the organism to mobilize enough energy to respond to the stress challenge, GC modulate the HPA axis and related brain structures via a negative feedback loop involving mineralocorticoid and glucocorticoid receptors. Corticotropin-releasing hormone is also expressed in the amygdala and hippocampus [16,17]. In these neuronal populations, it enhances memory consolidation and improves memory through long-term potentiation during acute and moderate stress [18,19], thus participating in a

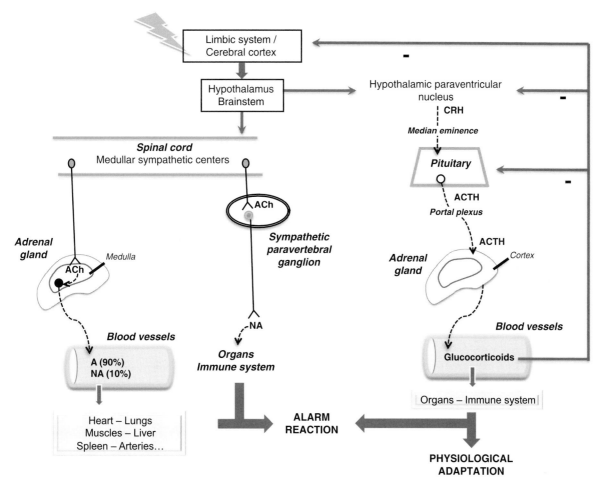

Figure 10.2 Schematic representation of the cross-talk between the hypothalamic-pituitary-adrenal axis (HPA) and the sympathetic nervous system (SNS) in an adapted stress response. A potential stressor is first perceived by the organism through various sensory modalities, which will inform superior integrative centers of the potential danger. A rapid conscious analysis of the potential threat involving the cerebral cortex and limbic structures such as the hippocampus will determine the reality of the danger. In such a case, the mobilization of the HPA axis through the hypothalamic paraventricular nucleus ultimately leads to the secretion of glucocorticoids by the adrenal cortex as detailed in Figure 10.1. Meanwhile, brainstem structures are also activated by limbic and cerebral afferent inputs. Such structures are thus able to mobilize medullar sympathetic centers from which efferent cholinergic outputs will target not only the adrenal medulla but also sympathetic paravertebral ganglions. The medullar sympathetic signals will induce the release of adrenaline (A) and noradrenaline (NA) in the bloodstream, whereas the activation of sympathetic paravertebral efferent noradrenergic fibers will directly act upon several organs and the immune system. The adrenergic mediators released in the blood will in turn act upon adrenergic receptors located on various targets such as the heart, lungs, muscles, liver, spleen, sweat glands, or arteries. Both the HPA activation and the mobilization of the SNS ultimately lead to an appropriate alarm reaction aimed at enabling the organism to face the stressful situation. AC: acetylcholine; ACTH: adrenocorticotropin hormone; CRH: cortico-tropin releasing hormone.

potential further recall of the stressful experience to better adjust the response of the HPA axis in a similar situation. Furthermore, through its action on noradrenergic neurons of the locus coeruleus located in the brainstem (Figures 10.3 and 10.4) [20], CRH also contributes to the release of NA throughout the brain thus centrally enhancing arousal and vigilance. Meanwhile, AVP may also modulate behavioral stress responses, emotional memory, and anxiety [17,21]. Thus, the CRH and locus coeruleus/NA/SNS systems

participate in a positive feedback loop including projections of CRH-secreting neurons from the lateral paraventricular nucleus of the hypothalamus to the hindbrain sympathetic system, and reciprocal projections of catecholaminergic fibers from the locus coeruleus/NA system, via the ascending noradrenergic bundle, into the hypothalamic paraventricular nucleus (Figure 10.4) [10].

Beyond this classical adaptive view of the stress response, one has to keep in mind that different types

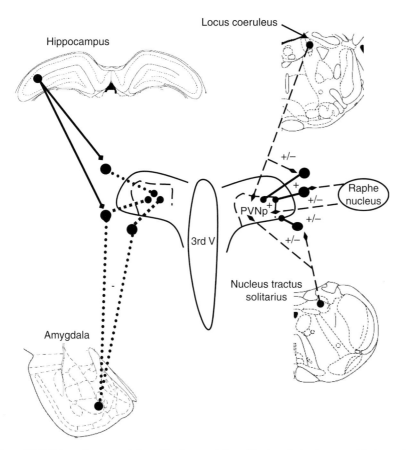

Figure 10.3 Schematic representation of the fine regulation of the hypothalamic paraventricular nucleus (PVN) based on frontal sections of the rat brain [58]. The parvocellular part of the PVN is controlled by a neuronal microenvironment composed of GABAergic and glutamatergic neurons. These interneurons as well as CRH neurons are the targets of regulatory inputs coming from the hippocampus (glutamatergic afferences), the amygdala (GABAergic afferences), the locus coeruleus and the nucleus tractus solitarius (NTS; noradrenergic afferences), as well as the raphe nucleus (serotoninergic afferences). Indeed, the hippocampus exerts a strong tonic regulatory modulation via the activation of mineralocorticoid receptors (MR) that bind plasma glucocorticoids (GC) with a high affinity. In basal condition, these receptors are mainly occupied when plasma levels of GC are low. In stressful situations, the rise in GC affects both hippocampal MR and GC receptors (GR), and thus inhibits the activity of PVN cells. Hippocampal GR are involved in the phasic inhibition of the PVN, thus participating in the feedback control of the HPA axis. The PVN is also targeted by noradrenergic inputs arising from the locus coeruleus and NTS; these noradrenergic fibers directly or indirectly modulate the activity of CRH cells. Among other brain areas known to modulate the PVN in stress situations, the amygdala and the prefrontal cortex project in or around the PVN, thus exerting inhibitory or excitatory stimulations on this structure. 3rd V: third ventricle; CRH: corticotropin-releasing hormone; PVNp: parvocellular part of the hypothalamic paraventricular nucleus. Full line: excitatory pathway; dotted line: inhibitory pathway; dashed line: inhibitory/excitatory pathway. Adapted from Viltart and Vanbesien-Mailliot [57].

of stressors will elicit different responses involving various neuronal populations and stress mediators. For example, physical stressors such as blood loss, trauma, or cold rapidly recruit the brainstem and hypothalamic regions [14], whereas psychological stressors such as social embarrassment, examinations, or deadlines primarily involve stress mediators in brain regions that subserve emotion and fear (the amygdala and the prefrontal cortex), learning and memory (the hippocampus), and decision making (the prefrontal cortex) [22–24].

Stress and fear: link with mood disorders

When a chronic stress occurs, a slightly different hypothalamic response is described with a hyperactivity of the HPA axis. In particular, a marked increase in AVP mRNA is paralleled by a decline in CRH mRNA in the hypothalamic paraventricular nucleus [25]. This results in a long-lasting release of circulating glucocorticoids [25]. As discussed above, the pattern and magnitude of stress responses are influenced by various

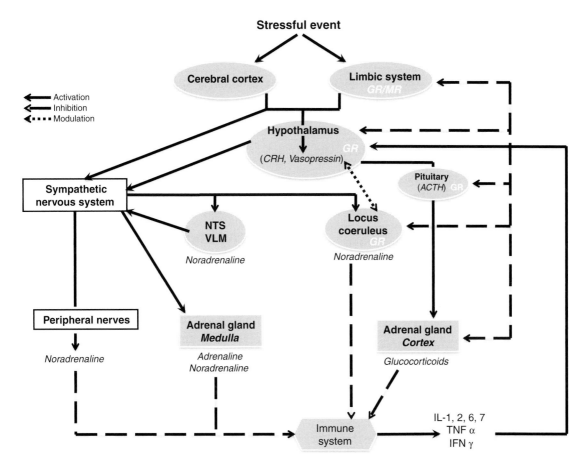

Figure 10.4 Integrated view of the adaptation of an organism to a stressor. The stress reaction mobilizes the autonomous nervous system, the central nervous system, and the immune system. The tight cross-talk between these three partners enables a short-term adaptation as well as a long-term adaptation mobilizing the release of arginine vasopressin (AVP) from the hypothalamic paraventricular nucleus. The regulation and modulation of these intricate systems are mediated via numerous compounds (neurotransmitters, neurohormones, cytokines ...). CRH, corticotropin-releasing hormone; GR, glucocorticoid receptors; IL, interleukin; IFNγ, interferon γ. MR, mineralocorticoid receptors; NTS, nucleus tractus solitarius; TNFα, tumor necrosis factor alpha; VLM, ventrolateral medulla. Adapted from Viltart [59].

factors, including the duration of exposure to the stressor (acute vs. chronic), the type of stressor (physical vs. psychological), the environment of the individual, the age, the gender, or even neonatal influences that can program alterations in the stress reactivity through epigenetic factors [26,27]. Stress hormones (CRH, AVP, GC, NA, A) and other mediators such as dopamine, serotonin, urocortin, orexin, dynorphin, or cytokines not only contribute to daily life challenges but are also associated to major life stressors. This process called *allostasis* [28] maintains stability, or homeostasis, through change. However, when these mediators are not down-regulated after the stress is over, or not adequately up-regulated during stress, or hypersecreted during a chronic stress, this may lead

over time to wear-and-tear, i.e., allostatic load on the body and brain. Thus, the organism switches from a short-term adaptation to a stressor to potential long-term damages that affect the function of the whole body including cardiovascular (atherosclerosis, heart diseases), metabolic (obesity, bone demineralization), and immune (chronic infections) systems, as well as the structure and function of the brain itself (neurodegeneration) (see Chapter 19, this volume). Many of these physiological alterations are characteristic of major depressive illnesses and may also be found in other chronic anxiety disorders (see Chapter 3, this volume). Thus, the development of psychiatric disorders ranging from generalized anxiety to major depression [29] can result from this allostatic load induced by unresolved stressful life events. Stress is now widely acknowledged as a predisposing and precipitating factor in psychiatric illnesses. The different anxiety disorders such as panic disorder, agoraphobia, posttraumatic stress disorder, social phobia, specific phobias, generalized anxiety disorder, or obsessive-compulsive disorder [29], share a common phenotype: excessive, unpredictable, irrational fear and avoidance of anxiety. The neuroanatomical circuits involved in anxiety are closely related to those activated by fear, and implicate the amygdala, the hypothalamus, and the brainstem. Likewise major depression is a common psychiatric disorder with a complex and multifactorial etiology, involving similar brain areas than those activated in chronic stress and anxiety disorders. The underlying mechanisms associated with the pathogenesis of major depression include monoamine deficits, HPA axis dysfunctions, inflammatory, and/or neurodegenerative alterations. The reported hyperactivity of the HPA axis in major depression is associated with an impairment of the GC-mediated negative feedback of this axis, a process commonly described as the GC resistance that it is currently a matter of debate in the literature. Similarly, when the dexamethasone suppression test is performed in patients suffering from major depression, the administration of this GC analog does not modify the elevated levels of circulating cortisol indicating the absence of a negative feedback [30]. An alteration in the function of GC receptors might play a major role in this resistance [31]. Furthermore, imaging studies of brain changes in major depression and anxiety disorders have reported changes in the volume of structures such as the hippocampus, the amygdala, and the prefrontal cortex [32,33]. Such changes must be considered as part of the neurobiological consequences of these illnesses and are likely to contribute to impaired cognitive functions. Indeed, these three brain structures are targets for stress hormones. In particular, the hippocampal formation, which expresses high levels of glucocorticoid and mineralocorticoid receptors, is important for learning and memory and is vulnerable to the effects of stress and trauma. Besides, the amygdala mediates physiological and behavioral responses associated with fear whereas the prefrontal cortex plays an important role in working memory, executive functions, and extinction of learning. It should also be noted that, in animal models of repeated stress, neurons in the hippocampus and prefrontal cortex respond to stress by atrophy and cell death, whereas neurons in the amygdala elicit a growth response [28]. Yet, these effects are not necessarily damaging for the organism and may be curable and reversible with accurate medications and/or environment. However, whether reversible or not, the effects of a chronic stress may predispose to a greater vulnerability to adverse consequences from other insults. This last point is particularly important in the case of sepsis; indeed, individuals with an altered stress response and/or psychiatric diseases may also exhibit a deregulation of stress hormones that might impact their physiological responses to pathogens.

Stress and immune reactivity

The adverse effects of stress on health and immune reactivity have been documented in numerous studies [34,35]. On the one hand, stress is classically known to suppress immune function and increase the susceptibility to infections and cancer. But on the other hand stress is also described to exacerbate asthma, allergy, autoimmune, and inflammatory diseases. In this view, the consequences of stress might as well be beneficial or harmful depending on the type of immune reactions elicited (see Chapter 22, this volume). Indeed, immune responses can be defined according to their end effects on health [36]. *Immunoprotective responses* promote efficient wound healing, eliminate viral infections and cancer, and mediate vaccine-induced immunological memory. The result of this rapid and robust response upon immune cell activation is an efficient clearance of pathogens and a rapid resolution of inflammation. Conversely, *immunopathological responses* correspond to autoimmune diseases or responses against innocuous agents (allergies, asthma). In this case, the inflammation remains chronic and non-resolved. Finally, *immunoregulatory/inhibitory responses* are defined as those that involve immune cells and factors inhibiting the function of other immune cells; this results in failure of proinflammatory, allergic, and autoimmune responses. Stress-induced immunoprotection would thus appear beneficial whereas stress-induced immunosuppression, enhancement of immunopathology, or lasting inflammation is more likely to be harmful in the long term. Thus, the activation of immunoregulation/inhibition processes by a stressor has a dual outcome: it may as well be beneficial in the case of autoimmune and proinflammatory disorders or harmful in the case of infections and cancer [36]. In humans, immune responses to stressors are affected by various factors such as the duration of the stress (short-term/acute vs. long-term/chronic), the age, the gender, differential effects of endogenous cortisol vs. synthetic glucocorticoids used as a therapeutic treatment, or the time of the day. Numerous studies have reported a biphasic effect of an acute stress on blood leukocytes. In particular, Dhabhar and McEwen [37] observed an initial increase in the number of blood leukocytes, occurring within minutes of the beginning of the stress response, that is correlated with the high levels of NA/A released through the activation of the SNS. In the later stages of a stress response, the activation of the HPA axis results in a decreased number of blood leukocytes paralleled by their extravasation from blood vessels to reach peripheral targets such as the skin, lungs, gastro-intestinal and urinary-genital tracts. This extravasation prepares the organism to potential lasting immune challenges that may be imposed by the stressor [37,38]; such a biphasic immune response is considered adaptive. However, a chronic stress is followed by a down-regulation of various components of the immune system and results in decreased B-cells, T-cells, and large granular lymphocytes, as well as reduced natural killer cell activity and proliferative responses to mitogens. Likewise, such a chronic stress alters the balance of Th1/Th2 cytokines with a strong deviation towards the Th2 component. Altogether, these immune alterations may enhance the susceptibility to various infections, ultimately increasing morbidity and mortality of SIRS patients (see Chapters 17 and 22, this volume) [39–41].

As discussed earlier, the HPA activation following acute stress results in the release of GC that can exert anti-inflammatory effects, being immunosuppressive and immunomodulatory [42,43]. However, the sustained release of GC occurring during a long-lasting stress might exert opposite effects depending on their targets. In the periphery, GC inhibit lymphocyte proliferation and dendritic cell maturation; they also induce the apoptosis of basophils, eosinophils, and T-cells [44]. In the central nervous system, GC are not systematically anti-inflammatory and can even be pro-inflammatory, promoting extravasation, migration of immune cells, and inducing the release and accumulation of nitric oxide, prostanoids, and cytokines (TNFα, IL-1β, IL-6, or IFNγ). Thus, GC also have opposite effects in the central nervous system, being either neuroprotective and anti-inflammatory, or neurotoxic and pro-inflammatory. This apparent glucocorticoid paradox depends on: (a) the type of GC

receptor activated, (b) the level of GC (physiological or supraphysiological), (c) the duration of exposure to GC, (d) the type of neural cells implicated (neurons or glial cells), and (e) the brain area targeted. Furthermore, in addition to these effects of GC, catecholamines released by the SNS mediate stress-induced increases in peripheral and central inflammatory cytokines [45]. Such pro-inflammatory actions of catecholamines have notably been demonstrated using pharmacologic agonists or antagonists of alpha- and beta-adrenergic receptors under acute stress, which respectively attenuate or prevent the stress-induced release of IL-1β and IL-6 in the hypothalamus [45].

In view of these data, one could expect that an ongoing depressive syndrome might durably impact the immune reactivity of an individual, thereby programming a deleterious vulnerability in the case of sepsis (Figure 10.5). Thus, a better understanding of the regulation of immune factors by GC and catecholamines is crucial to improve current therapeutic approaches, and ultimately the survival of patients discharged from the ICU with strong stress-related disorders, such as chronic stress or generalized anxiety and depression.

Consequences of depression on immune functions

As mentioned earlier, numerous studies have documented a hyperactivity of the HPA axis in depressed patients [46]. This hyperactivation is initiated by the hypersecretion of CRH and AVP followed by the subsequent increased secretion and reactivity of GC, which leads to an altered feedback inhibition of the HPA axis. In addition, depressed patients also show a decline in both enumerative and functional measures of immunity [47]; in particular, a significant reduction in natural killer effector cells and natural killer cell activity [48], as well as increased levels of circulating pro-inflammatory cytokines, have been reported in these patients [49]. Such a pro-inflammatory state in chronically depressed patients might appear contradictory with their high levels of circulating GC. However, this apparent contradiction is waived in the context of the GC resistance discussed above.

Moreover, such a chronic stressful situation also increases the SNS activity which, combined with the steroid resistance, might lead to the activation of brain microglia, as well as of macrophages and monocytes in

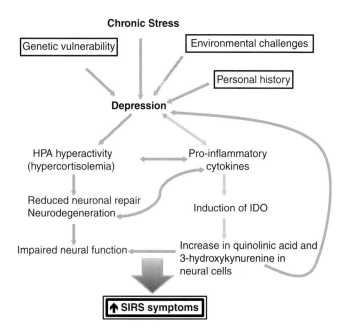

Chronic Stress

Genetic vulnerability

Environmental challenges

Personal history

Depression

HPA hyperactivity
(hypercortisolemia)

Pro-inflammatory
cytokines

Reduced neuronal repair
Neurodegeneration

Induction of IDO

Impaired neural function

Increase in quinolinic acid and
3-hydroxykynurenine in
neural cells

⬆ SIRS symptoms

Figure 10.5 Summary of the cascade of events linking stress, depression, and altered immune reactivity in sepsis. HPA, hypothalamic-pituitary-adrenal axis; IDO, indoleamine 2,3 dioxygenase; SIRS, systemic inflammatory response syndrome.

the periphery, thereby leading to a sustained inflammatory state [50]. Indeed, the Th1 immune pathway involving pro-inflammatory cytokines such as IFNγ is increased while the Th2 pathway involving anti-inflammatory cytokines such as IL-10 is decreased. In this view, depression can strongly impact the outcomes of SIRS survivors through its lasting effects on the immune function. A recent study conducted in an animal model of depression-like symptoms [51] supports the inflammatory/neurodegenerative hypothesis of depression initially proposed by Maes in 1993 [52]. In this experimental analog, external stress-induced depression-like behaviours are associated with increased levels of pro-inflammatory cytokines, cyclooxygenase-2 (an enzyme involved in the synthesis of prostaglandins), expression of Toll-like receptors, and lipid peroxidation; antineurogenic effects, reduced brain-derived neurotrophic factor levels, and apoptosis have also been described in this animal study [51]. Similarly, a treatment with the cytokine IFNα has been shown to induce depressive symptoms in humans [53]. These data underline the importance of the activation of the immune system and the subsequent neurodegeneration in depression. Furthermore, recurrently depressed patients exhibit significant reduction in the size of brain areas like the hippocampus [30]. The role of cytokines and GC in this depression-induced neurodegeneration has been addressed in several studies [30] that linked these

three parameters into the kynurenine hypothesis. In physiological conditions, the essential amino acid tryptophan, the limiting factor for the synthesis of the main regulator of mood, serotonin, can also be degraded by the enzyme indoleamine 2,3 dioxygenase (IDO). This generates kynurenic acid, a neuroprotective metabolite, but also neurotoxic metabolites such as quinolinic acid and 3-hydroxykynurenine. These two last compounds readily cross the blood–brain barrier and act as agonists of NMDA receptors. In pathological conditions, pro-inflammatory cytokines are known to enhance the activation of IDO and promote the synthesis of 3-hydroxykynurenine, thereby switching the kynurenine pathway towards neurotoxicity [30]. The resulting glutamate excitotoxicity is thus contributing to increased apoptosis of astrocytes, oligodendroglia, and neurons. Moreover, the elevation in IDO activity is further depleting brain serotonin contents, thereby sustaining the development of depression-like behavior. Thus, elevated cytokine levels and the GC resistance due to the depression-induced hyperactivation of the HPA axis might generate a vicious circle in which the released cytokines are likely to perpetuate the depressive symptoms.

The importance of depression-induced inflammation is highlighted by the use of antidepressants. In fact, selective serotonin reuptake inhibitors such as fluoxetine or paroxetine, tricyclic antidepressants such as imipramine, reversible inhibitors of monoamine oxidase such as moclobemide, noradrenergic antidepressants such as reboxetin, or even lithium and atypical antidepressants such as tianeptine, have anti-inflammatory effects. All these antidepressants reduce peripheral and central inflammatory pathways. In particular, they decrease pro-inflammatory cytokines such as IL-1β, IL-12, IL-6, TNFα, or IFNγ, and/or increase levels of IL-10, a major anti-inflammatory cytokine [54,55]. In addition, these psychoactive drugs stimulate neuronal differentiation, synaptic plasticity, axonal growth, and regeneration through stimulatory effects on the expression of different neurotrophic factors. They also attenuate apoptotic pathways through the activation of Bcl-2 and Bcl-xl proteins, and the inhibition of caspase-3. Thus, antidepressant treatments might have promising effects in the case of SIRS patients with comorbid depression. They could exert an anti-inflammatory action and may indirectly modulate the central monoamine dysfunction by correcting the changes in the immune and endocrine systems. Their neuroprotective action would also be highly beneficial for SIRS survivors.

Finally, one has to keep in mind that all stressors do not systematically produce identical changes in the immune system. Different types of stress produce different degrees of endocrine and sympathetic activation, and individual coping strategies can modify the impact of stress on these systems [39]. Furthermore, several data from the literature suggest an enhancement of immune competence when improving the coping capabilities of individuals. The implementation of interventional strategies such as hypnosis, relaxation, exercise, classical conditioning, or cognitive behavioral strategies has been shown to reduce stress-induced immunosuppression in individuals [39]. However, more attention has been paid to their outcomes on the immune system than on depressive states of individuals. Future research is thus needed to better understand how variations in affective state might be useful indicators of immunity.

Conclusion: impact of comorbid conditions on the survival of patients with sepsis

Altogether, the data and hypotheses reviewed in this chapter underline the severe impact of chronic stress and stress-related disorders ranging from anxiety to major depression on the immune reactivity. Both clinical and experimental studies indicate that chronic stress

increasing the activity of the HPA axis plays a major role in initiating anxiety and ultimately depression. Indeed, there is an increase in plasma and brain levels of critical molecules involved in the manifestation of the depressive syndrome, such as GC and pro-inflammatory cytokines, paralleling elevated concentrations of the acute phase protein. In particular, a dysfunction in the central regulation of GC, noradrenaline, glutamate, and serotonin signals is clearly documented. Moreover, the stress-induced hypersecretion of cytokines may reinforce depressive symptoms. All these central and peripheral changes add to the complexity of these biological responses, which is encompassed in the concept of relative adrenal insufficiency described in sepsis and may account not only for the difficulty of the clinical diagnosis but also for the conflicting results of the corticosteroid replacement therapy in severe sepsis/septic shock (see Chapters 19 and 20, this volume). Currently, treatments used in ICU for SIRS patients intend to modify the activity of the SNS (modulation of the action of catecholamines, pharmacological stimulation of vagus nerve) or the HPA axis (corticosteroid therapy). Such therapeutic strategies have however to be implemented keeping in mind that the emotional state in which patients reach the ICU can negatively impact the efficacy of the treatment. Biomarkers might help physicians to better evaluate the emotional state of their patients. In this view, copeptine has been recently proposed as a prognostic marker in the acute phase of illnesses. This peptide, derived from the pre-provasopressin, is released in an equimolar ratio to AVP and thus reflects the production of AVP and cortisol. The prognostic accuracy of copeptin has been analyzed in various diseases such as sepsis, pneumonia, lower respiratory tract infections, or stroke and was found to accurately reflect disease severity and to discriminate patients with adverse outcomes from those with better chances of survival [56]. An accurate prognostic assessment has the potential to enable clinicians to select more appropriate therapies and help them successfully plan and monitor the rehabilitation, thus optimizing the management of individual patients and the allocation of limited healthcare resources.

References

1. Selye H. A syndrome produced by diverse nocuous agents. *Nature* 1936;**138**:32.

2. Laborit H. [The inhibition of action. Interdisciplinary approach of its mechanisms and physiopathology]. *Ann Med Psychol (Paris)* 1988;**146**(6):503–22.

3. Bone RC, Balk RA, Cerra FB, *et al.* Definitions for sepsis and organ failure and guidelines for the use of innovative therapies in sepsis. The ACCP/SCCM Consensus Conference Committee. American College of Chest Physicians/Society of Critical Care Medicine. *Chest* 1992;**101**(6):1644–55.

4. Black PH. Stress and the inflammatory response: a review of neurogenic inflammation. *Brain Behav Immun* 2002;**16**(6):622–53.

5. Black PH. The inflammatory consequences of psychologic stress: relationship to insulin resistance, obesity, atherosclerosis and diabetes mellitus, type II. *Med Hypotheses* 2006;**67**(4):879–91.

6. Abrams TE, Vaughan-Sarrazin M, Rosenthal GE. Variations in the associations between psychiatric comorbidity and hospital mortality according to the method of identifying psychiatric diagnoses. *J Gen Intern Med* 2008;**23**(3):317–22.

7. Abrams TE, Vaughan-Sarrazin M, Rosenthal GE. Preexisting comorbid psychiatric conditions and mortality in nonsurgical intensive care patients. *Am J Crit Care* 2010;**19**(3):241–9.

8. Abrams TE, Vaughan-Sarrazin M, Rosenthal GE. Influence of psychiatric comorbidity on surgical mortality. *Arch Surg* 2010;**145**(10):947–53.

9. Davydow DS, Richardson LP, Zatzick DF, Katon WJ. Psychiatric morbidity in pediatric critical illness survivors: a comprehensive review of the literature. *Arch Pediatr Adolesc Med* 2010;**164**(4):377–85.

10. Chrousos GP, Gold PW. The concepts of stress and stress system disorders. Overview of physical and behavioral homeostasis. *JAMA* 1992;**267**: 1244–52.

11. Goldstein DS, McEwen B. Allostasis, homeostats, and the nature of stress. *Stress* 2002;**5**:55–8.

12. McEwen BS. *The End of Stress as We Know It.* Washington, DC: Dana Press; 2002.

13. Maier SF, Watkins LR. Cytokines for psychologists: implications for bidirectional immune-to-brain communication for understanding behavior, mood, and cognition. *Psychol Rev* 1998;**105**:83–107.

14. Ulrich-Lai YM, Herman JP. Neural regulation of endocrine and autonomic stress responses. *Nat Rev Neurosci* 2009;**10**(6):397–409.

15. Elenkov IJ, Wilder RL, Chrousos GP, Vizi ES. The sympathetic nerve – an integrative interface between two supersystems: the brain and the immune system. *Pharmacol Rev* 2000;**52**(4):595–638.

16. Swanson LW, Sawchenko PE, Rivier J, Vale WW. Organization of ovine corticotropin-releasing factor immunoreactive cells and fibers in the rat brain: an immunohistochemical study. *Neuroendocrinology* 1983;**36**:165–86.

17. Koob GF. A role for brain stress systems in addiction. *Neuron* 2008;**59**:11–34.

18. Blank T, Nijholt I, Eckart K, Spiess J. Priming of long-term potentiation in mouse hippocampus by corticotropin-releasing factor and acute stress: implications for hippocampus-dependent learning. *J Neurosci* 2002;**22**:3788–94.

19. Roozendaal B, Brunson KL, Holloway BL, McGaugh JL, Baram TZ. Involvement of stress-released corticotropin-releasing hormone in the basolateral amygdala in regulating memory consolidation. *Proc Natl Acad Sci USA* 2002;**99**:13908–13.

20. Reul JM, Labeur MS, Wiegers GJ, Linthorst AC. Altered neuroimmunoendocrine communication during a condition of chronically increased brain corticotropin-releasing hormone drive. *Ann N Y Acad Sci* 1998;**840**:444–55.

21. Joëls M, Baram TZ. The neuro-symphony of stress. *Nat Rev Neurosci* 2009;**10**(6):459–66.

22. De Kloet ER, Joëls M, Holsboer F. Stress and the brain: from adaptation to disease. *Nature Rev Neurosci* 2005;**6**:463–75.

23. McEwen BS. Physiology and neurobiology of stress and adaptation: central role of the brain. *Physiol Rev* 2007;**87**:873–904.

24. McGaugh JL. The amygdala modulates the consolidation of memories of emotionally arousing experiences. *Annu Rev Neurosci* 2004;**27**:1–28.

25. Lightman SL. The neuroendocrinology of stress: a never ending story. *J Neuroendocrinol* 2008;**20** (6):880–4.

26. Weaver IC, Cervoni N, Champagne FA, *et al.* Epigenetic programming by maternal behavior. *Nat Neurosci* 2004;**7**(8):847–54.

27. Champagne FA, Meaney MJ. Transgenerational effects of social environment on variations in maternal care and behavioral response to novelty. *Behav Neurosci* 2007;**121**(6):1353–63.

28. McEwen BS. Protection and damage from acute and chronic stress: allostasis and allostatic overload and relevance to the pathophysiology of psychiatric disorders. *Ann N Y Acad Sci* 2004;**1032**:1–7.

29. American Psychiatric Association. *Diagnostic and Statistical Manual of Mental Disorders, Fourth edition, Text Revision* (DSM–IV–TR). Washington, DC: American Psychiatric Association; 2000.

30. Zunszain PA, Anacker C, Cattaneo A, Carvalho LA, Pariante CM. Glucocorticoids, cytokines and brain abnormalities in depression. *Prog Neuropsychopharmacol Biol Psychiatry* 2011;**35** (3):722–9.

31. Carvalho LA, Pariante CM. In vitro modulation of the glucocorticoid receptor by antidepressants. *Stress* 2008;**11**(6):411–24.

32. Sexton CE, Mackay CE, Ebmeier KP. A systematic review and meta-analysis of magnetic resonance imaging studies in late-life depression. *Am J Geriatr Psychiatry* 2012 Feb 29. [Epub ahead of print].

33. Zeng LL, Shen H, Liu L, *et al.* Identifying major depression using whole-brain functional connectivity: a multivariate pattern analysis. *Brain* 2012; **135**(5):1498–507.

34. McEwen BS. Protective and damaging effects of stress mediators: allostasis and allostatic load. *N Engl J Med* 1998;**338**:171–9.

35. Ader R. *Psychoneuroimmunology*. 4th edn. San Diego, CA: Academic Press; 2006.

36. Dhabhar FS. Enhancing versus suppressive effects of stress on immune function: implications for immunoprotection and immunopathology. *Neuroimmunomodulation* 2009;**16**(5):300–17.

37. Dhabhar FS, McEwen BS. Bidirectional effects of stress and glucocorticoid hormones on immune function: possible explanations for paradoxal observations. In Ader R, Felten SF, Cohen N, editors. *Psychoneuroimmunology*. 3rd edn. San Francisco, CA: Academic Press; 2001.

38. Dhabhar FS, McEwen BS. Stress-induced enhancement of antigen-specific cell-mediated immunity. *J Immunol* 1996;**156**(7):2608–15.

39. Olff M. Stress, depression and immunity: the role of defense and coping styles. *Psychiatry Res* 1999;**85**(1):7–15.

40. Marshall GD. Neuroendocrine mechanisms of immune dysregulation: applications to allergy and asthma. *Ann Allergy Asthma Immunol* 2004;**93**(2 Suppl 1):S11–17.

41. Mitsonis CI, Potagas C, Zervas I, Sfagos K. The effects of stressful life events on the course of multiple sclerosis: a review. *Int J Neurosci* 2009;**119**:315–35.

42. Li M, Wang Y, Guo R, Bai Y, Yu Z. Glucocorticoids impair microglia ability to induce T cell proliferation and Th1 polarization. *Immunol Lett* 2007;**109**(2):129–37.

43. Nair A, Hunzeker J, Bonneau RH. Modulation of microglia and CD8(+) T cell activation during the development of stress-induced herpes simplex virus type-1 encephalitis. *Brain Behav Immun* 2007;**21**(6):791–806.

44. Sorrells SF, Sapolsky RM. An inflammatory review of glucocorticoid actions in the CNS. *Brain Behav Immun* 2007;**21**(3):259–72.

45. García-Bueno B, Caso JR, Leza JC. Stress as a neuroinflammatory condition in brain: damaging and protective mechanisms. *Neurosci Biobehav Rev* 2008; **32**(6):1136–51.

46. Arborelius L, Owens MJ, Plotsky PM, Nemeroff CB. The role of corticotropin-releasing factor in depression and anxiety disorders. *J Endocrinol* 1999;**160**(1): 1–12.

47. Herbert TB, Cohen S. Stress and immunity in humans: a meta-analytic review. *Psychosom Med* 1993;**55**(4):364–79.

48. Evans D, Petitto J, Leserman J, *et al.* Stress, depression and natural killer cells: potential clinical relevance. *Clin Neuropharmacol* 1992;**15** (Suppl 1 Pt A):656A–7A.

49. Raison CL, Capuron L, Miller AH. Cytokines sing the blues: inflammation and the pathogenesis of depression. *Trends Immunol* 2006;**27**(1):24–31.

50. Leonard BE. The concept of depression as a dysfunction of the immune system. *Curr Immunol Rev* 2010;**6**(3):205–12.

51. Kubera M, Obuchowicz E, Goehler L, Brzeszcz J, Maes M. In animal models, psychosocial stress-induced (neuro)inflammation, apoptosis and reduced neurogenesis are associated to the onset of depression. *Prog Neuropsychopharmacol Biol Psychiatry* 2011;**35** (3):744–59.

52. Maes M. A review on the acute phase response in major depression. *Rev Neurosci* 1993;**4**(4):407–16.

53. Capuron L, Miller AH. Cytokines and psychopathology: lessons from interferon-alpha. *Biol Psychiatry* 2004;**56**(11):819–24.

54. Connor TJ, Leonard BE. Depression, stress and immunological activation: the role of cytokines in depressive disorders. *Life Sci* 1998;**62**(7): 583–606.

55. Maes M. Depression is an inflammatory disease, but cell-mediated immune activation is the key component of depression. *Prog Neuropsychopharmacol Biol Psychiatry* 2011;**35**(3):664–75.

56. Katan M, Christ-Crain M. The stress hormone copeptin: a new prognostic biomarker in acute illness. *Swiss Med Wkly* 2010;**140**:w13101.

57. Viltart O, Vanbesien-Mailliot CC. Impact of prenatal stress on neuroendocrine programming. *Scientific World J* 2007;**7**:1493–537.

58. Paxinos G, Watson C. *The Rat Brain in Stereotaxic Coordinates*. Sydney: Academic Press; 1998.

59. Viltart O. *Système nerveux autonome et réponse à l'agression*. In *Actualité en réanimation et urgence*. Paris: Elsevier Masson; 2007:103–31.

Chapter 11

Experimental models of cognitive dysfunction in infection and critical illness

Colm Cunningham

SUMMARY

It is well accepted that critical illness frequently leads to delirium and that sepsis and major trauma have negative long-term consequences for brain function in the affected individual. Despite this, the cognitive sequelae of critical illness have been little studied in animal models. In this chapter we review the literature on cognitive dysfunction in animal models of sepsis. The most commonly used models of sepsis, cecal ligation and puncture (CLP), inoculation with *Escherichia coli*, and injection of the bacterial endotoxin (lipopolysaccharide, LPS) have not been widely used to study sepsis-induced cognitive dysfunction. Cecal ligation and puncture has been shown to induce deficits in inhibitory avoidance at 10 and 30 days post-sepsis but this returned to normal by 60 days. These deficits can be modulated by rivastigmine, epinephrine, MK-801, naloxone, and glucose, but it remains unclear whether the deficits reflect reversible neurochemical alteration or transient damage to the brain. Conversely experiments with LPS have shown neuronal apoptosis and synaptic loss in multiple brain regions, dependent on inducible nitric oxide synthase (iNOS), with impaired spatial working memory remaining at 12 weeks post-sepsis. Combining these data with acute imaging and EEG studies, there is evidence for acutely impaired brain function (EEG, PET) related to tissue perfusion (CBF) in the acute time frame, with inflammation significantly contributing to the neuronal death and denervation occurring during this period and leading to long-term deficits. This is congruent with other approaches suggesting that IL-1β can impair LTP, an electrophysiological correlate of learning, and experiments using both LPS and *E. coli* at lower doses have implicated IL-1β in cognitive impairments in aversively motivated tasks such as contextual fear conditioning. It is important, however, to integrate the influences from multiple factors that may contribute to both long- and short-term cognitive dysfunction during and following sepsis. It is now clear that age and prior cognitive status have a significant influence on whether systemic inflammatory insults will induce cognitive symptoms, and synaptic loss and microglial priming have been implicated in this increased susceptibility. In addition, it seems clear that sedation and anesthesia contribute to cognitive manifestations and ultimately these influences will also be integrated into animal models of critical illness. The pathophysiology of delirium and of post-sepsis cognitive dysfunction remains unclear and the failure of recent clinical trials emphasizes that further detailed, multifactorial, animal model studies are necessary to increase our understanding of the interface between inflammatory activation and neuronal dysfunction and death.

Introduction

Over the last number of years it has become obvious that critical illness frequently leads to delirium and/or long-term cognitive decline [1,2]. Indeed it seems relatively clear that delirium per se, whether experienced in the context of sepsis or major trauma in an otherwise healthy individual or in the context of a milder insult on a background of dementia or aging, has negative long-term consequences for the individual [3]. This has contributed to the growing conceptualization of delirium as a precipitous collapse of brain function that constitutes an emergency situation for the individual. One of the major triggers for episodes of delirium, both in the ICU and in a geriatric setting, is systemic inflammation or infection. Therefore, delirium caused by infection is, in a sense, critical illness irrespective of the severity of the infection that may precipitate it. In this chapter, I will discuss

Brain Disorders in Critical Illness, ed. Robert D. Stevens, Tarek Sharshar, and E. Wesley Ely. Published by Cambridge University Press. © Cambridge University Press 2013.

experimental animal approaches to studying delirium and long-term cognitive impairment in the setting of sepsis and infection. Animal models have provided valuable information on hypotension, hypoperfusion, blood–brain barrier disruption, and other key features that may underpin septic encephalopathy [4], but here we will focus on those studies modeling cognitive dysfunction arising from sepsis. Similarly there is not sufficient space to examine liver failure, malaria, meningitis, and other illnesses that can lead to encephalopathy.

Sepsis

The deleterious consequences of sepsis and, in particular, severe sepsis and septic shock can be broadly attributed to a hyperinflammatory state. Robust inflammatory and adaptive immune responses are required to eliminate an infectious agent that succeeds in escaping its initial site of local infection and becoming systemically disseminated. However in severe sepsis this inflammatory response may become extremely damaging for the individual and may lead to hypotension, organ failure, septic encephalopathy/delirium, and death. Even if patients survive the initial "cytokine storm" of acute sepsis, they frequently become immunosuppressed due to apoptosis of, and impaired chemotaxis for, lymphocytes and leukocytes, leading to further infections and complications. This delicate balance between mounting an immune response of sufficient strength to clear the pathogen and avoiding major bystander damage to the host tissue becomes important for interventions since many molecules may be key both in causing cognitive dysfunction and in coordinating the immune response. For example, IL-1β, tumor necrosis factor alpha (TNFα), and nitric oxide are key molecules in the coordination of the immune response and in elimination of pathogens but can produce a shock-like hypotensive state [5–7]. A number of preclinical studies (though not all) suggested that targeting these molecules could protect against sepsis-induced mortality, particularly in LPS-induced sepsis, but also in many studies using active infection. As a result, a number of clinical studies have targeted these molecules by the administration of the endogenous inhibitor IL-1 receptor antagonist (IL-1ra), monoclonal anti-TNFα antibodies, or soluble receptors or nitric oxide inhibitors. These strategies have shown very limited efficacy in preventing fatal septic shock and significant meta-analysis of immunomodulation in sepsis [8] indicated that inflammation should only

be tempered if it is likely to endanger the individual. Such a strategy may alter the way new therapies are assessed in the future but in the meantime the standard therapy remains antibiotic treatment to target any identified microbial species, fluid resuscitation and vasopressors to reverse hypotension, and removal or drainage of the source of the infection [9].

Sepsis induces CNS pathology and cognitive impairments

Typically, animal models of sepsis-associated cognitive dysfunction have either used relatively low, although still sickness inducing, doses in order to study acute effects of systemic inflammation, or very high doses to mimic severe sepsis in order to examine the long-term pathological and/or cognitive impact of these severe insults, and one probably has to separate these issues since the paradigms required to study them are not necessarily the same. It should be noted that there are ample studies showing that systemic LPS, infection, or indeed individual cytokines can induce brain inflammatory changes. Such studies have not been considered in this review unless combined with cognitive studies. Chapter 18, this volume, discusses some of the best characterized aspects of CNS effects of systemic stimulation.

Cecal ligation and puncture, in which rodents are exposed to polymicrobial sepsis, is one of the most clinically relevant models of sepsis and cognitive function, and has been assessed in rats undergoing this procedure. Animals were first shown to have impaired inhibitory avoidance and decreased open-field habituation at 10 days post-sepsis induction [10]. Although these effects may be difficult to disentangle from persisting sepsis effects on emotional state and locomotor activity in an open field, appropriate controls have generally been performed. The authors subsequently showed that the open-field habituation impairments at 10 days post-sepsis can be prevented by multiple dosing with the cholinesterase inhibitor rivastigmine [11]. However, failure to habituate in an open field does not necessarily represent impaired memory function, and in any case does not persist beyond 10 days in those studies. Conversely, inhibitory avoidance appears to persist at 30 days post-CLP, but not at 60 days [12]. In the step-down inhibitory avoidance task, animals are exposed to a foot shock when stepping onto a wire grid in the training session and, when re-exposed to this context 24 hours later, typically show a much longer latency to step down. Animals 10 days or 30 days after CLP show significantly shorter latencies to step down than sham-operated animals, suggesting a failure to remember the foot shock or the context in which it was experienced. The authors show that learning in this task can be improved using a number of cognitive-enhancing drugs including epinephrine, naloxone, dexamethasone, glucose [13], cannabidiol [14], and MK-801 [15], perhaps related to increased brain-derived neurotrophic factor (BDNF) production. However, most of these treatments also improve learning in sham-operated animals and thus may operate by entirely different mechanisms, perhaps compensating for a memory system that is showing deficits rather than reversing those deficits. Since these animals are not re-tested after drug wash-out there is also no evidence for a stable 'reversal' of sepsis-induced impairment. Given that the authors suggest that the memory impairments are not due to neuronal death it is unfortunate that the authors have made no assessment of pathology in these cognitive studies. Reversible changes in presynaptic terminal density, dendritic branching, or indeed neurotransmitter receptor localization may contribute to the observed deficits, but these avenues have not been investigated and the nature of the deficit remains unclear despite numerous publications with this paradigm. Importantly, the deficits do not reflect long-term cognitive impairment as observed in clinical survivors, since these rodents spontaneously recover by 30 or 60 days, depending on the task assessed, perhaps arguing for disturbed growth factor activity as a key mechanism.

Long-term cognitive decline, associated with neuronal death, has been observed in a series of rat studies. In these studies, LPS (10 mg/kg) has been administered intraperitoneally to induce severe sepsis, as evidenced by mortality of 17–40%. Collectively these studies show that severe LPS-induced sepsis induces significant apoptosis and neuronal loss in multiple regions of the rat brain, and significant glial activation, including iNOS activation [16]. Associated with this, they describe spatial working memory deficits in a radial arm maze at 12 weeks post-sepsis and neuronal loss in the hippocampus and prefrontal cortex, as well as decreased cholinergic enervation of the parietal association and barrel field cortices [17]. They do not observe significant impairments on a passive avoidance task similar to that in which CLP rats showed impairments [10]. While these cognitive tests have been demonstrative of long-term cognitive deficits,

the authors have also shown, at 24 hours post-sepsis induction, markedly decreased cerebral metabolism using microPET imaging of glucose uptake (^{18}FDG) associated with decreased cerebral blood flow and decreased alpha activity in EEG [18]. More recent studies from this group showed that similar challenges in mice, allowing use of transgenic animals, demonstrate a key role for iNOS in both cognitive deficits and changes in both presynaptic and postsynaptic molecules [19]. Collectively these data point towards acutely impaired brain function (EEG, PET) related to tissue perfusion (CBF) in the acute phase, with inflammation significantly contributing to neuronal death, and denervation occurring during this period and leading to long-term deficits as measured, much later, by working memory deficits. This is also consistent with MRI studies of CLP showing vasogenic edema and N-acetylaspartate/choline ratios indicative of neuronal damage [20]. However, the acute cognitive deficits, prevalent *during* sepsis have not been addressed in these studies of severe sepsis. A schematic of a number of these cognitive studies is shown in Figure 11.1.

Studies from other laboratories also suggest that inflammatory mediators produced during the acute phase contribute to cognitive deficits. Activity-dependent, long-term potentiation (LTP) is thought to underlie some forms of learning and memory. Cecal ligation and puncture prevented the induction of LTP in vitro in hippocampal slices taken 24 hours after sepsis induction and IL-1ra could protect against this LTP-induction deficit in CLP-treated animals [21]. IL-1β was significantly elevated and temporally related to septic encephalopathy in sepsis patients and in the same study was shown to increase GABA$_A$ receptor insertion at the cell surface, leading to increased GABAergic tone [22], potentially decreasing synaptic strength and contributing to cognitive deficits. Mice treated with LPS (1 mg/kg) showed impairments in contextual fear-conditioning experiments and these were ameliorated by prior treatment with IL-1ra [23]. In this task animals are exposed to a context, which they explore for some time, and are then exposed to an auditory cue (a tone) and a foot shock and are then returned to their home cage. The consolidation of the memory of the context in which they received the shock is impaired by sepsis, induced by LPS, immediately after exposure to this context, as measured by decreased freezing on subsequent exposure

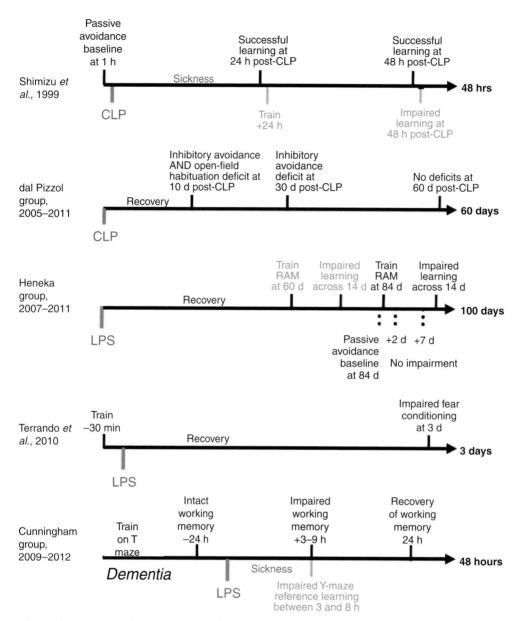

Figure 11.1 A schematic depiction of timelines for animal studies of sepsis-induced cognitive impairment. Each timeline shows the timing of sepsis induction relative to when animals were trained and when they were tested on various cognitive tasks. Where animals were tested while still experiencing sickness, this is indicated by "sickness" on the timeline, while those who have emerged from sickness behavior are labeled "recovery." Each experimental design may encompass several studies by the same research group and the group is shown on the extreme left of the scheme. The final timeline was performed on animals that had existing neurodegenerative disease at the time of LPS challenge. The studies from which these timelines are taken are all identifiable in the reference list [23,25,27,28]. CLP, cecal ligation and puncture; LPS, lipopolysaccharide; RAM, radial arm maze.

to the same context (see Figure 11.1). The authors also report that these deficits are absent in animals lacking the functional IL-1RI, although they do not discuss the disparity between their data, showing inhibition of all LPS-induced responses, and previous data indicating

that the IL-1RI−/− mice show fully robust acute phase and behavioral responses to LPS (http://jaxmice.jax.org/strain/003245.html). It is also our experience of these mice that LPS-induced working memory deficits were identical in wild-type and IL-1RI mice (Skelly and

Cunningham, unpublished observations), albeit in a working memory task and at significantly lower doses of LPS. Although IL-1 is consistently implicated, TNFα remains an important sepsis-induced mediator that has been implicated in encephalopathy [24] but little studied in the context of sepsis-associated cognitive dysfunction.

It is also important to note that the contextual fear-conditioning task cannot inform on long-term cognitive dysfunction/decline. Since animals are exposed to the context and sepsis was then induced a short time afterwards, what these experiments demonstrate is that sepsis prevents the initial consolidation of the memory of the context. Testing days, weeks, or months later should all demonstrate the same thing: that the memory was never consolidated to begin with. Therefore, these studies show that learning is impaired during sepsis and, similar to the CLP studies of the dal Pizzol group, the only deficit shown is on an aversive task. There are a number of caveats that come with contextual fear conditioning that make it difficult to generalize to hippocampal function or indeed memory function (see [25] for review). To the credit of these authors, the test phase was conducted after animals had returned to a state in which they did not manifest sickness behavior, but given the profoundly aversive nature of sepsis itself, recent illness may significantly diminish the nature or degree of the aversion to the context in which the shock was experienced, potentially altering the behavior of the animals in this apparatus. Importantly, while the hippocampus is known to have a role in contextual fear conditioning, the amygdala is also crucial, and thus using this task as the sole means of assessing hippocampal memory function runs the risk of mistaking alterations in amygdala function for a hippocampal deficit. To emphasize this point, investigators using the Morris water maze (MWM) test of hippocampal-dependent visuospatial learning found no effect of CLP on retention of previously acquired learning in this maze [26].

There is limited information from animal studies on the confusional state *during* sepsis. One older study examined passive avoidance 24 and 48 hours after induction of CLP sepsis [27]. Animals that were trained on this task, immediately before sepsis, showed intact memory when tested 24 hours after sepsis induction (Figure 11.1). Conversely, animals that were trained *during* sepsis (i.e. 24 hours post-sepsis induction) did show impairments 24 hours later (48 hours post-sepsis induction). These findings

argue that inflammation, even in profound sepsis, affects consolidation rather than retention of memory and this is consistent with the MWM data mentioned above [26]. Most investigators interested in the acute effects of immune stimulation on learning and memory have used much lower doses of immune stimulators or pathogens. These studies, broadly, report that immune stimulation has negative consequences for learning and memory but these findings must be read with caution. Even at lower doses, the acute sickness-inducing effects of these immune activators have profound effects on mood, motivation, locomotor activity, locomotor speed, interest in food rewards, stress responses, and consequent exploratory patterns in mazes [27]. Therefore, the very activities that one typically uses to assess cognitive function in rodents are profoundly altered in animals during sickness. Therefore, we must be extremely cautious to avoid mistaking emotional and behavioral differences for cognitive impairments. This subject has been reviewed in considerable detail recently [28] and the details will not be revisited here. However, a couple of examples will be examined in order to summarize what one can say with confidence.

Visuospatial learning and memory in the Morris water maze has been reported to be affected by LPS or IL-1β injections (see [28] for review). However, these impairments frequently assessed only latency to reach the hidden platform. Distance traveled, route taken, and probe trials are important measures that facilitate robust conclusions about whether rodents actually show locomotor, emotional, or cognitive deficits. More recent studies accounting for these parameters show very limited effects of systemic LPS [29], IL-1β [30], or other inflammatory stimuli. Thus the previously reported systemic inflammation-induced visuospatial learning deficits have not stood up to multiple repetitions and confounding factors may explain many of the positive results.

Impairments in contextual fear conditioning seem more robust [31,32] and it appears that IL-1β may have a key role in disrupting consolidation of the memory for context. It is probably significant that this is the most sensitive to inflammatory stimulation and is aversive, contains a strong amygdala involvement, and where examined in sepsis models has been found to be sensitive. Thus inflammation can significantly impair consolidation of new memory, but this seems particularly true in this aversive paradigm.

Finally it is worth emphasizing that the paucity of studies showing genuinely long-term cognitive impairment after sepsis in rodents is at odds with the now accepted long-term effects in patients. In this context it may be significant that patients receive significant doses of both analgesics and sedatives and these may contribute significantly to the deficits observed. Clinically, the use of GABAergic sedatives such as the benzodiazepines midazolam and lorazepam may contribute to the incidence of delirium in the ICU. Recent studies with the alpha-2 adrenergic receptor agonist dexmedetomidine showed decreased prevalence of delirium compared with benzodiazepine use [33,34]. This may be linked with reported immunosuppressive effects of GABA agonists [35], or may result from the unfortunate combination of sepsis-induced derangements with the well-described direct effects of benzodiazepines on memory function via GABA$_A$ receptors [36–38]. There are some basic studies incorporating anesthesia with isoflurane and buprenorphine with the sterile inflammation that is characteristic of surgery [39], but none to my knowledge combining benzodiazepines and sepsis to examine cognitive outcomes. Moving towards modeling of the full complexity of ICU delirium and long-term cognitive decline, some of these factors will need to be integrated into animal studies.

The interaction between insult severity and subject predisposition

In attempting to understand inflammation-induced delirium pathophysiology we have found it helpful to think of a continuum of systemic inflammation from severe sepsis in the ICU to milder inflammation in susceptible populations (Figure 11.2). There is clinical evidence that severe insults can produce delirium in an otherwise healthy population while much milder insults may be sufficient in a population that is cognitively vulnerable due to prior cognitive impairment. How this works at a pathophysiological level is not clear. A number of years ago we provided the first evidence that microglia are primed by neurodegenerative pathology such that they now produced exaggerated CNS inflammatory responses to systemic inflammatory insults [40]. This results in selective amplification of IL-1β responses in areas of prior pathology and this has obvious relevance for inflammation-induced delirium in susceptible populations [41] (see also Chapter 19, this volume). Recent clinical hypotheses in delirium have drawn on

this idea since it provides a mechanism by which inflammation might selectively be amplified in areas of the brain with prior pathology [42,43]. We have recently demonstrated its relevance in acute cognitive dysfunction: we showed that a low dose of the bacterial endotoxin, LPS, has no impact on spatial reference memory or working memory performance in normal animals, but if the treated animals are in the early pre-symptomatic stages of progressive neurodegenerative disease, this insult is now sufficient to impair learning of a Y-maze spatial reference memory task and to induce acute and transient working memory deficits akin to delirium [44,45] in a novel T-maze alternation task. Furthermore, progression to more advanced stages of neurodegeneration, such that the animals are now on the cusp of disease-associated cognitive impairments, increases the incidence, severity, and duration of LPS-induced cognitive deficits (Skelly & Cunningham, unpublished data). This susceptibility is associated with decreasing density of presynaptic terminals, offering a very tangible loss of cognitive reserve that may directly predispose individuals to inflammation-induced delirium. The priming of microglia appears to persist and indeed increase as neurodegenerative disease progresses [40,44,46] (months in mice, and therefore probably many years in chronic human neurodegenerative disease) and, when induced by acute CNS injury in mice, lasts for at least 1 month [47]. The further activation of these primed microglia, induced by

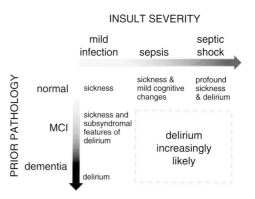

Figure 11.2 A schematic prediction for how severity of insult and prior pathology interact to increase the likelihood of delirium during sepsis. While mild infection is likely to induce only symptoms of sickness behavior in individuals who have no pathology at baseline, similar insults may produce subsyndromal delirium in individuals with mild cognitive impairment at baseline, and may produce florid delirium in those with existing dementia. Thus, as severity of sepsis and severity of underlying pathology increase, so increases the probability of delirium. MCI, mild cognitive impairment. This figure is presented in color in the color plate section.

systemic inflammatory insults such as infection, injury, or surgery, is transient and appears to last only as long as the secondary insult can exert its influence [45,47]. This interaction between severity of systemic inflammation and prior predisposition is also seen in the association between pro-inflammatory cytokines induced by hip fracture and replacement surgery and the occurrence of delirium: elevated pro-inflammatory cytokines predict delirium, but this association is lost upon adjustment for prior cognitive impairment [48]. There is also evidence that cognitive impairments arising from the superimposition of CLP upon traumatic brain injury are significantly greater than those produced by either insult alone [26]. Acute cognitive impairments induced by systemic LPS or infection with *E. coli* have also been observed to be more prominent in aged rodents with respect to young rodents [49,50], and although some of these studies come with similar caveats about reliance on aversive tasks and failure only to consolidate new memories, it is significant that IL-1β has once again been implicated as an important molecule in disturbance of memory function [51]. Though IL-1β can act directly on neurons and can impair LTP [52], it has been shown that the prostaglandin PGE2 is necessary and sufficient for the production of the CFC memory impairment in young animals [53], and we have recently shown that cyclooxygenase inhibition, and reduction of blood and brain PGE2 levels, can provide protection against the acute working memory deficits produced by low-dose systemic LPS on a background of dementia (Griffin *et al.,* submitted). Possible mechanisms of cognitive dysfunction are shown in Figure 11.3.

The role of acetylcholine in delirium – sepsis vs. dementia

A recent clinical trial of the acetylcholinesterase inhibitor rivastigmine as a treatment for ICU delirium was stopped prematurely due to a number of deaths and no evidence of improvement in the other treated patients [54]. Cholinergic hypofunction is a key feature of the proposed "final common pathway" for delirium and cholinergic inhibition using atropine has been used to mimic delirium in rats [55] on the basis that changes in medication increasing anticholinergic function can lead to episodes of delirium [56]. These data suggest that cholinergic neuromodulation is important in normal cognitive function and loss of this can lead to cognitive deficits. There are prior data

linking IL-1β elevation to PGE2 production [57], inhibition of acetylcholine outflow [58], and cognitive dysfunction [57,59]. Apart from a direct neuromodulatory role, work from the laboratory of Kevin Tracey has shown that cholinergic activation of the viscera via the vagal nerve suppresses peripheral macrophage function by interaction with the nicotinic alpha-7 receptor [60]. However, despite the fact that these receptors have been shown on microglia and can down-regulate microglial activation [61], inhibition of microglial activation by endogenous acetylcholine has not been assessed in a biological context relevant to sepsis. We have recently used the ribosomal toxin saporin linked to an antibody against the p75 neurotrophin receptor, which is enriched on basal forebrain cholinergic neurons of the medial septum and ventral diagonal band, to produce partial lesions of the basal forebrain cholinergic nuclei. Approximately 25% loss of cholinergic ennervation of the hippocampus did not alter the hippocampal transcription of pro-inflammatory cytokines in response to systemic LPS [62]. However, systemic LPS (100 μg/kg) produced acute and transient working deficits, in a cholinergic-dependent task, in these lesioned animals, but had no impact in normal animals. Furthermore, pretreatment with the acetylcholinesterase inhibitor donepezil provides partial, but incomplete protection. What these data suggest is that with a pre-existing cholinergic deficit, cholinesterase inhibition is partially protective against infection-induced cognitive dysfunction. The importance of such inhibition may be substantially less when the brain is confronted with septic shock and all of the physiological derangement that entails. Furthermore, suppression of systemic immune function at that time may be deleterious, as the rivastigmine clinical trial suggests [54]. Future investigations in preventing or treating ICU delirium will need considerably more knowledge of delirium pathophysiology before such interventions can be made with confidence of success.

Conclusion

One may have to look at lower-grade infection to have any chance to cognitively interrogate the question of acute dysfunction, but could perhaps use MRI and EEG analysis in rodents to assess interventions in the acute status change when using robust sepsis. Since long-term cognitive impairment can be assessed long after the acute sickness, higher doses can be used to

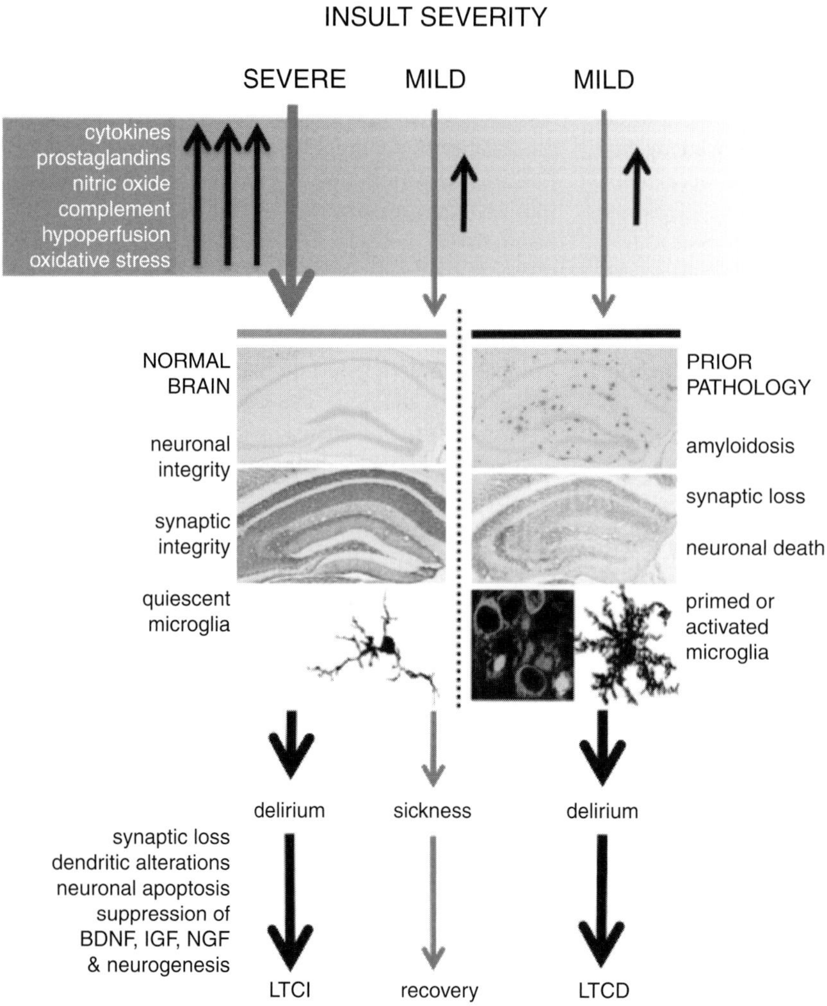

Figure 11.3 Possible routes to delirium and long-term cognitive impairment resulting from infection. The concentrations of cytokines, prostaglandins, nitric oxide, complement factors, and the degree of hypoperfusion and oxidative stress increase as a function of the severity of sepsis ($\uparrow\uparrow\uparrow$ versus $\uparrow$). This will influence the severity of the cognitive symptoms. Compared with the normal brain, the aged or neurodegenerative brain may show increased amyloid pathology, decreased presynaptic terminal density, and increased numbers of dying neurons and primed microglia. Systemic inflammatory mediators and tissue perfusion will have fundamentally different consequences in the brain, depending on the pathological state of that brain at baseline. Mild insults may produce nothing more than reversible sickness symptoms in the normal brain. However, even moderate inflammation may have effects on synaptic function, dendritic structure, growth factor synthesis and maturation, and indeed on neurogenesis. The impacts of these changes will be considerable in a brain that is functioning with limited cognitive reserve. Furthermore, in those with overt pathology, microglia may be primed to produce exaggerated CNS inflammatory responses, effectively amplifying the severity of the systemic insult. Interleukin-1β, TNFα, prostaglandin E2, and nitric oxide have been directly implicated in the cognitive deficits in animal models. In addition to acute cognitive changes, more severe inflammatory responses are likely to induce neuronal damage and death. In pathologically normal patients who experience severe sepsis this is likely to lead to *de novo* inflammatory damage and long-term cognitive impairment (LTCI). For those with existing progressive disease, these patients are likely to suffer accelerated long-term cognitive decline (LTCD). BDNF, brain-derived neurotrophic factor; IGF, insulin-like growth factor; NGF, nerve growth factor. This figure is presented in color in the color plate section.

study this phenomenon. In both instances however, researchers must remain mindful of the importance of key inflammatory molecules in the clearing of infection. Thus, a demonstration that IL-1β, TNFα, nitric oxide (NO), or PGE2 are important in producing these long- or short-term deficits will not necessarily imply that these are valid targets in the clinical setting. In this regard, such treatments will need to jump all of the hurdles at which many promising anti-septic shock treatments have already fallen.

References

1. Ebersoldt M, Sharshar T, Annane D. Sepsis-associated delirium. *Intensive Care Med* 2007;**33**:941–50.

2. Iwashyna TJ, Ely EW, Smith DM, *et al*. Long-term cognitive impairment and functional disability among survivors of severe sepsis. *JAMA* 2010;**304**:1787–94.

3. Witlox J, Eurelings LS, De Jonghe JF, *et al*. Delirium in elderly patients and the risk of postdischarge mortality, institutionalization, and dementia: a meta-analysis. *JAMA* 2010;**304**:443–51.

4. Papadopoulos MC, Davies DC, Moss RF, *et al*. Pathophysiology of septic encephalopathy: a review. *Crit Care Med* 2000;**28**:3019–24.

5. Macmicking JD, Nathan C, Hom G, *et al*. Altered responses to bacterial infection and endotoxic shock in mice lacking inducible nitric oxide synthase. *Cell* 1995;**81**:641–50.

6. Okusawa S., Gelfand JA, Ikejima T, *et al*. Interleukin 1 induces a shock-like state in rabbits. Synergism with tumor necrosis factor and the effect of cyclooxygenase inhibition. *J Clin Invest* 1988;**81**:1162–72.

7. Tracey KJ, Lowry SF, Cerami A. Cachectin: a hormone that triggers acute shock and chronic cachexia. *J Infect Dis* 1988;**157**:413–20.

8. Eichacker PQ, Parent C, Kalil A, *et al*. Risk and the efficacy of antiinflammatory agents: retrospective and confirmatory studies of sepsis. *Am J Respir Crit Care Med* 2002;**166**:1197–205.

9. Suffredini AF, Munford RS. Novel therapies for septic shock over the past 4 decades. *JAMA* 2011;**306**:194–9.

10. Barichello T, Martins MR, Reinke A, *et al*. Cognitive impairment in sepsis survivors from cecal ligation and perforation. *Crit Care Med* 2005;**33**:221–3; discussion 262–3.

11. Comim CM, Pereira JG, Steckert A, *et al*. Rivastigmine reverses habituation memory impairment observed in sepsis survivor rats. *Shock* 2009;**32**:270–1.

12. Tuon L, Comim CM, Petronilho F, *et al*. Time-dependent behavioral recovery after sepsis in rats. *Intensive Care Med* 2008;**34**:1724–31.

13. Tuon L, Comim CM, Petronilho F, *et al*. Memory-enhancing treatments reverse the impairment of inhibitory avoidance retention in sepsis-surviving rats. *Crit Care* 2008;**12**:R133.

14. Cassol-Jr OJ, Comim CM, Silva BR, *et al*. Treatment with cannabidiol reverses oxidative stress parameters, cognitive impairment and mortality in rats submitted to sepsis by cecal ligation and puncture. *Brain Res* 2010;**1348**:128–38.

15. Cassol-Jr OJ, Comim CM, Constantino LS, *et al*. Acute low dose of MK-801 prevents memory deficits without altering hippocampal DARPP-32 expression and

BDNF levels in sepsis survivor rats. *J Neuroimmunol* 2011;**230**:48–51.

16. Semmler A, Okulla T, Sastre M, *et al*. Systemic inflammation induces apoptosis with variable vulnerability of different brain regions. *J Chem Neuroanat* 2005;**30**:144–57.

17. Semmler A, Frisch C, Debeir T, *et al*. Long-term cognitive impairment, neuronal loss and reduced cortical cholinergic innervation after recovery from sepsis in a rodent model. *Exp Neurol* 2007;**204**:733–40.

18. Semmler A, Hermann S, Mormann F, *et al*. Sepsis causes neuroinflammation and concomitant decrease of cerebral metabolism. *J Neuroinflammation* 2008;**5**:38.

19. Weberpals M, Hermes M, Hermann S, *et al*. NOS2 gene deficiency protects from sepsis-induced long-term cognitive deficits. *J Neurosci* 2009;**29**:14177–84.

20. Bozza FA, Garteiser P, Oliveira MF, *et al*. Sepsis-associated encephalopathy: a magnetic resonance imaging and spectroscopy study. *J Cereb Blood Flow Metab* 2010;**30**:440–8.

21. Imamura Y, Wang H, Matsumoto N, *et al*. Interleukin-1beta causes long-term potentiation deficiency in a mouse model of septic encephalopathy. *Neuroscience* 2011;**187**:63–9.

22. Serantes R, Arnalich F, Figueroa M, *et al*. Interleukin-1beta enhances GABAA receptor cell-surface expression by a phosphatidylinositol 3-kinase/Akt pathway: relevance to sepsis-associated encephalopathy. *J Biol Chem* 2006;**281**:14632–43.

23. Terrando N, Rei Fidalgo A, Vizcaychipi M, *et al*. The impact of IL-1 modulation on the development of lipopolysaccharide-induced cognitive dysfunction. *Crit Care* 2010;**14**:R88.

24. Alexander JJ, Jacob A, Cunningham P, *et al*. TNF is a key mediator of septic encephalopathy acting through its receptor, TNF receptor-1. *Neurochem Int* 2008;**52**:447–56.

25. Maren S. Pavlovian fear conditioning as a behavioral assay for hippocampus and amygdala function: cautions and caveats. *Eur J Neurosci* 2008;**28**:1661–6.

26. Venturi L, Miranda M, Selmi V, *et al*. Systemic sepsis exacerbates mild post-traumatic brain injury in the rat. *J Neurotrauma* 2009;**26**:1547–56.

27. Shimizu I, Adachi N, Liu K, *et al*. Sepsis facilitates brain serotonin activity and impairs learning ability in rats. *Brain Res* 1999;**830**:94–100.

28. Cunningham C, Sanderson DJ. Malaise in the water maze: untangling the effects of LPS and IL-1beta on learning and memory. *Brain Behav Immun* 2008;**22**(8):1117–27.

29. Sparkman NL, Kohman RA, Scott VJ, *et al*. Bacterial endotoxin-induced behavioral alterations in two

variations of the Morris water maze. *Physiol Behav* 2005;**86**:244–51.

30. Thomson LM, Sutherland RJ. Interleukin-1beta induces anorexia but not spatial learning and memory deficits in the rat. *Behav Brain Res* 2006;**170**:302–7.

31. Pugh CR, Kumagawa K, Fleshner M, *et al.* Selective effects of peripheral lipopolysaccharide administration on contextual and auditory-cue fear conditioning. *Brain Behav Immun* 1998;**12**:212–29.

32. Thomson LM, Sutherland RJ. Systemic administration of lipopolysaccharide and interleukin-1beta have different effects on memory consolidation. *Brain Res Bull* 2005;**67**:24–9.

33. Pandharipande PP, Sanders RD, Girard TD, *et al.* Effect of dexmedetomidine versus lorazepam on outcome in patients with sepsis: an a priori-designed analysis of the MENDS randomized controlled trial. *Crit Care* 2010;**14**:R38.

34. Riker RR, Shehabi Y, Bokesch PM, *et al.* Dexmedetomidine vs midazolam for sedation of critically ill patients: a randomized trial. *JAMA* 2009;**301**:489–99.

35. Bhat R, Axtell R, Mitra A, *et al.* Inhibitory role for GABA in autoimmune inflammation. *Proc Natl Acad Sci USA* 2010;**107**:2580–5.

36. Brioni JD, Arolfo MP. Diazepam impairs retention of spatial information without affecting retrieval or cue learning. *Pharmacol Biochem Behav* 1992;**41**:1–5.

37. Kant GJ, Wylie RM, Vasilakis AA, *et al.* Effects of triazolam and diazepam on learning and memory as assessed using a water maze. *Pharmacol Biochem Behav* 1996;**53**:317–22.

38. Nabeshima T, Tohyama K, Ichihara K, *et al.* Effects of benzodiazepines on passive avoidance response and latent learning in mice: relationship to benzodiazepine receptors and the cholinergic neuronal system. *J Pharmacol Exp Ther* 1990;**255**:789–94.

39. Cibelli M, Fidalgo AR, Terrando N, *et al.* Role of interleukin-1beta in postoperative cognitive dysfunction. *Ann Neurol* 2010;**68**:360–8.

40. Cunningham C, Wilcockson DC, Campion S, *et al.* Central and systemic endotoxin challenges exacerbate the local inflammatory response and increase neuronal death during chronic neurodegeneration. *J Neurosci* 2005;**25**:9275–84.

41. MacLullich AM, Ferguson KJ, Miller T, *et al.* Unravelling the pathophysiology of delirium: a focus on the role of aberrant stress responses. *J Psychosom Res* 2008;**65**:229–38.

42. Cerejeira J, Firmino H, Vaz-Serra A, *et al.* The neuroinflammatory hypothesis of delirium. *Acta Neuropathol* 2010;**119**:737–54.

43. Van Gool WA, Van De Beek D, Eikelenboom P. Systemic infection and delirium: when cytokines and acetylcholine collide. *Lancet* 2010;**375**:773–5.

44. Cunningham C, Campion S, Lunnon K, *et al.* Systemic inflammation induces acute behavioral and cognitive changes and accelerates neurodegenerative disease. *Biol Psychiatry* 2009;**65**:304–12.

45. Murray C, Sanderson DJ, Barkus C, *et al.* Systemic inflammation induces acute working memory deficits in the primed brain: relevance for delirium. *Neurobiol Aging* 2012; **33**(3):603–16.e3.

46. Combrinck MI, Perry VH, Cunningham C. Peripheral infection evokes exaggerated sickness behaviour in pre-clinical murine prion disease. *Neuroscience* 2002;**112**:7–11.

47. Palin K, Cunningham C, Forse P, *et al.* Systemic inflammation switches the inflammatory cytokine profile in CNS Wallerian degeneration. *Neurobiol Dis* 2008;**30**:19–29.

48. Van Munster BC, Bisschop PH, Zwinderman AH, *et al.* Cortisol, interleukins and S100B in delirium in the elderly. *Brain Cogn* 2010;**74**:18–23.

49. Barrientos RM, Higgins EA, Biedenkapp JC, *et al.* Peripheral infection and aging interact to impair hippocampal memory consolidation. *Neurobiol Aging* 2006;**27**:723–32.

50. Chen J, Buchanan JB, Sparkman NL, *et al.* Neuroinflammation and disruption in working memory in aged mice after acute stimulation of the peripheral innate immune system. *Brain Behav Immun* 2008;**22**:301–11.

51. Frank MG, Barrientos RM, Hein AM, *et al.* IL-1RA blocks *E. coli*-induced suppression of Arc and long-term memory in aged F344xBN F1 rats. *Brain Behav Immun* 2010;**24**:254–62.

52. Vereker E, O'Donnell E, Lynch A, *et al.* Evidence that interleukin-1beta and reactive oxygen species production play a pivotal role in stress-induced impairment of LTP in the rat dentate gyrus. *Eur J Neurosci* 2001;**14**:1809–19.

53. Hein AM, Stutzman DL, Bland ST, *et al.* Prostaglandins are necessary and sufficient to induce contextual fear learning impairments after interleukin-1 beta injections into the dorsal hippocampus. *Neuroscience* 2007;**150**:754–63.

54. Van Eijk MM, Roes KC, Honing ML, *et al.* Effect of rivastigmine as an adjunct to usual care with haloperidol on duration of delirium and mortality in critically ill patients: a multicentre, double-blind, placebo-controlled randomised trial. *Lancet* 2010;**376**:1829–37.

55. Trzepacz PT, Leavitt M, Ciongoli K. An animal model for delirium. *Psychosomatics* 1992;**33**:404–15.

56. Tune LE. Serum anticholinergic activity levels and delirium in the elderly. *Semin Clin Neuropsychiatry* 2000;**5**:149–53.

57. Matsumoto Y, Yamaguchi T, Watanabe S, *et al.* Involvement of arachidonic acid cascade in working memory impairment induced by interleukin-1 beta. *Neuropharmacology* 2004;**46**:1195–200.

58. Rada P, Mark GP, Vitek MP, *et al.* Interleukin-1 beta decreases acetylcholine measured by microdialysis in the hippocampus of freely moving rats. *Brain Res* 1991;**550**:287–90.

59. Taepavarapruk P, Song C. Reductions of acetylcholine release and nerve growth factor expression are correlated with memory impairment induced by interleukin-1beta administrations: effects of omega-3 fatty acid EPA treatment. *J Neurochem* 2010;**112**:1054–64.

60. Tracey KJ. Physiology and immunology of the cholinergic antiinflammatory pathway. *J Clin Invest* 2007;**117**:289–296.

61. De Simone R, Ajmone-Cat MA, Carnevale D, *et al.* Activation of alpha7 nicotinic acetylcholine receptor by nicotine selectively up-regulates cyclooxygenase-2 and prostaglandin E2 in rat microglial cultures. *J Neuroinflammation* 2005;**2**:4.

62. Field RH, Gossen A, Cunningham C. Prior pathology in the basal forebrain cholinergic system predisposes to inflammation-induced working memory deficits: reconciling inflammatory and cholinergic hypotheses of delirium. *J Neurosci* 2012;**32**:6288–94.

Chapter 12

Neurobiological effects of systemic physiological and metabolic insults

Jean-Francois Payen, Gérard Audibert, and Nicolas Bruder

SUMMARY

Several systemic factors have been found to affect the brain in patients with traumatic brain injury (TBI) and in stroke. Primary injury is the anatomic damage caused at the time of insult. This produces vulnerable cells that are further compromised by secondary brain injury, which includes excitotoxicity, oxidative stress, inflammation, apoptosis, and mitochondrial dysfunction. In this context, systemic physiological and metabolic insults should be considered as strong contributors to aggravate the neurological outcome. All these factors have in common the potential to compromise the balance between brain oxygen delivery and consumption, then to favor brain tissue hypoxia. Their biochemical pathways to account for this cerebral deterioration are numerous, complex, and not fully understood. This review summarizes the neurological impact of these systemic factors in injured brain as well as in the setting of non-neurological critical illness. These systemic factors can be schematically divided into those reducing oxygen supply to the brain tissue, i.e., arterial hypotension, low cardiac output, hypocapnia, systemic hypoxia, anemia, and hyperthermia, and those favoring brain metabolic disturbances, i.e., arterial hypotension and blood glucose abnormalities.

Introduction

Cerebral ischemia and TBI have similar mechanisms contributing to loss of cellular integrity and tissue destruction [1]. Both injuries are considered to be a dual insult composed of primary and secondary processes. Primary injury is the anatomic damage caused at the time of insult. This produces vulnerable cells that are further compromised by secondary brain injury. Secondary brain damage occurs at the cellular level and results from a complex biochemical cascade, including excitotoxicity, oxidative stress, inflammation, apoptosis, and mitochondrial dysfunction. Secondary brain damage is a major factor in determining patient outcome following primary brain insult. Several systemic factors have been found to worsen secondary brain damage [2,3]. All have in common the potential to compromise the balance between brain oxygen delivery and consumption, then to favor brain tissue hypoxia (Figure 12.1). These systemic factors can be schematically divided into those reducing oxygen supply to the brain tissue, i.e., arterial hypotension, low cardiac output, hypocapnia, systemic hypoxia, anemia, and hyperthermia, and those favoring brain metabolic disturbances, i.e., arterial hypotension and blood glucose abnormalities.

Arterial hypotension

A close association between hypotension and outcome has been established for years. In 717 severe TBI patients, systolic blood pressure (SBP) of less than 90 mmHg in the field occurred in 34.6% of patients, and was a major determinant of outcome [2]. Out- and in-hospital hypotensive events doubled the mortality rate after brain trauma. A recent analysis found a U-shaped relationship between outcome and SBP or mean arterial blood pressure (MBP), with no evidence of an abrupt threshold effect [4]. Best outcomes were observed for SBP values of the order of 135 mmHg (or MBP 90 mmHg). The association between high arterial blood pressure and poorer outcome disappeared after adjustment for age, motor Glasgow Coma Scale (GCS) score, and pupil response, because of a possible concomitant elevation of intracranial pressure (ICP) in patients with altered autoregulation. This U-shaped relationship between blood pressure and mortality rate was also shown in patients with

Brain Disorders in Critical Illness, ed. Robert D. Stevens, Tarek Sharshar, and E. Wesley Ely. Published by Cambridge University Press. © Cambridge University Press 2013.

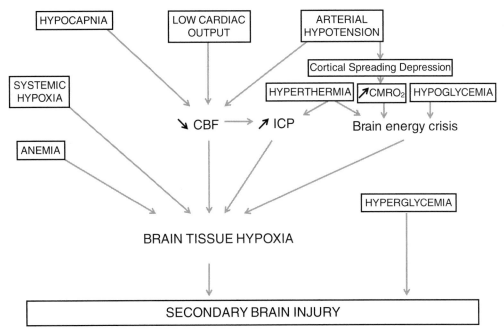

Figure 12.1 Systemic factors involved in secondary brain damage. CBF, cerebral blood flow; CMRO$_2$, cerebral metabolic rate in oxygen; ICP, intracranial pressure.

acute ischemic or hemorrhagic stroke [5,6]. A large variability in blood pressure values is detrimental for the brain as well.

Traumatic brain injury experimentally reduces cerebral blood flow (CBF) to approximately 60% from baseline. Posttrauma hypotension further decreases CBF to increase contusion areas and cortical neuronal damage [7]. Episodes of arterial hypotension did not aggravate tissue injury or neurological deficits following brain trauma, but delayed cognitive recovery [8]. In models of stroke, the extension of brain lesion is closely linked with the occurrence of arterial hypotension. Conversely, mild induced hypertension (30% above baseline values) increases CBF and cerebral metabolic rate in oxygen (CMRO$_2$) in the core ischemic area as well as in the penumbra, resulting in a 50% decrease in infarct volume. Brain metabolism after TBI is characterized by a depressed CMRO$_2$ to 45% of normal values and by a decreased cerebral arterio-venous difference for oxygen and glucose [9]. This is aggravated by arterial hypotension or low cerebral perfusion pressure, leading to brain tissue hypoxia. Arterial hypotension can also worsen brain injury by suppressing the expression of neuroprotective genes, e.g., brain-derived neutrophic factor (BDNF), glutathione peroxidase 1 (GPX-1) and heme oxygenase-1 (HO-1) [10].

There is also a growing interest about cortical spreading depression (CSD) and its possible relationship with arterial hypotension. Cortical spreading depression is a slow propagating wave of neuronal and glial depolarization that develops after trauma, stroke, and subarachnoid hemorrhage. Spreading depolarization is characterized by breakdown of cell ion gradients and neuronal swelling after sustained depolarization of neurons [11]. Cortical spreading depression coincides with a failure of brain ion homeostasis including an extracellular increase in K$^+$ concentration, an extracellular decrease in Ca^{++} and Cl$^-$ concentrations, and a decline in pH. At the same time, the neuronal uptake of water leads to neuronal swelling and a massive release of amino acids, especially glutamate and aspartate, which play a role in the spreading mechanism of CSD [12]. Restoration of the ionic gradients after CSD is energetically demanding. The normal hemodynamic response to spreading depolarization is an increased CBF to meet the metabolic demand (preserved neurovascular coupling). However, repeated episodes of CSD may allow insufficient time for cells to recover. This induces an inverse hemodynamic response with arteriolar constriction, then a prolonged hypoperfusion (inverse neurovascular coupling). Therefore, CSD leads to spreading ischemia. This phenomenon can be monitored using a brain tissue oxygen pressure ($PtiO_2$) probe showing a biphasic $PtiO_2$ pattern, i.e., a hypoxic then hyperoxic phase. Accordingly, the hyperoxic phase disappears with clusters of CSD at the expense of the hypoxic response. This mechanism has been suggested to play a crucial role in the development of delayed ischemia after subarachnoid hemorrhage [13].

Cortical spreading depression can be related to the peri-infarct depolarization (PID) in boundary zones of brain ischemia that contributes to infarct expansion. Preliminary data suggest that CSD could be associated with poor outcome at 6 months after TBI. In this context, arterial hypotension should contribute to aggravate cerebral ischemia through the development of CSD. Indeed, arterial hypotension increased the duration of CSD and delayed the restoration of ionic shifts associated with CSD [14]. Hyperoxia failed to reverse the effect of hypotension, while arterial hypertension accelerated brain recovery after CSD. Therefore, arterial hypotension could also impact on the neurological outcome of brain-injured patients by facilitating the development of CSD. Arterial hypertension could hasten the recovery from CSD regardless of its effects on cerebral perfusion pressure (CPP) or the status of autoregulation.

Low cardiac output

The possible role of low cardiac output as a contributing factor to influence cerebral perfusion has been neglected for decades. In subjecting 35 severely head-injured patients to manipulation of arterial blood pressure, Bouma et al. concluded that CBF was not related to cardiac output regardless of the status of autoregulation [15]. However, CBF remained unchanged within less than 20% changes of cardiac output from baseline in that study. The statement that CBF was fully independent of changes of cardiac output has been questioned by studies with volunteers during dynamic exercise. Using transcranial Doppler to estimate CBF by measuring blood flow velocity in the mean cerebral artery, the exercise-induced increased cardiac output was associated with a parallel increase in CBF, independently of arterial carbon dioxide pressure [16]. A cardio-selective beta-1 adrenergic blockade affected comparably cardiac output and cerebral blood flow velocity. Moreover, the relationship between changes in cerebral blood flow velocity and in cardiac output at rest and during exercise during gradual manipulation of central blood volume was linear, even at the plateau of cerebral

autoregulation [17]. Collectively these results suggest that cardiac output is one important factor in regulating the cerebral blood flow velocity in volunteers.

Whether increasing cardiac output could result in improved brain perfusion in brain-injured patients has received little attention. Early hemodynamic exploration following brain insult showed that TBI patients had signs of increased sympathetic activation, i.e., elevated cardiac index, mild tachycardia and hypertension, and high systemic vascular resistance with concomitant reduced tissue perfusion and oxygenation during the first 24 hours after injury [18]. In addition, a high pulmonary vascular resistance as a reflection of heart failure was found in patients with elevated ICP [19]. Interestingly, non-survivors had initially lower cardiac index and oxygen tissue delivery values, as well as more peripheral vasoconstriction compared with survivors [18]. In that study, authors concluded that "early hemodynamic therapy directed toward improving cardiac output and tissue perfusion may be a useful approach to prevention of additional neurological deterioration." In line with this assumption are studies exploring the use of inotropic agents in brain-injured patients. In patients with symptomatic vasospasm after subarachnoid hemorrhage (SAH), an improvement of CBF and reversal of vasospasm was indeed obtained with dobutamine with a concomitant increased cardiac output and no changes in arterial blood pressure [20]. An early goal-directed hemodynamic management to optimize cardiac output and volume status in post-SAH vasospasm was associated with better clinical course and fewer cardiopulmonary complications compared with conventional methods [21]. The possible reasons for myocardial dysfunction are numerous after brain injury. High pulmonary vascular resistance possibly reflects pulmonary vasoconstriction centrally mediated by brain damage. The Cushing response to increased ICP with systemic hypertension and sinus bradycardia may play a role as well. Associated extra cranial lesions can alter cardiac function through the development of hypovolemia or direct myocardial lesions. In addition, these patients are given large doses of sedatives as part of treatment for intracranial hypertension, that requires more vasoactive agents to overcome cardiac depressor effects, as shown elsewhere [22]. Taken together, these findings suggest that the injured brain is at risk of ischemia from reduced CBF not only by increased ICP but also by reduced cardiac index. More attention should be paid to exploring and potentially restoring normal cardiac function in patients with severe brain injury.

Respiratory disturbances

Systemic hypoxia

An association between systemic hypoxia and both higher mortality rates and long-term adverse cognitive outcomes after TBI is well documented. Episodes of brain tissue hypoxia defined by $PtiO_2$ less than 20 mmHg are associated with poor functional outcome [23]. Conversely, studies suggest that a goal-directed therapy based on maintaining $PtiO_2$ values above 20 mmHg might be associated with improved patient outcome [24]. Physiologically, CBF increases when arterial PO_2 falls under 60 mmHg. In normal subjects, middle cerebral artery flow velocity increased by 13% in response to a 10% decrease in arterial O_2 saturation. However, the response to systemic hypoxia in CBF is not uniform throughout the overall brain: the most prominent response in CBF can be seen in the nuclei of the basal ganglia and in the brainstem, while the lowest increase in hypoxia-induced CBF response comes from cortical regions [25]. The CBF response to mild systemic hypoxia is variable among subjects as well. This should explain why the cerebral cortex is particularly susceptible to systemic hypoxia and why the amplitude of hypoxia-induced tissue injury can vary among patients. Systemic hypoxia not only reduces oxygen availability for aerobic metabolism but also increases the neuro-inflammatory response to TBI, reduces apoptosis inhibitor proteins and activates caspases, that in turn increases contusion size and cell death [26]. Finally, the combination of systemic hypoxia and arterial hypotension is particularly detrimental: mortality after TBI increased from 22.9% to 54.6% and from 36.6% to 75% in patients with both insults [2,27–29].

Hypo- and hypercapnia

Cerebral blood flow is linearly linked with arterial carbon dioxide pressure ($PaCO_2$) as it varies by 4–6% per mmHg of $PaCO_2$ changes. Changes in cerebral blood volume (CBV) induced by $PaCO_2$ are of less amplitude than changes in CBF. In TBI patients, hypocapnia decreases CBF and slightly increases $CMRO_2$, representing a detrimental challenge to the injured brain [30]. Spontaneous hyperventilation is also associated with an increased risk of brain tissue hypoxia. The effect of prolonged hypocapnia on CBF and CBV cannot be sustained because a progressive buffering of perivascular alkalosis occurs. Return to normocapnia after a prolonged period of hypocapnia causes rebound of cerebral hyperemia, ICP increase, or cerebral hemorrhage. Although hypercapnia increases CBF in normal subjects, the vasodilatory effect of hypercapnia can raise ICP in injured brain with low compliance that decreases brain perfusion. Both hypocapnia and hypercapnia have been associated with poor clinical outcome after TBI [31–33]. Although mild to moderate hypercapnia ($PaCO_2$ 60–100 mmHg) was neuroprotective along with a reduced apoptosis in a model of transient cerebral ischemia [34], further studies are warranted to confirm these findings. Meanwhile, current guidelines recommend maintaining $PaCO_2$ within normal range ($PaCO_2$ 35–40 mmHg) after brain injury. If indicated, therapeutic hyperventilation requires dedicated monitoring of brain metabolism, i.e., brain tissue oxygen pressure or jugular venous bulb saturation in oxygen.

Blood glucose abnormalities

Hyperglycemia has been identified for years as a risk factor for mortality and morbidity in the intensive care unit (ICU) as well as perioperative settings [35,36]. There is also a large body of evidence that hyperglycemia is independently associated with poorer neurological outcomes and higher risk of death in stroke and TBI patients. In stroke models, animals with hyperglycemia had poorer outcomes than controls; this was likely due to greater intracellular acidosis and tissue accumulation of lactate and glutamate, higher production of oxygen free radicals, and an intracellular calcium overload [37]. A lower survival rate of the potentially salvageable ischemic penumbra was also found. In a rodent model of intracerebral hemorrhage, hyperglycemia promoted the expansion of hematoma through the plasma kallikrein-mediated inhibition of platelet-vessel wall interaction [38]. In patients who died from septic shock, hyperglycemia was associated with microglial apoptosis [39]. All these findings indicate that hyperglycemia is deleterious for the injured brain although the exact mechanisms for this effect are not fully understood.

It became logical to conduct clinical studies about whether tight glycemic control, i.e., blood glucose between 4.4 and 6.1 mmol/l, could improve patient outcomes. In critically ill patients, intensive insulin therapy was shown originally to reduce mortality and morbidity, including bloodstream infections, acute renal failure, and critical illness neuropathy [40]. Similar benefits were found after cardiac surgery, acute myocardial infarction, and acute neurological injury. However, other studies were not able to replicate these findings, raising considerable debate over the safety and efficacy of tight glycemic control. In a large randomized trial, intensive insulin therapy increased mortality among critically ill patients, which was partly related to a higher incidence of severe hypoglycemia, i.e., blood glucose level ≤ 2.2 mmol/l (40 mg/dl) in the intervention group [41]. In the population of brain-injured patients, studies in which glucose concentrations were reduced early after the onset of cerebral insult constantly failed to show neurological improvement. Treatment with glucose-potassium-insulin infusions to maintain capillary glucose at 4–7 mmol/l did not reduce the incidence of death 90 days after acute stroke [42]. No benefit in patient outcomes was found when intensive insulin therapy was randomly allocated to severe TBI patients, while the incidence of hypoglycemia significantly increased in this group [43].

Studies with cerebral microdialysis found no association between hyperglycemia and cerebral glucose metabolism. In TBI patients, tight glycemic control even increased the incidence of cerebral microdialysis markers of metabolic distress, i.e., elevated glutamate and lactate/pyruvate ratio and low levels of microdialysis glucose (< 0.2 mmol/l), together with increased oxygen extraction fraction [44]. In other terms, injured brain behaved as if it was ischemic, even with no reduction of CBF. Decreased extracellular cerebral glucose measured by cerebral microdialysis actually reflects an increase in the utilization of cerebral glucose to supply restorative pathways in the injured brain, particularly ionic pumps and neurochemical cascades. This cerebral hyperglycolysis was considered as a pathophysiological response to brain insult in numerous animal studies. In humans, regional and global cerebral hyperglycolysis was found within the first week after severe head injury using [^{18}F] fluorodeoxyglucose-positron emission tomography (FDG-PET) [45]. Because there was no evidence of concomitant reduction in CBF, cerebral hyperglycolysis was considered as reflecting excessive metabolic demand (brain energy crisis), e.g., electrographic seizures and/or episodes of cortical spreading depression (CSD, see above). Using rapid extracellular glucose sampling in experimental stroke, a gradual depletion of the extracellular glucose was found to develop in the ischemic penumbra along with the propagation of peri-infarct depolarization [46]. In addition, the reduced plasma glucose (hypoglycemia) contributed to increase the frequency of depolarization. Taken together, these findings suggest that glucose depletion may occur in the injured brain through an excessive metabolic demand, even during non-ischemic conditions. Given that low levels of microdialysis glucose are associated with poor neurological outcome, the advantages of further reducing blood glucose supply for the injured brain is legitimately questioned.

In clinical practice, hyperglycemia on admission should be considered as a marker of the brain injury severity. Avoidance of hyperglycemia (>10 mmol/l) must be recommended for brain-injured patients. A reduction of blood glucose less than 6 mmol/l with intensive insulin therapy increases the risk of severe hypoglycemia and exacerbates brain metabolic distress. Recent data suggest that high glucose variability during the ICU stay, i.e., mean absolute glucose change per hour, would be independently associated with higher ICU and in-hospital mortality, and might be more important than hyperglycemia at clinical level [47]. It appears then reasonable to target blood glucose between 8 and 10 mmol/l and to avoid large glucose variability for brain-injured patients. Whether this strategy per se can improve neurological outcome awaits further clarification.

Anemia

Anemia is traditionally considered as an aggravating factor after brain injury. However, the relationships between blood hemoglobin concentration and cerebral injury are still unclear in the clinical setting. In volunteers subjected to acute isovolemic hemodilution, no cerebral effect was detectable until hemoglobin concentration was reduced to 7 g/dl, but further reduction of hemoglobin levels to 6 and 5 g/dl impaired their cognitive function and memory [48]. This detrimental effect of anemia increases with age. In a large cohort of 10,949 patients undergoing cardiac surgery, nadir hematocrit during cardiopulmonary bypass was an independent predictor of perioperative stroke [49]. Following experimental neurotrauma, acute hemodilutional anemia to target hemoglobin concentrations between 5 and 7 g/dl increased cerebral injury [50]. In patients with moderate to severe TBI, maintenance of hemoglobin concentration between 7 and 9 g/dl was not associated with higher mortality rate compared with a more liberal strategy, i.e., hemoglobin concentration between 10 and 12 g/dl

[51]. These results can be related to some mechanisms of brain response to acute anemia.

The acute reduction in arterial oxygen content increases cardiac output to maintain oxygen delivery to tissue. The corresponding increase in CBF is accompanied by elevated brain tissue oxygen extraction that can reach a maximum of 75% before cerebral hypoxia occurs. Increased CBF is the consequence of both cerebral vasodilation and a lower blood viscosity. The brain vasodilation is mainly the result of enhanced production of nitric oxide (NO) by perivascular neurons and vascular smooth muscle. Anemia-induced vasodilation was blunted by 7-nitroindazole, a NO synthase inhibitor, and an increase in neuronal NO synthase (NOS) gene expression was detected in the cerebral cortex of anemic rats [52]. An up-regulation of the endothelial and inducible forms of NOS was found during anemia. In addition, hemoglobin itself plays a role in the regulation of cerebral oxygen delivery. In normal conditions, NO binds to the heme to form S-nitroso-hemoglobin (SNO-Hb) located in the center of the molecule. If oxygen is unloaded, the structure of the heme is modified allowing the exposure of SNO-Hb and the release of NO, allowing the matching of microcirculatory blood flow to oxygen demand [53].

Acute anemia activates also intracellular pathways in the brain, which may be either protective or harmful [54]. Hypoxia inducible factor (HIF) is a key protein of the cellular response to hypoxia. Expressed in neurons, astrocytes, and endothelial cells, HIF production is also increased during anemia to act as a transcription factor and promote the synthesis of several molecules including erythropoietin and vascular endothelial growth factor (VEGF) [55]. Erythropoietin has numerous protective effects including the down-regulation of apoptotic mediators, stimulation of neural progenitor cell proliferation, and limitation of blood–brain barrier permeability [56]. Vascular endothelial growth factor promotes angiogenesis and neurogenesis. These effects are, however, counterbalanced by the anemia-induced generation of reactive oxygen species and the activation of neuronal apoptosis. The increased cortical inducible NOS form is responsible for enhanced adhesion molecule expression and leukocyte adhesion, reflecting brain inflammation.

Should acute anemia be actively corrected in brain-injured patients? This point is difficult to address because anemia can be a surrogate marker of the illness severity and blood transfusion is required for the most severely ill patients. In a retrospective study, poorer outcome in TBI patients was more likely associated with blood transfusion than with anemia [57]. In patients with subarachnoid hemorrhage without vasospasm, blood transfusion was associated with higher risk of adverse outcomes [58]. Conversely, red blood cell transfusion reduced brain tissue oxygen extraction fraction in vulnerable brain regions of anemic patients with subarachnoid hemorrhage [59]. Further prospective studies are needed to evaluate the effects of anemia in brain-injured patients, as well as to confirm the benefit of blood transfusion on cerebral ischemia with balancing systemic and cerebral risks of transfusion [60,61].

Hyperthermia and sepsis

Hyperthermia

Fever per se has deleterious effects on normal brain. Febrile seizures are classical complications that may result in severe encephalopathy for some patients. Fever-induced refractory epileptic encephalopathy in school-aged children (FIRES), idiopathic hemiconvulsion-hemiplegia syndrome (IHHS) in infancy, and new-onset refractory status epilepticus (NORSE) in adults are severe conditions triggered by fever [62]. Etiology of these conditions could involve brain inflammation, in particular pro-inflammatory cytokines. Among candidates, interleukin-1β (Il-1β) affects neuronal excitability by inhibiting the astrocytic reuptake of glutamate. Because glutamate is massively released from injured astrocytes and neurons during brain injuries, this release would be exacerbated with hyperthermia. In addition, Il-1β inhibits the $GABA_A$ receptor that increases neuron excitability. Finally, seizures induce pro-inflammatory reactions, which aggravate seizure severity.

Brain trauma induces the release of pro-inflammatory cytokines, including Il-1, Il-6, and tumor necrosis factor alpha (TNFα). The levels of cytokines reach their maximum at 4–8 hours after insult. Levels of TNFα return to baseline within 24 hours while IL-1 remains increased. This may explain the early febrile response after TBI in the absence of infection. However, the exact role of cytokines in this context is still unclear. Mice deficient in TNFα had improved cognitive functions at 7 days post-TBI by comparison with wild-type animals, but this effect disappeared at 2–3 weeks post-injury [63]. In addition, hyperthermia up-regulates the inducible form of NOS.

This may increase the permeability of the blood–brain barrier and contribute to the development of vasogenic edema after TBI [64].

Hyperthermia occurs in at least 70% of patients after stroke, SAH, or TBI and should be considered as a secondary brain injury. Clinical studies have shown an association between fever and poor outcome, but a cause–effect relationship has not been proven yet. Indeed, hyperthermia denotes various physiological reactions including that to cerebral inflammation, direct hypothalamic damage, and/or secondary infection. Whatever the mechanism, hyperthermia is closely associated with elevated ICP and poor outcome in brain-injured patients [65,66]. Both CBF and CBV increase with the rise in brain temperature, and may cause an elevation of ICP in brain with low compliance. However, there is no evidence of a temperature threshold to target for those patients. Although antipyretics are often ineffective in brain-injured patients, hyperthermia should be managed aggressively to maintain normothermia. In the Paracetamol (Acetaminophen) In Stroke (PAIS) trial, paracetamol improved outcome in patients with baseline body temperature 37–39 °C [67].

Increased brain metabolism is accompanied by heat production that keeps brain tissue warmer than body core. However, core temperature is not a reliable surrogate for brain temperature because the difference between the sites fluctuates with the core temperature [65]. In addition, the elevation of brain temperature is not uniform across the cerebral structures: a dorso-ventral temperature gradient has been described with cooler temperature in the dorsally located structures [68]. After brain injury, hyperthermia is associated with an extension of neuronal damage. In stroke models, warming the brain at the time or after the ischemia was associated with a higher rate of mortality and an increase in the volume of infarct, the basal ganglia being the most vulnerable region. In patients with TBI, measured brain temperature within the range 36.5–38.0 °C was associated with the lowest probability of death [69]. Comparably to arterial hypotension, a U-shaped curve could describe the relationship between brain temperature and outcome.

Sepsis

Sepsis-associated encephalopathy is a frequent complication of severe sepsis and is associated with increased mortality, morbidity, and a long-term cognitive impairment [70]. Uncontrolled activation of the microglia induced by the pro-inflammatory cytokines and cholinergic inhibition may create a neuroinflammatory response and eventually neurodegeneration [71] (Figure 12.2). Sepsis-related brain dysfunction involves alteration of neurotransmission, brain mitochondrial dysfunction, oxidative stress, and cell apoptosis [70]. At the microcirculatory level, endothelial activation and disruption of the blood–brain barrier result in diffuse ischemic

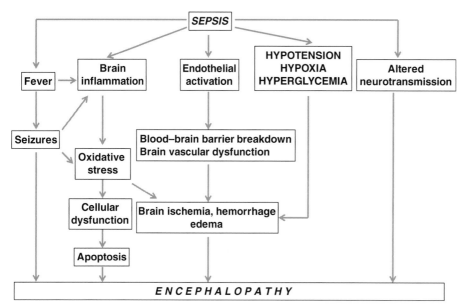

Figure 12.2 Possible mechanisms involved in the sepsis-associated encephalopathy.

Table 12.1 Brain consequences of secondary brain injuries, according to sources [5,6,28,29,31–33,39].

Secondary brain injury	Impact on prognosis	Mechanism	Frequency in hospital
Arterial hypotension	Stroke: +18% mortality for every 10 mmHg decrease in SAP < 120 mmHg; TBI: SAP < 90 mmHg → Mortality × 2	Decreased CB; increased metabolic demand via CSD; decreased expression of neuroprotective genes	Emergency unit: 9–24%; ICU: > 25%
Low cardiac output	?	Decreased CBF; contributes to pulmonary edema and hypoxia	7–15% global cardiac hypokinesia after SAH
Hypoxia	TBI: Mortality × 2	Decreased O_2 available for brain metabolism; increased neuroinflammatory response; apoptosis	Prehospital: 25–50%
Hypocapnia	TBI: Mortality × 2	Decreased CBF; brain ischemia	Prehospital: 25–40%
Hypercapnia	TBI: Mortality × 2	Increased ICP; brain herniation	Prehospital: 10–43%
Hyperglycemia		Microglial apoptosis	
Anemia	?		
Fever	?	Brain inflammation	40–80% in ICU
Sepsis	Delirium; encephalopathy; brain ischemia	Brain inflammation; endothelial activation; apoptosis; microvascular dysfunction; altered neurotransmission	10–60% in ICU

CBF, cerebral blood flow; CSD, cortical spreading depression; ICP, intracranial pressure; ICU, intensive care unit; SAH, subarachnoid hemorrhage; SAP, systolic arterial pressure; TBI, traumatic brain injury.

damage and microhemorrhages. The cortical capillary density is progressively decreased [72]. These changes were confirmed by MRI studies and postmortem examination of patients with septic shock displaying ischemic brain lesions in the white matter, and a neuronal and microglial apoptosis in cardiovascular autonomic centers [73,74]. Thus, brain damage due to sepsis results from complex interactions between the immune system, neurons, glial, and microglial cells. The clinical features range from reversible symptoms of delirium, posterior reversible encephalopathy syndrome, or leuco-encephalopathy to long-term neurological disability related to brain infarction or hemorrhage [70]. No specific treatment exists yet, but it is recommended to rule out meningitis, brain abscess, or encephalitis, and to avoid neurotoxic drugs.

In conclusion, several systemic factors can aggravate neurological outcome following primary brain insult, as summarized in Table 12.1. The biochemical pathways to account for this cerebral deterioration are numerous, complex, and not fully understood. Nevertheless, more attention should be given in clinical practice toward the detection, prevention, and treatment of conditions associated with high risk of brain hypoxia.

References

1. Bramlett HM, Dietrich WD. Pathophysiology of cerebral ischemia and brain trauma: similarities and differences. *J Cereb Blood Flow Metab* 2004;**24**:133–50.

2. Chesnut RM, Marshall LF, Klauber MR, *et al.* The role of secondary brain injury in determining outcome from severe head injury. *J Trauma* 1993;**34**:216–22.

3. Jeremitsky E, Omert L, Dunham CM, *et al.* Harbingers of poor outcome the day after severe brain injury: hypothermia, hypoxia, and hypoperfusion. *J Trauma* 2003;**54**:312–19.

4. Butcher I, Maas AI, Lu J, *et al.* Prognostic value of admission blood pressure in traumatic brain injury: results from the IMPACT study. *J Neurotrauma* 2007;**24**:294–302.

5. Leonardi-Bee J, Bath PM, Phillips SJ, *et al.* Blood pressure and clinical outcomes in the International Stroke Trial. *Stroke* 2002;**33**:1315–20.

6. Vemmos KN, Tsivgoulis G, Spengos K, *et al.* U-shaped relationship between mortality and admission blood pressure in patients with acute stroke. *J Intern Med* 2004;**255**:257–65.

7. Matsushita Y, Bramlett HM, Kuluz JW, *et al.* Delayed hemorrhagic hypotension exacerbates the hemodynamic and histopathologic consequences of traumatic brain injury in rats. *J Cereb Blood Flow Metab* 2001;**21**:847–56.

8. Schutz C, Stover JF, Thompson HJ, et al. Acute, transient hemorrhagic hypotension does not aggravate structural damage or neurologic motor deficits but delays the long-term cognitive recovery following mild to moderate traumatic brain injury. *Crit Care Med* 2006;**34**:492–501.

9. Glenn TC, Kelly DF, Boscardin WJ, et al. Energy dysfunction as a predictor of outcome after moderate or severe head injury: indices of oxygen, glucose, and lactate metabolism. *J Cereb Blood Flow Metab* 2003;**23**:1239–50.

10. Hellmich HL, Garcia JM, Shimamura M, et al. Traumatic brain injury and hemorrhagic hypotension suppress neuroprotective gene expression in injured hippocampal neurons. *Anesthesiology* 2005;**102**:806–14.

11. Dreier JP. The role of spreading depression, spreading depolarization and spreading ischemia in neurological disease. *Nat Med* 2011;**17**:439–47.

12. Lauritzen M, Dreier JP, Fabricius M, et al. Clinical relevance of cortical spreading depression in neurological disorders: migraine, malignant stroke, subarachnoid and intracranial hemorrhage, and traumatic brain injury. *J Cereb Blood Flow Metab* 2011;**31**:17–35.

13. Bosche B, Graf R, Ernestus RI, et al. Recurrent spreading depolarizations after subarachnoid hemorrhage decreases oxygen availability in human cerebral cortex. *Ann Neurol* 2010;**67**:607–17.

14. Sukhotinsky I, Yaseen MA, Sakadzic S, et al. Perfusion pressure-dependent recovery of cortical spreading depression is independent of tissue oxygenation over a wide physiologic range. *J Cereb Blood Flow Metab* 2010;**30**:1168–77.

15. Bouma GJ, Muizelaar JP. Relationship between cardiac output and cerebral blood flow in patients with intact and with impaired autoregulation. *J Neurosurg* 1990;**73**:368–74.

16. Ide K, Pott F, Van Lieshout JJ, et al. Middle cerebral artery blood velocity depends on cardiac output during exercise with a large muscle mass. *Acta Physiol Scand* 1998;**162**:13–20.

17. Ogoh S, Brothers RM, Barnes Q, et al. The effect of changes in cardiac output on middle cerebral artery mean blood velocity at rest and during exercise. *J Physiol* 2005;**569**:697–704.

18. Nicholls TP, Shoemaker WC, Wo CC, et al. Survival, hemodynamics, and tissue oxygenation after head trauma. *J Am Coll Surg* 2006;**202**:120–30.

19. Tamaki T, Isayama K, Yamamoto Y, et al. Cardiopulmonary haemodynamic changes after severe head injury. *Br J Neurosurg* 2004;**18**:158–63.

20. Joseph M, Ziadi S, Nates J, et al. Increases in cardiac output can reverse flow deficits from vasospasm independent of blood pressure: a study using xenon computed tomographic measurement of cerebral blood flow. *Neurosurgery* 2003;**53**:1044–51.

21. Mutoh T, Kazumata K, Ishikawa T, et al. Performance of bedside transpulmonary thermodilution monitoring for goal-directed hemodynamic management after subarachnoid hemorrhage. *Stroke* 2009;**40**:2368–74.

22. Payen JF, Chanques G, Mantz J, et al. Current practices in sedation and analgesia for mechanically ventilated critically ill patients: a prospective multicenter patient-based study. *Anesthesiology* 2007;**106**:687–95.

23. Chang JJ, Youn TS, Benson D, et al. Physiologic and functional outcome correlates of brain tissue hypoxia in traumatic brain injury. *Crit Care Med* 2009;**37**:283–90.

24. Spiotta AM, Stiefel MF, Gracias VH, et al. Brain tissue oxygen-directed management and outcome in patients with severe traumatic brain injury. *J Neurosurg* 2010;**113**:571–80.

25. Binks AP, Cunningham VJ, Adams L, et al. Gray matter blood flow change is unevenly distributed during moderate isocapnic hypoxia in humans. *J Appl Physiol* 2008;**104**:212–17.

26. Goodman MD, Makley AT, Huber NL, et al. Hypobaric hypoxia exacerbates the neuroinflammatory response to traumatic brain injury. *J Surg Res* 2011;**165**:30–7.

27. McHugh GS, Engel DC, Butcher I, et al. Prognostic value of secondary insults in traumatic brain injury: results from the IMPACT study. *J Neurotrauma* 2007;**24**:287–93.

28. Chi JH, Knudson MM, Vassar MJ, et al. Prehospital hypoxia affects outcome in patients with traumatic brain injury: a prospective multicenter study. *J Trauma* 2006;**61**:1134–41.

29. Stocchetti N, Furlan A, Volta F. Hypoxemia and arterial hypotension at the accident scene in head injury. *J Trauma* 1996;**40**:764–7.

30. Coles JP, Fryer TD, Coleman MR, et al. Hyperventilation following head injury: effect on ischemic burden and cerebral oxidative metabolism. *Crit Care Med* 2007;**35**:568–78.

31. Davis DP, Idris AH, Sise MJ, et al. Early ventilation and outcome in patients with moderate to severe traumatic brain injury. *Crit Care Med* 2006;**34**:1202–8.

32. Dumont TM, Visioni AJ, Rughani AI, et al. Inappropriate prehospital ventilation in severe traumatic brain injury increases in-hospital mortality. *J Neurotrauma* 2010;**27**:1233–41.

33. Helm M, Hauke J, Lampl L. A prospective study of the quality of pre-hospital emergency ventilation in

patients with severe head injury. *Br J Anaesth* 2002;**88**:345–9.

34. Zhou Q, Cao B, Niu L, *et al*. Effects of permissive hypercapnia on transient global cerebral ischemia-reperfusion injury in rats. *Anesthesiology* 2010;**112**:288–97.

35. Rovlias A, Kotsou S. The influence of hyperglycemia on neurological outcome in patients with severe head injury. *Neurosurgery* 2000;**46**:335–42; discussion 42–3.

36. Lipshutz AK, Gropper MA. Perioperative glycemic control: an evidence-based review. *Anesthesiology* 2009;**110**:408–21.

37. Anderson RE, Tan WK, Martin HS, *et al*. Effects of glucose and PaO_2 modulation on cortical intracellular acidosis, NADH redox state, and infarction in the ischemic penumbra. *Stroke* 1999;**30**:160–70.

38. Liu J, Gao BB, Clermont AC, *et al*. Hyperglycemia-induced cerebral hematoma expansion is mediated by plasma kallikrein. *Nat Med* 2011;**17**:206–10.

39. Polito A, Brouland JP, Porcher R, *et al*. Hyperglycaemia and apoptosis of microglial cells in human septic shock. *Crit Care* 2011;**15**:R131.

40. van den Berghe G, Wouters P, Weekers F, *et al*. Intensive insulin therapy in the critically ill patients. *N Engl J Med* 2001;**345**:1359–67.

41. Finfer S, Chittock DR, Su SY, *et al*. Intensive versus conventional glucose control in critically ill patients. *N Engl J Med* 2009;**360**:1283–97.

42. Gray CS, Hildreth AJ, Sandercock PA, *et al*. Glucose-potassium-insulin infusions in the management of post-stroke hyperglycaemia: the UK Glucose Insulin in Stroke Trial (GIST-UK). *Lancet Neurol* 2007;**6**:397–406.

43. Bilotta F, Caramia R, Cernak I, *et al*. Intensive insulin therapy after severe traumatic brain injury: a randomized clinical trial. *Neurocrit Care* 2008;**9**:159–66.

44. Vespa P, Boonyaputthikul R, McArthur DL, *et al*. Intensive insulin therapy reduces microdialysis glucose values without altering glucose utilization or improving the lactate/pyruvate ratio after traumatic brain injury. *Crit Care Med* 2006;**34**:850–6.

45. Bergsneider M, Hovda DA, Shalmon E, *et al*. Cerebral hyperglycolysis following severe traumatic brain injury in humans: a positron emission tomography study. *J Neurosurg* 1997;**86**:241–51.

46. Hopwood SE, Parkin MC, Bezzina EL, *et al*. Transient changes in cortical glucose and lactate levels associated with peri-infarct depolarisations, studied with rapid-sampling microdialysis. *J Cereb Blood Flow Metab* 2005;**25**:391–401.

47. Egi M, Finfer S, Bellomo R. Glycemic control in the ICU. *Chest* 2011;**140**:212–20.

48. Weiskopf RB, Kramer JH, Viele M, *et al*. Acute severe isovolemic anemia impairs cognitive function and memory in humans. *Anesthesiology* 2000;**92**:1646–52.

49. Karkouti K, Djaiani G, Borger MA, *et al*. Low hematocrit during cardiopulmonary bypass is associated with increased risk of perioperative stroke in cardiac surgery. *Ann Thorac Surg* 2005;**80**:1381–7.

50. Hare GM, Mazer CD, Hutchison JS, *et al*. Severe hemodilutional anemia increases cerebral tissue injury following acute neurotrauma. *J Appl Physiol* 2007;**103**:1021–9.

51. McIntyre LA, Fergusson DA, Hutchison JS, *et al*. Effect of a liberal versus restrictive transfusion strategy on mortality in patients with moderate to severe head injury. *Neurocrit Care* 2006;**5**:4–9.

52. Hare GM, Mazer CD, Mak W, *et al*. Hemodilutional anemia is associated with increased cerebral neuronal nitric oxide synthase gene expression. *J Appl Physiol* 2003;**94**:2058–67.

53. Pawloski JR, Hess DT, Stamler JS. Export by red blood cells of nitric oxide bioactivity. *Nature* 2001;**409**:622–6.

54. Hare GM, Tsui AK, McLaren AT, *et al*. Anemia and cerebral outcomes: many questions, fewer answers. *Anesth Analg* 2008;**107**:1356–70.

55. McLaren AT, Marsden PA, Mazer CD, *et al*. Increased expression of HIF-1alpha, nNOS, and VEGF in the cerebral cortex of anemic rats. *Am J Physiol Regul Integr Comp Physiol* 2007;**292**:R403–14.

56. Velly L, Pellegrini L, Guillet B, *et al*. Erythropoietin 2nd cerebral protection after acute injuries: a double-edged sword? *Pharmacol Ther* 2010;**128**:445–59.

57. Carlson AP, Schermer CR, Lu SW. Retrospective evaluation of anemia and transfusion in traumatic brain injury. *J Trauma* 2006;**61**:567–71.

58. Kramer AH, Gurka MJ, Nathan B, *et al*. Complications associated with anemia and blood transfusion in patients with aneurysmal subarachnoid hemorrhage. *Crit Care Med* 2008;**36**:2070–5.

59. Dhar R, Zazulia AR, Videen TO, *et al*. Red blood cell transfusion increases cerebral oxygen delivery in anemic patients with subarachnoid hemorrhage. *Stroke* 2009;**40**:3039–44.

60. Le Roux PD. Anemia and transfusion after subarachnoid hemorrhage. *Neurocrit Care* 2011;**15**:342–53.

61. Utter GH, Shahlaie K, Zwienenberg-Lee M, *et al*. Anemia in the setting of traumatic brain injury: the arguments for and against liberal transfusion. *J Neurotrauma* 2011;**28**:155–65.

62. Nabbout R, Vezzani A, Dulac O, *et al.* Acute encephalopathy with inflammation-mediated status epilepticus. *Lancet Neurol* 2011;**10**:99–108.

63. Scherbel U, Raghupathi R, Nakamura M, *et al.* Differential acute and chronic responses of tumor necrosis factor-deficient mice to experimental brain injury. *Proc Natl Acad Sci USA* 1999;**96**: 8721–6.

64. Thompson HJ, Tkacs NC, Saatman KE, *et al.* Hyperthermia following traumatic brain injury: a critical evaluation. *Neurobiol Dis* 2003;**12**: 163–73.

65. Rossi S, Zanier ER, Mauri I, *et al.* Brain temperature, body core temperature, and intracranial pressure in acute cerebral damage. *J Neurol Neurosurg Psychiatry* 2001;**71**:448–54.

66. Greer DM, Funk SE, Reaven NL, *et al.* Impact of fever on outcome in patients with stroke and neurologic injury: a comprehensive meta-analysis. *Stroke* 2008;**39**:3029–35.

67. den Hertog HM, van der Worp HB, van Gemert HM, *et al.* The Paracetamol (Acetaminophen) In Stroke (PAIS) trial: a multicentre, randomised, placebo-controlled, phase III trial. *Lancet Neurol* 2009;**8**:434–40.

68. Kiyatkin EA. Brain temperature homeostasis: physiological fluctuations and pathological shifts. *Front Biosci* 2010;**15**:73–92.

69. Sacho RH, Vail A, Rainey T, *et al.* The effect of spontaneous alterations in brain temperature on outcome: a prospective observational cohort study in patients with severe traumatic brain injury. *J Neurotrauma* 2010;**27**:2157–64.

70. Iacobone E, Bailly-Salin J, Polito A, *et al.* Sepsis-associated encephalopathy and its differential diagnosis. *Crit Care Med* 2009;**37**:S331–6.

71. van Gool WA, van de Beek D, Eikelenboom P. Systemic infection and delirium: when cytokines and acetylcholine collide. *Lancet* 2010;**375**:773–5.

72. Taccone FS, Su F, Pierrakos C, *et al.* Cerebral microcirculation is impaired during sepsis: an experimental study. *Crit Care* 2010;**14**:R140.

73. Sharshar T, Gray F, Lorin de la Grandmaison G, *et al.* Apoptosis of neurons in cardiovascular autonomic centres triggered by inducible nitric oxide synthase after death from septic shock. *Lancet* 2003;**362**:1799–805.

74. Sharshar T, Carlier R, Bernard F, *et al.* Brain lesions in septic shock: a magnetic resonance imaging study. *Intensive Care Med* 2007;**33**:798–806.

Cerebral ischemia and reperfusion

Raymond C. Koehler

SUMMARY

Neuronal injury arising from cerebral ischemia depends on the severity and duration of ischemia. With complete cerebral ischemia due to cardiac arrest, different populations of neurons are selectively vulnerable to different durations of arrest based on their input from other neuronal populations, their neurotransmitter receptor profile, and internal signaling cascade. With focal cerebral ischemia, vulnerability depends on the severity of blood flow reduction. Early changes include decreased protein synthesis with moderate reductions in blood flow, decreased oxygen consumption and electrical activity with more severe reductions in blood flow, and neuronal depolarization and large-scale release of neurotransmitters with very severe reductions in blood flow. In general, the amount of tissue that can be salvaged by reperfusion and neuroprotective agents decreases dramatically as the duration of ischemia is extended over a period of several hours. Recurrent waves of depolarization spreading over cortex metabolically tax compromised neurons in the ischemic border region. Even with restoration of blood flow and recovery of energy metabolism, neurons can undergo delayed cell death due to calcium homeostatic dysfunction, altered lipid signaling, generation of reactive oxygen species, stress in the endoplasmic reticulum, delayed impairment of mitochondrial respiration, mitochondrial depolarization, activation of inflammatory cells, and a milieu of pro-inflammatory cytokines. Demise of the cell can occur not only as a result of loss of ATP and bursting of cell membranes, but also by execution of caspase-dependent and caspase-independent cell signaling pathways. Evidence indicates that translocation of apoptosis-inducing factor from the mitochondria to the nucleus is a major caspase-independent pathway of neuronal cell death after ischemia and reperfusion. New research is being directed at protecting all components of the integrated neurovascular unit, determining how adult neural stem cells, cell therapy, and promotion of growth factors can aid in angiogenesis, reorganizing synaptic connections and neural networks, and improving functional outcome after cerebral ischemia. Finally, vascular risk factors not only increase the incidence of stroke, but also might worsen the severity of injury and interfere with repair of the brain after ischemia.

The brain consumes relatively large amounts of oxygen and glucose and is highly vulnerable to reductions in their supply. In this chapter, the concepts of how the severity and duration of cerebral ischemia influence the magnitude of injury will be addressed, and the sequence of mechanisms that lead to neuronal injury during ischemia and reperfusion will be discussed.

Blood flow thresholds

When perfusion pressure decreases, vasodilation helps to limit the reduction in cerebral blood flow (CBF; see Chapter 14, this volume, on autoregulation). As vasodilatory reserve becomes exhausted, increases in O_2 extraction help to maintain the global cerebral metabolic rate of oxygen ($CMRO_2$). However, the extraction reserve is limited, and reductions in $CMRO_2$ generally become apparent when CBF decreases by more than 50%. The reduction in $CMRO_2$ is not uniform on a microcirculatory scale. Images of tissue oxygenation markers can reveal spatial gradients spreading away from cortical penetrating arterioles and cortical capillaries. Thus, as O_2 supply becomes impaired, neurons furthest from arterioles and capillaries are most at risk of suffering impaired oxidative metabolism.

Brain Disorders in Critical Illness, ed. Robert D. Stevens, Tarek Sharshar, and E. Wesley Ely. Published by Cambridge University Press. © Cambridge University Press 2013.

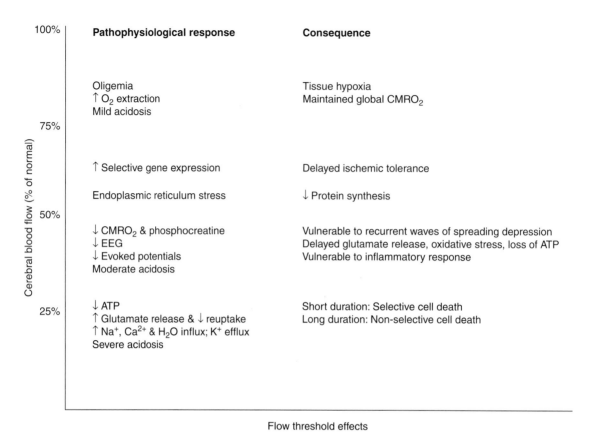

Flow threshold effects

Figure 13.1 Schematic of cerebral blood flow thresholds that produce pathophysiological responses and associated consequences to the tissue over different ranges of blood flow reductions.

On a macroscopic scale, the concept of flow thresholds has emerged over the past 30 years as summarized in Figure 13.1 [1]. Protein synthesis becomes impaired when CBF decreases below 50–60% of normal. Electroencephalographic activity and evoked potentials become impaired when CBF decreases below 40–50% of normal and when $CMRO_2$ is reduced (see Chapter 25, this volume, on electroencephalography and evoked potentials). Transmembrane ionic gradients are lost as neurons depolarize when CBF is decreased below 25–30% of normal. Loss of transmembrane ionic gradients causes water to shift from the extracellular compartment to the intracellular compartment. Because the unimpaired diffusion distances for water are smaller inside the cell, the apparent diffusion distances on MRI diffusion-weighted images (DWI) decrease in brain regions that have undergone anoxic depolarization. Prolonged loss of transmembrane ionic gradients leads to cell death. Likewise, regions with persistent changes in DWI are destined to undergo massive cell death. In contrast,

regions of brain with impaired electrical activity or protein synthesis have the potential to survive if CBF is restored. However, if CBF remains below 50–60% of normal for an extended period of time, neurons in these regions will eventually die.

When focal cerebral ischemia is produced by occlusion of a major cerebral artery, a macroscopic spatial gradient of CBF arises as a result of anastomoses between pial arteries supplied by the anterior, middle, and posterior cerebral arteries. Collateral blood flow through these anastomoses is thought to be diminished in experimental models of chronic hypertension. The spatial gradient of CBF can produce a patchwork of areas that undergoes rapid anoxic depolarization and that is often referred to as the ischemic core. The ischemic core is surrounded by regions that have intermediate reductions in CBF and associated impaired electrical activity and protein synthesis. These regions of potentially salvageable tissue are often called the penumbra. Finally, the penumbra can be surrounded by regions with mild reductions of CBF that will not result in eventual infarction. Such mild reductions in CBF are referred to as oligemia.

From a clinical perspective, knowledge of which regions are destined to die and which are potentially salvageable would be useful for tailoring individual therapy and for enrollment of patients in neuroprotective clinical trials. Perfusion-weighted imaging (PWI) with MRI is often used to define the volume of tissue in which blood flow is reduced to levels below the oligemic range. The difference between volume demarcated by PWI and that demarcated by DWI can be used to assess a salvageable penumbral tissue volume. However, this assessment of penumbra is a rough estimate since the transition from oligemia to penumbra is not precise and because the thresholds used to demarcate vulnerable regions in PWI and DWI may not be optimal for a particular patient [2]. Consequently, the PWI/DWI mismatch can overestimate the penumbra defined by other measures [1]. Moreover, functional outcome is highly dependent on the location of the injury, and rescuing a small volume of tissue in a critical region could have a disproportionate effect on outcome. Thus, location can be as important as volume when assessing the mismatch between PWI and DWI.

Duration of ischemia

Neuronal injury depends on both the severity and duration of reduced CBF. In the case of complete cerebral ischemia produced by cardiac arrest, ATP is depleted within a few minutes. As ATP decreases, large influxes of sodium and calcium ions and an efflux of potassium ions cause neurons to undergo anoxic depolarization. Return of spontaneous circulation can often result in rapid recovery of ATP production by mitochondria and restoration of transcellular ion gradients. However, oxidative stress and mitochondrial dysfunction can lead to metabolic disturbances hours or even days after resuscitation from cardiac arrest and produce delayed neurodegeneration. The magnitude and the delay of neurodegeneration depend on the duration of complete ischemia. In general, as the duration of complete ischemia is extended over an approximate range of 3–30 minutes, more neurons undergo secondary metabolic failure, and the delay becomes progressively shorter. As the duration of complete ischemia lengthens, mitochondrial dysfunction becomes so severe that an increasing number of cells are unable to restore transcellular ionic gradients and undergo rapid necrotic cell death.

If ischemia is incomplete, the time to reach critically low levels of ATP decreases exponentially with increased severity of CBF reduction. Thus, neurons in the ischemic core may undergo depolarization over a period of tens of minutes, whereas those in the penumbra may require several hours. Electrical silence in penumbral neurons helps to decrease metabolic demand and conserve ATP for maintenance of ionic gradients. Rapid loss of dendritic spines in neurons has been observed and may contribute to decreased connectivity. Using hypothermia and barbiturates to decrease intraischemic metabolic demand can also extend the time that brain ATP is sustained during incomplete ischemia. On the other hand, recurrent spreading waves of depolarization occur in cerebral cortex during ischemic stroke. Restoration of ionic gradients after repetitive depolarization taxes the limited availability of ATP and may push neurons in the penumbra that are on the metabolic cusp into a state of irreversible depolarization. Thus, spreading waves of depolarization are thought to accelerate the conversion of penumbra into regions of irreversible injury [3]. Because the reduction in CBF during ischemic stroke is highly variable, the time during which penumbral tissue can be salvaged is also highly heterogeneous among patients. Figure 13.2 summarizes the sequence of major events occurring during ischemic stroke, including the transition from penumbral tissue to infarcted tissue and subsequent brain repair processes.

Injury during reperfusion

Because the degree of neuronal injury is critically dependent on ischemic duration, rapid restoration of CBF is a major goal for patients who have undergone cardiac arrest or ischemic stroke (see Chapter 37, this volume, for further discussion of hypoxic-ischemic encephalopathy). However, restoration of CBF does not necessarily halt the injury process. Damage to cell organelles impairs normal cellular function and decreases the ability of the cell to handle additional oxidative stress. Calcium entry during ischemia overloads the intracellular calcium buffering capacity of the endoplasmic reticulum (ER) and mitochondria and may limit the capabilities of this safety mechanism during early reperfusion. Removal of excess intracellular sodium by sodium-calcium exchangers results in additional calcium influx during early reperfusion. Extracellular glutamate increases during ischemia as a result of synaptic release and impaired reuptake by glial and neuronal glutamate

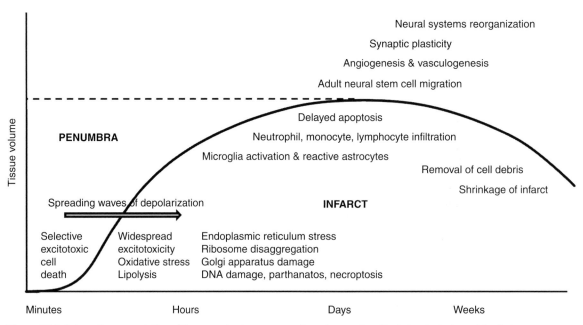

Figure 13.2 Schematic representation of the approximate sequence of events occurring after ischemic stroke and the factors that play a role in the transition of salvageable tissue in the penumbra to eventual infarction.

transporters that depend on a normal sodium gradient. Persistent elevations of extracellular glutamate during early reperfusion will stimulate sodium and calcium entry through AMPA and NMDA receptors and lead to excitotoxicity. After extracellular glutamate is restored, excitotoxicity can persist because glutamate receptor phosphorylation can cause alterations in calcium influx and receptor trafficking to the membrane. Such phosphorylation can be modulated by other neurotransmitters [4]. Sodium and calcium also can enter cells through acid-sensitive ion channels that are activated at pH below 7.0. Persistent acidosis in brain during reperfusion is thought to enhance intracellular calcium by this and possibly other mechanisms [5]. Thus, multiple mechanisms contribute to calcium dyshomeostasis during reperfusion. Calcium dyshomeostasis has many adverse consequences, including stimulation of calcium-dependent phopholipase-A_2, calcium/calmodulin stimulation of neuronal nitric oxide (NO) synthase and calcium-activated proteases such as calpains, and increased formation of reactive oxygen species (ROS).

Phospholipase A_2-generated eicosanoids

Stimulation of phospholipases during ischemia mobilizes arachidonic acids and other fatty acids.

Reoxygenation permits metabolism of fatty acids by various oxygenase enzymes, the metabolites of which can have adverse or protective actions. For example, the cyclooxygenase metabolite PGE2 exerts adverse effects via stimulation of EP1 and EP3 receptors and beneficial effects via EP2 receptors and possibly EP4 receptors [6]. Furthermore, the cyclooxygenase products PGD_2 and PGI_2 can exert protective effects via their actions on DP1 and IP receptors, respectively, whereas PGD_2 may also act on DP2 receptors to promote neuronal death. The net effect of inhibiting cyclooxygenase-1 and cyclooxygenase-2 activity during ischemia is neuroprotection. The lipoxygenase pathway is generally considered to exert adverse effects, but these effects appear to be less profound than those arising from the cyclooxygenase pathway. Arachidonic acid is also metabolized by specific cytochrome P450 enzymes to produce 20-hydroxyeicosatetraenoic acid (20-HETE) and epoxyeicosatrienoic acids (EETs). 20-HETE contributes to cerebral vasoconstriction during hypertension and subarachnoid hemorrhage, but it also exerts direct neuronal effects that contribute to ischemic injury [7]. In contrast, EETs contribute to cerebral vasodilation during neuronal activation[8] and ischemia [9]. They may also exert ischemic neuroprotection by their anti-inflammatory properties. Therefore, arachidonic acid metabolites exert diverse effects, but the over-abundance of arachidonic acid during ischemia and reperfusion leads to a preponderance of adverse cell signaling that contributes to neuronal injury. On the other hand, metabolites of docosahexaenoic acid are generally considered to have beneficial effects.

Reactive oxygen species

The increased calcium load, together with impaired oxidative phosphorylation in mitochondria, provides a source of superoxide anion, which can then be converted to hydrogen peroxide by superoxide dismutase (SOD). Up-regulation of NADPH oxidase activity has taken on increasing importance as another source of superoxide during reperfusion. Other sources that are thought to be particularly important in endothelium are xanthine oxidase and NO synthase, the latter of which can become uncoupled and generate superoxide instead of NO. Because ischemic injury varies inversely with expression of SOD, superoxide is considered to play an important role in oxidative stress during reoxygenation [10]. Nitric oxide is another important player. Neuronal NO synthase associates with postsynaptic density-95 protein near NMDA receptors and is stimulated by the influx of calcium. Superoxide and NO rapidly combine to form highly reactive peroxynitrite, which can damage DNA, RNA, lipids, and proteins. Superoxide can also enter into other pathways, augment release of free iron, and produce hydroxyl radicals. Lipid peroxidation chain reactions are initiated by rearrangement of double bonds in polyunsaturated fatty acids to form conjugated dienes, lipid peroxyl radicals, a lipid hydroperoxide, and a lipid alkoxyl radical that propagates additional lipid peroxidation. Furthermore, the increases in protein carbonyl formation and nitration of tyrosine moieties by peroxynitrite are thought to alter the function of certain proteins. The combination of lipid peroxidation, protein carbonyl formation, and protein nitration during reoxygenation is thought to alter membrane function in the cell membrane, ER, Golgi apparatus, and nuclear envelope.

Endoplasmic reticulum stress

Severe ischemia impairs protein synthesis as a result of decreased ATP availability. However, protein synthesis can also be impaired with normal levels of ATP during moderate ischemia or during reperfusion from severe ischemia. Oxidative damage to ER lipid membrane and proteins and depletion of ER calcium stores causes unfolded proteins to accumulate. During ischemia and reperfusion, an ER stress signaling system is activated that triggers a response to unfolded proteins accumulating in the ER lumen [11]. Ordinarily, this response induces the synthesis of chaperone proteins to assist in proper folding and increases phosphorylation of eukaryotic initiation factor 2α (eIF2α) to slow overall protein translation and accumulation of unfolded proteins. The protein glucose-regulated protein-78 (GRP-78) is normally bound in the ER membrane to two kinases: RNA-dependent protein kinase-like ER eIF2α kinase (PERK) and inositol-requiring enzyme (IRE1). When unfolded proteins accumulate, GRP-78 dissociates from these two kinases and binds to the unfolded proteins. Upon dissociation, PERK phosphorylates eIF2α to suppress protein synthesis, and IRE1 is activated to cut X-box binding protein-1 (xbp1) mRNA. The spliced xbp1 mRNA then induces transcription of ER chaperone proteins. However, the unfolded protein response may not resolve after ischemia because ER damage is too severe to express the spliced xbp1 protein or the chaperone proteins. Moreover, PERK is normally dephosphorylated by GADD34, but its protein expression may also be impaired after ischemia. Severe damage to the ER may limit its ability to repair itself. Furthermore, cross-talk between the ER and apoptotic signaling molecules can augment apoptosis. In general, neurons with a prolonged ER stress response are destined to die from apoptosis or from an inability to replenish the normal turnover of proteins. Because overexpression of SOD attenuates the ER stress response, early administration of antioxidants is postulated to provide neuroprotection, in part, by ameliorating ER stress.

Mechanisms of cell death

Secondary injury takes place in mitochondria where opening of the mitochondrial transition pore results in loss of the membrane potential that is necessary for normal respiration. Activity of the tricarboxylic cycle becomes limited by loss of pyruvate dehydrogenase activity. Alternative substrates that bypass this bottleneck, such as ketones and acetyl-L-carnitine, have been shown to provide protection in some models of global and focal ischemia. However, neurons without sufficient ATP to maintain ionic gradients during severe ischemia swell and die by necrosis. Neurons with sufficient ATP to maintain ionic gradients during moderate ischemia or during reperfusion after severe or moderate ischemia may still die by some form of regulated cell death.

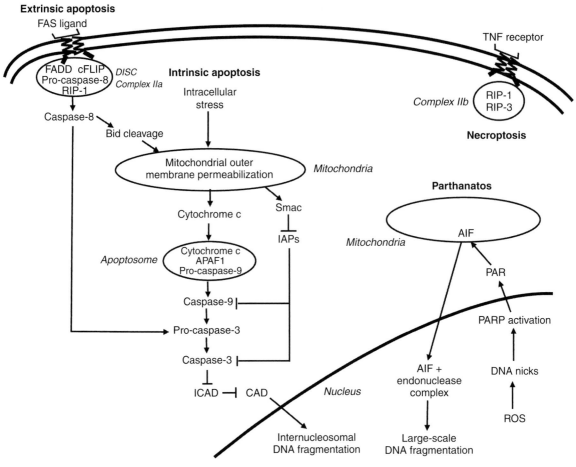

Figure 13.3 Schematic diagram of the major ischemic cell death signaling pathways for extrinsic apoptosis, intrinsic apoptosis, pathanatos, and necroptosis. AIF, apoptosis-inducing factor; APAF1, apoptosis protease activating factor; Bid, BH3-interacting domain death agonist; CAD, caspase-activated deoxyribonuclease; cFLIP, [FADD-like interleukin-1β-converting enzyme]-inhibitory protein; DISC, death-inducing signal complex; FADD, FAS-associated death domain; IAPs, inhibitors of apoptosis protein; ICAD, inhibitor of CAD; PAR, PARP, poly(ADP-ribose) polymerase; poly(ADP-ribose) polymers; RIP, receptor interacting protein kinase; ROS, reactive oxygen species; Smac, second mitochondria-derived activator of caspases; TNF receptor, tumor necrosis factor receptor.

Many forms of regulated cell death exist [12], but those involved in cerebral ischemia are broadly categorized into intrinsic and extrinsic caspase-dependent cell death and intrinsic and extrinsic caspase-independent cell death. Key features of these pathways are summarized in Figure 13.3. Classical apoptosis requires caspases. Intrinsic apoptosis involves mitochondrial outer membrane permeabilization and loss of membrane potential in a large portion of the cell's mitochondria, release of cytochrome c from mitochondria, and a molecular interaction of cytochrome c with pro-caspase-9 and the adapter protein APAF1 to form the apoptosome. The apoptosome platform stimulates activation of caspase-9 and consequent cleavage of pro-caspase-3 to active caspase-3.

Caspase-3 then stimulates a specific caspase-activated endonuclease to degrade genomic DNA. This pathway is well regulated at each step. Various inhibitory proteins can act as brakes on the formation of activated caspase-9 and caspase-3. Moreover, mitochondrial permeabilization and release of cytochrome c from the mitochondria is influenced by the balance of pro-apoptotic (Bax, Bak) and anti-apoptotic (Bcl-2) members of the Bcl-2 family. In addition, oxidative damage to DNA activates p53, which produces a truncated form of Bid that then promotes mitochondrial depolarization and cytochrome c release.

One of the major caspase-independent intrinsic pathways of cell death after cerebral ischemia involves poly(ADP-ribose) polymerase (PARP) and apoptosis-inducing factor (AIF). Oxidative damage to DNA normally activates PARP, which adds poly(ADP-ribose) polymer chains onto histones to expand the double helix and allow the operation of the DNA repair machinery. However, after ischemia and reperfusion, widespread oxidative damage to DNA can lead to robust activation of PARP. A portion of the poly(ADP-ribose) polymers exit the nucleus on a binding partner and trigger release of AIF from the mitochondria. The released AIF translocates to the nucleus and activates a different endonuclease to produce large-scale DNA degradation. This PARP-dependent cell death pathway has been denoted as parthanatos [13]. In cultured neurons, cell death from NMDA exposure occurs primarily by parthanatos, whereas cell death from AMPA exposure occurs primarily by caspase-dependent apoptosis.

In extrinsic apoptosis, extracellular ligands of the FAS, tumor necrosis factor alpha (TNFα), and TNF-related apoptosis inducing ligand (TRAIL) receptors on the plasma membrane lead to recruitment of receptor interacting protein-1 (RIP-1) and other proteins to form complex I. This complex can lead to formation of a death-inducing signal complex (DISC or complex IIa), which includes RIP-1, pro-caspase-8, and the FAS-associated protein with a death domain (FADD). Formation of DISC leads to activation of caspase-8, which then cleaves pro-caspase-3 to stimulate the caspase-activated endonuclease. Activation of caspase-8 also increases formation of truncated Bid, which then amplifies the intrinsic apoptotic pathway. Under some conditions, the binding of TNFα to its receptor is associated with ubiquitination of RIP-1 in complex I and leads to activation of nuclear factor kB instead of DISC formation.

A caspase-independent pathway also involves stimulation of FAS, TNFα, or TRAIL receptors and formation of complex I. However, in this case a different complex is formed in the cytosol. This complex, denoted complex IIb, is formed by an interaction between RIP-1 and RIP-3 through the kinase activity of RIP-1. Complex IIb induces cell death by a mechanism that is not entirely clear but which morphologically resembles necrosis rather than apoptosis. This form of cell death has been denoted as RIP-1-dependent regulated necrosis (necroptosis).

Experiments in which male animals have been subjected to ischemic stroke have shown that PARP inhibitors, PARP-1 gene deletion, and decreased AIF expression produce substantial reductions in infarct volume. Thus, parthanatos serves as a major cell death pathway in ischemic stroke, at least in males. Interestingly, a small molecule inhibitor of RIP-1 kinase activity also reduces infarct volume in male animals, thereby indicating that necroptosis also contributes to cell death from ischemic stroke. The infarct volume in young, healthy female animals is generally smaller than that in their male counterparts within 1 day of experimental transient focal ischemia. The smaller infarct size in female animals is partly attributable to estrogen effects on collateral blood flow. Surprisingly, experimental evidence indicates that the primary pathways responsible for cell death differ between male and female animals, and this difference is independent of estrogen levels. Infarct volume reduction in females is more sensitive to caspase inhibitors than to PARP inhibitors or gene deletion. Furthermore, females have a greater activation of caspase-8 and a down-regulation of the X-chromosome-linked inhibitory apoptotic protein that normally suppresses caspase-3 activation [14]. Thus, female animals appear to utilize canonical apoptotic signaling to a greater degree than do males after transient focal cerebral ischemia. However, the morphology of most dying neurons does not resemble that of pure apoptosis, and hybrid pathways of cell death are likely to be recruited.

Selective vulnerability

Global ischemia and reperfusion do not produce neuronal loss in a random fashion. Rather, subpopulations of neurons are selectively vulnerable. Brief global ischemia followed by reperfusion produces selective injury in hippocampal CA1 pyramidal neurons, and the delay in cell death is inversely related to the duration of ischemia. With increasing ischemic durations, cell death becomes increasingly evident in cerebellar Purkinje neurons, striatal medium spiny neurons, neocortical neurons, CA2 and CA3 regions of hippocampus, thalamic sensory nuclei, and some brainstem nuclei. In immature brain, the CA1 region of hippocampus is not more vulnerable than other hippocampal regions, and portions of non-primary sensorimotor cortex that are not fully metabolically active are more resistant to ischemia than are active regions. Delayed subclinical seizure activity may eventually develop in association with propagated injury in limbic structures.

In experimental models of proximal middle cerebral artery occlusion, cell death becomes evident in striatum with as little as 15–30 minutes of occlusion followed by reperfusion, whereas cortical injury usually requires longer durations of occlusion. The striatum is considered to be more vulnerable than cortex to focal ischemia because its collateral blood flow is less than that of cortex during middle cerebral artery occlusion. In addition, medium spiny neurons may have greater intrinsic vulnerability than some populations of cortical neurons.

Selective vulnerability is generally attributable to the balance of excitatory and inhibitory inputs. Neurons with high densities of glutamate receptors are considered particularly vulnerable. Loss of GABA-releasing neurons shifts the balance in neuronal circuits and may lead to increased excitability in remaining neurons. Thus, vulnerability depends on the expression of excitatory neurotransmitter receptors in the cell membrane, the particular neuronal circuitry, and how the strength of neurotransmission changes over time. Slow neurotransmitters that modulate the function and internalization of glutamate receptors presumably are also important. Thus, dopaminergic receptors in the striatum of newborns appear to modulate excitotoxic damage in this region and contribute to its selective vulnerability in term neonatal hypoxic-ischemic encephalopathy [15].

Blood–brain barrier

Prolonged cerebral ischemia leads to increased permeability across the blood–brain barrier. Instituting reperfusion can accelerate damage to the barrier. When the duration of focal ischemia exceeds several hours, reperfusion can result in petechial hemorrhage. Hemorrhage is more likely to occur in ischemic core where neurons are already undergoing cell death. Gross disruption of the barrier is mediated by activation of matrix metalloproteinases (MMPs), such as MMP-9.

Tissue plasminogen activator (tPA) is used to dissolve clots and restore perfusion. Although it was originally approved for use within 3 hours of the onset of stroke symptoms, a more recent European trial with tPA demonstrated significant benefit to stroke victims when used within 4.5 hours from the onset of symptoms [16]. With reperfusion beyond 4.5 hours, the amount of remaining tissue that can be salvaged presumably becomes relatively small and, in most patients, will not have a substantial effect on neurological outcome. In addition, tPA has adverse effects that may negate the benefit of reoxygenation. For example, tPA can augment excitotoxicity via NMDA receptors and increase the activation of MMPs during reperfusion. The latter effect promotes barrier disruption and hemorrhagic transformation. Several experimental studies have tested a variety of adjunct therapies to limit the adverse effects of delayed tPA administration with the hope of extending the therapeutic time window for its administration.

Inflammation

Severe oxidative stress and neuronal injury generate an inflammatory response (see also Chapter 18, this volume, on inflammatory mechanisms) [17]. Dying cells release molecules, such as advanced glycation endproducts (AGE), high mobility group B1 (HMGB1), and hyaluronic acid. These molecules provide a danger signal that is sensed by a variety of receptors, including receptors for AGE (RAGE) and Toll-like receptors, and serve to activate nuclear factor κB and other transcription factors, which then induce an inflammatory response. In the case of focal cerebral ischemia, microglia become activated and transform into a macrophage state within several hours. Cytokines released by vascular cells and microglia stimulate expression of adhesion molecules and integrins on the endothelial wall. Rolling and sticking leukocytes can be observed within a few hours of the onset of ischemia and reperfusion. In general, neutrophil transmigration into the ischemic zone begins within the first day, monocytes within the second day, and lymphocytes 2 days after ischemia. This profile may be accelerated with severe ischemia. Recent evidence suggests that the spleen may serve as a source for cytokines and inflammatory cells in stroke (see also Chapter 17, this volume, on neuro-immunological cross-talk).

In the ischemic border regions, some neurons die rapidly while others remain temporarily viable. As the infarction process proceeds, these remaining neurons in the border region succumb for a variety of reasons related to impaired energy metabolism and protein synthesis; oxidative stress; loss of trophic factors; and the milieu of cytokines, chemokines, and other inflammatory molecules. Activated microglia and blood-borne macrophages migrate to the border zone and phagocytose dying cells and debris. Numerous strategies have been tested in experimental stroke models to blunt various components of the inflammatory response and the spread of infarction.

However, none has yet been successfully translated into clinical practice. At later recovery times, the inflammatory response may help set the stage for the repair process.

Brain repair

The brain retains some capacity to rewire itself and compensate for lost cortical function. Functional MRI, optical imaging, and electrophysiology indicate dynamic changes in peri-infarct neuronal circuits. Neuronal plasticity is presumed to depend on repeated use and release of trophic factors that lead to reorganization of neuronal dendrites, spines, and synapses. Because the effect of growth factors on neurons can depend on co-activation of NMDA receptors, functioning NMDA receptors are thought to play a positive role in the repair process. Astrocytes, which sense and integrate the activity of many synapses, release brain-derived neurotrophic factor (BDNF), which promotes connectivity. Increases in vascular endothelial growth factor stimulate sprouting of new blood vessels in the peri-infarct region. Activated MMPs degrade the extracellular matrix and permit sprouting of new blood vessels and neuronal dendrites. The nuclear protein HMGB1 normally stimulates inflammation when released from dying neurons in the acute injury phase, but its release from reactive astrocytes in the repair phase is thought to help promote angiogenesis. Microglia may release BDNF and glial-derived neurotrophic factor during the repair phase of recovery. Thus, specific treatments designed to inhibit inflammation may need to be limited to the acute phase of injury so as not to impair functional recovery [17].

Cortical reorganization during the repair process relies on integrated signaling among neurons, astrocytes, microglia, oligodendrocytes, endothelial cells, pericytes, and smooth muscle. Thus, enhancing the repair process depends on the health of individual components of the neurovascular unit. Consequently, increasing efforts have been made at protecting the neurovascular unit during the acute phase and promoting positive interactive signaling during the repair phase of injury. In addition to pharmacological approaches with erythropoietin and phosphodiesterase inhibitors, cell therapy strategies have been successfully applied in experimental stroke models. Interestingly, chemoattractants in injured brain are sufficient to recruit systemically administered bone marrow-derived mesenchymal cells and endothelial progenitor cells to the injured site. Although these cells are not transformed into neurons, the interstitial milieu of the injured brain is thought to stimulate these transplanted cells to generate trophic factors that then improve the health of endogenous astrocytes and vascular cells and promote their own production of trophic factors. Indeed, exogenous cell therapy administered after experimental stroke provides long-term improvements in functional recovery [18]. In addition, endogenous adult neural stem cells migrate to the injured site where they also are thought to provide a source of trophic factors for repair mechanisms. Ways to augment stem cell migration and function are under investigation.

Vascular risk factors

Hypertension, hypercholesterolemia, diabetes, cigarette smoking, aging, and hyperhomocysteinemia represent vascular risk factors for stroke [17]. They can also exacerbate injury once stroke occurs. Chronic hypertension produces inward remodeling of large cerebral arteries, rarefaction of small vessels, and limited collateral blood flow. In general, the risk factors produce a pro-oxidant state that can augment the inflammatory response in cerebral vessels. Mitochondrial production of ROS can be increased in the endothelium. In addition, angiotensin-2 and β-amyloid promote superoxide production by NADPH oxidase. The increased superoxide combines with NO to form peroxynitrite and reduces bioavailability of NO. Risk factors may also reduce endothelial NO production by changes in NO synthase expression and trafficking to caveolae, rho-kinase induced suppression of NO synthase activity, post-translational modifications, and arginine and tetrahydrobiopterin availability. Statins, exercise, and activation of peroxisome proliferator-activated receptor γ can improve endothelial NO synthase function and may counter some of the adverse effects of risk factors. Suppression of NO synthase function not only impairs smooth muscle relaxation but can increase platelet aggregation and limit angiogenesis and collateral formation; it may also have secondary effects on the endothelial niche for neurogenesis and oligodendrocyte precursors after stroke. Thus, vascular risk factors may also influence the repair process during recovery from stroke by impeding protection of the neurovascular unit.

Conclusion

Ischemia and reperfusion initiate a complex cascade of events in neurons, glia, vascular cells, and extracellular matrix that together comprise the neurovascular unit. The injury process is highly dynamic and depends on complex signaling within cells and cross-talk among various types of cells. Therapeutic strategies need to consider the timing of the various steps in the injury cascade and repair process and the integrated response among elements of the neurovascular unit. Thus, emphasis is now being placed on strategies that acutely protect the neurovascular unit as a whole and that chronically enhance brain repair and restoration of neurological function.

References

1. Heiss WD. The ischemic penumbra: correlates in imaging and implications for treatment of ischemic stroke. The Johann Jacob Wepfer Award 2011. *Cerebrovasc Dis* 2011;**32**:307–20.

2. Dani KA, Thomas RG, Chappell FM, *et al.* Computed tomography and magnetic resonance perfusion imaging in ischemic stroke: definitions and thresholds. *Ann Neurol* 2011;**70**:384–401.

3. Lauritzen M, Dreier JP, Fabricius M, *et al.* Clinical relevance of cortical spreading depression in neurological disorders: migraine, malignant stroke, subarachnoid and intracranial hemorrhage, and traumatic brain injury. *J Cereb Blood Flow Metab* 2011;**31**:17–35.

4. Greengard P. The neurobiology of slow synaptic transmission. *Science* 2001;**294**:1024–30.

5. Pignataro G, Simon RP, Xiong ZG. Prolonged activation of ASIC1a and the time window for neuroprotection in cerebral ischaemia. *Brain* 2007;**130**:151–8.

6. Andreasson K. Emerging roles of PGE2 receptors in models of neurological disease. *Prostaglandins Other Lipid Mediat* 2010;**91**:104–12.

7. Renic M, Kumar SN, Gebremedhin D, *et al.* Protective effect of 20-HETE inhibition in a model of oxygen-glucose deprivation in hippocampal slice cultures. *Am J Physiol Heart Circ Physiol* 2012;**302**(6):H1285–93.

8. Koehler RC, Roman RJ, Harder DR. Astrocytes and the regulation of cerebral blood flow. *Trends Neurosci* 2009;**32**:160–9.

9. Zhang W, Otsuka T, Sugo N, *et al.* Soluble epoxide hydrolase gene deletion is protective against experimental cerebral ischemia. *Stroke* 2008;**39**: 2073–8.

10. Chen H, Yoshioka H, Kim GS, *et al.* Oxidative stress in ischemic brain damage: mechanisms of cell death and potential molecular targets for neuroprotection. *Antioxid Redox Signal* 2011;**14**:1505–17.

11. Paschen W, Mengesdorf T. Endoplasmic reticulum stress response and neurodegeneration. *Cell Calcium* 2005;**38**:409–15.

12. Galluzzi L, Vitale I, Abrams JM, *et al.* Molecular definitions of cell death subroutines: recommendations of the Nomenclature Committee on Cell Death 2012. *Cell Death Differ* 2012;**19**:107–20.

13. Wang Y, Kim NS, Haince JF, *et al.* Poly(ADP-ribose) (PAR) binding to apoptosis-inducing factor is critical for PAR polymerase-1-dependent cell death (parthanatos). *Sci Signal* 2011;**4**:ra20.

14. Siegel C, Li J, Liu F, Benashski SE, McCullough LD. miR-23a regulation of X-linked inhibitor of apoptosis (XIAP) contributes to sex differences in the response to cerebral ischemia. *Proc Natl Acad Sci USA* 2011;**108**:11662–7.

15. Yang ZJ, Torbey M, Li X, *et al.* Dopamine receptor modulation of hypoxic-ischemic neuronal injury in striatum of newborn piglets. *J Cereb Blood Flow Metab* 2007;**27**:1339–51.

16. Hacke W, Kaste M, Bluhmki E, *et al.* Thrombolysis with alteplase 3 to 4.5 hours after acute ischemic stroke. *N Engl J Med* 2008;**359**:1317–29.

17. Moskowitz MA, Lo EH, Iadecola C. The science of stroke: mechanisms in search of treatments. *Neuron* 2010;**67**:181–98.

18. Shen LH, Li Y, Chen J, *et al.* One-year follow-up after bone marrow stromal cell treatment in middle-aged female rats with stroke. *Stroke* 2007;**38**:2150–6.

Brain perfusion and autoregulation in systemic critical illness

Martin Siegemund and Luzius A. Steiner

SUMMARY

In systemic critical illnes, brain perfusion and auto-regulation may be profoundly affected. Changes in vascular tone and endothelial dysfunction are thought to play a key role in the development of alterations in cerebral perfusion, and blood–brain barrier dysfunction may further aggravate these effects. Data from animal models suggest that the cerebral microcirculation is not affected by hemorrhagic or cardiogenic but markedly by septic shock. In patients with septic shock, cerebral ischemia has been demonstrated. Homeostatic mechanisms such as cerebrovascular pressure autoregulation or CO_2-reactivity may be altered in systemic critical illness. However, only a few studies are available on this topic and their conclusions are often contradictory, as only small numbers of subjects recruited from different patient populations were investigated. Furthermore, in critically ill patients the effects on the cerebral circulation of vasopressors and other therapeutic interventions may be changed due to dysfunction of the blood–brain barrier. Despite the fact that alterations in cerebral perfusion are documented in several studies, based on the currently available data it is not possible to establish a clear link between brain dysfunction and altered cerebral perfusion in systemic critical illness.

Introduction

With increasing interest in brain dysfunction in critically ill patients, interest in cerebral perfusion and its role in brain dysfunction in critical care medicine is growing. However, most clinical studies on cerebral perfusion have been performed in brain-injured patients and extrapolation of the results of such studies to patients without neurological or neurosurgical disorders are of limited value. Nevertheless, there is a growing number of publications on cerebral perfusion, particularly in sepsis. For other forms of systemic critical illness such as the adult respiratory distress syndrome (ARDS) or hemorrhagic or cardiogenic shock, data are scarce despite the fact that any form of shock may profoundly influence cerebral perfusion and function due to hypotension and a reduction in oxygen transport. Apart from the underlying disease, some of our management strategies, e.g., those incorporating the use of vasopressors or permissive hypercapnia, may have an impact on cerebral perfusion. In this chapter we summarize the current literature on how cerebral perfusion and vascular reactivity may be changed in non-neurological and non-neurosurgical critically ill patients with or without clinically manifest brain dysfunction. Table 14.1 gives an overview of mechanisms potentially influencing cerebral perfusion in this group of patients.

Molecular mechanisms affecting cerebral perfusion in systemic critical illness

Vascular tone

Under normal conditions blood flow in the cerebral microcirculation is relatively heterogeneous. With increased oxygen and glucose demand of neurons and astrocytes, functional recruitment augments flow in normally slowly perfused capillaries through the release of diffusible vasodilators such as prostaglandin E2, arachidonic acid, and potassium. During acute critical illness this direct metabolic feedback may be altered [1].

Brain Disorders in Critical Illness, ed. Robert D. Stevens, Tarek Sharshar, and E. Wesley Ely. Published by Cambridge University Press. © Cambridge University Press 2013.

Table 14.1 Overview of factors potentially influencing cerebral perfusion in systemic critical illness.

Factor	Mechanism	Comments
Critical illness	Various forms of shock and vascular dysfunction	Different forms of shock seem to influence cerebral perfusion to a different extent
Physiological mechanisms	Cerebrovascular autoregulation	Determines effects of MAP on CBF. May be impaired
	CO_2-reactivity	Very strong influence of $PaCO_2$ on CBF
	O_2-reactivity	Hypoxia < 8 kPa increases CBF
	Flow-metabolism coupling	Governs effect of sedation on CBF
Therapy	Vasopressors	Integrity of blood–brain barrier and autoregulation will influence effects. May change pharmacokinetics of sedation
	Sedation	Reduces cerebral metabolism and blood flow. May affect autoregulation
	Permissive hypercapnia	Interferes with autoregulation

CBF: cerebral blood flow; MAP: mean arterial pressure; $PaCO_2$: arterial partial pressure of CO_2.

Blood–brain barrier and SIRS

The blood–brain barrier is a physical and metabolic barrier, constituted of cerebral microvascular endothelial cells, astrocytic foot processes, and pericytes, that restricts the passage of substances from the blood to the brain and helps maintain brain homeostasis and microvascular blood flow. In sepsis, cerebral endothelial cells are activated by microbial factors and pro-inflammatory cytokines. Leukocytes cross the endothelial layer and enter the brain. In a rat model of peritonitis by cecal ligation and puncture the increased leukocyte rolling and adherence directly altered microvascular flow, and increased local cytokine and chemokine levels [2]. Inflammatory processes also increase local activation of thrombocytes and coagulation factors. These local processes promote endothelial dysfunction and result in blood–brain barrier breakdown leading to perivascular edema as

well as ischemia due to microthrombosis [3]. The disturbed microvascular blood flow and the increased production of nitric oxide (NO) lead to an increase in reactive oxygen and nitrogen species (ROS/RNS) leading to lipid and endothelial peroxidation, inflammation, mitochondrial dysfunction, and apoptosis [4]. Reactive oxygen or nitrogen species either from activated leucocytes during inflammation or from ischemia and reperfusion alter the blood–brain barrier during critical illness. Hypoxia and reoxygenation as in stroke, cardiac arrest, and ARDS increase oxidative stress and blood–brain barrier permeability by an alteration of the intercellular tight junctions. Much of the cellular damage caused by a hypoxic insult is thought to occur during the reperfusion and oxygenation phase by alteration of the oligomeric assembly of the critical transmembrane tight junction protein occludine [5]. A synopsis of documented factors influencing the cerebral microcirculation and the blood–brain barrier is shown in Figure 14.1.

Any form of circulatory shock may be accompanied by severe brain dysfunction. The effect of different types of shock on the cerebral microcirculation has recently been characterized in animal models. In a rat model of *hemorrhagic* shock, cerebral microvascular flow was preserved during moderate and severe blood losses despite systemic decreases in pressure and flow, including decreased microcirculatory blood flow in the buccal mucosa [6]. In a rat model of *cardiogenic* shock, in contrast to a striking reduction in cardiac output, arterial pressure, and buccal microcirculatory flow, cerebral cortical microcirculatory flow was also fully preserved [7]. In contrast, in a sheep model of peritonitis, cerebral microcirculation was impaired during sepsis, with a significant reduction in perfused small vessels at the onset of septic shock [8] (Figure 14.2).

Cerebral blood flow and cerebral perfusion in systemic critical illness

Monitoring cerebral perfusion in critically ill patients is difficult. The gold standard for the determination of cerebral perfusion and metabolism is positron emission tomography. However, this costly and complex method must be considered a research tool in this setting. Magnetic resonance imaging and Xenon computed tomography scans or the [133]Xenon clearance methods are able to quantify CBF. However, they are also rarely used in this patient group as they only provide information at a specific time point and

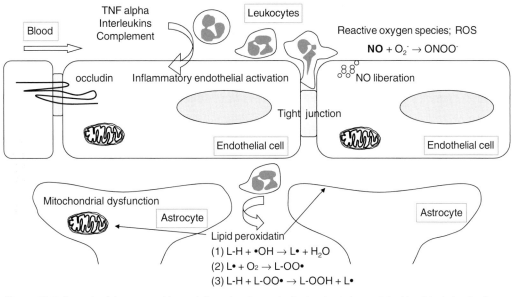

Figure 14.1 Synopsis of documented factors influencing the cerebral microcirculation and the blood–brain barrier. Some of the factors (e.g., nitric oxide, NO) influence cerebral perfusion at different levels of the brain circulation and have positive (e.g., vasodilation) or negative (e.g., production of reactive oxygen or nitrogen species) effects. The cytokines and chemokines liberated during acute illness activate cerebral endothelial cells and promote the rolling, sticking, and migration of leukocytes. L, Lipid; L-OO, lipid alkylperoxyl radical; L-OOH, Lipid hydroxyperoxide; O_2^-, superoxide; OH: hydroxyl radical; $ONOO^-$, hydroxyperoxide; TNF alpha, tumor necrosis factor alpha.

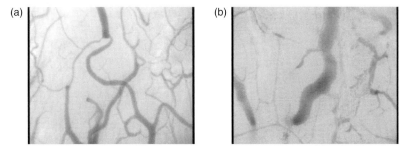

Figure 14.2 Microcirculation in septic shock. Digital microphotographs of the cerebral cortical microcirculation of a sheep at baseline (left) and onset of septic shock (right). Previously published by BioMed Central in: Taccone FS, Su F, Pierrakos C, et al. Cerebral microcirculation is impaired during sepsis: an experimental study. Crit Care 2010;**14**:R140. Reproduced with permission.

necessitate the transfer of the patient to the scanner. Transcranial Doppler is the simplest way to non-invasively obtain repeated real-time estimates of CBF. Transcranial Doppler measures *blood flow velocity* in the basal cerebral arteries, not CBF, and the linear relationship between CBF and mean flow velocity is only present if neither the diameter of the insonated vessel, nor the angle of insonation change during the examination. This assumption is probably fulfilled for most situations where examinations of the basal cerebral arteries are performed in systemic critically ill patients. The clinical usefulness of transcranial Doppler lies mostly in its ability to quantify cerebrovascular pressure autoregulation and CO_2-reactivity. While interesting, invasive methods such as brain tissue oxymetry and cerebral microdialysis are not suitable for patients with non-neurological

critical illness. Cerebral hemoglobin saturation measured non-invasively by near-infrared spectroscopy is a surrogate marker of cerebral venous saturation and hence oxygen extraction. Newer devices have been shown to have a good specificity and sensitivity for intracranial changes. However, the precise location and size of the monitored brain volume remains unclear. Despite the advantage of being non-invasive and increasing evidence that NIRS may also allow non-invasive monitoring of cerebral blood volume [9] and cerebrovascular autoregulation [10], this technology has yet to find its place in the management of critically ill patients.

Cerebral ischemia is a reality in many critically ill patients. In a post mortem analysis of the brains of patients who died from sepsis, multiple small ischemic lesions could be identified in different areas of the brain [11]. Possible explanations are the hypotension seen in sepsis, especially when concurrent with pre-existing cerebrovascular disease or autoregulatory failure. However, also thrombotic mechanisms due to a high hematocrit and increased viscosity of blood in sepsis may lead to watershed infarction, as has been described in a septic patient with prolonged hypotension [12]. However, extensive cerebral lesions have also been described in a septic patient without hypotension [13]. Cerebral ischemia and reperfusion are covered extensively in Chapter 13, this volume.

Several studies show a reduction of cerebral blood flow (CBF) in sepsis. Using the ^{133}Xe clearance technique, Bowton et al. demonstrated that CBF was reduced in nine patients with sepsis independent from changes in blood pressure or cardiac output [14]. Similarly, Maekawa et al. found significantly lower CBF in six patients with sepsis-associated delirium than in conscious controls [15]. In healthy volunteers, Moller and colleagues reported a reduction in CBF after an intravenous bolus of endotoxin [16]. Although they did not measure CO_2-reactivity in their subjects, these authors assumed that CO_2-reactivity was intact in their volunteers and explained the CBF reduction with hyperventilation due to the general symptoms of malaise following endotoxin administration. This result underscores the importance of CO_2 control in studies investigating the cerebral circulation. With normal CO_2-reactivity CBF will change by approximately 15% per kPa change in the arterial partial pressure of CO_2 ($PaCO_2$). Hence, even small changes of $PaCO_2$ during studies exploring cerebral perfusion may obscure the effects of any investigated intervention or mechanism.

Several studies investigate the cerebral effects of different resuscitation strategies in animal models of hemorrhagic shock [17,18]. In such experiments mean arterial blood pressure, cerebral perfusion pressure (CPP), and cerebral oxygenation decrease significantly. Also changes of cerebral energy metabolism indicating anaerobic glycolysis were described. Various regimens of fluid therapy were only in part successful in improving cerebral perfusion. So far, the results of such studies have not had an impact on the clinical management of hemorrhagic shock.

Intracranial pressure in systemic critical illness

Mean arterial pressure (MAP) is low in many patients with systemic critical illness. Accordingly, CPP is low as well. There are data suggesting that brain edema may occur in some patients with sepsis. Hence the influence of intracranial pressure (ICP) on CPP must be considered. Pfister et al. measured ICP non-invasively in 16 patients with sepsis and reported moderate elevations of ICP > 15 mmHg in half of the patients [19]. An ICP > 20 mmHg was not observed in that group of patients. CPP < 50 mmHg was found in 20% of the patients. Assuming that cerebrovascular pressure autoregulation is intact and the plateau of the autoregulatory curve is not shifted, these results suggest that CPP in the majority of the investigated patients was likely to be in the lower range of the autoregulatory plateau (Figure 14.3).

In severe hepatic failure, cerebral edema and increased ICP may be observed. It has been recommended to monitor ICP in selected cases and to stabilize CPP in the range > 60 mmHg [20].

Cerebrovascular reactivity in systemic critical illness

Cerebrovascular reactivity refers to homeostatic and protective mechanisms which may play an important role in patients with severely perturbed physiology. Clinically, the most relevant are CO_2-reactivity and pressure autoregulation.

CO_2-reactivity

The data on CO_2-reactivity in systemic critical illness are inconclusive. Various methods were used, and, apart from the extensive data on neurosurgical and neurological patients, data are only available for patients with sepsis. Over the range of $PaCO_2$ levels between 3.0 and 7.0 kPa, Matta and Stow found relative CO_2-reactivity to be within normal limits in 10 patients in the early stages of sepsis, i.e., < 24 h after admission to the intensive care unit (ICU) [21]. All their patients were mechanically ventilated and sedated with midazolam and fentanyl. Absolute CO_2-reactivity was lower than that reported in awake subjects but consistent with values obtained during sedation and anesthesia. Similarly, Thees and colleagues reported a normal response to a decrease in $PaCO_2$ in 10 patients with sepsis using transcranial Doppler (TCD) and cardiac output measurement by thermodilution [22]. Again all patients were mechanically ventilated, but sepsis had been established for > 48 h. Bowton and colleagues also reported normal cerebrovascular CO_2-reactivity in

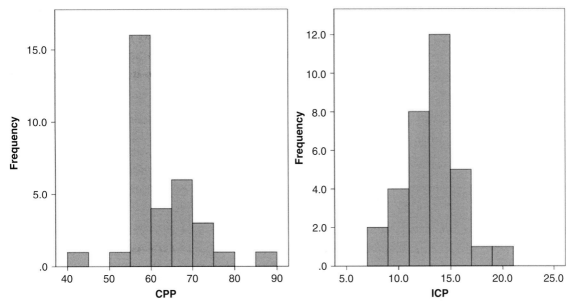

Figure 14.3 Non-invasive determination of cerebral perfusion pressure (CPP) and intracranial pressure (ICP) in patients with sepsis, severe sepsis, or septic shock. Fifty-two daily measurements in 16 patients with sepsis, severe sepsis, or septic shock are shown. Keeping in mind the limitations of non-invasive determinations (here transcranial Doppler) of ICP, moderate elevations of ICP seem to occur in patients with sepsis. In the majority of these patients CPP was in a range close to the lower threshold of cerebrovascular pressure autoregulation.

nine septic patients [14]. In contrast, Terborg and colleagues reported impaired CO_2-reactivity in septic patients, independent of changes in MAP [23]. They used TCD and near-infrared spectroscopy (NIRS) to assess CO_2-induced vasomotor reactivity by inducing hypercapnia through reductions in the ventilatory minute volume in eight mechanically ventilated septic patients. However, all their patients suffered from a neurological or neurosurgical illness, which may have affected the results. Bowie and colleagues observed significantly impaired cerebral CO_2-reactivity in septic patients in a study of 12 sedated and ventilated patients who had sepsis for > 24 h using TCD at normocapnia, hypocapnia, and hypercapnia [24]. Finally, a recent study found a reduced vasodilatory response to acetazolamide in patients with sepsis-associated delirium [25] (Figure 14.4). The conflicting findings of the available studies are most likely a consequence of the small sample sizes, differing methods, differences in timing of the measurements of CO_2-reactivity, and in the severity of illness between groups, which is reflected by the significant differences in mortality as well as in some of the drugs used in the management of these patients.

Pressure autoregulation

Autoregulation is a key defensive mechanism against hypo- and hyperperfusion and is therefore of considerable interest not only in patients with brain injury but any patient who is likely to go through periods of marked hypo- or hypertension. Physiologically, cerebrovascular pressure autoregulation is expected to keep CBF more or less constant in the range of MAP 60–160 mmHg or CPP 50–150 mmHg. These thresholds may be changed by physiological alterations such as changes in $PaCO_2$ or sympathetic tone and certain drugs, but also by pathological processes interfering with the complex regulation of cerebrovascular tone outlined in the first part of this chapter.

Autoregulation is influenced by $PaCO_2$ due to the fact that CO_2 dilates or constricts the same part of the vascular bed that is responsible for autoregulation. With increasing $PaCO_2$, autoregulation deteriorates, i.e., the plateau of the autoregulatory curve is shortened or with values of $PaCO_2$ > 10 kPa most likely abolished. This is not only of theoretical interest, as Taccone *et al.* recently confirmed this in patients with septic shock [26] and it is probably safe to assume that

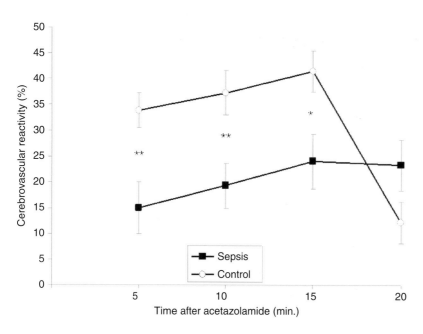

Figure 14.4 Carbon dioxide-reactivity in patients with septic encephalopathy. Percentage increase of the middle cerebral artery mean blood flow velocity in patients with sepsis-associated encephalopathy and in controls at 5, 10, 15, and 20 minutes after injection of acetazolamide. In patients with encephalopathy the increase in flow velocity is significantly lower than in controls, i.e., CO_2-reactivity is impaired. Means and standard errors are shown. Previously published by BioMed Central in Szatmari S, Vegh T, Csomos A, *et al.* Impaired cerebrovascular reactivity in sepsis-associated encephalopathy studied by acetazolamide test. *Crit Care* 2010; **14**:R50. Reproduced with permission.

with high levels of $PaCO_2$, such as in permissive hypercapnia, cerebrovascular autoregulation is lost. Whether this is of clinical importance remains to be proven. A further factor that may influence the upper and lower thresholds of autoregulation in critically ill patients is sympathetic tone. The larger "inflow tract" vessels of the brain are innervated by adrenergic fibers and the sympathetic tone therefore influences the limits of autoregulation: the plateau of the autoregulatory curve is shifted towards lower pressure thresholds with low sympathetic tone and towards higher pressure thresholds with increasing sympathetic tone.

Only a few studies have addressed the effects of systemic critical illness on cerebral autoregulation. Matta and Stow reported intact pressure autoregulation in 10 mechanically ventilated patients with sepsis, not in septic shock, using a phenylephrine infusion to increase MAP by 20 mmHg [21]. In contrast, Smith and colleagues reported loss of cerebrovascular autoregulation in 15 patients with septic shock as they were able to demonstrate a correlation between cardiac index and CBF using TCD and cardiac output measured by thermodilution [27]. In a more recent study, Pfister and colleagues found disturbed cerebral autoregulation in patients with sepsis-associated delirium, but not in patients with plain sepsis, using TCD [28]. This suggests that cerebral autoregulation is possibly intact in patients with sepsis but disturbed with more severe disease or complications manifesting as septic

shock or sepsis-associated delirium. Their data also suggest a possible link between disturbed autoregulation and dysfunction of the blood–brain barrier.

Several drugs interfere with cerebrovascular autoregulation. Any cerebral vasodilator such as nitroglycerine or sodium nitroprusside will reduce the efficiency of this mechanism [29]. Recently, volatile anesthetics have been introduced for sedation into intensive care medicine. All volatile anesthetics interfere with autoregulation in a dose-dependent manner. However, there are differences between the individual substances, and sevoflurane is thought to be the substance with the least influence on autoregulation [30].

In patients with cardiogenic shock, ventricular assist devices and intraaortic balloon pumps have been suspected to change cerebral perfusion and interfere with autoregulation. However, so far this has not been clearly demonstrated. It has been shown that with intraaortic balloon pumps, CBF dynamics change but autoregulation is preserved [31]. With pulsatile ventricular devices it is unclear whether autoregulation is influenced [32].

Flow-metabolism coupling

A further important characteristic of the cerebral circulation is the adaptation of CBF in relation to metabolic demand, i.e., neuronal activity. This is of clinical relevance, as for example the effect of sedation on CBF is affected by this mechanism. In head-injured patients this mechanism may be disrupted, in patients with systemic critical illness there are no data available on this topic. Impaired cerebral microvascular blood flow in sepsis disrupts normal flow-metabolism coupling and causes a delay in sensory evoked potentials. In a rat model of septic shock, neither sepsis treatment with norepinephrine nor the blockade of the inducible nitric oxide synthase could prevent this effect [33].

Clinical aspects

Neurobiological effects of systemic physiological and metabolic insults are covered in Chapter 12, this volume. In the following sections we will address some of the effects of intensive care treatment on cerebral perfusion.

Cerebrovascular effects of vasopressors

Systemically applied catecholamines typically cause a small reduction in normocapnic CBF (approximately 5–15%) [34]. Several factors need to be considered when interactions between catecholamines and cerebral blood vessels are studied [34]. Instability in $PaCO_2$ during studies on cerebrovascular effects of vasoactive drugs, may influence CBF measurements profoundly. The presence or absence of autoregulation or an intervention exceeding the range of autoregulation will also strongly influence the reaction of CBF to a change in MAP.

The blood–brain barrier should be thought of not only as a structural barrier but also as an enzymatic barrier: cerebral microvessels contain monoamine oxidase, hence catecholamines are unlikely to cross the blood–brain barrier in their intact form. Furthermore, intrinsic adrenergic nerves that innervate cerebral microvessels seem to modulate the permeability of the blood–brain barrier. Some studies suggest that there is metabolic stimulation of the brain through beta-adrenoceptors [34], for example, a study in conscious rats without brain injury investigated systemic infusions of phenylephrine, norepinephrine, and epinephrine. The achieved changes in MAP were within the range of autoregulation, and only epinephrine led to an increase in CBF. This was interpreted as a metabolic effect due to a beta-adrenoreceptor stimulation. In contrast, in an intact physiological sheep model, hypertension induced by epinephrine and norepinephrine was associated with neither global changes in CBF nor

with cerebral oxygen utilization, both of which remained constant. In contrast, at equivalent doses, dopamine caused cerebral hyperemia and increased global cerebral oxygen utilization. Most likely a disturbance in the function of the blood–brain barrier will change the response of cerebral perfusion and metabolism to catecholamines. The available data suggest that the cerebrovascular response to our management may be highly variable and depends on a large number of interacting variables. Possibly protocols using NIRS to non-invasively measure the effects of systemic changes on cerebral oxygenation could give us further insight into this topic. Recent studies have addressed this issue in healthy volunteers but are difficult to interpret due to changes in $PaCO_2$ during measurements.

Cerebrovascular effects of other drugs

In human and animal studies on cerebral perfusion, background effects of sedatives and interactions between catecholamines and sedatives need to be considered [34]. All intravenous sedatives will decrease cerebral metabolism and, if flow-metabolism coupling is intact, also CBF. In an ovine model comparing animals without an intracranial pathology in the awake state and anesthetized with either propofol or isoflurane, epinephrine, norepinephrine, and dopamine did not change pressure autoregulation [35,36]. Work by Strebel and colleagues in patients without cerebral pathology indicates that norepinephrine and phenylephrine do not directly affect intracranial hemodynamics in patients anesthetized with isoflurane or propofol [37]. Rather, the hemodynamic changes observed with vasoconstrictors reflect the effect of the background anesthetic agents on cerebral pressure autoregulation. A very interesting study in sheep showed that epinephrine, norepinephrine, and dopamine significantly reduced mean arterial propofol concentrations [38]. There were parallel reductions of concentrations in sagittal sinus blood leaving the brain. The data are consistent with a mechanism based on increased first-pass dilution and clearance of propofol, secondary to an increased cardiac output. Such changes in propofol concentration may directly affect CBF. Finally, statins have been reported to have cerebroprotective effects. However, it is unknown whether this group of drugs has a clinically relevant impact on cerebral perfusion.

Effects of body temperature on cerebral perfusion

Hypothermia reduces cerebral metabolism and CBF. In a pediatric model of cardiac arrest and resuscitation, delayed induction of hypothermia decreased cerebral perfusion and decreased the lower limit of autoregulation [39]. The effects of fever and elevated brain temperature on cerebral perfusion are not well described. In brain-injured patients, brain tissue oxygen partial pressure increases and cerebral oxygen extraction fracture decreases suggesting hyperperfusion [40]. However, it is unclear whether such changes are of clinical relevance in patients without brain injury.

Areas of uncertainty and direction of future research

Data, particularly clinical data on cerebral perfusion in systemic critical illness, are scarce. Important areas of uncertainty are the impact of the severity and type of the critical illness on cerebral (microcirculatory) perfusion and cerebrovascular homeostatic mechanisms, the influence of the underlying disease on the response to treatment, and most importantly, the question regarding the role of cerebral perfusion in the development of brain dysfunction. In our opinion the following questions should have a high priority in future clinical research agendas on this topic: In which groups of patients suffering from systemic critical illness has an altered cerebral perfusion an influence on outcome? Does inclusion of therapeutic targets regarding cerebral perfusion into treatment algorithms confer any benefit to critically ill patients? Despite the difficulties associated with neuroimaging in critically ill patients these methods, particularly PET scanning, could in our opinion significantly enhance our understanding of cerebral perfusion and metabolism and their role in the development of brain dysfunction in critical illness. This method potentially allows imaging not only of cerebral perfusion and metabolism but of other mechanisms which may play a role such as activation of microglia.

Conclusions

Systemic critical illness may profoundly influence the cerebral microvasculature, the blood–brain barrier, cerebral perfusion, and physiological protective or compensatory mechanisms such as autoregulation or CO_2-reactivity. It is unclear whether decreased consciousness in non-sedated critically ill patients is a protective mechanism against or a consequence of inadequate substrate and oxygen delivery due to altered cerebral microcirculatory perfusion and flow-metabolism coupling. Only very little work has been performed on the difficult topic of whether there is a link between cerebral perfusion and cerebral dysfunction. So far, apart from obvious perturbations such as severe hypotension or insufficient oxygen delivery, data suggest that brain dysfunction in systemic critical illness is not simply a consequence of inadequate cerebral perfusion despite the fact that changes in cerebral perfusion may be observed. To complicate matters, most clinical studies focus on small groups of patients with sepsis and differ substantially in regard to methods and patient characteristics, making interpretation very difficult. The complex interaction of a systemic inflammatory response with the blood–brain barrier, the cerebral microcirculation as well as effects of drugs and management strategies used in critically ill patients need to be studied in more detail to untangle their intricate relationships.

References

1. Paulson OB, Hasselbalch SG, Rostrup E, Knudsen GM, Pelligrino D. Cerebral blood flow response to functional activation. *J Cerebr Blood Flow Metab* 2010;**30**:2–14.

2. Comim CM, Vilela MC, Constantino LS, *et al.* Traffic of leukocytes and cytokine up-regulation in the central nervous system in sepsis. *Intensive Care Med* 2011;**37**:711–18.

3. Burkhart CS, Siegemund M, Steiner LA. Cerebral perfusion in sepsis. *Crit Care* 2010;**14**:215.

4. Berg RM, Moller K, Bailey DM. Neuro-oxidative-nitrosative stress in sepsis. *J Cerebral Blood Flow Metab* 2011;**31**:1532–44.

5. Lochhead JJ, McCaffrey G, Quigley CE, *et al.* Oxidative stress increases blood–brain barrier permeability and induces alterations in occludin during hypoxia-reoxygenation. *J Cerebral Blood Flow Metab* 2010;**30**:1625–36.

6. Wan Z, Sun S, Ristagno G, Weil MH, Tang W. The cerebral microcirculation is protected during experimental hemorrhagic shock. *Crit Care Med* 2010;**38**:928–32.

7. Wan Z, Ristagno G, Sun S, Li Y, Weil MH, Tang W. Preserved cerebral microcirculation during cardiogenic shock. *Crit Care Med* 2009;**37**:2333–7.

8. Taccone FS, Su F, Pierrakos C, *et al.* Cerebral microcirculation is impaired during sepsis: an experimental study. *Crit Care* 2010;**14**:R140.

9. Calderon-Arnulphi M, Alaraj A, Slavin KV. Near infrared technology in neuroscience: past, present and future. *Neurol Res* 2009;**31**:605–14.

10. Steiner LA, Pfister D, Strebel SP, *et al.* Near-infrared spectroscopy can monitor dynamic cerebral autoregulation in adults. *Neurocrit Care* 2009;**10**(1):122–8.

11. Sharshar T, Annane D, de la Grandmaison GL, *et al.* The neuropathology of septic shock. *Brain Pathol* 2004;**14**:21–33.

12. Nagaratnam N, Brakoulias V, Ng K. Multiple cerebral infarcts following septic shock. *J Clin Neurosci* 2002;**9**:473–6.

13. Finelli PF, Uphoff DF. Magnetic resonance imaging abnormalities with septic encephalopathy. *J Neurol Neurosurg Psychiatry* 2004;**75**:1189–91.

14. Bowton DL, Bertels NH, Prough DS, Stump DA. Cerebral blood flow is reduced in patients with sepsis syndrome. *Crit Care Med* 1989;**17**:399–403.

15. Maekawa T, Fujii Y, Sadamitsu D, *et al.* Cerebral circulation and metabolism in patients with septic encephalopathy. *Am J Emerg Med* 1991;**9**:139–43.

16. Moller K, Strauss GI, Qvist J, *et al.* Cerebral blood flow and oxidative metabolism during human endotoxemia. *J Cereb Blood Flow Metab* 2002;**22**:1262–70.

17. Cavus E, Meybohm P, Doerges V, *et al.* Cerebral effects of three resuscitation protocols in uncontrolled haemorrhagic shock: a randomised controlled experimental study. *Resuscitation* 2009;**80**:567–72.

18. Cavus E, Meybohm P, Dorges V, *et al.* Regional and local brain oxygenation during hemorrhagic shock: a prospective experimental study on the effects of small-volume resuscitation with norepinephrine. *J Trauma* 2008;**64**:641–8; discussion 648–9.

19. Pfister D, Schmidt B, Smielewski P, *et al.* Intracranial pressure in patients with sepsis. *Acta Neurochir Suppl* 2008;**102**:71–5.

20. Han MK, Hyzy R. Advances in critical care management of hepatic failure and insufficiency. *Crit Care Med* 2006;**34**:S225–31.

21. Matta BF, Stow PJ. Sepsis-induced vasoparalysis does not involve the cerebral vasculature: indirect evidence from autoregulation and carbon dioxide reactivity studies. *Br J Anaesth* 1996;**76**:790–4.

22. Thees C, Kaiser M, Scholz M, *et al.* Cerebral haemodynamics and CO_2-reactivity during sepsis syndrome. *Crit Care* 2007;**11**:R123.

23. Terborg C, Schummer W, Albrecht M, *et al.* Dysfunction of vasomotor reactivity in severe sepsis and septic shock. *Intensive Care Med* 2001;**27**:1231–4.

24. Bowie RA, O'Connor PJ, Mahajan RP. Cerebrovascular reactivity to carbon dioxide in sepsis syndrome. *Anaesthesia* 2003;**58**:261–5.

25. Szatmari S, Vegh T, Csomos A, *et al.* Impaired cerebrovascular reactivity in sepsis-associated encephalopathy studied by acetazolamide test. *Crit Care* 2010;**14**:R50.

26. Taccone FS, Castanares-Zapatero D, Peres-Bota D, *et al.* Cerebral autoregulation is influenced by carbon dioxide levels in patients with septic shock. *Neurocrit Care* 2010;**12**:35–42.

27. Smith SM, Padayachee S, Modaresi KB, Smithies MN, Bihari DJ. Cerebral blood flow is proportional to cardiac index in patients with septic shock. *J Crit Care* 1998;**13**:104–9.

28. Pfister D, Siegemund M, Dell-Kuster S, *et al.* Cerebral perfusion in sepsis-associated delirium. *Crit Care* 2008;**12**:R63.

29. Paulson OB, Strandgaard S, Edvinsson L. Cerebral autoregulation. *Cerebrovasc Brain Metab Rev* 1990;**2**:161–92.

30. Engelhard K, Werner C. Inhalational or intravenous anesthetics for craniotomies? Pro inhalational. *Curr Opin Anaesthesiol* 2006;**19**:504–8.

31. Bellapart J, Geng S, Dunster K, *et al.* Intraaortic balloon pump counterpulsation and cerebral autoregulation: an observational study. *BMC Anesthesiology* 2010;**10**:3.

32. Bellapart J, Chan GS, Tzeng YC, *et al.* The effect of ventricular assist devices on cerebral autoregulation: a preliminary study. *BMC Anesthesiology* 2011;**11**:4.

33. Rosengarten B, Wolff S, Klatt S, Schermuly RT. Effects of inducible nitric oxide synthase inhibition or norepinephrine on the neurovascular coupling in an endotoxic rat shock model. *Crit Care* 2009;**13**:R139.

34. Pfister D, Strebel SP, Steiner LA. Effects of catecholamines on cerebral blood vessels in patients with traumatic brain injury. *Eur J Anaesthesiol Suppl* 2008;**42**:98–103.

35. Myburgh JA, Upton RN, Grant C, Martinez A. The effect of infusions of adrenaline, noradrenaline and dopamine on cerebral autoregulation under isoflurane anaesthesia in an ovine model. *Anaesth Intensive Care* 2003;**31**:259–66.

36. Myburgh JA, Upton RN, Grant C, Martinez A. The effect of infusions of adrenaline, noradrenaline and dopamine on cerebral autoregulation under propofol anaesthesia in an ovine model. *Intensive Care Med* 2003;**29**:817–24.

37. Strebel SP, Kindler C, Bissonnette B, Tschaler G, Deanovic D. The impact of systemic vasoconstrictors on the cerebral circulation of anesthetized patients. *Anesthesiology* 1998;**89**:67–72.

38. Myburgh JA, Upton RN, Grant C, Martinez A. Epinephrine, norepinephrine and dopamine infusions decrease propofol concentrations during continuous propofol infusion in an ovine model. *Intensive Care Med* 2001;**27**:276–82.

39. Lee JK, Brady KM, Mytar JO, *et al.* Cerebral blood flow and cerebrovascular autoregulation in a swine model of pediatric cardiac arrest and hypothermia. *Crit Care Med* 2011;**39**(10): 2337–45.

40. Stocchetti N, Protti A, Lattuada M, *et al.* Impact of pyrexia on neurochemistry and cerebral oxygenation after acute brain injury. *J Neurol Neurosurg Psychiatry* 2005;**76**:1135–9.

Chapter 15

Delirium and neurotransmitter dysfunction

Willem A. van Gool

SUMMARY

Delirium is one of the clinical manifestations of encephalopathy in critical illness. During delirium multiple, complex, and non-linear interacting systems in the brain are out of order. This chapter reviews changes in neurotransmitter systems that are associated with delirium. After discussing the "classical" neurotransmitters: acetylcholine and the three mono-amine transmitters, dopamine, noradrenaline, and serotonin (5-hydroxytryptamine) in critical illness, the chapter continues with a discussion of the amino acids that have been established as neurotransmitters: gamma-aminobutyric acid (GABA), glycine, glutamate, and aspartate. The chapter concludes with a brief discussion of the role of serine and nitric oxide and the implications of the "false neurotransmitter" hypothesis in critical illness encephalopathy.

Whereas all neurotransmitter systems will be prone to imbalances before, during, and shortly after delirium, changes in the cholinergic system are identified as having a unique combination of potential explanatory power. Cholinergic deficiency combines a potential explanation for the impairments of attention that are crucial in the symptoms of delirium, with a possible link with the role of innate immunity in the brain that seems to play in critical illness encephalopathy. Moreover, the cholinergic deficiency hypothesis can be put to test by investigating the effects of the various drugs that affect cholinergic functions, for their effects on the alleviation of symptoms or the prevention of delirium or its long-term sequelae.

Introduction

Delirium is a clinical syndrome that is characterized by a varying set of concurrent neuropsychiatric symptoms. During a delirious episode patients suffer from different combinations of symptoms including cognitive impairments, abnormalities of attention, altered levels of psychomotor activity, and sleep–wake changes. Thus, delirium is intrinsically heterogeneous from a phenomenological point of view and there are large variations in the clinical picture and the severity of symptoms between patients and even within an individual patient during a single period with delirium. Most probably, these variations in delirium symptoms and severity should be attributed to differences in the underlying impairments of multiple, complex, and non-linear interacting systems in the brain. Changes in neurotransmitter systems play a pivotal role in these derangements.

In this chapter the changes in neurotransmitter systems that are associated with delirium will be explored. The focus will be first on the "classical" neurotransmitter systems: the cholinergic system and the three monoamine transmitters, dopamine, noradrenaline, and serotonin (5-hydroxytryptamine), followed by a discussion of the amino acids that have been established as neurotransmitters: gamma-aminobutyric acid (GABA), glycine, glutamate, and aspartate. The chapter concludes with a brief discussion of the roles of serine and nitric oxide and the implications of the "false neurotransmitter" hypothesis in critical illness encephalopathy.

Cholinergic neurotransmission

Cholinergic network

The cell bodies of brain cholinergic neurons are located in the basal forebrain, striatum (caudate nucleus, putamen, and nucleus accumbens), meso-pontine tegmental nuclei, cranial motor nuclei, and spinal motor neurons (Figure 15.1) [1,2]. Cholinergic neurons and their ramifications form a widespread

Brain Disorders in Critical Illness, ed. Robert D. Stevens, Tarek Sharshar, and E. Wesley Ely. Published by Cambridge University Press. © Cambridge University Press 2013.

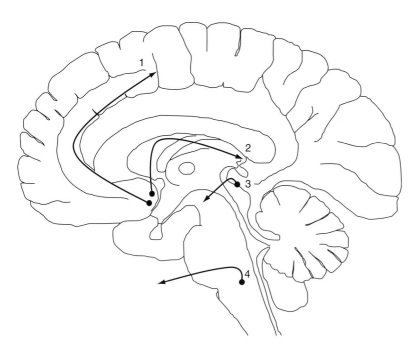

Figure 15.1 Schematic representation of the most important cholinergic projections: (1) from the basal forebrain widespread to the cortex, (2) from the septum via the fornix to the hippocampus, (3) from the habenular nuclei to the interpeduncular nucleus, (4) cranial nerve to the motor nuclei.

network of ascending and descending projections, although the former exceed the latter. Acetylcholine itself binds to two major subtypes of receptors that are indicated as either muscarinic or nicotinic, based on differential binding affinities for these substances. The nicotinic receptor is a pentameric ligand-gated membrane channel, whereas muscarinic receptors are G-protein linked [1,2]. Nicotinic receptors are mainly involved in mediating the effects of acetylcholine in autonomic ganglia and the neuromuscular junction, but these receptors are also expressed in the central nervous system. There are five muscarinic subtypes of cholinergic receptors of which M1 is the most abundant subtype in cortex and hippocampus, M2 in brainstem, cerebellum, and thalamus, and M4 is most often found in the striatum.

The role of the cholinergic system in cognitive functions is widely documented in animal and human research [1,2]. This work received much impetus in the 1980s from findings indicating that Alzheimer's disease is associated with an important loss of cholinergic neurons. A variety of animal experimental paradigms that indicate that antimuscarinic agents, such as scopolamine and atropine, impair memory performance have lent further support for the "cholinergic hypothesis" in Alzheimer's disease [3]. Moreover, cholinergic agonists tend to reverse these impairments again, stimulating hope for cholinomimetic therapy in this disease. Since then, it has

become increasingly clear that the pathology of Alzheimer's disease is not restricted to degeneration of a single neurotransmitter system, but that beta-amyloid and presenilins are important factors in the process that leads to widespread degeneration of cortical networks underlying dementia in Alzheimer's disease. Currently it is widely acknowledged that loss of cholinergic transmission alone cannot account for the whole clinicopathological picture of Alzheimer's disease. The lack of robust clinical benefit in most patients treated with cholinergic drugs is consistent with this insight [3].

As the clinical dementia syndrome may not be fully explained by selective cholinergic impairments, the clinical signs that occur as a result of cholinergic deficiency are much more relevant in the context of delirium [3]. Clinical descriptions from older literature at the time that atropine coma was advocated as a safe alternative for insulin coma in the treatment of psychosis, documented that "restlessness, occasionally mild excitement, confusion" can result from anticholinergic treatment and that at higher doses, "memory disturbance, disorientation, clouded consciousness, illusions and most frequently visual hallucinations" are manifested [4,5]. Others have reported depression, impaired consciousness, perceptual distortion, disturbances of thought and association, severe anxiety, and restlessness. Interestingly, upon administration of the cholinesterase inhibitor tetrahydroaminoacridine, currently better known as tacrine, this neuropsychiatric cholinergic deficiency syndrome completely reversed within minutes. At that time, "broadening of attention" indicating difficulties with filtering out distracting stimuli was identified as the most salient effect of anticholinergic treatment [3]. These clinical descriptions of the cholinergic deficiency syndrome (CDS) caused by anticholinergic treatment resemble very closely the state of delirium [3]. Apparently, cholinergic deficiency can fully account for the clinical picture of delirium. Evidence from experiments using new techniques for measuring rapid changes in cholinergic neurotransmission indicates that changes in cholinergic modulation on a timescale of seconds is triggered by sensory input cues and serves to facilitate cue detection and attentional performance [1,2]. Whereas cholinergic mechanisms normally facilitate active maintenance of sensory input and planned responses, functional impairments in the cholinergic network may very well explain the spectrum of neuropsychiatric symptoms observed in delirium.

Acetylcholine and inflammation

In addition to its network role, cholinergic signal transduction most probably also plays a role in the inflammatory component of clinical conditions that are usually associated with delirium, such as sepsis or other forms of critical illness [6]. In systemic inflammation and/or infection, the peripheral immune system strongly affects the brain. Pro-inflammatory cytokines generated in the periphery communicate with the brain. Peripheral administration of lipopolysaccharide, for example, may cause a rapid and steep rise in concentrations of tumor necrosis factor alpha (TNFα) in the brain of rodents. Whereas peripheral TNFα levels gradually subside over a period of several hours to days, increased amounts of TNFα in the brain may persist for months after just a single challenge [7]. This increased brain TNFα is associated with microglial activation and further cytokine release in the brain. Whereas microglia are usually in a quiescent state, their activation seems to be pivotal in the innate immune response of the brain. Microglia can play a role in phagocytosis and antigen presentation, and these cells can proliferate rapidly. They have the potential to secrete a range of inflammatory mediators (such as cytokines, chemokines, and proteases) [8,9].

Cytotoxic substances released by activated microglia may play a role in causing the acute behavioral changes in delirium associated with systemic

infections. Franceschi and colleagues noted age-related up-regulation of inflammatory responses of innate immunity, which accords with clinical wisdom that elderly patients in particular are prone to delirium, even after stimuli that appear to be innocuous [10]. The same observation applies to individuals with (incipient) neurodegenerative diseases that are associated with microglial activation in the early stages.

The cholinergic network and neuroinflammation

Systemic infection and anticholinergic side effects are both well recognized risk factors for delirium. Vagus nerve stimulation inhibits systemic inflammation, and acetylcholine can inhibit release of the pro-inflammatory cytokines TNFα and interleukins-1 and -6 in human endotoxin-stimulated macrophages. These and related experiments have paved the way for hypotheses on the role of cholinergic mechanisms in anti-inflammatory processes [11]. Analogous to what has been noted in peripheral tissues, acetylcholine seems to also have a role in control of brain inflammation: microglia express nicotinic receptors and activation of these cholinergic receptors attenuates the pro-inflammatory response in vitro [5]. Based on these considerations, it has been suggested that impaired cholinergic inhibitory control of microglia in elderly people, and to a greater extent in patients with (incipient) neurodegenerative diseases, contributes to an uncontrolled neuroinflammatory reaction of excessively activated microglia [6]. This hypothesis directly connects the alleged network effects of cholinergic neurotransmission as an explanation for most of the neuropsychiatric symptoms in delirium with a role of failing cholinergic control of microglia upon cytokine stimulation (Figure 15.2). This hypothesis resembles an echo of the age-old controversy disputing the "soup versus sparks" mechanisms concerning the question of how neurons communicate: failing cholinergic control may unite cytokine "soup" effects with network "spark" mechanisms in the generation of delirium. Restoring cholinergic control or other means that inhibit microglia might play a role in preventing delirium or limiting its duration under this hypothesis [6].

In several clinical studies the alleged role of deficient cholinergic neurotransmission in delirium has been put to the test. Gamberini *et al.* examined

Inhibitory cholinergic control

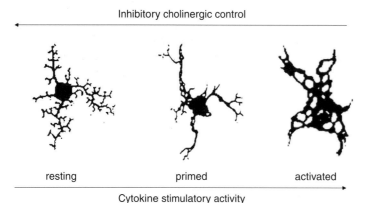

resting   primed   activated

Cytokine stimulatory activity

Figure 15.2 Schematic representation of different degrees of microglial activation, increasing from left to right. The upper arrow depicts the inhibitory control of the cholinergic system on microglia, whereas the lower arrow represents the stimulatory effect of cytokines.

the effects of low-dose oral rivastigmine in preventing postoperative delirium in elderly patients undergoing elective cardiac surgery in a randomized clinical trial [12]. With rates of delirium of 30% and 32% of patients in the placebo and rivastigmine groups, respectively, this study did not support a decisive role of cholinergic deficiency in causing delirium. However, as noted by the investigators, interpretation of this study is hampered by the low dose of rivastigmine (3 doses of 1.5 mg) that was used, the limited power of the study, and the possibility that cases of subsyndromal delirium may have been missed [12]. Another possibility is that cholinergic depletion does play a more important role in sepsis-associated delirium and not so much in other forms of delirium, such as perioperative delirium for instance. Increasing cholinergic tone may not offer further protection in subjects who do not suffer cholinergic deficiency, and this may also explain the absence of a protective effect of a cholinesterase inhibitor in another clinical trial probing the effects of rivastigmine, as an add-on in addition to haloperidol, to treat delirium in a heterogeneous group of patients admitted to the intensive care unit (ICU) [13]. Perhaps the post-acute phase is more appropriate to investigate a potential role of cholinesterase inhibitors in stimulating recovery after delirium, alleviating persistent subsyndromal delirium, and/or in preventing new episodes of delirium.

Dopamine

The dopamine-releasing neurons in the ventral midbrain (in the pars compacta of the substantia nigra) and ventral tegmental area are the major sources of this neurotransmitter in the cerebral cortex and in most subcortical areas. These projections form the nigrostriatal and mesocorticolimbic dopaminergic pathways that end in the dorsal and ventral striatum (including prefrontal cortex), respectively (Figure 15.3). These two groups of neurons in the substantia nigra and the ventral tegmental area of the midbrain release dopamine in "tonic" and "phasic" mode [14]. Tonic dopamine neurons fuel a steady, baseline level of dopamine and in their phasic, releasing mode, dopamine levels sharply increase or decrease for several seconds.

The midbrain dopaminergic nuclei and their target areas serve a critical role in voluntary motor control and reward-motivated behaviors and cognitive functions. Dopamine transmission is associated with establishing memories of cue-reward associations and the motivation to seek rewards [14]. As such it plays an important role in reinforcement and motivation of actions. Antidopaminergic drugs interfere with reinforcement learning, while dopaminergic stimulation acts as reinforcer. It appears that dopamine release fulfils a necessary condition for motivation of actions in order to achieve the desired goals.

Nicotinic and muscarinic acetylcholine receptors within the substantia nigra and ventral tegmental area modulate dopamine transmission in the dorsal/ventral striatum and prefrontal cortex. Further cholinergic modulation of forebrain dopaminergic transmission is attributed to cholinergic interneurons in the striatum. These dopaminergic and cholinergic interactions are mediated through stimulation of the dopaminergic D1 and D5 receptors, leading to increased secretion of acetylcholine and D2, D3, and D4 receptors lowering levels of acetylcholine. Steiner suggested that age-related changes in the balance between several subtypes of dopamine receptors and their respective effects on cholinergic transmission, may explain the

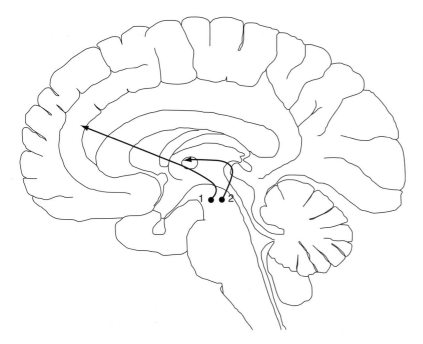

Figure 15.3 Schematic representation of the projections of dopaminergic mesotelencephalic system: (1) from the substantia nigra to the striatum and (2) from the ventral tegmentum and the substantia nigra to the cortex (medial frontal, anterior cingulated, and entorhinal cortex).

strong age effects on the incidence of delirium in association with severe illness [15].

Symptoms of delirium are frequent and disabling complications of Parkinson's disease. Excess of levodopa pharmacotherapy is usually presumed to cause hallucinations. However, several observations cast doubt on this straightforward explanation: hallucinations in Parkinson's disease have been known from the time before dopamine therapy was available, the exclusive causal role of high levels of l-dopa in causing neuropsychiatric manifestations has not been documented convincingly, and a high-dose intravenous challenge with levodopa in Parkinson's disease patients failed to provoke hallucinations [3].

Apart from presynaptic characteristics, postsynaptic variations also may be relevant in pathways leading to delirium. In an international validation study among elderly hospital patients, van Munster and colleagues found that specific alleles of the SLC6A3 and possibly the DRD2 genes protect for delirium [16]. The SLC6A3 gene is coding for the dopamine transporter affecting extracellular dopamine concentrations, and the DRD2 gene has been studied before in attention deficit hyperactivity disorder, schizophrenia, and movement disorders. The specific single nucleotide polymorphism that was studied in the DRD2 gene in relation to delirium might be associated with lower transcription/translation rate, resulting in decreased

D2 receptor availability and, as a consequence, a lower incidence of delirium [16].

Noradrenalin

Most of the brain noradrenergic neurons are concentrated in the locus coeruleus, a cluster of noradrenalin-containing neurons located adjacent to the fourth ventricle in the pontine brainstem, as the primary source of an extensive noradrenergic innervation of the forebrain (Figure 15.4). Neurons in the locus coeruleus provide the sole source of noradrenalin to the hippocampus and neocortex. Noradrenalin acts at multiple receptors traditionally divided in three receptor subtypes [17]. In all laminae of the neocortex, beta-receptors are coupled to the Gs/cAMP second messenger system, whereas alpha-1 and alpha-2 receptors are concentrated in the superficial layers and are coupled to the phosphoinositol and Gi/cAMP systems, respectively. Recent findings suggest that these divisions may be even more complicated since multiple subtypes have been identified.

In the context of delirium it is interesting that locus coeruleus activation, produced by the cholinergic agonist, bethanechol, is associated with activation of cortical EEG [18]. This effect is most probably a causal relationship, because increased locus coeruleus neuronal discharge always preceded EEG activation, and

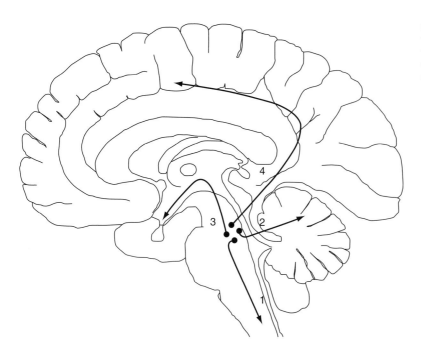

Figure 15.4 Schematic representation of the noradrenergic locus coeruleus system with projection to: (1) the spinal cord, (2) cerebellum, (3) hypothalamus, and (4) the entire cortex.

pretreatment with a beta-receptor antagonist prevented EEG activation following bethanechol-induced LC activation.

Analogous to the dual effects of cholinergic modulators that have direct effects on neuronal networks as well as on inflammatory processes, it is interesting to note also that the central alpha-2 adrenoceptor agonists have the potential to enhance macrophage phagocytosis and bacterial clearance resulting in improved outcomes in animal models of bacterial sepsis [19]. One of the most interesting recent developments relating to noradrenergic mechanisms in delirium concerns the alpha-2 agonist dexmedetomidine, which is a highly selective and potent agonist. Dexmedetomidine provides sedation with modest analgesic and possible antidelirium effects with little respiratory depression [20]. The drug could provide some advantages over commonly used sedatives and analgesics perioperatively such as GABA agonists, since dexmedetomidine combines analgesic effects with a lack of respiratory depression, sympatholytic blunting of the stress response, preservation of neutrophil function, and the drug may establish a more natural sleep-like state. Indeed, several studies suggest that dexmedetomidine has a promising role in prevention of delirium in critically ill patients, but study outcomes have not always been conclusive [21,22]. Steiner concluded that despite its effects on mortality, duration of mechanical ventilation, and length of stay

in intensive care, currently it remains unclear whether dexmedetomidine reduces incidence or severity of delirium in the ICU [23].

Serotonin

Serotonin is a neurotransmitter synthesized in both peripheral tissues and the brain. A relatively small number of neurons produce all of the serotonin (5-hydroxytryptamine) and there is a high density of terminals throughout the central nervous system. Cell bodies of serotonergic neurons are located primarily within the midline raphe nuclei of the midbrain, pons, and medulla (Figure 15.5). Most of the forebrain, thalamic, striatal, and cortical projections originate from the more rostrally positioned raphe nuclei, whereas the more caudally located nuclei project primarily to the spinal cord, medulla, pons, midbrain, and cerebellum. Variations in serotonin receptor genes have been identified which give rise to a wide repertoire of receptor isoforms, mostly G-protein-coupled, grouped into seven families based upon sequence homology and second messenger systems [24]. Brain serotonin has been implicated in many physiological processes and behavioral mechanisms, for example temperature regulation, sleep–wake rhythms, sexual behavior, aggression, nociception, and mood.

Alterations in serotonergic activity have been associated with delirium, but these changes concern

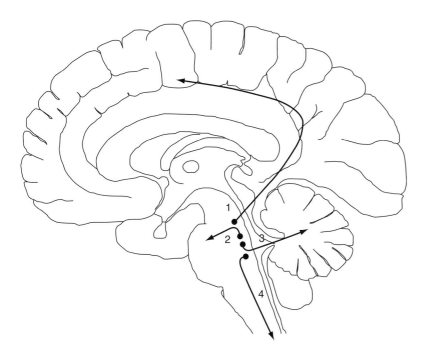

Figure 15.5 Schematic representation of serotonergic projections from the raphe nuclei in the reticular formation: (1) to the hemispheres, (2) intrinsically to the brainstem, (3) to the cerebellum, and (4) through the raphespinal tract.

both increased as well as decreased activity. Van der Mast and Fekkes suggest that common risk factors for delirium such as severe illness, surgery, and trauma act through their effects on plasma amino acid concentrations including the serotonin precursor tryptophan [25]. Indeed, extremely low and high plasma tryptophan and tyrosine levels are associated with incident delirium in mechanically ventilated patients, suggesting that alterations of these amino acids may be important in the pathogenesis of delirium in the ICU. Based on these findings it has been suggested that the association of delirium with alterations in tryptophan concentrations can be explained by the production of neurotoxic metabolites of tryptophan, fluctuations of serotonin or its downstream neurotransmitter, melatonin, or a combination of these factors [26]. The former explanation may involve kynurenine (and associated metabolites), since this pathway may be activated during the systemic inflammatory response seen in critical illness. Under these circumstances kynurenine may be metabolized to the neurotoxin quinolinic acid, potentially having detrimental bystander effects.

Amino acid neurotranmitters

Gamma-aminobutyric acid

Gamma-aminobutyric acid (GABA) is the most important inhibitory neurotransmitter in the brain.

Gamma-aminobutyric acid is released by Purkinje cells in the cerebellum – striatal neurons projecting to the substantia nigra thus inhibiting dopamine release; stellate neurons in the cerebral cortex – and by hippocampal basket cells both affecting local cortical circuits. Gamma-aminobutyric acid's actions concern: (1) fast, phasic inhibitory postsynaptic potentials that are transiently mediated by low-affinity receptors; (2) a more persistent, tonic, form of receptor-mediated inhibition, mediated through high-affinity extrasynaptic receptors; and finally (3) a slowly rising and slowly decaying phasic inhibitory activity [27].

After prolonged episodes of GABA agonism by the use of benzodiazepines or drugs like baclofen, withdrawal of these drugs causes a sudden release of GABAergic inhibitory activity in the nervous system [28]. This may induce delirium associated with tachycardia, autonomic changes, and even seizures and spasticity, possibly through disinhibition of previously suppressed monoamine pathways.

Glycine

The amino acid neurotransmitter glycine mediates inhibitory effects at the synapse in motor and sensory reflex circuits of the spinal cord, but it can also be found in the brainstem, cerebellum, and retina. There it exerts its effects through synaptic ligand-gated ion chloride-channel receptors that belong to the cysteine-loop

145

family [29]. Outside the synapse, glycine receptors are not only widely distributed through the nervous system but also, for example, on macrophages. Neuronal glycine receptors have been implicated in both ethanol- and propofol-induced hypnosis, explaining that the glycine receptor antagonist, strychnine, may dose-dependently counteract some of the propofol effects in animal experiments [30]. Therefore, the role that glycine receptors in the brain apparently play in hypnotic states may be of relevance to the pathogenesis of hypoactive delirium [31].

Glutamate

As the most abundant and dominant excitatory neurotransmitter in the nervous system, glutaminergic neurons project from the cerebral cortex to the caudate nucleus via a corticostriatal path. Glutaminergic neurons also project on Purkinje cells in the cerebellum, neurons in the olfactory bulb, and the pyriform lobe. From the entorhinal cortex they project to the hippocampus (perforant path), and finally glutaminergic neurons connect the hippocampus with the septal area. At the postsynaptic membrane, glutamate activates AMPA (a-amino-3-hydroxy-5-methyl-4-isoxazolepropionic acid), N-methyl-D-aspartate (NMDA), and kainate ligand-gated ion channels [29,32]. In the context of delirium the alleged role of glutamate in learning and memory may be of relevance as it is implicated in the capacity of NMDA receptors to induce hippocampal long-term potentiation (LTP); a bioelectric phenomenon linked to synaptic plasticity and viewed as a cellular model for learning and memory.

Potentially related to the effects of alcohol intake specifically on the NMDA receptors, glutaminergic neurotransmission has been implicated in alcohol withdrawal syndrome [33]. N-methyl-D-aspartate receptor supersensitivity and its activation during periods of withdrawal from ethanol may explain the autonomic instability, behavioral agitation, and psychosis that can be seen in alcohol withdrawal delirium [34]. While various studies examined different polymorphisms of glutamate receptors, only one significant association has been reported of a specific allele coding for a subunit of the glutamatergic kainate receptor in alcoholic subjects suffering from withdrawal delirium [35].

Aspartate

After its abundant presence in the brain during embryonic development and the perinatal phase, levels of aspartate decrease sharply in adulthood. However, these reductions do not hold for restricted areas of the olfactory bulb, cerebellum, and hypothalamus [36]. Aspartate presence in the latter region points to its regulatory role in neuroendocrine functions in the hypothalamus. Aspartate can bind to NMDA receptors because of its affinity for the glutamate binding site [36].

In rodent models the aspartate-dependent potentiation of hippocampal synaptic plasticity is associated with a selective enhancement of spatial memory. Aspartate, by serving as an endogenous modulator of NMDA receptors, has been suggested to possess antipsychotic properties, thus it is tempting to speculate that impairments of aspartate neurotransmission may lead to decreased thresholds for delirium. The observation of symptoms resembling delirium in patients harboring auto antibodies against the NMDA receptor seems to support such a contention [37].

Miscellaneous neurotransmitters and "false neurotransmitter" hypothesis

Consistent with the notion that mainly astrocytes produce serine, recent evidence indicates that high amounts of serine are found in areas of mammalian brain harboring glia [38]. After its release, serine seems to act as an endogenous ligand of NMDA receptors, thus potentially affecting glutamatergic neurotransmission. In this respect there might be a functional link with nitric oxide (NO) since neuronal NO synthase can also be found in the same cells. Darra and colleagues have reviewed the cross-talk between serine and NO (nNOS) in astrocytes and the resulting interaction between astrocytes and neurons in the regulation of glutamatergic neurotransmission [38]. These authors conclude that under physiological conditions glutamate might act on either postsynaptic neurons or neighboring astrocytes through the NMDA or specific receptors, respectively. In astrocytes this can lead to increase in the levels of serine which subsequently inhibits nNOS activity, whereas in neurons the glutamate induces results in activation of nNOS. The NOS that is produced as a result of this activation is hypothesized to reach adjacent astrocytes and there to lead to a decrease in astrocytic serine contents [38]. Darra and colleagues propose that this serine-NO interaction between neurons and astrocytes may serve to achieve a glutamate-induced increase in serine content in astrocytes and that in this sequence of events the moderate amounts of NO act beneficially. Under inflammatory conditions in critical illness however, the action of pro-inflammatory cytokines is suggested to induce a decrease of NO contents in astrocytes and this ultimately gives rise to increased levels of serine. Upon increased release of serine from astrocytes, the calcium influx will increase in postsynaptic neurons also as a result of enhanced glutamate release from presynaptic neurons. In this way, the role of NO in the cross-talk between astrocytes and neurons may have deleterious effects under inflammatory conditions [38].

Hepatic encephalopathy is a serious and complex neuropsychiatric syndrome that shares features with the hypoactive delirium. In a classic paper, Fischer and Baldessarini, who were inspired in part by the effects of large doses of metaraminol or other alpha-adrenergic amines in the treatment of the hepatorenal syndrome, suggested that some of the neurological and also the cardiovascular complications of hepatic failure should be attributed to accumulation of false neurochemical transmitters, originally mainly focusing on adrenergic neurotransmitters [39].

Based on a more generic interpretation of this hypothesis, the competitive action on amino acid transport across the blood–brain barrier, branched-chain amino acids (BCAAs) have been extensively studied in hepatic encephalopathy. A Cochrane review confirmed that BCAAs significantly tend to improve functioning in patients suffering from hepatic encephalopathy [40].

Concluding remarks

As indicated in the introduction the clinical connotation "delirium" refers to many different phenomena. Also, the boundaries of this clinical syndrome are not always perfectly clear. Sometimes it is difficult to delineate delirium from related clinical syndromes like dementia, subsyndromal delirium, acute psychosis, or even from normality. Despite its intrinsically heterogeneous character, its large variations in clinical symptoms and severity, its poorly defined clinical boundaries, and its complex etiology, delirium often falls prone to the fallacy of reification. Reification is, in the words of the philosopher Alfred North Whitehead, the mistake of taking an abstract concept (or belief or opinion) for a physical or "concrete" reality [41]. This fallacy of misplaced concreteness occurs often in

research on delirium, because it is very tempting to consider delirium as a well-defined, homogeneous condition; both from a phenomenological and etiological point of view this is attractive for clinicians as well as basic researchers (and their funding agencies). Delirium taken as a concrete reality, almost as a "thing," invites the search for genetic markers, the ultimate delirium biomarker or the single causative culprit, either a specific metabolite, protein, or neurotransmitter that accounts for all symptoms in delirious states. Given its intrinsically heterogeneous nature such attempts are deemed to fail. Delirium associated with sepsis, in alcohol abstinence, in neurodegenerative disease, or delirium induced by use of specific drugs, will be fundamentally different. It is not likely at all that there will be a one and only magic bullet to explain, prevent, and cure delirium.

On the other hand, listing and studying all possible deranged mechanisms, neurotransmitters, and metabolites will not be very helpful either to students of delirium. Considering the profound abnormalities in the central nervous system underlying delirium, almost all measures are prone to marked abnormalities, therefore it will be next to impossible to definitely refute any specific metabolite, protein, or neurotransmitter system to be possibly involved. Although a multitude of mechanisms may play a role, some of these may be more important than others in causing delirium, to paraphrase George Orwell.

The field of research into encephalopathy in critical illness has much to gain from theoretical rigor. In the past the field may have been too open for reasoning based on circumstantial evidence only. In reviewing the possible role of specific neurotransmitter systems in delirium, many of the substances discussed above are not only implicated in delirium, but also in many other conditions, such as addiction, schizophrenia, or stroke, to give some examples of the speculations that have been made in relation to excitatory neurotransmitters. Obviously, that cannot be true. Analyzed in terms of diagnostic test research, researchers may be too sensitive in their attempts to identify critical factors in the pathogenesis of critical illness encephalopathy. If any given substance that can be loosely connected to delirium is immediately acknowledged as an important key player, the specificity of this process of identification will be too low and there will be too many false positives on the research agenda. In the long term this will be problematic, especially if researchers fail to subject their favorite molecule to the most critical test: if a specific mechanism, neurotransmitter, or metabolite is hypothesized to a play a role in mediating certain effects, it should be subjected to the most critical test or experiment as early as possible, because the research community gains most by excluding such candidate key mechanisms, neurotransmitters, or metabolites.

In this chapter, the specific role of the cholinergic system in the etiology of delirium was emphasized. This is not to claim that acetylcholine is the one and only neurotransmitter that is important in the etiopathogenesis of delirium [2,5]. As indicated above, all neurotransmitter systems will be prone to imbalances before, during, and shortly after delirium. However, changes in the cholinergic system possess a unique combination of explanatory power.

Cholinergic deficiency offers a potential explanation for the impairments of attention that are crucial in the symptoms of delirium [2]. In delirious states the cholinergic system may be the link between neurotransmitter abnormalities and the role of innate immunity in the brain [5]. Moreover, the cholinergic deficiency hypothesis can be put to the test by investigating the various drugs that affect cholinergic functions, for their effects on the alleviation of symptoms or the prevention of delirium or its long-term sequelae.

References

1. Hasselmo ME, Sarter M. Modes and models of forebrain cholinergic neuromodulation of cognition. *Neuropsychopharmacology* 2011;**36**:52–73.

2. Graef S, Schönknecht P, Sabri O, Hegerl U. Cholinergic receptor subtypes and their role in cognition, emotion, and vigilance control: an overview of preclinical and clinical findings. *Psychopharmacology (Berl)* 2011;**215**:205–29.

3. Lemstra AW, Eikelenboom P, Van Gool WA. The cholinergic deficiency syndrome and its therapeutic implications. *Gerontology* 2003;**49**:55–60.

4. Forrer GRMJJ. Atropine coma: a somatic therapy in psychiatry. *Am J Psychiatry* 1958;**115**:455–8.

5. Itil TFM. Anticholinergic drug-induced delirium: experimental modification, quantitative EEG and behavioral correlations. *J Nerv Ment Dis* 1966;**143**:492–507.

6. Van Gool WA, van de Beek D, Eikelenboom P. Systemic infection and delirium: when cytokines and acetylcholine collide. *Lancet* 2010;**375**:773–5.

7. Qin L, Wu X, Block ML, *et al.* Systemic LPS causes chronic neuroinflammation and progressive neurodegeneration. *Glia* 2007;**55**:453–62.

8. Teeling JL, Perry VH. Systemic infection and inflammation in acute CNS injury and chronic neurodegeneration: underlying mechanisms. *Neuroscience* 2009;**158**:1062–73.

9. Perry VH. The influence of systemic inflammation in the brain: implications for chronic neurodegenerative disease. *Brain Behav Immun* 2004;**18**:407–13.

10. Franceschi C, Capri M, Monti D, *et al.* Inflammaging and anti-inflammaging: a systemic perspective on ageing and longevity emerged from studies in humans. *Mech Ageing Dev* 2007;**128**:92–105.

11. Tracey KJ. The inflammatory reflex. *Nature* 2002;**420**:853–9.

12. Gamberini M, Bolliger D, Lurati Buse GA, *et al.* Rivastigmine for the prevention of postoperative delirium in elderly patients undergoing elective cardiac surgery – a randomized controlled trial. *Crit Care Med* 2009;**37**:1762–8.

13. van Eijk MM, Roes KC, Honing ML, *et al.* Effect of rivastigmine as an adjunct to usual care with haloperidol on duration of delirium and mortality in critically ill patients: a multicentre, double-blind, placebo-controlled randomised trial. *Lancet* 2010;**376**:1829–37.

14. Bromberg-Martin ES, Matsumoto M, Hikosaka O. Dopamine in motivational control: rewarding, aversive, and alerting. *Neuron* 2010;**68**:815–34.

15. Steiner LA. Postoperative delirium. Part 1: pathophysiology and risk factors. *Eur J Anaesthesiol* 2011;**28**:628–36.

16. van Munster BC, de Rooij SE, Yazdanpanah M, *et al.* The association of the dopamine transporter gene and the dopamine receptor 2 gene with delirium, a meta-analysis. *Am J Med Genet B Neuropsychiatr Genet* 2010;**153B**:648–55.

17. Berridge CW, Waterhouse BD. The locus coeruleus-noradrenergic system: modulation of behavioral state and state-dependent cognitive processes. *Brain Res Brain Res Rev* 2003;**42**:33–84.

18. Lester DB, Rogers TD, Blaha CD. Acetylcholine-dopamine interactions in the pathophysiology and treatment of CNS disorders. *CNS Neurosci Ther* 2010;**16**:137–62.

19. Hofer S, Steppan J, Wagner T, *et al.* Central sympatholytics prolong survival in experimental sepsis. *Crit Care* 2009;**13**:133.

20. Mantz J, Josserand J, Hamada S. Dexmedetomidine: new insights. *Eur J Anaesthesiol* 2011;**28**:3–6.

21. Pandharipande PP, Sanders RD, Girard TD, *et al.* Effect of dexmedetomidine versus lorazepam on outcome in patients with sepsis: an a priori-designed analysis of the MENDS randomized controlled trial. *Crit Care* 2010;**14**:R38.

22. Riker RR, Shehabi Y, Bokesch PM, *et al.* Dexmedetomidine vs. midazolam for sedation of critically ill patients: a randomized trial. *JAMA* 2009;**301**:489–99.

23. Steiner LA. Postoperative delirium. Part 2: detection, prevention and treatment. *Eur J Anaesthesiol* 2011;**28**:723–32.

24. Carr GV, Lucki I. The role of serotonin receptor subtypes in treating depression: a review of animal studies. *Psychopharmacology (Berl)* 2011;**213**:265–87.

25. Van der Mast RC, Fekkes D. Serotonin and amino acids: partners in delirium pathophysiology? *Semin Clin Neuropsychiatry* 2000;**5**:125–31.

26. Pandharipande PP, Morandi A, Adams JR, *et al.* Plasma tryptophan and tyrosine levels are independent risk factors for delirium in critically ill patients. *Intensive Care Med* 2009;**35**:1886–92.

27. Capogna M, Pearce RA. GABA (A, slow): causes and consequences. *Trends Neurosci* 2011;**34**:101–12.

28. Leo RJ, Baer D. Delirium associated with baclofen withdrawal: a review of common presentations and management strategies. *Psychosomatics* 2005;**46**:503–7.

29. Foster AC, Kemp JA. Glutamate- and GABA-based CNS therapeutics. *Curr Opin Pharmacol* 2006;**6**:7–17.

30. Nguyen HT, Li KY, daGraca RL, *et al.* Behavior and cellular evidence for propofol-induced hypnosis involving brain glycine receptors. *Anesthesiology* 2009;**110**:326–32.

31. Ye JH, Sokol KA, Bhavsar U. Glycine receptors contribute to hypnosis induced by ethanol. *Alcohol Clin Exp Res* 2009;**33**:1069–74.

32. Traynelis SF, Wollmuth LP, McBain CJ, *et al.* Glutamate receptor ion channels: structure, regulation, and function. *Pharmacol Rev* 2010;**62**:405–96.

33. Adamis D, Van Munster BC, Macdonald AJ. The genetics of deliria. *Int Rev Psychiatry* 2009;**21**:20–9.

34. Tsai G, Coyle JT. The role of glutamatergic neurotransmission in the pathophysiology of alcoholism. *Annu Rev Med* 1998;**49**:173–84.

35. Preuss UW, Zill P, Koller G, *et al.* Ionotropic glutamate receptor gene GRIK3 SER310ALA functional polymorphism is related to delirium tremens in alcoholics. *Pharmacogenomics J* 2006;**6**:34–41.

36. Errico F, Napolitano F, Nisticò R, Centonze D, Usiello A. D-aspartate: an atypical amino acid with neuromodulatory activity in mammals. *Rev Neurosci* 2009;**20**:429–40.

37. Irani SR, Vincent A. NMDA receptor antibody encephalitis. *Curr Neurol Neurosci Rep* 2011;**11**:298–304.

38. Darra E, Ebner FH, Shoji K, Suzuki H, Mariotto S. Dual cross-talk between nitric oxide and D-serine in astrocytes and neurons in the brain. *Cent Nerv Syst Agents Med Chem* 2009;**9**:289–94.

39. Fischer JE, Baldessarini RJ. False neurotransmitters and hepatic failure. *Lancet* 1971;**298**:75–80.

40. Als-Nielsen B, Koretz RL, Kjaergard LL, Gluud C. Branched-chain amino acids for hepatic encephalopathy. *Cochrane Database Syst Rev* 2003;**2**: CD001939.

41. Whitehead, AN. *Science and the Modern World*. Old Tappan, NJ: Free Press (Simon & Schuster); 1925 (reissue 1997).

Neuromodulatory and neurotoxic effects of sedative agents

Jean Mantz and Souhayl Dahmani

SUMMARY

Sedatives and analgesics aim at ensuring comfort and safety in the mechanically ventilated, critically ill patient. Whilst these drugs potently modulate neurotransmission in the central nervous system (CNS) to provide their beneficial effects, a body of recent work suggests that some of them may contribute to the impairment of cognitive recovery after intensive care. The most frequently used sedatives (propofol, benzodiazepines, etomidate, thiopental, but also volatile anesthetics) produce their hypnotic effects via enhancement of the inhibitory transmission mediated via the gamma-aminobutyric acid A ($GABA_A$) receptors. Ketamine and xenon exhibit exclusive antagonistic properties toward the excitatory transmission mediated via the N-methyl-D-aspartate receptors. Opioids act on G-protein-coupled receptors (mu and delta) to produce their analgesic effects. When repeatedly exposed to agonists, opioid receptors undergo a complex internalization/degradation process called "desensitization," which accounts in part for the mechanisms of opioid tolerance. Of the other drug categories that have proven their utility as additional sedatives, particularly in case of dangerous agitation, neuroleptics (blockers of the dopamine D2 receptors) and alpha-2 adrenoceptor agonists (clonidine, dexmedetomidine) represent interesting solutions. Toxicity of some drugs (i.e., volatile anesthetics or ketamine at high concentrations), but also neuroprotection by others, has been reported in vitro. However, there is no evidence of clinical neurotoxicity of these agents when used as sedatives in critically ill patients in the intensive care unit (ICU). Recently, dexmedetomidine has been developed as a primary sedative for mechanically ventilated patients in the ICU. This agent exerts its effects via a unique mechanism (agonist of the alpha-2 adrenoceptors) which confers some favorable properties with respect to the goals to be achieved in a sedated, mechanically ventilated patient. Its sedation profile preserves rousability and its mechanism of action preserves non-REM sleep, which may contribute to its delirium-sparing effects. The need for drugs acting on the CNS, such as sedatives and analgesics, has to be carefully evaluated on a daily basis at the bedside to limit the potential detrimental effects associated with oversedation in critically ill patients.

Introduction

Critical care is associated with a hostile environment. For several decades, there has been general agreement that the comfort and safety of critically ill, mechanically ventilated patients was facilitated by deep pharmacological sedation. This view of sedation and analgesia for ICU patients has completely changed because it has been suspected that a deep level of sedation was unnecessary in most of ICU patients, and even resulted in an increased rate of complications. Prolongation of the duration of mechanical ventilation and an increased length in ICU stay are most likely to contribute to the morbidity induced by oversedation. For example, it has been well documented that continuous intravenous sedation with benzodiazepines and opioids is a predictor of ventilator-acquired pneumonia. A large body of recent work has unambiguously shown that alleviation of an unnecessary deep level of sedation improves outcome in ICU patients. By either discontinuing sedation daily, or titrating sedatives and analgesics to target levels corresponding to a calm, comfortable, and communicative patient, it is possible to decrease the duration of mechanical ventilation and length of stay, which results in a decreased morbidity. The availability of a large panel of clinical sedation and pain scales validated for ICU patients provides a unique opportunity to target sedation and analgesia via nurse-driven algorithms at the bedside.

Whilst sedatives and analgesics have been considered neuroprotective for decades, mainly because of their ability to decrease brain oxygen consumption, this view has been challenged by a growing body of evidence obtained both from the clinical and experimental setting, which suggests that sedation may harm brain function in ICU patients [1,2]. As an example of this, benzodiazepines, which are commonly used as the primary regimen for sedation of mechanically ventilated patients in the ICU, are a risk factor for delirium in these patients [3,4]. In the present chapter, we will briefly review the main molecular mechanisms by which sedatives, anesthetics, opioid analgesics, and antipsychotics modulate neurotransmission in the CNS. We will discuss a possible toxicity of these agents for the brain and examine the relevance of these findings to some subpopulations of ICU patients. Finally, special emphasis will be put on the original profile of dexmedetomidine, a potentially brain-protective alpha-2 adrenoceptor which has been licensed in Europe recently (Table 16.1).

Table 16.1 Main target receptors of the neuronal cell membrane for sedatives/analgesics used in the intensive care unit.

Target receptors	Drugs	Action
$GABA_A$ receptor	Benzodiazepines, thiopental, propofol, etomidate, volatile anesthetics	Agonist
NMDA receptors	Ketamine, xenon	Antagonist
Dopamine D2 receptors	Neuroleptics	Antagonist
Opioid receptors (mu, delta)	Opioids	Agonist
Alpha-2 adrenoceptors	Clonidine, dexmedetomidine	Agonist

GABA, Gamma-aminobutyric acid; NMDA, N-methyl-D-aspartate.

Modulation of neurotransmission by sedatives, anesthetics, opioid analgesics, and antipsychotics

Sedatives and anesthetics

The majority of intravenous sedatives or anesthetic agents, including barbiturates, propofol, and benzodiazepines, selectively modulate the $GABA_A$ receptor by potentiating and prolonging the binding of GABA released by presynaptic neurons [5]. Thus, they increase the duration of the opening of the channel. At higher concentrations, some intravenous anesthetics may also elicit opening of the $GABA_A$ channel without the need for the endogenous neurotransmitter. Propofol delays desensitization of the $GABA_A$ receptor, a mechanism which plays an important role if inhibitory synapses are rapidly and repetitively activated.

It is now commonly acknowledged that most inhaled agents act by enhancing the chloride conductance of the $GABA_A$ receptor, thereby reinforcing inhibitory synaptic and extrasynaptic transmission. In addition to their predominant action on $GABA_A$ receptors, halogenated volatile anesthetics inhibit excitatory neurotransmission at the presynaptic level, mainly by decreasing the release of glutamate. On the other hand, non-halogenated volatile anesthetics like xenon, nitric oxide, cyclopropane, as well as some intravenous agents, i.e., ketamine, have little if any effect on the different subtypes of $GABA_A$ receptors tested to date. They mainly depress the excitatory neurotransmission at the postsynaptic level by blunting the activation of NMDA receptors by glutamate. Ketamine acts by entering and blocking the channel itself in a non-competitive manner. Numerous volatile anesthetics, as well as propofol, applied at subclinical concentrations, inhibit nicotinic acetylcholine receptors (nAChR). This latter mechanism is likely to be involved in the antinociceptive, rather than immobilizing effects of anesthetic agents.

Molecular genetic techniques (like targeted mutagenesis or the engineering of chimeric receptors) have enabled determination of the precise location of some regions and/or sites critical for the action of anesthetics and sedatives. The current literature on this field is extremely important and still growing. Some of the main findings in this area may be summarized as follows. First, experiments conducted on the glycine and the $GABA_A$ receptor have identified some amino acid residues located between transmembrane domains TM2 and TM3, which are mandatory for volatile anesthetics to potentiate these receptors in the presence of their endogenous agonists. Second, the potentiation of the $GABA_A$ receptor by propofol is altered by the targeted mutation of specific amino acids located within the TM2 domain on the beta subunit. Third, the sensitivity of NMDA receptors to ketamine is dependent on arginine residues located at the level of the NR2B and NR1 subunits. These arginine residues are part of the Mg^{2+} – blockade sensitive site of the NMDA channel. These landmark works point out the high specificity of the interactions between anesthetic/sedative agents and neurotransmitter receptors. They demonstrate the complexity of such interactions since, for example, two anesthetics modulating the activity of a given receptor may act at different sites of this receptor.

Cortical $GABA_A$ receptors seem to play a critical role in sedation/hypnosis induced by anesthetics and sedatives. This was corroborated by results of functional neuroimaging studies conducted in the human. Subhypnotic, sedative, concentrations of anesthetics reduce cortical metabolism by 30–50%, while the metabolism of subcortical structures is not much altered. Taken together, these different results suggest that the hypnotic effects of sedatives given to ICU patients largely involve cortical $GABA_A$ receptors. The $alpha_1$ subunit of $GABA_A$ receptors plays an important role as well, notably in sedation and amnesia elicited by diazepam [6]. It must be emphasized that, at the protein level, $beta_2$ and $alpha_1$ subunits of $GABA_A$ receptors are most frequently associated with $gamma_2$ subunits and that $beta_2$ subunit-containing $GABA_A$ receptors are the most widely distributed isoforms in the CNS.

Opioids

Opioids are the most effective analgesic compounds known, but their clinical use is limited by significant adverse effects. Respiratory depression is the most severe short-term adverse effect of opioids, whilst development of tolerance and dependence occurs after repeated opioid administration. Critically ill patients under continuous infusion of opioids during a sufficient period of time (1 week at 20 µg/hour sufentanil) should be considered at risk to develop a withdrawal syndrome [7]. Receptor desensitization is

the pharmacological substrate underlying receptor drug tolerance. Three main mechanisms are associated with G-protein-coupled receptor (such as the opioid receptors) desensitization: receptor phosphorylation, receptor internalization and/or sequestration, and receptor down-regulation (reduction in the total number of receptors). The signaling pathways of opioid receptors are well characterized. After the ligand binds the receptor, conformational changes allow cellular coupling of many Gi/o proteins to the C-terminal part of the opioid receptor. The activated subunits may inhibit adenylate cyclase, or directly act with ion channels in the membrane [8]. All three opioid receptor subtypes suppress the activity of various Ca^{2+} channels, thereby reducing cell excitability. At the postsynaptic level, opioid receptors mediate hyperpolarization by opening K^+ channels, thereby preventing action potential propagation [8]. Like many other G-protein-coupled receptors, opioid receptor activation is associated with a number of conformational changes that trigger signaling and regulation. Regulatory steps usually start with phosphorylation of the receptor followed by beta-arrestin recruitment and disruption of receptor signaling by G-protein-coupled effectors. Since arrestins bind to the coat-structure of clathrin-coated pits, a great majority of opioid ligands that promote functional desensitization also enhance sequestration [9]. The main steps of homologous desensitization of G-protein-coupled receptors are provided in Figure 16.1. A recent body of evidence has shown the effects of opioids on specific immune signaling, some of them having potential therapeutic implications [10]. Opioid agonists may activate glial cells via an agonist activity at the glial Toll-like receptor (TLR4), which plays a role in the development of opioid tolerance [11]. This suggests that attenuation of central glial activation by selective antagonism of TLR may be a clinical method to distinguish between beneficial (analgesic) and undesirable (tolerance) effects of opioids. Besides, depression of the immune system by opioids is a well-recognized phenomenon, and many mechanisms have been proposed to account for this finding. For example, it is well established that a variety of cell types, including mature and immature B-cells, T-cells, and macrophages, express opioid receptors or mRNA for these receptors [12]. Therefore, it is not surprising that a huge number of papers have shown that opioids induce functional changes in immune cells which may result in alteration of the immune function [12,13].

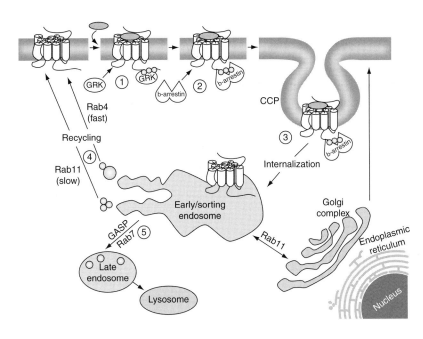

Figure 16.1 Steps involved in the homologous desensitization process of G-protein-coupled receptors. (1) Phosphorylation of the opioid receptor by GRK; (2) Receptor phosphorylation increases its affinity for beta-arrestin, which promotes interaction between the two proteins; and (3) receptor internalization. Internalized receptors are then directed to early/sorting endosomes where interaction with different regulatory proteins will allow them to recycle back to the membrane (4), or will be directed toward degradation (5). From Nagi K, Pineyro G. Regulation of opioid receptor signaling: implication for the development of analgesic tolerance. *Mol Brain* 2011;**4**:25, with permission [9].

Antipsychotics

When facing an agitated, mechanically ventilated ICU patient, the additional use of antipsychotics such as neuroleptics can be considered. These drugs are the cornerstone of the treatment of psychiatric disorders such as schizophrenia, reducing the activity of the mesolimbic dopaminergic system, which is thought to be responsible for the positive symptoms of this disease. They exhibit, however, a broad and complex pattern of cellular effects at the receptor and post-receptor level. All antipsychotic drugs, either from the first (haloperidol, chlorpromazine) or the second generation (quetiapine), share in common the ability to act as dopamine D2 receptor antagonists [14]. Second-generation neuroleptics are also 5-HT$_{2A}$ receptor antagonists, which may contribute to reduce extrapyramidal side effects when combined with reduced D2 receptor blockade. Chronic neuroleptic administration also results in profound changes in the expression/activity of glutamate receptors in various brain structures, as well as changes in the expression of growth factors. Besides, recent reports have also revealed antimicrobial, antiprionic, and anticancerous activities for certain members of the phenothiazine group [15].

Several lines of evidence suggest that treatment with neuroleptics may attenuate or prevent the occurrence of delirium, a major complication occurring in the ICU, under certain circumstances. In a randomized controlled trial, Girard and co-workers found no difference in the ability of the neuroleptics haloperidol and ziprasidone to reduce the incidence of delirium in ICU mechanically ventilated patients [16]. In another RCT, Devlin *et al.* reported the efficacy of quetiapine to reduce the time spent with delirium in ICU patients [17]. Recently, risperidone given for treatment in subsyndromal delirium was associated with reduced clinical delirium after cardiac surgery [18]. Altogether, these results suggest that there may be space for targeted neuroleptic prophylaxis in some subpopulations of ICU patients. These populations remain, however, to be clarified.

Are sedatives neurotoxic?

Experimental data

Experimental neurotoxicity of sedatives and anesthetics has been examined in animal models at the extremes of age, but most of the studies have been conducted in the rodent neonate and primate [19]. In the rodent neonate, the optimal window for the expression of sedative- and anesthetic-induced neurotoxicity ranges between postnatal days 5 and 14, which corresponds to the peak of neurogenesis in this species. Systemic administration of repeated supratherapeutic 20 mg/kg doses of ketamine in the newborn rat induced neuronal death and abnormalities of synaptogenesis. In some studies, these disorders have been associated with the occurrence of cognitive dysfunction in the adult rat. Ketamine-induced neurotoxicity has also been reported in vitro for therapeutic concentrations (5 mg/kg). This ketamine concentration has been shown to alter dendritic growth in cell cultures. In the primate, ketamine neurotoxicity has also been observed for doses ranging from 20 to 50 mg/kg, provided that continuous i.v. administration has been maintained for 24 hours. Altogether, these results suggest that ketamine at supratherapeutic doses may induce neurotoxicity in the mammalian brain.

Direct neurotoxicity of volatile anesthetics such as isoflurane has been demonstrated in vitro. Isoflurane (2%) increases the protein expression of beta-amyloid substance and caspase-3 in the rat brain [20]. A recent study performed in the primate indicates that at least 5 hours of exposure to isoflurane (0.7–1.5%) is required to elicit isoflurane-induced apoptosis [19]. Importantly, co-administration of midazolam and isoflurane in the newborn rat enhances neuronal death, which suggests synergy between sedatives in the production of experimental neurotoxicity. On the other hand, there is now compelling evidence that the inflammatory response is likely to play an exacerbating role in the neurotoxic phenomena. Recent evidence suggests that beside their possible neurotoxic effects, such agents as propofol may also exert a protective action against the neurotoxic lesions produced by septic or non-septic inflammatory response [21].

Several hypotheses may account for the mechanisms of the neurotoxic effects of sedatives and anesthetics observed experimentally. An inversion of the chloride current observed in the developing brain may explain that activation of the $GABA_A$ receptor by sedatives may induce excitotoxicity, as is the case for stimulation of the NMDA receptors following cerebral ischemia. Both the production of NGF and a decrease in the activation of the survival protein Akt have been observed following propofol administration in rats at postnatal day 7. Recent data indicate that sedatives/anesthetics may slow down cell proliferation and dendritogenesis without inducing immediate neuronal death [19]. These results are important, since neurogenesis remains active all the life. Therefore, exposure to anesthetics/sedatives in the early postnatal period may lead to an impairment of cognitive functions in the elderly. Finally, the accelerating effect of apoptosis (which is a physiological phenomenon) may also be considered.

Clinical implications

Stroke represents a major undesirable adverse event experienced by some critically ill patients. However, no data are available to support any protective or aggravating role played by sedatives or analgesics in the occurrence of stroke in any clinical setting. Therefore, other end points are necessary to examine the effects of these pharmacological agents on brain function in the critically ill. Both delirium and long-term cognitive dysfunction post-ICU are the witness of cerebral dysfunction in these patients. Delirium represents a serious adverse event occurring in mechanically ventilated ICU patients. Critically ill patients who have experienced at least one episode of delirium during their stay exhibit an increased risk of mortality after intensive care [22]. Besides, several lines of evidence suggest that delirium may predict long-term cognitive deterioration after ICU discharge. Older persons admitted into the ICU are at high risk to develop delirium and accelerated cognitive dysfunction after intensive care. Patients' status, severity of illness, inflammatory response to sepsis, sleep deterioration, and a huge number of medications, including sedatives and analgesics, are likely to contribute to the deterioration of cognitive function. Whilst sedatives were considered, so far, as more or less brain protective, because they decrease brain oxygen consumption, they clearly appear to date as potential causes for acute and chronic brain dysfunction in ICU patients. As a matter of fact, benzodiazepines and opioids have been identified as independent risk factors for delirium in this patient population [4]. Data obtained from a large database of critically ill patients indicate that the administration of benzodiazepines is an independent risk factor of mortality in comparison with propofol [4]. On the other hand, experimental evidence suggests that a number of sedatives (and anesthetics) may cause cerebral toxicity in vitro and impair long-term cognitive functions, at least in at-risk patient subpopulations such as the elderly critically ill. At the opposite, whether sedatives, analgesics, and anesthetics may cause brain toxicity in the pediatric population remains a matter of debate. Therefore, it can be accepted that some sedatives not only modulate neurotransmission but may also contribute to impair recovery of cognitive function and quality of life after intensive care.

A recent body of evidence suggests that volatile anesthetics could represent an interesting alternative to i.v. agents such as propofol or midazolam for ICU sedation, at least when weaning from the ventilator is considered. Intravenous sedation is associated with depression of rousability and ventilator drive. Moreover, prolonged periods of sedation >7 days with administration of at least 5 mg/hour midazolam and 20 μg/kg sufentanil is a risk factor for the occurrence of weaning syndromes, which consist of delirium and dangerous agitation developed after cessation of intravenous sedation [7]. Volatile anesthetics such as isoflurane or sevoflurane provide sedation, analgesia, and some degree of myorelaxation. In contrast to midazolam or long-acting opioids, they are short-acting agents with minimal (sevoflurane) to moderate (isoflurane) accumulation when low-inspired concentrations are delivered over a prolonged period of time. Their use allows rapid recovery of spontaneous ventilation after stopping its administration to the patient. A recent randomized controlled trial performed in ICU patients sedated with sevoflurane indicates that administration of low-inspired concentrations of sevoflurane was associated with a reduction of the duration of mechanical ventilation and weaning period, ICU stay, and in the incidence of respiratory complications. Interestingly, the incidence of delirium after weaning from the ventilator was found significantly decreased in comparison with patients sedated with i.v. agents [23]. The explanations which may account for this finding are either the sedative and opioid-sparing effect of sevoflurane or specific properties of volatile anesthetics on neurotransmission, or both.

Role of dexmedetomidine in mechanically ventilated ICU patients

General considerations

There is growing interest for the role of alpha-2 adrenoceptor agonists in anesthesia and intensive care. Indeed, these agents exhibit a wide pattern of properties including sedative, anesthetic-sparing, analgesic, and sympatholytic properties. Clonidine is the most popular agent in this category of pharmacology agents in Europe and it has been used in a large number of situations such as ICU sedation, facilitation of regional anesthesia, or control of opioid or alcohol withdrawal syndrome [24]. However, clonidine is a long-acting agent and its use is often associated with a rebound in blood pressure following its discontinuation. Dexmedetomidine is a potent and much more selective agonist of the alpha-2 adrenergic receptors

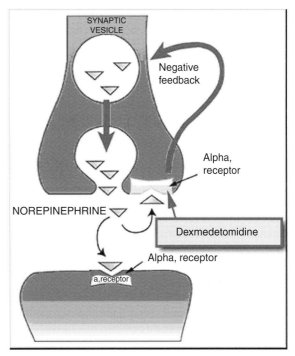

Figure 16.2 Action of dexmedetomidine at the noradrenergic synapse. Dexmedetomidine acts as an agonist of the presynaptic agonist of the alpha-2 adrenoceptors, which exerts a negative feedback on norepinephrine release into the central noradrenergic and peripheral sympathetic noradrenergic synapse.

than clonidine, with a broad pattern of actions on the mammalian brain (Figure 16.2). A large body of recent work supports that this agent exhibits a favorable profile in anesthesia and intensive care [24]. Cellular effects mediated via other signaling pathways than those triggered by stimulation of the alpha-2 adrenoceptors have been reported. Some of them have been shown to be involved in dexmedetomidine's neuroprotective properties both in vitro and in vivo. Interestingly, these brain-protective effects might, for the first time, be relevant to the clinical setting, since dexmedetomidine reduces the number of days with delirium or coma in mechanically ventilated patients in the ICU [25–27]. Also, it does not exert significant depression on the ventilatory drive and may preserve physiological sleep better than any other sedative in ICU patients. Preliminary data suggest that dexmedetomidine may reduce mortality in septic ICU patients via attenuation of immunosuppression [28]. Although reduction by alpha-2 adrenoceptor agonists in the incidence of postoperative major adverse cardiac events has been shown in patients undergoing vascular surgery, severe mishaps due to uncontrollable hypotension and bradycardia have been reported with dexmedetomidine in patients with compromised left ventricular function or heart conduction blocks.

Basic non-alpha-2 adrenoceptor-mediated mechanisms of action of dexmedetomidine and their relevance to neuroprotection

Dexmedetomidine's effects in the CNS were classically thought to proceed via stimulation of the alpha-2 adrenoceptor inhibitory pathway. This has been extensively demonstrated in the past, with interesting applications, particularly in neuroprotection. Dexmedetomidine increases the phosphorylation of focal adhesion kinase, a key non-receptor tyrosine kinase cellular enzyme which may couple rapid events, such as action potentials and transmitter release, to long-lasting effects in the brain, such as plasticity and survival [29]. This effect provides neuroprotection in experimental models, including neonatal cerebral excitotoxic injury. Elegant experiments indicate that this neuroprotective effect is mediated via stimulation of the alpha-2A adrenoceptor subtype. Several lines of evidence support that dexmedetomidine exerts some important cellular effects via signaling pathways other than the alpha-2 -adrenoceptor adenylate cyclase complex. Dexmedetomidine inhibits neuronal sodium and delays potassium inward rectifier currents. This mechanism also accounts for the inhibitory action of dexmedetomidine on neuronal activity. Dexmedetomidine increases ERK1/2 phosphorylation, a key MAP kinase involved in cell survival and memory. This effect is mediated via activation of protein kinase C, and most likely imidazoline receptors [30]. Dexmedetomidine also increases the expression of growth factors such as epidermal growth factor and brain-derived neurotrophic factors, which participate in neuroprotection. Recently, we have shown that dexmedetomidine exerts both pre- and postconditioning effects against ischemic injury in hippocampal organotypic slice cultures [24]. Both tyrosine kinase and ERK1/2 phosphorylation participate in these protective effects. This may open new perspectives for the clinical use of dexmedetomidine since, theoretically, brain damage may even be attenuated when this agent is administered post-injury. Unlike other agents such as volatile

anesthetics, dexmedetomidine was not found to facilitate the apoptotic cascade [24]. Preliminary experimental data in a rabbit model of spine trauma failed, however, to show any benefit from dexmedetomidine (1 µg/kg) in terms of recovery.

Role of dexmedetomidine for sedation and analgesia in mechanically ventilated ICU patients

The goals and standard of care of analgesia and sedation of mechanically ventilated ICU patients have undergone considerable changes in the last 10 years. There is now convincing evidence that an excessively deep level of sedation results in increased morbidity and perhaps mortality, due to the prolongation of mechanical ventilation and ICU stay. On the other hand, undersedation is associated with severe adverse effects such as an increased risk of accidental extubation or major cardiac adverse events in patients at risk for coronary syndrome. To date, except in specific situations such as severe head trauma, or severe acute respiratory distress syndrome, the optimal level of sedation in ICU patients should target a calm, but rousable patient, who should be able to communicate his needs, particularly for analgesia. Algorithms for sedation and analgesia based on re-evaluation of comfort and pain by nurses using specific sedation and pain scales have proved to be efficacious in accelerating recovery. Noteworthy, both daily awakening trials and active physiotherapy reduce the duration of mechanical ventilation and ICU stay, and perhaps mortality [31,32].

Currently, propofol and benzodiazepines are the most frequently used agents for continuous ICU sedation in the USA and Europe, respectively. Dexmedetomidine has become available in the USA, Asia, Middle East, Japan, Australia, and recently in Europe. However, it represents only 4% of the drugs used in the USA for ICU sedation. The specific profile of this agent is very interesting from the intensivist's point of view, since it preserves rousability and does not depress spontaneous ventilation, which may facilitate weaning from the ventilator. Further supporting this statement, bispectral index (BIS) values associated with an Observer Assessment of Alertness/ Sedation (OAA/S) score ≤ 2 in volunteers were significantly lower with dexmedetomidine compared with propofol (46 vs. 67). On the other hand, dexmedetomidine exhibits favorable properties towards brain protection, which have been confirmed in two recent major trials on ICU sedation (MENDS [25] and SEDCOM [26]). In these prospective, controlled, randomized trials, dexmedetomidine was compared with lorazepam (midazolam, respectively) for ICU sedation. Although no difference in overall mortality was found, the number of days free of coma or delirium was markedly decreased in the dexmedetomidine group. A recent meta-analysis of five studies confirms and extends these findings by showing a significant reduction in the risk of delirium with dexmedetomidine compared with control (relative risk 0.45; 95% confidence interval 0.32 to 0.64). Further, in the MENDS trial, a closer analysis of the group of septic patients was carried out. This subgroup analysis included 39 septic patients (19 in the dexmedetomidine group, 20 in the lorazepam group). Baseline demographics, ICU type, and admission diagnosis of the sepsis were similar in both groups. Dexmedetomidine-treated patients had more days that were free of delirium or ventilatory support. In septic patients, the risk of death at 28 days was reduced by 70% in the dexmedetomidine group compared with the lorazepam group (p = 0.04). Although these results are preliminary and need confirmation in large prospective studies, it is possible that dexmedetomidine improves survival in septic patients by either specific immunological mechanisms or by avoidance of lorazepam or both. Interestingly, several lines of evidence suggest that dexmedetomidine prolongs survival in experimental models of sepsis. This effect may be mediated via reduction in the inflammatory process and cytokine production [28]. Lack of apoptosis induction by dexmedetomidine in comparison with other sedatives/anesthetics, and improved macrophage function represent possible contributive factors as well. In a pilot study conducted in ICU patients with postoperative abdominal complications, blood levels of tumor necrosis factor alpha (TNFα), and interleukin-1 and -6 were found to be decreased at 24 hours post-surgery in patients sedated with dexmedetomidine compared with those who had received propofol. Large differences were also observed in intra-abdominal pressure at 24 hours (12.4 ± 5.8 vs. 18.1 ± 2.8 mmHg, p < 0.05) and 48 hours (13.9 ± 6.2 vs. 18.7 ± 3.5 mmHg, p < 0.05) in favor of the dexmedetomidine group [33]. A follow-up study has recently shown that in comparison with midazolam, patients sedated with dexmedetomidine had fewer secondary infections in the ICU [13].

Sleep is severely disturbed in mechanically ventilated ICU patients [34]. The ICU environment participates in a disorganization of the sleep pattern, together with specific drugs and mechanical ventilation. Sleep deprivation is one of the most undesirable events reported by patients after discharge from the ICU. Sleep fragmentation represents another problem in mechanically ventilated ICU patients. Indeed, it has been shown that multiple episodes of awakening occur during one single night in these patients, leading to frequent sleep interruptions. Persistent sleep disturbances have been reported in a significant number of ICU patients even several weeks after discharge. Whether sleep disturbances impact on the outcome of ICU patients by increasing morbidity or even mortality remains to be shown. However, there is indirect experimental and clinical evidence that this may be the case, and that sleep disorders may contribute to alter weaning from the ventilator or may favor the occurrence of post-ICU cognitive dysfunction. Quality and quantity of sleep seems to be more preserved by dexmedetomidine than with other sedative regimens. There is clinical evidence that the EEG pattern associated with dexmedetomidine sedation mimics that of non-REM sleep [35]. This unique property makes this agent an excellent candidate for the attenuation of sleep disturbance and its putative consequences on long-term cognitive functions in ICU patients. The relationship between sleep deprivation and delirium has been studied for many years, and has been regarded as reciprocal. Therefore, it may be speculated that dexmedetomidine may also tackle delirium by restoring, at least in part, sleep quality in ICU patients. Dexmedetomidine may have a potential to be an agent particularly appropriate for sedation and analgesia in the pediatric ICU. Lack of experimental neurotoxicity and presence of neuroprotection in experimental models of perinatal excitotoxic injury make dexmedetomidine particularly interesting for the pediatric population. It has been successfully used for analgesia and sedation of preterm infants. The sedation target concentration is similar to that in adults; however, changes in clearance in the first years of life dictate infusion rates that change with age.

Conclusion

Practices in ICU sedation have moved towards alleviation of the level of sedation in ICU patients. It appears that oversedation, and particularly the use of benzodiazepines as primary agents for ICU sedation, may increase mortality and impair cognitive functions at a distance from the ICU in some categories of ICU patients such as elderly patients. Conversely, the use of physical and cognitive rehabilitation programs together with the use of dexmedetomidine, a new sedative with brain protective and possibly anti-inflammatory properties, represents a promising approach to improve brain function after intensive care in the critically ill.

References

1. Hughes CG, Pandharipande PP. Review articles: the effect of perioperative and intensive care unit sedation and brain organ dysfunction. *Anesth Analg* 2011;**112**:1212–17.

2. Sanders RD, Pandharipande PP, Davidson AJ *et al.* Anticipating and managing delirium and cognitive decline in adults. *Br Med J* 2011;**343**:d4331.

3. Pandharipande P, Shintani A, Peterson J *et al.* Lorazepam is an independent risk factor for transitioning to delirium in intensive care unit patients. *Anesthesiology* 2006;**104**:21–6.

4. Pisani MA, Murphy TE, Araujo KL. *et al.* Benzodiazepine and opioid use and the duration of intensive care unit delirium in an older population. *Crit Care Med* 2009;**37**:177–83.

5. Jurd R, Arras M, Lambert S, *et al.* General anesthetic actions in vivo strongly attenuated by a point mutation in the GABA(A) receptor beta3 subunit. *FASEB J* 2003;**17**:250–2.

6. Rudolph UF, Crestani D, Benke D, *et al.* Benzodiazepine actions mediated by specific gamma-aminobutyric acid(A) receptor subtypes. *Nature* 1999;**401**:796–800.

7. Cammarano WB, Pittet JF, Weitz S *et al.* Acute withdrawal syndrome related to administration of sedative and analgesic medications in adult intensive care unit patients. *Crit Care Med* 2000;**26**:676–84.

8. Busch-Dienstfertig M, Stein C. Opioid receptors and opioid peptide-producing leukocytes in inflammatory pain: basic and therapeutic aspects. *Brain, Behav Immunity* 2010;**24**:683–94.

9. Nagi K, Pineyro G. Regulation of opioid receptor signaling: implication for the development of analgesic tolerance. *Mol Brain* 2011;**4**:25.

10. Hutchinson MR, Shavit Y, Grace PM. *et al.* Exploring the neuroimmunopharmacology of opioids: an integrative review of central immune signaling and their implications for opioid analgesia. *Pharmacol. Rev* 2011;**63**:772–810.

11. Hutchison MR, Bland ST, Johnson KW *et al.* Opioid induced glial activation: mechanisms of activation and implications for opioid analgesia, dependence and reward. *Sci World J* 2007;**7**(Suppl 2):98–111.

12. Eisenstein TK. Opioids and the immune system: what is their mechanism of action? *Br J Pharmacol* 2011;**164**:126–8.

13. Zhang EI, Xiong J, Parker BL *et al.* Depletion and recovery of lymphoid subsets following morphine administration. *Br J Pharmacol* 2011;**164**:1829–44.

14. Molteni R, Calabrese F, Racagni G *et al.* Antipsychotic drug actions on gene modulation and signaling mechanisms. *Pharmacol Therapeut* 2009;**124**:74–85.

15. Sudeshna G, Parimal K. Multiple non-psychiatric effects of phenothiazines: a review. *Eur J Pharmacol* 2010;**648**:6–14.

16. Girard TD, Pandharipande P, Carson S *et al.* Feasibility, efficacy and safety of antipsychotics for intensive care unit delirium: the MIND, randomized, placebo-controlled trial. *Crit Care Med* 2010;**38**:428–37.

17. Devlin J, Roberts R, Fong J *et al.* Efficacy and safety of quetiapine in critically ill patients with delirium: a prospective, multicenter, randomized, double-blind, placebo-controlled pilot study. *Crit Care Med* 2010;**38**:419–27.

18. Hakim S, Othman A, Naoum D. Early treatment with risperidone for subsyndromal delirium after on-pump cardiac surgery in the elderly: a randomized trial. *Anesthesiology* 2012;**116**:987–97.

19. Loepke AW, Soriano SG. An assessment of the effects of general anesthetics on developing brain structure and neurocognitive function. *Anesth Analg* 2008;**106**:1681–707.

20. Xie Z, Dong Y, Maeda U. *et al.* The common inhalation anesthetic isoflurane induces apoptosis and increases amyloid beta protein levels. *Anesthesiology* 2006;**104**:988–94.

21. Dahmani S, Chhor V, Mantz J *et al.* Effects of cerebral inflammation on propofol-induced neurotoxicity in an in vitro rodent model of neuron and microglial cell cultures. *American Society Anesthesiologists Annual Meeting;* 2011: A 694 (abstract).

22. Ely EW, Shintani A, Truman B *et al.* Delirium as a predictor of mortality in mechanically ventilated patients in the intensive care unit. *JAMA* 2004;**291**:1753–62.

23. Mesnil M, Capdevila X, Bringuier S *et al.* Long term sedation in intensive care unit: a randomized comparison between inhaled sevoflurane and intravenous propofol or midazolam. *Intensive Care Med* 2011;**37**:933–41.

24. Mantz J, Josser J, Hamada S. Dexmedetomidine: new insights. *Eur J Anaesthesiol* 2011;**28**:3–6.

25. Pandharipande PP, Pun BT, Herr DL, *et al.* Effect of sedation with dexmedetomidine vs lorazepam on acute brain dysfunction in mechanically ventilated patients: the MENDS randomized controlled trial. *JAMA* 2007;**298**:2644–53.

26. Riker RR, Shehabi Y, Bokesch P, *et al.* Dexmedetomidine vs midazolam for sedation in critically ill patients: a randomized trial. *JAMA* 2009;**301**:489–99.

27. Jakob S, Rukuonen E, Grounds M, *et al.* Dexmedetomidine versus midazolam or propofol for sedation during prolonged mechanical ventilation two randomized controlled trials. *JAMA* 2012;**307**:1151–60.

28. Sanders R, Hussel T, Maze M. Sedation and immnunomodulation. *Crit Care Clin* 2009;**25**:551–70.

29. Dahmani S, Tesniere A, Rouelle D, *et al.* Effects of anesthetic agents on focal adhesion kinase (pp125FAK) tyrosine phosphorylation in rat hippocampal slices. *Anesthesiology* 2004;**101**:344–53.

30. Dahmani S, Paris A, Jannier V, *et al.* Dexmedetomidine increases hippocampal phosphorylated extracellular signal-regulated protein kinase 1 and 2 content by an alpha2-adrenoceptor-independent mechanism: evidence for the involvement of imidazoline I1 receptors. *Anesthesiology* 2008;**108**:457–66.

31. Girard TD, Kress JP, Fuchs BD, *et al.* Efficacy and safety of a paired sedation and ventilator weaning protocol for mechanically ventilated patients in intensive care (Awakening and Breathing Controlled Trial): a randomised controlled trial. *Lancet* 2008;**371**:126–34.

32. Schweickert WD, Pohlman MC, Pohlman AS, *et al.* Early physical and occupational therapy in mechanically ventilated, critically ill patients: a randomized controlled trial. *Lancet* 2009;**373**:1874–82.

33. Tasdogan M, Memis D, Sut N, *et al.* Results of a pilot study on the effect of propofol and dexmedetomidine on inflammatory responses and intraabdominal pressure in severe sepsis. *J Clin Anesth* 2009;**21**:394–40.

34. Roche Campo F, Drout X, Thille AW, *et al.* Poor sleep quality is associated with late non-invasive ventilation failure in patients with acute hypercapnic respiratory failure. *Crit Care Med* 2010;**38**:477–85.

35. Huuponen F, Maksimow A, Lapinlampi P, *et al.* Electroencephalogram spindle activity during dexmedetomidine sedation and physiological sleep. *Acta Anaesthesiol Scand* 2008;**52**:289–94.

Neuroimmunological cross-talk in critical illness

Robert Dantzer and Keith W. Kelley

SUMMARY

There is evidence that systemic inflammation can propagate to the brain and induce profound changes in brain functions that culminate in delirium. Our understanding of how events originating in the peripheral immune system can ultimately impact on the brain has benefited from the discovery that cytokines and their receptors are expressed in the brain. Furthermore, it is now known that peripherally produced cytokines induce the expression of brain cytokines by brain myeloid cells, including perivascular macrophages and microglia. The brain is therefore able to form a cellular and molecular representation of the peripheral inflammatory response and this occurs in the absence of a breakdown of the blood–brain barrier. Activation of immune-to-brain communication pathways is at the origin of the central components of the host response to infection, including fever, activation of the hypothalamic-pituitary-adrenal axis, and sickness behavior. Communication pathways from the innate immune system to the brain involve the sensory nerves that innervate the site of the body in which the inflammatory response is taking place. Sickness behavior is the normal response of the host to an infection just like fear is an adaptive response to a danger. In addition to their pivotal role in the elicitation of sickness behavior, brain cytokines are also involved in the regulation of learning and memory. Their overexpression during peripheral inflammation is responsible for cognitive dysfunction and alterations in hippocampus-dependent memory. Inflammation is also associated with alterations in mood that can culminate in the development of symptoms of depression. Pro-inflammatory cytokines activate the tryptophan-degrading enzyme indoleamine 2,3 dioxygenase. This results in the formation of kynurenine metabolites, some of which are neurotoxic and can contribute to inflammation-associated depression and cognitive dysfunction. Understanding the way immune-to-brain communication pathways are recruited during surgery and infection should help not only to better understand the pathophysiology of delirium in the intensive care unit (ICU) but also to propose appropriate therapeutic means to prevent or treat postoperative delirium.

Introduction

Systemic inflammation is well known to be a risk factor for longer length of stay in the ICU. Systemic inflammation is also a risk factor for delirium or acute brain dysfunction in the ICU, although the number of studies that document this last relationship is still limited. In a study carried out at the Department of Anesthesiology at Vanderbilt University School of Medicine, Pratik Pandharipande and his collaborators showed that higher levels of procalcitonin, a biomarker of infection with Gram-negative bacteria, and C-reactive protein, a biomarker of inflammation, were associated with more days of delirium/coma regardless of the presence of sepsis [1]. This study included 87 medical and surgical ICU patients from two tertiary care centers, with a median age of 60 years. Procalcitonin and CRP were assayed on plasma collected within 24 hours of enrollment. In another study carried out by Konstance Plaschke and collaborators at the Department of Pathology of the University of Heidelberg in Germany, open-heart cardiac surgery patients who showed delirium on the first postoperative day had higher interleukin-6 (IL-6) levels than non-delirious patients [2]. In a group of 185 consecutive patients aged 65 years and older and acutely admitted to the Department of Internal Medicine at the Academic Medical Center in Amsterdam, the Netherlands, those patients with delirium had

Brain Disorders in Critical Illness, ed. Robert D. Stevens, Tarek Sharshar, and E. Wesley Ely. Published by Cambridge University Press. © Cambridge University Press 2013.

significantly more IL-6 and IL-8 levels above the detection limit as compared with patients who did not have delirium, independently of infection [3]. Although these clinical studies are very limited in their scope they all attest to a link between delirium and biomarkers of inflammation. At the preclinical level, several studies carried out on laboratory rodents show that surgery-induced inflammation can lead to cognitive dysfunction independently of the possible remnants of anesthesia.

All these findings indicate that systemic inflammation can propagate to the brain and induce profound changes in brain functions that culminate in delirium. The objective of this chapter is to discuss how events originating in the peripheral immune system can ultimately impact on the brain. This knowledge should help not only to better understand the pathophysiology of delirium in the ICU but also to propose appropriate therapeutic means.

Propagation of peripheral inflammation to the brain

In 1984, Adriano Fontana published the first evidence that the pro-inflammatory cytokine IL-1 is synthesized in the brain of mice injected intraperitoneally with lipopolysaccharide from *Escherichia coli* [4]. Lipopolysaccharide was already known to induce the production of cytokines by peripheral macrophages and monocytes. Because of their large molecular weight, peripherally produced cytokines cannot invade the brain unless there is a breach in the blood–brain barrier, which does not occur at the subseptic dose of lipopolysaccharide that was used by Fontana and his colleagues. In their experiments, mice were killed 1–5 hours after the injection of lipopolysaccharide. Their brains were perfused to avoid retaining any blood cells and extracted for assaying bioactive IL-1, using a bioassay represented by proliferation of thymocytes in presence of a suboptimal dose of the mitogen phytohemagglutinin. Extracts of brains from mice treated with endotoxin increased the proliferative response of thymocytes to phytohemagglutinin in a dose-dependent matter. To show that this was not due to just some contaminating factor contained in brain extracts, Fontana *et al.* did the same experiment in mice genetically resistant to lipopolysaccharide. As expected, brain extracts from these mice had no effect. Furthermore, naïve mice injected with brain extracts from lipopolysaccharide-treated,

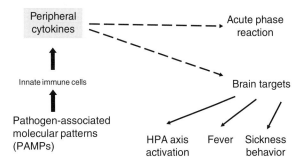

Figure 17.1 Peripheral cytokines such as interleukin-1 are released by innate immune cells in response to pathogen-associated molecular patterns that bind Toll-like receptors. These cytokines ultimately act in the brain to increase the set point for temperature regulation, resulting in fever, to activate the hypothalamic-pituitary-adrenal (HPA) axis, and to allow the organism to adjust its behavior to cope with the energetic requirements of the fever response and the immune response (the so-called sickness behavior).

endotoxin-responsive mice developed a fever response, indicating that IL-1 produced in the brain acts as a pyrogen and is probably similar to macrophage-derived IL-1.

At the time of the experiments carried out by Fontana, IL-1 had not yet been fully characterized at the molecular level and it was therefore difficult to go further. The cloning, sequencing, and expression of IL-1 gene products took place in 1985. This enabled researchers to intensify investigation of the brain effects of this cytokine in various physiological and pathological conditions (Figure 17.1). IL-1 actually refers to two different cytokines, IL-1α and IL-1β. IL-1α exists mainly in a membrane-bound form whereas IL-1β is released extracellularly. Working at Tufts University in Boston, Massachussets, Charles Dinarello demonstrated in 1986 that recombinant human IL-1β injected intravenously into rabbits or endotoxin-resistant mice induces a fever response [5]. Hugo Besedovsky who was at the time at the Schweizerisches Forschungsinstitut in Davos, Switzerland, was searching for the molecular identity of the endogenous factor that was produced by leukocytes during the course of an adaptive response and was able to signal the brain to activate the pituitary-adrenal axis so as to regulate the immune response. Hypothesizing that IL-1β could be the candidate, he teamed with Charles Dinarello to gain access to sufficient quantities of recombinant human IL-1β to inject into mice. He showed that subpyrogenic doses of IL-1β increased circulating levels of the pituitary-adrenal hormones ACTH and corticosterone even when injected into athymic nude mice, an indication that this effect was not mediated by the secondary release of products from mature T-lymphocytes [6]. In association with Frank Berkenbosch in the group of Fred Tilders at the Free University in Amsterdam, the Netherlands, Besedovsky then went on to show that the pituitary-adrenal activity of IL-1β is mediated by the release of corticotropin-releasing hormone (CRH) from parvocellular neurons of the paraventricular nucleus of the hypothalamus [7]. This was done in a series of three different experiments. In the first experiment, the pituitary-adrenal activity of IL-1β was abrogated by immunoneutralization of CRH. In a second experiment, administration of colchicine that blocks fast axonal transport of neurotransmitters and neuropeptides in neurons decreased the accumulation of CRH in the median eminence in response to IL-1β, confirming that CRH is transported from cell bodies in the paraventricular nucleus of the hypothalamus to terminals in the median eminence in order to be released. Finally, primary cultures of anterior pituitary cells that normally release adrenocorticotropin hormone in response to CRH did not respond to IL-1β. These three series of results were important since they were the first ones to demonstrate that peripherally injected IL-1β ultimately acts in the brain.

In the second half of the 1980s, the polymorphic nature of the brain effects of IL-1α and IL-1β became quickly apparent as the number of studies on various endpoints, including behavior, increased exponentially. In 1988, Benjamin Hart at the School of Veterinary Medicine at the University of California at Davis, proposed that all the metabolic and behavioral effects of IL-1β are actually part of an adaptive response of the host to fight infection [8]. He termed this adaptive response sickness behavior to emphasize that it occurs in the context of a sickness episode. To cope with viral and bacterial infections, a sick individual must mount a fever that, because of its very high metabolic cost, precludes any other energy-demanding activity, including exploratory behavior, self-grooming, and searching for food. In 1989, Dantzer and Kelley independently proposed to term sickness behavior the diverse behavioral changes that develop in response to activation of the innate immune system and they put this sickness response in the context of the regulatory network of interactions between the brain and the immune system [9]. They

pointed out the fact that it is important for the brain to be informed about an infection via cytokines produced by the immune system in order to regulate the development and amplitude of the peripheral immune response. Sickness behavior was therefore viewed as only one example of the various means that are amenable to the brain for regulating the host response to infection.

An important step forward for the understanding of immune-to-brain communication pathways was the demonstration that cytokines, including IL-1β, are actually produced in the brain during a systemic immune response. Partial evidence for this was already available thanks to the work carried out by Fontana that was mentioned earlier in this section. However, the ultimate demonstration had to wait for the move to molecular biology techniques by neuroendocrinologists, which opened the way for the measurement of transcripts for peptides at the level of mRNA. This became possible with the introduction of the first thermocyclers for the polymerase chain reaction after reverse transcription of RNA into DNA in the early 1990s. Within a few years, several groups showed that peripherally administered lipopolysaccharide induces expression of transcripts for pro-inflammatory cytokines in rodent brain [10–12]. Coupled with the observation that direct injections of very small amounts of cytokines into the brain recapitulate most of the effects of cytokines administered at the periphery, these findings confirmed that cytokines act directly into the brain to induce fever, pituitary-adrenal activation, and sickness behavior.

At the same time, the first neuronatomical studies on the expression and distribution of cytokines and their receptors in the brain brought supplementary evidence to the existence of a brain compartment of cytokines [13]. Cytokines and their receptors are present in the brain in two forms: a constitutive form that is mainly expressed in neurons; and an inducible form that is mainly expressed in myeloid-derived cells, including microglia and brain macrophages. To take just one example, expression of IL-1β, IL-6, and TNFα, mRNA was found to be increased in the hippocampus and hypothalamus of mice injected peripherally with lipopolysaccharide or IL-1β. The time course of this brain expression was delayed compared with the one observed in peripheral organs, such as the spleen and pituitary, with a maximum around 2–4 hours post LPS [12]. Immunocytochemistry with an antibody raised against rat IL-1β showed that the expression of

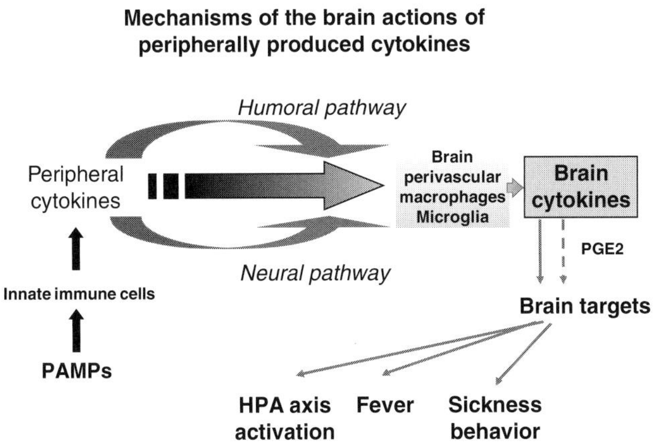

Mechanisms of the brain actions of peripherally produced cytokines

Figure 17.2 Peripherally produced cytokines do not act directly on brain targets to induce fever, activation of the hypothalamic-pituitary-adrenal axis, and sickness behavior. The peripheral immune message is transmitted to the brain via several immune-to-brain communication pathways involving a humoral pathway and a neural pathway. This results in the activation of brain perivascular macrophages and microglia and the production of brain cytokines by these brain cells. Brain cytokines act directly or indirectly, via the production of prostaglandins (e.g., PGE2), on brain functions. PAMPs, pathogen-associated molecular patterns.

immunoreactive IL-1β in the brain of rats injected intravenously or intraperitoneally with lipopolysaccharide was mostly restricted to macrophages in the meninges and choroid plexus and to microglia in the brain parenchyma [14]. It was proposed that IL-1β produced by these cells serves as a communication signal for adjacent or more distant targets (neurons, endothelial cells, microglial cells) to play a role in the induction of non-specific symptoms of sickness. This hypothesis was supported by the observation that administration of the interleukin-1 receptor antagonist IL-1ra into the lateral ventricle of the brain blocked the behavioral effects of peripherally injected IL-1β in rats [15]. These sickness behaviors occurred independently of fever and the IL-1β-induced increase in metabolic rate. Sickness behavior in response to lipopolysaccharide was however unaltered in IL-1β-deficient mice [16], probably because of the redundancy of the cytokine network. This last aspect was further explored in mice that were made genetically deficient for the type I IL-1 receptor. Administration of IL-1β to these mice either intraperitoneally or into the lateral cerebral ventricle had no effect on behavior, whereas administration of lipopolysaccharide was still able to elicit a full-blown sickness behavior [17,18]. However, blockade of TNFα action in the brain by administration of TNF binding protein resulted in the abrogation of lipopolysaccharide-induced sickness behavior in mice deficient for IL-1R1 but not in wild-type mice. These results indicate that TNFα that is also induced in response to lipopolysaccharide takes over in the absence of a functional IL-1 system.

All the experiments described above unequivocally show that cytokines are produced in the brain during a systemic immune response and act in the brain to induce their behavioral effects. However, they provide no information on the mechanisms by which cytokines that are produced and released at the periphery ultimately propagate to the brain. The current views on the ways peripherally produced cytokines act in the brain are represented in Figure 17.2. The initial hypothesis that was formulated to account for the pyrogenic effects of IL-1β when injected intravenously postulated that this cytokine acts on the circumventricular organs of the brain that are devoid of a fully functional blood–brain barrier response. There, IL-1β would induce the synthesis and release of lipophilic prostaglandins E2 that would diffuse freely on the brain side of the blood–brain barrier and ultimately reach their target in the medial preoptic area of the hypothalamus [18]. This hypothesis was formulated at a time when little information was available on the biology of cytokines. However, in contrast to what was proposed at the time for endogenous pyrogens, most cytokines including IL-1β do not behave as hormones. They are not released in the general circulation to reach distant targets but are geared to act as paracrine or autocrine communication signals in the immediate cellular environment in which they are produced. Another problem was that this hypothesis did not predict the existence of a central compartment of cytokines relaying the peripheral compartment.

In the context of inflammation, an obvious pathway of communication from the immune system to the brain is the neural route, since the four cardinal features of inflammation include two sensory components, *dolor* (pain) and *calor* (heat). The body site at which inflammation takes place feels painful and warm, and this is dependent on neural conduction via the afferent nerves that innervate it. When IL-1β or the cytokine inducer lipopolysaccharide is injected intraperitoneally, the obvious route of communication from the peritoneal cavity to the brain is represented by the spinal nerves innervating the peritoneum and visceral organs and the vagus nerves. Neuroendocrinologists had already demonstrated in the late 1970s that the gastrointestinal peptide chole-cystokinin inhibits feeding by stimulating the vagus nerves, since its satiety-inducing effect was abrogated by the subdiaphragmatic section of the vagus nerves [19]. It was therefore logical to assess whether sub-diaphragmatic vagotomy also abrogated the central effects of IL-1β and lipopolysaccharide. The first evidence in favor of this hypothesis was the observation that subdiaphragmatic vagotomy blocked expression of the early activation gene c-Fos in the primary and secondary projection areas of the vagus nerves in response to intraperitoneal administration of lipopolysaccharide to rats [20]. The same surgical procedure was found to abrogate both hyperalgia [21] and the sickness behavior response to peripheral cytokines [22]. This effect was not due to any uncontrolled consequence of vagotomy since it was not associated with any alteration of the peripheral inflammatory response. The subdiaphragmatic section of the vagus nerves also abrogated the inducible expression of IL-1β mRNA in the hypothalamus in response to intra-peritoneal lipopolysacccharide. This means that in the absence of vagal afferent information, the brain becomes blind and deaf to immune stimuli that are initiated in the peritoneal cavity.

The results obtained after vagotomy have been essentially confirmed by a much more selective approach consisting of reversibly blocking afferent nerve conduction in the vagus nerves by application of a locally acting anesthetic agent on the dorsal vagus nucleus [23]. Transmission of the immune message to the brain is not restricted to the vagus nerves. Sections of the glossopharyngeal nerve in rats injected with lipopolysaccharide into the soft palate were both able to block inflammation-induced sickness [24].

An important feature of subdiaphragmatic vagot-omy is that it reliably blocks the behavioral response to peripheral immune stimulation but has little or very limited effects on the fever and the pituitary-adrenal response to cytokines. An illustration of this difference is provided by an experiment in which sickness behavior and changes in body temperature were measured in the same rats that had been vagotomized or submitted to sham surgery before being injected with lipopolysaccharide or IL-1β intraperitoneally [25]. Vagotomy abrogated the development of sickness behavior but not of fever. These findings mean that different immune-to-brain communication pathways probably operate in parallel to trigger the various components of the host response to infection. This observation has led to a re-examination of the old humoral theory of communication in which circulating cytokines were supposed to act on the brain via circumventricular areas of the brain. Detailed neuro-anatomical studies of the expression of IL-1β in the brain in response to intraperitoneal IL-1β showed that the first wave of IL-1β expression occurs in macrophage-like cells in circumventricular organs such as the area postrema. From there the cytokine message gradually propagates to microglial cells in the adjacent brain parenchyma in the nucleus tractus sol-itarius. Endothelial cells of brain vessels are also involved in the initial response to peripheral cytokines, as shown by their ability to express the inducible cyclo-oxygenase enzyme COX2 as well as immunoreactive IL-1β and NFκB [26–28]. The existence of intricate interactions between perivascular macrophages and endothelial cells in response to circulating lipopolysac-charide and IL-1β has been demonstrated recently. However, these interactions impact only the pituitary-adrenal response to cytokines but not sickness behavior [29].

Another route of communication from the periphery to the brain is represented by cytokine transporters [30]. Although their exact molecular nature is still unknown, they are likely to correspond to cytokine receptors that undergo internalization upon binding of their ligand before dissociation of the ligand receptor complex. The existence of such receptors has been demonstrated for IL-1α, TNFα, and IL-2. A physiological role for the transport of IL-1α into the brain has been demonstrated in an experiment in which human recombinant IL-1α was injected into mice at a dose that impaired retention of a discrim-inative avoidance response, and this effect was abol-ished by intracerebral administration of an antibody specific to human but not to mouse IL-1α [31].

How the three different routes of immune-to-brain communication pathways interact with each other has not yet been investigated. In situations of systemic inflammation, the humoral route of communication is likely to predominate together with cytokine trans-porters, with the neural route playing little role. In situations of localized inflammation, the neural route is the most important pathway. Transmission via afferent nerves bypasses the humoral route and cytokine transporters [32].

Pro-inflammatory cytokines alter cognition

The possible impact of cytokines on cognition was examined relatively late in time in comparison to the pyrogenic, neuroendocrine, and behavioral effects of cytokines. One of the reasons for this is that sick animals have obvious difficulties performing in the type of task that is used to assess memory and learning. Their motor abilities are impaired and their appetence for positive rewards is strongly reduced. The first article on IL-1β and learning was published in 1993 and described the impairing effects of intraperitoneal administration of IL-1β on acquisition in the Morris water maze [33]. More systematic studies of the effects of lipopolysaccharide, IL-1β, and other pro-inflammatory cytokines were published in the years after. The emphasis shifted gradually from peripherally administered recombinant cytokines to endogenously produced cytokines.

The two main aspects that emerge from this literature are the privileged role of IL-1β in hippocampal-dependent learning and the different roles of constitutive and inducible IL-1β for learning and memory, with the former facilitating and the latter impairing learning and memory.

A series of experiments carried out by the group of Steve Maier at the University of Colorado at Boulder illustrates very well the first aspect [34]. In these experiments, the production and release of endogenous IL-1β was triggered by exposure of rats to inescapable electric foot shocks. This resulted in a selective deficit in the learning of context-dependent conditioned fear. In this task, rats were placed into a new chamber. After being allowed free exploration of the chamber they received a few inescapable electric shocks preceded or not by a tone. They were then returned to their home cage and 1–3 days later replaced into the chamber but with no shock. In this situation, the rats usually display a defensive freezing response to the chamber that is further increased if they are also re-exposed to the tone associated with shock. The freezing response to the chamber is mediated by a conditioned fear circuit involving the hippocampus, whereas the response to the sound is mediated by a conditioned fear circuit involving the amygdala. Blockade of the endogenous IL-1β response

to shock by administration of IL-1ra during the conditioning phase of the procedure abrogated the fear response to the chamber but not to the tone. Conversely, further induction of IL-1β in the brain by administration of lipopolysaccharide following exposure to electric shocks impaired the contextual fear response but not the fear response to the tone associated with shock.

The role of constitutive versus inducible IL-1β in learning is well illustrated by a series of experiments carried out by Raz Yirmiya at the Hebrew University in Jerusalem, Israel [35]. Learning was assessed by speed of swimming to the immersed platform in the Morris water maze task. In this task, mice are placed in a circular pool filled with water in which they must first swim to a visible platform in order to escape. The platform is then immersed so it becomes invisible and the animals have to use extra-maze navigational cues to reach the now hidden platform. Once they have learned the task, the platform is moved to a different location and the time spent investigating the previous location of the platform provides an indication of the strength of learning. Transgenic mice in which the type I IL-1 receptor IL-1R1 had been knocked out were impaired in their acquisition of the task. The same deficit was observed in transgenic mice with an overexpression of the IL-1 receptor antagonist IL-1ra in the brain and in wild-type mice chronically injected with IL-1ra into the lateral ventricle of their brains. Conversely, mice injected chronically into the lateral ventricle of the brain with IL-1β displayed a deficit in the acquisition of the task. Similar effects were observed in the hippocampal-dependent version of the fear-conditioning task.

The impairing effects of inflammation on cognition are exacerbated during aging. This is due to the fact that aging is associated with an imbalance between the innate immune system and the adaptive immune system, to the advantage of the innate immune system. The importance of inflammation in aging-related disorders is such that a neologism has been forged to describe it, in the form of "inflammaging" [36]. As can be expected based on the propagation of inflammation from the periphery to the brain, inflammaging is also present in the brain. Brain macrophage-like cells are primed. They respond to inflammatory stimuli by producing and releasing more cytokines. As a consequence, inflammation-associated cognitive disorders are exacerbated in aged individuals. This can be demonstrated in various ways. In a typical experiment, aged mice were compared with young adult mice in their response to a relatively small dose of lipopolysaccharide. This dose had no effect on acquisition of the Morris water maze by young adult mice, but significantly impaired behavioral performance in aged mice [37].

There have been a few studies carried out in volunteers injected with a subseptic dose of lipopolysaccharide to determine the possible occurrence of cognitive alterations in addition to the symptoms of sickness that are invariably induced by this treatment. Administration of 0.8 ng/kg lipopolysaccharide from *Salmonella* impaired declarative memory but improved working memory 3–9 hours after treatment [38]. Improvement of working memory and psychomotor speed capacity was observed in association with increased alertness in subjects injected with 2 ng/kg lipopolysaccharide from *E. coli* [39]. In another study in which subjects received a sufficient dose of lipopolysaccharide from *E. coli* (0.4 ng/kg) to induce elevations in body temperature and circulating pro-inflammatory cytokines, no effect on altertness, memory performance, and executive functions was observed [40]. These disparate findings show that not all forms of memory are sensitive to an acute surge of pro-inflammatory cytokines in humans, and that seemingly paradoxical improvements in working memory are probably accounted for by the increased arousal that is associated with the anxiety caused by the perception of the interoceptive feelings induced by endotoxin.

Postoperative cognitive dysfunction is mediated by propagation of inflammation to the brain

The possibility that pro-inflammatory cytokines mediate the cognitive alterations that develop after surgery has been investigated in a systematic manner over the last 5 years. In one of the first papers in this field, adult rats were submitted to splenectomy under neuroleptic anesthesia and their ability to alternate in a Y maze that assesses working memory was evaluated 1–7 days after surgery. Behavioral performance was impaired at day 1 and 3 post-surgery and back to normal at day 7. This impairment was not due to anesthesia, since anesthetized rats that were not submitted to surgery were not different from control rats. The impairment in working memory was associated with an increase in hippocampal IL-1β measured at the mRNA and protein level [41].

Further evidence for a causal role of pro-inflammatory cytokines in post-surgery cognitive alterations is provided by intervention studies, in which expression of the candidate cytokines is blocked by a cytokine antagonist or absent because of deletion of the corresponding gene. The impairment in hippocampal-dependent fear conditioning caused by tibia surgery in adult rats was prevented by pretreatment with the anti-inflammatory agent minocycline, as well as by antagonism of IL-1, using either administration of IL-1ra or IL-1R1 knockout mice [42]. Similar results were obtained when TNFα was blocked by prophylactic administration of a neutralizing antibody against TNFα in mice submitted to an open tibial fracture under isoflurane anesthesia and buprenorphine analgesia [43]. In this last model, TNFα appeared much earlier in the general circulation than IL-1β and IL-6, at 30 minutes instead of 6 h.

The inflammaging hypothesis predicts that aged subjects should be more prone to postoperative cognitive dysfunction than adults. This prediction was verified when aged mice were submitted to laporotomy under ketamine anesthesia and tested in a variant of the Morris water maze 24 h later. In this task, mice had to swim to a new location of the hidden platform after they had previously learned the maze. Aged but not adult mice were impaired in their ability to change strategy and learn the new version of the task, and this was associated with a higher expression of IL-1β mRNA in their hippocampus [44].

Mechanisms of neuroimmune interactions in postoperative cognitive dysfunction

It is beyond the scope of this chapter to discuss the mechanisms that are responsible for the systemic inflammatory response syndrome that develops in surgery patients (see [45] for a recent review). As mentioned above, *de novo* activation of the cytokine network is mediated by recognition of pathogen-associated molecular patterns by pattern-recognition receptors. Pattern-recognition receptors include Toll-like receptors, that are present at the cell membrane, and intracellular receptors, known as NOD-like receptors. These latter receptors interact with multi-protein complexes that form the inflammasome. The inflammasome cooperates with Toll-like receptors to enhance and prolong the innate immune response. Infectious micro-organisms are not always needed as ligands of pattern-recognition factors. Endogenous factors released by injured cells have the same role. In particular, alarmins represent an important category of endogenous danger signals that are released in response to pathogen-associated molecular patterns but also to tissue damage and stressors. The high mobility group (HMG) proteins are alarmins that signal through the receptor for advanced glycation end-products (RAGE) and Toll-like receptors. Knowing that high mobility group box-1 protein can be released actively by innate immune cells in response to pathogen-associated molecular patterns or passively from dying cells, it is interesting to note that this protein has the same pro-inflammatory activity in the brain as IL-1β [46]. Whether alarmins play a role in the propagation of inflammation from the periphery to the brain remains to be determined. Other endogenous danger signals include heat shock proteins, hyaluronanic acid, ATP, and uric acid.

The mechanisms of action of cytokines on brain functions are not fully understood. There are cytokine receptors on neurons. Patch clamp experiments show that IL-1β and TNFα can increase excitatory synaptic transmission or decrease inhibitory synaptic transmission. However, these effects are usually rapid (a few seconds) and relatively short lasting (a few minutes), which does not fit the time course of the effects of cytokines on brain functions. Some of the effects of cytokines on synaptic transmission are mediated by prostaglandins. However, most of the brain effects of cytokines are probably secondary to alterations in neuron-glia interactions. These alterations have mainly been studied in the context of inflammation-induced neuropathic pain [47,48].

Cytokines do not always act on the brain directly. Many brain effects of cytokines are actually mediated by downstream intermediates. One of them is represented by activation of the tryptophan-degrading enzyme, indoleamine 2,3 dioxygenase (Figure 17.3). By metabolizing tryptophan along the kynurenine pathway that generates cytotoxic compounds, activation of this enzyme in macrophages and dendritic cells

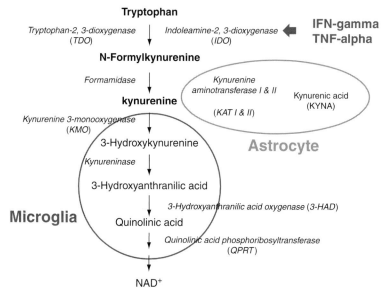

Immune stimuli activate the tryptophan degrading pathway, which ultimately results in the formation of neurotoxic compounds by activated microglial cells

Figure 17.3 Peripherally produced cytokines including inteferon-gamma and tumor necrosis factor-alpha can activate the tryptophan-degrading enzyme indoleamine 2,3 dioxygenase. Kynurenine can be transported into the brain by the same transporter that carries tryptophan. The fate of kynurenine depends on the enzymatic equipment of the cell. In astrocytes, kynurenine is further metabolized in kynurenic acid that acts as an antagonist of the N-methyl-D-aspartate (NMDA) receptor. In microglia, kynurenine is metabolized in 3-hydroxykynurenine and quinolinic acid. Both compounds are able to generate free radicals. In addition, quinolinic acid acts as an agonist of the NMDA receptor

Possible therapeutic strategies:

1. Down-regulate macrophage/microglia activation: e.g., minocycline

2. **Abrogate inflammation:**

    2.1. Anti-cytokines strategies: Anti-inflammatory cytokines (e.g., IL-10) or cytokine antagonists (e.g., etanercept)

    2.2. Anti-inflammatory agents: ketamine (activation of heme oxygenase?)

3. Antagonize downstream metabolites of kynurenine by blocking indoleamine 2,3 dioxygenase activation

Figure 17.4 Possible therapeutic strategies in critical illness. Note that inflammation can be targeted at the level of innate immune cells or at the level of the pro-inflammatory cytokines and their receptors. Another possible target is represented by the activation of indoleamine 2,3 dioxygenase.

contributes to development of immunotolerance [49]. Depletion of tryptophan in the local milieu renders cytotoxic T-lymphocytes unable to proliferate and to exert their cytotoxic activity. In addition, generation of cytotoxic kynurenine metabolites is detrimental to lymphocytes. This important mechanism for regulating the immune response has important side effects in the brain. Kynurenine can be transported into the brain using the same amino acid transporter as tryptophan. Activated microglia have the necessary enzymatic equipment to transform kynurenine into 3-hydroxykynurenine and quinolinic acid [50]. These compounds are potent free radical donors and act as agonists of the NMDA receptor. Astrocytes have the necessary enzymatic equipment to transform kynurenine into kynurenic acid which acts as an antagonist of the alpha-7 nicotinic receptor and the NMDA receptor. Since microglial cells are activated following surgery and during systemic inflammation, the production of kynurenine metabolites is likely to be biased toward the production of 3-hydroxykynurenine and quinolinic acid. This mechanism has already been shown to mediate development of symptoms of depression [51].

Translational aspects of neuroimmune interactions in postoperative cognitive dysfunction

The evidence provided so far indicates that the systemic inflammatory response that occurs during the course of an infection or in response to surgery propagates to the brain via immune-to-brain communication pathways and causes cognitive dysfunction. If this sequence of events is clinically relevant, it should be sufficient to prevent the inflammatory response in order to treat postoperative cognitive dysfunction

(Figure 17.4). The problem with this strategy is that the inflammatory process per se is certainly useful at least in part to promote healing. This holds true even for endogenous danger signals. For instance antagonism of RAGE has been found to suppress peripheral nerve regeneration due to the importance of this receptor for inflammatory and axonal outgrowth pathways [52]. This means that administration of cytokine or cytokine receptor antagonists should be restricted to cases of chronic inflammation in which the deleterious component of the inflammatory response overcomes its potential benefit.

Another strategy consists of targeting propagation of the inflammatory response from the periphery to the brain or acting directly into the brain in order to down-regulate neuroinflammation. Local anesthesia, especially if carried out at the level of the first synaptic relay of sensory afferents, can block the neuroimmune consequences of peripheral activation of the innate immune system. Administration of the local anesthetic bupivacaine into the dorsal nucleus of the vagus nerves temporarily blocked the activating effects of intraperitoneal lipopolysaccharide on c-Fos labeling in the brain as well as the social withdrawal response to lipopolysaccharide [23]. Pretreatment with the second-generation tetracycline minocyline that has marked down-regulatory effects on microglia was found to prevent the neuroinflammatory effects of surgery in a mouse model of post-surgery cognitive dysfunction [42]. In addition to its antagonist activity at the level of the NMDA receptor, ketamine has anti-inflammatory properties due in particular to its ability to activate heme oxygenase-1. This enzyme that catalyzes the degradation of heme into biliverdin plays an important role in down-regulating inflammation. The activation of heme oxygenase-1 by ketamine could explain the positive results obtained on patients submitted to cardiac surgery by Judith Hudetz at the Veterans Administration Medical Center in Milwaukee, Wisconsin [53]. If the kynurenine degradation pathway of tryptophan proves to be activated in patients with postoperative cognitive dysfunction, it will certainly be important to limit its activation by agents acting as antagonists of indoleamine 2,3 dioxygenase or the downstream enzymes.

Whatever the strategy selected for preventing or treating postoperative cognitive dysfunction, it is important that clinicians work in close interaction with neuroimmunologists in order to select the most appropriate biomarkers of the pathophysiological pathway of interest and the agents that are the most likely to interfere with this pathway.

References

1. McGrane S, Girard TD, Thompson JL, et al. Procalcitonin and C-reactive protein levels at admission as predictors of duration of acute brain dysfunction in critically ill patients. Crit Care 15(2):R78.

2. Plaschke K, Fichtenkamm P, Schramm C, et al. Early postoperative delirium after open-heart cardiac surgery is associated with decreased bispectral EEG and increased cortisol and interleukin-6. Intensive Care Med 36(12):2081–9.

3. de Rooij SE, van Munster BC, Korevaar JC, Levi M. Cytokines and acute phase response in delirium. J Psychosom Res 2007;62(5):521–5.

4. Fontana A, Weber E, Dayer JM. Synthesis of interleukin 1/endogenous pyrogen in the brain of endotoxin-treated mice: a step in fever induction? J Immunol 1984;133(4):1696–8.

5. Dinarello CA, Cannon JG, Mier JW, et al. Multiple biological activities of human recombinant interleukin 1. J Clin Invest 1986;77(6):1734–9.

6. Besedovsky H, del Rey A, Sorkin E, Dinarello CA. Immunoregulatory feedback between interleukin-1 and glucocorticoid hormones. Science 1986;233(4764):652–4.

7. Berkenbosch F, van Oers J, del Rey A, Tilders F, Besedovsky H. Corticotropin-releasing factor-producing neurons in the rat activated by interleukin-1. Science 1987;238(4826):524–6.

8. Hart BL. Biological basis of the behavior of sick animals. Neurosci Biobehav Rev 1988;12(2):123–37.

9. Dantzer R, Kelley KW. Stress and immunity: an integrated view of relationships between the brain and the immune system. Life Sci 1989;44(26):1995–2008.

10. Ban E, Haour F, Lenstra R. Brain interleukin 1 gene expression induced by peripheral lipopolysaccharide administration. Cytokine 1992;4(1):48–54.

11. Gatti S, Bartfai T. Induction of tumor necrosis factor-alpha mRNA in the brain after peripheral endotoxin treatment: comparison with interleukin-1 family and interleukin-6. Brain Res 1993;624(1–2):291–4.

12. Laye S, Parnet P, Goujon E, Dantzer R. Peripheral administration of lipopolysaccharide induces the expression of cytokine transcripts in the brain and pituitary of mice. Brain Res Mol Brain Res 1994;27(1):157–62.

13. Breder CD, Dinarello CA, Saper CB. Interleukin-1 immunoreactive innervation of the human hypothalamus. Science 1988;240(4850):321–4.

14. Van Dam AM, Bauer J, Tilders FJ, Berkenbosch F. Endotoxin-induced appearance of immunoreactive interleukin-1 beta in ramified microglia in rat brain: a light and electron microscopic study. Neuroscience 1995;65(3):815–26.

15. Kent S, Bluthe RM, Dantzer R, et al. Different receptor mechanisms mediate the pyrogenic and behavioral effects of interleukin 1. Proc Natl Acad Sci USA 1992;89(19):9117–20.

16. Kozak W, Zheng H, Conn CA, et al. Thermal and behavioral effects of lipopolysaccharide and influenza in interleukin-1 beta-deficient mice. Am J Physiol 1995;269(5 Pt 2):R969–77.

17. Bluthe RM, Laye S, Michaud B, et al. Role of interleukin-1beta and tumour necrosis factor-alpha in lipopolysaccharide-induced sickness behaviour: a study with interleukin-1 type I receptor-deficient mice. Eur J Neurosci 2000;12(12):4447–56.

18. Saper CB, Breder CD. The neurologic basis of fever. N Engl J Med 1994;330(26):1880–6.

19. Anika SM, Houpt TR, Houpt KA. Satiety elicited by cholecystokinin in intact and vagotomized rats. Physiol Behav 1977;19(6):761–6.

20. Wan W, Wetmore L, Sorensen CM, Greenberg AH, Nance DM. Neural and biochemical mediators of endotoxin and stress-induced c-fos expression in the rat brain. Brain Res Bull 1994;34(1):7–14.

21. Watkins LR, Wiertelak EP, Goehler LE, et al. Neurocircuitry of illness-induced hyperalgesia. Brain Res 1994;639(2):283–99.

22. Bluthe RM, Walter V, Parnet P, et al. Lipopolysaccharide induces sickness behaviour in rats by a vagal mediated mechanism. C R Acad Sci III 1994;317(6):499–503.

23. Marvel FA, Chen CC, Badr N, Gaykema RP, Goehler LE. Reversible inactivation of the dorsal vagal complex blocks lipopolysaccharide-induced social withdrawal and c-Fos expression in central autonomic nuclei. Brain Behav Immun 2004;18(2):123–34.

24. Romeo HE, Tio DL, Taylor AN. Effects of glossopharyngeal nerve transection on central and peripheral cytokines and serum corticosterone induced by localized inflammation. *J Neuroimmunol* 2003;**136**(1–2):104–11.

25. Luheshi GN, Bluthe RM, Rushforth D, *et al.* Vagotomy attenuates the behavioural but not the pyrogenic effects of interleukin-1 in rats. *Auton Neurosci* 2000;**85**(1–3):127–32.

26. Quan N, Whiteside M, Kim L, Herkenham M. Induction of inhibitory factor kappaB alpha mRNA in the central nervous system after peripheral lipopolysaccharide administration: an in situ hybridization histochemistry study in the rat. *Proc Natl Acad Sci USA* 1997;**94**(20):10985–90.

27. Konsman JP, Tridon V, Dantzer R. Diffusion and action of intracerebroventricularly injected interleukin-1 in the CNS. *Neuroscience* 2000;**101**(4):957–67.

28. Nadjar A, Combe C, Laye S, *et al.* Nuclear factor kappaB nuclear translocation as a crucial marker of brain response to interleukin-1. A study in rat and interleukin-1 type I deficient mouse. *J Neurochem* 2003;**87**(4):1024–36.

29. Serrats J, Schiltz JC, Garcia-Bueno B, *et al.* Dual roles for perivascular macrophages in immune-to-brain signaling. *Neuron* **65**(1):94–106.

30. Quan N, Banks WA. Brain-immune communication pathways. *Brain Behav Immun* 2007;**21**(6):727–35.

31. Banks WA, Farr SA, La Scola ME, Morley JE. Intravenous human interleukin-1alpha impairs memory processing in mice: dependence on blood–brain barrier transport into posterior division of the septum. *J Pharmacol Exp Ther* 2001;**299**(2):536–41.

32. Quan N. Immune-to-brain signaling: how important are the blood-brain barrier-independent pathways? *Mol Neurobiol* 2008;**37**(2–3):142–52.

33. Oitzl MS, van Oers H, Schobitz B, de Kloet ER. Interleukin-1 beta, but not interleukin-6, impairs spatial navigation learning. *Brain Res* 1993;**613**(1):160–3.

34. Rachal Pugh C, Fleshner M, Watkins LR, Maier SF, Rudy JW. The immune system and memory consolidation: a role for the cytokine IL-1beta. *Neurosci Biobehav Rev* 2001;**25**(1):29–41.

35. Goshen I, Kreisel T, Ounallah-Saad H, *et al.* A dual role for interleukin-1 in hippocampal-dependent memory processes. *Psychoneuroendocrinology* 2007;**32**(8–10):1106–15.

36. Franceschi C, Capri M, Monti D, *et al.* Inflammaging and anti-inflammaging: a systemic perspective on aging and longevity emerged from studies in humans. *Mech Ageing Dev* 2007;**128**(1):92–105.

37. Godbout JP, Chen J, Abraham J, *et al.* Exaggerated neuroinflammation and sickness behavior in aged mice following activation of the peripheral innate immune system. *FASEB J* 2005;**19**(10):1329–31.

38. Cohen O, Reichenberg A, Perry C, *et al.* Endotoxin-induced changes in human working and declarative memory associate with cleavage of plasma "readthrough" acetylcholinesterase. *J Mol Neurosci* 2003;**21**(3):199–212.

39. van den Boogaard M, Ramakers BP, van Alfen N, *et al.* Endotoxemia-induced inflammation and the effect on the human brain. *Crit Care* **14**(3):R81.

40. Grigoleit JS, Oberbeck JR, Lichte P, *et al.* Lipopolysaccharide-induced experimental immune activation does not impair memory functions in humans. *Neurobiol Learn Mem* **94**(4):561–7.

41. Wan Y, Xu J, Ma D, *et al.* Postoperative impairment of cognitive function in rats: a possible role for cytokine-mediated inflammation in the hippocampus. *Anesthesiology* 2007;**106**(3):436–43.

42. Cibelli M, Fidalgo AR, Terrando N, *et al.* Role of interleukin-1beta in postoperative cognitive dysfunction. *Ann Neurol* **68**(3):360–8.

43. Terrando N, Rei Fidalgo A, Vizcaychipi M, *et al.* The impact of IL-1 modulation on the development of lipopolysaccharide-induced cognitive dysfunction. *Crit Care* **14**(3):R88.

44. Rosczyk HA, Sparkman NL, Johnson RW. Neuroinflammation and cognitive function in aged mice following minor surgery. *Exp Gerontol* 2008;**43**(9):840–6.

45. Lowry SF. The stressed host response to infection: the disruptive signals and rhythms of systemic inflammation. *Surg Clin North Am* 2009;**89**(2):311–26,vii.

46. O'Connor KA, Hansen MK, Rachal Pugh C, *et al.* Further characterization of high mobility group box 1 (HMGB1) as a proinflammatory cytokine: central nervous system effects. *Cytokine* 2003;**24**(6):254–65.

47. Miller RJ, Jung H, Bhangoo SK, White FA. Cytokine and chemokine regulation of sensory neuron function. *Handb Exp Pharmacol* **2009**(194):417–49.

48. Wieseler-Frank J, Maier SF, Watkins LR. Immune-to-brain communication dynamically modulates pain: physiological and pathological consequences. *Brain Behav Immun* 2009;**19**(2):104–11.

49. Grohmann U, Fallarino F, Puccetti P. Tolerance, DCs and tryptophan: much ado about IDO. *Trends Immunol* 2003;**24**(5):242–8.

50. Schwarcz R. The kynurenine pathway of tryptophan degradation as a drug target. *Curr Opin Pharmacol* 2004;**4**(1):12–17.

51. Dantzer R, O'Connor JC, Freund GG, Johnson RW, Kelley KW. From inflammation to sickness and depression: when the immune system subjugates the brain. *Nat Rev Neurosci* 2008;**9**(1):46–56.

52. Rong LL, Yan SF, Wendt T, *et al.* RAGE modulates peripheral nerve regeneration via recruitment of both inflammatory and axonal outgrowth pathways. *FASEB J* 2004;**18**(15):1818–25.

53. Hudetz JA, Iqbal Z, Gandhi SD, *et al.* Ketamine attenuates post-operative cognitive dysfunction after cardiac surgery. *Acta Anaesthesiol Scand* 2009;**53**(7):864–72.

Inflammatory mechanisms in chronic neurodegenerative disease: the impact of microglia priming

V. Hugh Perry

SUMMARY

Microglia, the resident macrophages of the central nervous system (CNS), have a relatively down-regulated phenotype when compared with other tissue macrophages. The CNS exerts an inhibitory influence on the microglia phenotype via neuronal expression of ligands which impact on receptors on the microglia. The loss or degeneration of neurons leads to activation of microglia as detected by changes in morphology and up-regulation, or *de novo* synthesis, of a spectrum of myeloid-related molecules. During chronic neurodegenerative disease in animal models the microglia are increased in number, have an activated morphology, but express an anti-inflammatory phenotype. In naïve animals a systemic inflammatory challenge leads to communication with the brain and is part of our defense against injury and infection. The macrophage populations of the brain are involved in signaling from the peripheral immune system to CNS neurons. A systemic inflammatory challenge in an animal with ongoing chronic neurodegeneration leads to switching of the microglia to a pro-inflammatory phenotype with the capacity to disrupt neuronal function and cause tissue degeneration. We propose that the impact of systemic inflammation on microglia primed by prior pathology, and their switching to an aggressive tissue-damaging phenotype, may underlie clinical observations that systemic inflammation in patients with Alzheimer's disease is associated with exacerbation of symptoms and acceleration in cognitive decline. The concept of microglia priming and secondary activation by systemic inflammation may have relevance to diverse neurological conditions and highlights the importance of prompt treatment of systemic infection and inflammation in patients with acute or chronic neurodegeneration.

Introduction

It is now well recognized that as people live longer than ever before, so the prevalence of those suffering from chronic neurodegenerative diseases of the brain is increasing. Old age is the single biggest risk factor for the development of chronic neurodegeneration and dementia. This is not just a problem for the northern hemisphere but a global problem that will have profound social and economic consequences for many decades to come [1]. At the present time there are no effective therapeutic interventions that arrest the onset or progression of diseases such as Alzheimer's disease, Parkinson's disease, motor neuron disease, or Huntington's disease. The diagnosis of these diseases is not straightforward, particularly in the early stages, and a considerable amount of research is devoted to the development of neurological, psychological, imaging, and biochemical techniques that will permit accurate and early diagnosis, a necessity for understanding the factors that trigger onset and drive progression of the disease. It is also apparent that even in the absence of clinical disease there are elderly subjects who may have significant pathology in the brain that has yet to reach a threshold to provoke overt clinical symptoms [2]. One area that offers potential for modulating disease onset and progression is by targeting the inflammatory processes associated with chronic neurodegeneration [3]. Recent research into the innate immune response in the brain during chronic neurodegenerative disease has highlighted how interactions with systemic inflammation may have profound consequences for both the expression of acute symptoms, and also for the progression of the neurodegenerative disease.

Brain Disorders in Critical Illness, ed. Robert D. Stevens, Tarek Sharshar, and E. Wesley Ely. Published by Cambridge University Press. © Cambridge University Press 2013.

Innate immune cells of the brain

The CNS, in common with other organs of the body, has a population of resident macrophages. Microglia are the resident macrophages of the brain parenchyma and there are other macrophage populations, including the perivascular macrophages (PVMs), adjacent to the cerebral endothelium, macrophages in the circumventricular organs, the choroid plexus, and meninges. Microglia are present throughout the neuraxis and although they differ in their density, with variations in their morphology, from one region to the next, they show little heterogeneity in the expression of myeloid-related molecules [4,5]. Recent evidence shows that a significant proportion of microglia are derived from a myeloid precursor cell in the yolk sac during embryogenesis [6]: these cells invade the embryonic nervous system playing a role in the removal of apoptotic cells and their processes and perhaps other functions as well. In rodents the microglia represent as many as 12% of all the cells in the substantia nigra, one of the most densely populated regions [4], but in the human brain the microglia in gray matter are a smaller percentage of the total cell population and the density is greater in white than in gray matter [7]. In the normal healthy brain the microglia are characterized by a highly branched morphology (Figures 18.1A, 18.2) and low levels of expression of myeloid antigens relative to other macrophages. There is evidence that ligands expressed by (e.g., CD200) or secreted by (e.g., CX3CL1) neurons bind their receptors on microglia (CD200R, CX3CRI) that lead to down-regulation of macrophage activation [8,9]. These molecules provide the inhibitory tone to microglia, which may be lost during neurodegenerative disease. The microglia may be very long-lived cells with a low rate of local division [10]: there is little recruitment of circulating monocytes into the microglia pool [11,12], although other brain macrophages may be replaced from the blood over periods of months. In vivo imaging studies of fluorescently labeled microglia show that they continually move their processes to palpate their local microenvironment, and it is calculated that they make contact with all the tissue within their territory within a few hours [13].

The functions of microglia in the normal healthy brain are poorly understood, but a number have been proposed. Since these are cells of the macrophage lineage we would expect these cells to be the first line of defense against injury and infection, and indeed the microglia are exquisitely sensitive to disturbances of brain homeostasis and injury [14]. We would thus expect them to play a role in the initiation of the immune response to injury and infection. It has been argued that microglia may play a role in monitoring synaptic function in development [15,16], in the adult brain [17], and in pathological conditions [15]. Although there is indirect evidence to support these proposed roles in the context of synaptic function, direct evidence for the active involvement of microglia in selectively modifying synaptic number or function in each of these conditions is at present lacking [18].

A key function of microglia is in the signaling from systemic immune responses to the brain. Following infection, and an immune response in peripheral tissue, signals are generated that communicate with the brain leading to changes in metabolism, fever, and changes in behavior such as anorexia, adipsia, lethargy, and depression. It has been highlighted elsewhere how important this response is to protect us against infection and aid recovery [19]. It is hard to imagine humans' survival in the absence of the CNS response to systemic injury and infection, and there are potentially useful parallels in the devastating consequences of the absence of the perception of pain [20]. The pathways by which systemic inflammation communicates with the CNS have been shown to involve both neural and humoral routes [19,21]. Inflammation in the thoracic abdominal cavity will activate sensory afferent fibers of the vagus nerve leading to activation of the nucleus of the solitary tract and connected brain regions [21]. The generation of circulating cytokines and other inflammatory mediators activates macrophage populations in the circumventricular organs, with spread of the signals into the brain parenchyma [22]. There is also signaling across the endothelial cells of the intact blood–brain barrier, which in turn signal to PVMs and microglia. Since no neuron is more than about 20 μm from the cerebral endothelium, this is likely to be a critical pathway [23]. The full complement of signaling pathways across the blood–brain barrier from different inflammatory conditions is yet to be defined and trans-blood–brain barrier signaling is a potentially critical target for modulation of immune-to-brain communication.

If the communication between systemic inflammation and the brain is regulated by the cerebral endothelium and the resident macrophages of the brain, then this raises the important question as to how this signaling might be affected by changes in these cell populations that accompany CNS degenerative disease and aging.

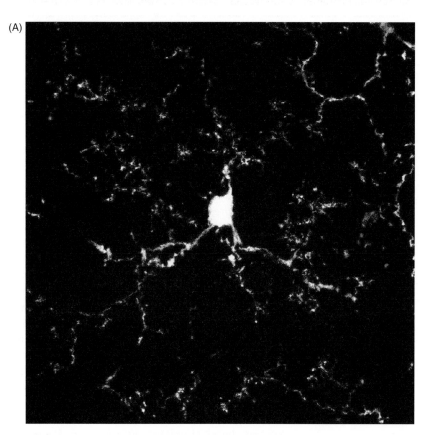

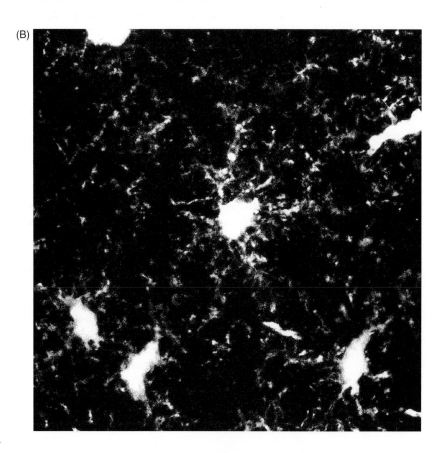

Figure 18.1 The morphology of microglia revealed by the expression of macrophage colony-stimulating factor receptor-green fluorescent protein transgene [49]: resident microglia in a normal mouse brain (A) and activated microglia in the brain of a mouse with prion disease (B).

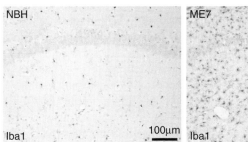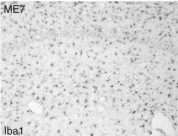

Figure 18.2 In the normal mouse hippocampus the microglia, as revealed by immunocytochemistry for the calcium binding protein Iba1, have a ramified morphology and appear regularly spaced at a low density across the hippocampus in a control mouse brain injected with normal brain homogenate (NBH). In the brain of a mouse with ME7-induced prion disease the microglia have greatly increased in density and have an activated morphology (ME7). Despite their proliferation and activated morphology the cells have an anti-inflammatory phenotype, they are primed by the ongoing neuropathology.

Innate immune response to chronic neurodegeneration

In the brains from patients who have died with chronic neurodegenerative disease such as Alzheimer's disease, Parkinson's disease, and others, the microglia are described as "activated" [8]. They have morphological features distinct from those seen in the normally healthy brain, a hypertrophied cell body, retracted and highly branched processes (Figures 18.1B, 18.2), and they express higher levels of diverse myeloid-related antigens [8,9]. A number of studies have also shown that these cells synthesize pro-inflammatory cytokines suggestive of a pro-inflammatory response associated with ongoing chronic neurodegeneration. The presence of these cytokines is of interest since studies in experimental models of stroke and traumatic brain injury have shown that inflammatory cytokines, such as interleukin-1ß, exacerbate an acute brain injury and that blocking the activity of this cytokine reduces the size of the lesion [24]. It is not, of course, immediately clear whether the innate immune response in diseases such as Alzheimer's or Parkinson's disease is simply a consequence of the ongoing accumulation of a mis-folded protein, and the degeneration of neurons and their processes, or whether this innate inflammatory response contributes to disease progression.

An important contribution to this debate came from epidemiology studies examining the impact of taking non-steroidal anti-inflammatory drugs (NSAIDs) on the onset or progression of Alzheimer's disease and subsequently in other neurodegenerative diseases such as Parkinson's disease. Although there is variability in the data, and a number of the studies involved only a small number of individuals, the data support the idea that taking NSAIDs for long periods of time, over several years, may lead to protection from the onset or progression to disease [25]. A similar finding has been reported in Parkinson's disease demonstrating an association between taking NSAIDs and some protection from disease onset or progression [26]. Clinical trials were initiated to test whether NSAIDs could be used to treat patients with Alzheimer's disease [27]. The trials demonstrated no significant impact on disease progression but suffered from a number of shortcomings, including the use of cyclooxygenase-2 inhibitors rather than NSAIDs with a broader specificity, initiating treatment during rather than prior to disease, and a relatively short time span.

Whatever the shortcomings of the neuropathological and epidemiological studies, the concept that the innate immune response in the brain, or neuroinflammation, may play a role in the pathogenesis of diseases such as Alzheimer's and Parkinson's disease is now an active area of research. The modulation of neuroinflammation offers a route to therapeutic intervention in diseases that have so far been refractory to treatment with therapeutic agents that target other components of the pathology, such as the degradation of amyloid, or interfere with the generation of the amyloidogenic proteins [28,29]. The goal of a significant research effort is to understand the role of inflammation in these diseases, and this requires that we understand more about this unusual innate immune response. The innate immune response in protein misfolding diseases of the CNS is dominated by cells of the myeloid macrophage lineage, may evolve over many years, and is likely a combination of the response to the accumulation of misfolded protein and the slow degeneration of neuronal processes and ultimately their cell bodies. The slow progressive nature of the disease raises interesting questions as to the extent microglia become adapted or tolerant to the presence of these potentially activating agents, or whether they become activated or primed by these signals. To learn more about the nature of the inflammatory response in chronic progressive neurodegeneration and how it evolves with disease progression requires relevant animal models.

Innate immune response in animal models of chronic neurodegeneration

The generation of transgenic mice that carry human genes coding for proteins that lead to protein misfolding diseases in the brain has had a major impact on the study of neurodegenerative diseases [30]. However, despite their value in understanding some aspects of the pathogenesis of diseases such as Alzheimer's and Parkinson's disease the majority of these models lack an essential ingredient, namely, the progressive and widespread degeneration of neurons. One laboratory model of chronic neurodegeneration, which directly mimics the human disease, and also has similarities with other protein misfolding diseases, is mouse prion disease. There are numerous models of mouse prion disease using different strains of mice and different agents, the combination of which lead to the accumulation of protease resistant PrP^{Sc} amyloid deposits in the brain, derived from a normal host protein PrP^{c}, and the progressive and widespread degeneration of neuronal processes and their cell bodies.

Studies on the ME7 model of prion disease, an agent that leads to the death of the mouse at 165 days post-infection, has revealed a number of components of the microglia response to chronic progressive neurodegeneration [31]. The microglia first take on an activated morphology several months before there is evidence of overt neuronal degeneration and then they increase in number during disease progression (Figure 18.1B and 18.2). The increase in microglia is predominantly a consequence of local proliferation. The inflammatory profile of these microglia is characterized not by typical pro-inflammatory cytokines but by the synthesis of the anti-inflammatory cytokine transforming growth factor-beta (TGF-ß), macrophage chemotactic protein-1 (MCP-1/CCL2), and raised levels of prostaglandin E2 [32,33,34]. This phenotype persists from the earliest onset of behavioral impairments and loss of synapses from the dorsal hippocampus, at approximately 12 weeks post disease initiation, up to the time when

there is widespread neurodegeneration and overt clinical symptoms at 20 weeks. The earliest stages of the degeneration process in the hippocampus involve the degeneration of synapses in the stratum radiatum and, perhaps somewhat contrary to expectations, the microglia do not engage in synaptic stripping and phagocytose the degenerating profiles [15]: instead the presynaptic elements are enveloped by the postsynaptic density (PSD) of the dendritic spine, although it is not clear whether this leads to internalization of either the degenerating presynaptic terminal or the postsynaptic density [35].

The observation that the microglia may adopt an activated morphology but with an apparently anti-inflammatory phenotype was somewhat surprising given the observations on postmortem material from studies of both Alzheimer's and Parkinson's disease patients. However, one clear difference between the patient groups and mice used in these studies is that the patient populations commonly suffer from diverse comorbidities, including both systemic inflammatory conditions and common systemic infections. We investigated whether systemic inflammation may impact on the innate immune response in the diseased brain in a manner that is different from that seen in the normal healthy brain.

Impact of systemic inflammation on the diseased brain

We challenged mice with ME7-induced prion disease with an intraperitoneal injection of lipopolysaccharide (LPS) to mimic aspects of a systemic bacterial infection [36,37]. The resulting production of peripheral inflammatory mediators led to sickness behaviors in these mice, as we would expect, except that the sickness behavior was much exaggerated when compared with naïve mice. Associated with the exaggerated sickness behaviors was enhanced production of pro-inflammatory cytokines in the brain when compared with naïve mice. We suggested that in the course of prion disease the microglia not only increase in number and are activated but they become "primed" by either the ongoing accumulation of misfolded protein, or the neurodegeneration, or perhaps both, and that the systemic signals switch the phenotype of the microglia from a benign anti-inflammatory phenotype to a pro-inflammatory phenotype [3,38]. Subsequent studies have shown that systemic challenge with LPS, or with double-stranded RNA to mimic a viral infection [39], leads to a switch in the cytokine production in the brain [36,37,39] and a dramatic up-regulation of macrophage receptors such as the IgG Fc receptors [40] with potentially important functional consequences.

The switch in phenotype of the primed microglia has both acute consequences, with exaggerated sickness behaviors and enhanced cytokine synthesis in the brain, and also chronic consequences, namely increased neuronal degeneration and early onset of symptoms of disease progression such as cognitive and motor deficits [36,37,39].

These experiments show that signaling from systemic inflammation to the brain, caused perhaps by systemic inflammatory disease or infection, has a profound effect on the diseased brain that is distinct from that seen in a healthy brain. A normally homeostatic response that provokes metabolic and behavioral changes that serve to protect us from infection becomes maladaptive in individuals with a diseased brain and exacerbates both disease symptoms and progression. The concept that microglia priming might underpin the response to systemic inflammation in other disease states such as brain trauma, stroke, or multiple sclerosis has been studied in animal models. In animal models of stroke systemic inflammation exacerbates lesion outcome [41]. It has long been recognized that a proportion of relapses in multiple sclerosis patients are associated with systemic infection [42], and our recent studies on an animal model of multiple sclerosis demonstrate that axon injury, an irreversible component of the disease, is exacerbated by systemic inflammation [43].

Systemic inflammation in Alzheimer's disease

There is a wealth of anecdotal evidence and clinical experience to suggest that systemic infection or inflammation exacerbates the symptoms of Alzheimer's disease. However, although it is known that systemic inflammation sufficient to cause delirium in elderly subjects or those with Alzheimer's disease indicates a poor prognosis, there is little evidence to ascertain whether systemic inflammation might itself have an impact on disease progression and symptoms in the absence of delirium. Our recent studies on a cohort of patients with Alzheimer's disease show that systemic inflammation, with sustained raised serum levels of tumor necrosis factor alpha (TNFα), and acute systemic infections are associated with accelerated cognitive

decline and exacerbation of symptoms of sickness behavior, such as depression, agitation, and apathy, typically seen in patients with Alzheimer's disease [44,45]. The studies described above in preclinical models provide a cellular and molecular basis by which systemic inflammation may impact on the diseased brain of patients with Alzheimer's disease and also perhaps with other chronic progressive neurodegenerative diseases.

Macrophage priming

The concept of macrophage priming has long been recognized in the context of in vitro studies. These studies show that priming of macrophages by a first stimulus, such as the cytokine γ-interferon, leads to the synthesis of receptors and signaling pathways so that a second triggering stimulus, for example LPS, leads to a more robust and exaggerated response when compared with the response of a naïve cell exposed to either stimulus alone [46]. The demonstration that microglia in the brain can be first primed by a stimulus such as neurodegeneration or the accumulation of a misfolded protein, by aging of the brain [47], or by a prior systemic infection [48] leading to an exaggerated response to a secondary systemic stimulus (Figure 18.3) has important implications for the care and treatment of individuals in an intensive care or other medical setting. The microglia present in the diseased brain in a relatively benign but primed state may be subsequently activated or triggered by signaling molecules, from acute or chronic systemic inflammation, leading to the generation of cytokines and other molecules with the capacity to either cause dysfunction or degeneration of the neurons, and acute exacerbation of symptoms. This phenomenon of microglia switching from a benign state to a tissue-damaging phenotype by systemic inflammation was first described in murine prion disease [31] but has now been described in diverse animal models [3] and may underpin the clinical decline associated with systemic inflammation [44,45]. If, however, the secondary stimulus is sufficiently powerful this may lead to excessive and prolonged activation of the microglia leading to delirium or sepsis-associated encephalopathy, as discussed in Chapters 11 and 38, this volume. The recognition and prompt treatment of even relatively common infections may have considerable benefit to patients in diverse medical settings suffering from degenerative diseases of the brain.

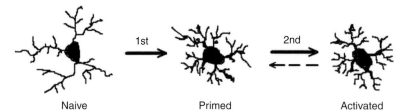

Naive   Primed   Activated

Figure 18.3 Microglia priming. In the naïve brain the microglia have fine, delicate, ramified processes that cover their own territory. These cells act as the first line of defence against tissue injury and infection and play a role in tissue homeostasis and communication between the immune system and the brain. A first stimulus such as acute or chronic neurodegeneration, accumulation of a misfolded protein, systemic infection, or decreased levels of expression of molecules that inhibit microglia activation will lead to the priming of the microglia. The primed microglia may have a morphologically activated appearance but do not synthesize pro-inflammatory molecules. A second stimulus such as a brain injury or a systemic inflammatory event will then trigger microglia activation leading to switching to a pro-inflammatory phenotype with the capacity to disrupt neuronal function or induce neurodegeneration. The activated phenotype may revert to the primed phenotype to be triggered by further secondary stimuli (see text).

Acknowledgments

The Medical Research Council UK, the Wellcome Trust, Alzheimer's Disease Society, Alzheimer's Research Trust, and the EU fund the work in the author's laboratory. I am grateful to Dr. Diego Gomez-Nicola for the images illustrated in Figures 18.1 and 18.2.

References

1. Ferri CP, Prince M, Brayne C, *et al.* Alzheimer's Disease International. Global prevalence of dementia: a Delphi consensus study. *Lancet* 2005;**366**:2112–17.

2. Neuropathology Group. Medical Research Council Cognitive Function and Aging Study. Pathological correlates of late-onset dementia in a multicentre, community-based population in England and Wales. Neuropathology Group of the Medical Research Council Cognitive Function and Ageing Study (MRC CFAS). *Lancet* 2001;**357**:169–75.

3. Perry VH, Nicoll JA, Holmes C. Microglia in neurodegenerative disease. *Nat Rev Neurol* 2010;**6**:193–201.

4. Lawson LJ, Perry VH, Dri P, *et al.* Heterogeneity in the distribution and morphology of microglia in the normal adult mouse brain. *Neuroscience* 1990;**39**:151–70.

5. de Haas AH, Boddeke HW, Biber K. Region-specific expression of immunoregulatory proteins on microglia in the healthy CNS. *Glia* 2008;**56**:888–94.

6. Ginhoux F, Greter M, Leboeuf M, *et al.* Fate mapping analysis reveals that adult microglia derive from primitive macrophages. *Science* 2010;**330**:841–5.

7. Mittelbronn M, Dietz K, Schluesener HJ, *et al.* Local distribution of microglia in the normal adult human central nervous system differs by up to one order of magnitude. *Acta Neuropathol* 2001;**101**:249–55.

8. Ransohoff RM, Perry VH. Microglial physiology: unique stimuli, specialized responses. *Annu Rev Immunol* 2009;**27**:119–45.

9. Kettenmann H, Hanisch UK, Noda M, *et al.* Physiology of microglia. *Physiol Rev* 2011;**91**:461–553.

10. Lawson LJ, Perry VH, Gordon S. Turnover of resident microglia in the normal adult mouse brain. *Neuroscience* 1992;**48**:405–15.

11. Mildner A, Schmidt H, Nitsche M, *et al.* Microglia in the adult brain arise from Ly-6ChiCCR2+ monocytes only under defined host conditions. *Nat Neurosci* 2007;**10**:1544–53.

12. Ajami B, Bennett JL, Krieger C, *et al.* Local self-renewal can sustain CNS microglia maintenance and function throughout adult life. *Nat Neurosci* 2007;**10**:1538–43.

13. Nimmerjahn A, Kirchhoff F, Helmchen F. Resting microglial cells are highly dynamic surveillants of brain parenchyma in vivo. *Science* 2005;**308**:1314–18.

14. Kreutzberg GW. Microglia: a sensor for pathological events in the CNS. *Trends Neurosci* 1996;**19**:312–18.

15. Stevens B, Allen NJ, Vazquez LE, *et al.* The classical complement cascade mediates CNS synapse elimination. *Cell* 200;**131**:1164–78.

16. Paolicelli RC, Bolasco G, Pagani F, *et al.* Synaptic pruning by microglia is necessary for normal brain development. *Science* 2011;**333**:1456–8.

17. Tremblay MÈ, Lowery RL, Majewska AK. Microglial interactions with synapses are modulated by visual experience. *PLoS Biol* 2010;**8**(11):e1000527.

18. Perry VH, O'Connor V. The role of microglia in synaptic stripping and synaptic degeneration: a revised perspective. *ASN Neuro* 2010;**2**(5). pii: e00047.

19. Dantzer R, O'Connor JC, Freund GG, *et al.* From inflammation to sickness and depression: when the immune system subjugates the brain. *Nat Rev Neurosci* 2008;**9**:46–56.

20. Drenth JP, Waxman SG. Mutations in sodium-channel gene SCN9A cause a spectrum of human genetic pain disorders. *J Clin Invest* 2007;**117**:3603–9.

21. Tracey KJ. The inflammatory reflex. *Nature* 2002;**420**(6917):853–9.

22. Lacroix S, Feinstein D, Rivest S. The bacterial endotoxin lipopolysaccharide has the ability to target the brain in upregulating its membrane CD14 receptor within specific cellular populations. *Brain Pathol* 1998;**8**:625–40.

23. Abbott NJ, Rönnbäck L, Hansson E. Astrocyte-endothelial interactions at the blood-brain barrier. *Nat Rev Neurosci* 2006;**7**:41–53.

24. Allan SM, Tyrrell PJ, Rothwell NJ. Interleukin-1 and neuronal injury. *Nat Rev Immunol* 2005;**5**:629–40.

25. Hoozemans JJ, Veerhuis R, Rozemuller JM *et al.* Soothing the inflamed brain: effect of non-steroidal anti-inflammatory drugs on Alzheimer's disease pathology. *CNS Neurol Disord Drug Targets* 2011;**10**:57–67.

26. Gao X, Chen H, Schwarzschild MA, Ascherio A. Use of ibuprofen and risk of Parkinson disease. *Neurology* 2011;**76**(10):863–9.

27. Lichtenstein MP, Carriba P, Masgrau R, *et al.* Staging anti-inflammatory therapy in Alzheimer's disease. *Front Aging Neurosci* 2010;**2**:142.

28. Miners JS, Barua N, Kehoe PG, *et al.* Aβ-degrading enzymes: potential for treatment of Alzheimer disease. *J Neuropathol Exp Neurol* 2011;**70**:944–59.

29. Frisardi V, Solfrizzi V, Imbimbo PB, *et al.* Towards disease-modifying treatment of Alzheimer's disease: drugs targeting beta-amyloid. *Curr Alzheimer Res* 2010;**7**:40–55.

30. Duyckaerts C, Potier MC, Delatour B. Alzheimer disease models and human neuropathology: similarities and differences. *Acta Neuropathol* 2008;**115**:5–38.

31. Perry VH. Contribution of systemic inflammation to chronic neurodegeneration. *Acta Neuropathol* 2010;**120**:277–86.

32. Boche D, Cunningham C, Docagne F, *et al.* TGFbeta1 regulates the inflammatory response during chronic neurodegeneration. *Neurobiol Dis* 2006;**22**:638–50.

33. Felton LM, Cunningham C, Rankine EL, *et al.* MCP-1 and murine prion disease: separation of early behavioural dysfunction from overt clinical disease. *Neurobiol Dis* 2005;**20**:283–95.

34. Minghetti L, Greco AF, Cardone F, *et al.* Increased brain synthesis of prostaglandin E2 and F2-isoprostane in human and experimental transmissible spongiform encephalopathies. *J Neuropathol Exp Neurol* 2000;**59**:866–71.

35. Siskova Z, Page A, O'Connor V, *et al.* Degenerating synaptic boutons in prion disease: microglia activation without synaptic stripping. *Am J Pathol* 2009;**175**:1610–21.

36. Cunningham C, Wilcockson DC, Campion S, *et al.* Central and systemic endotoxin challenges exacerbate the local inflammatory response and increase neuronal death during chronic neurodegeneration. *J Neurosci* 2005;**25**:9275–84.

37. Cunningham C, Campion S, Lunnon K, *et al.* Systemic inflammation induces acute behavioral and cognitive changes and accelerates neurodegenerative disease. *Biol Psychiatry* 2009;**65**:304–12.

38. Perry VH, Cunningham C, Holmes C. Systemic infections and inflammation affect chronic neurodegeneration. *Nat Rev Immunol* 2007;**7**:161–7.

39. Field R, Campion S, Warren C, *et al.* Systemic challenge with the TLR3 agonist poly I:C induces amplified IFNalpha/beta and IL-1beta responses in the diseased brain and exacerbates chronic neurodegeneration. *Brain Behav Immun* 2010;**24**:996–1007.

40. Lunnon K, Teeling JL, Tutt AL, *et al.* Systemic inflammation modulates Fc receptor expression on microglia during chronic neurodegeneration. *J Immunol* 2011;**186**:7215–24.

41. Buljevac D, Flach HZ, Hop WC, *et al.* Prospective study on the relationship between infections and multiple sclerosis exacerbations. *Brain* 2002;**125**:952–60.

42. McColl BW, Allan SM, Rothwell NJ. Systemic infection, inflammation and acute ischemic stroke. *Neuroscience* 2009;**158**:1049–61.

43. Moreno B, Jukes J-P, Vergara-Irigaray N, *et al.* Systemic inflammation induces axon injury during brain inflammation. *Ann Neurol* 2011;**70**: 932–42.

44. Holmes C, Cunningham C, Zotova E, *et al.* Systemic inflammation and disease progression in Alzheimer disease. *Neurology* 2009;**73**:768–74.

45. Holmes C, Cunningham C, Zotova E, *et al.* Proinflammatory cytokines, sickness behavior, and Alzheimer disease. *Neurology* 2011;**77**:212–18.

46. Schroder K, Sweet MJ, Hume DA. Signal integration between IFNgamma and TLR signalling pathways in macrophages. *Immunobiology* 2006;**211**:511–24.

47. Godbout JP, Chen J, Abraham J, *et al.* Exaggerated neuroinflammation and sickness behavior in aged mice

following activation of the peripheral innate immune system. *FASEB J* 2005;**19**:1329–31.

48. Ohmoto Y, Wood MJ, Charlton HM, *et al.* Variation in the immune response to adenoviral vectors in the brain: influence of mouse strain, environmental conditions and priming. *Gene Ther* 1999;**6**:471–81.

49. Sasmono RT, Oceandy D, Pollard JW, *et al.* A macrophage colony-stimulating factor receptor-green fluorescent protein transgene is expressed throughout the mononuclear phagocyte system of the mouse. *Blood* 2003;**101**:1155–63.

The neuroendocrine response to critical illness

David Luis and Djillali Annane

SUMMARY

Acute response to lipopolysaccharides (LPS) includes the release of a number of pro-inflammatory mediators that reach the brain in areas free of blood–brain barrier, or via specific transport systems. The hypothalamic-pituitary axis is also activated via neural routes. Then, infection is characterized by high circulating levels of adrenocorticotropin hormone (ACTH) and cortisol, which remain in plateau as long as the stressful condition is maintained. Circulating vasopressin levels follow a biphasic response with high concentrations, followed by relative vasopressin insufficiency in about one third of cases. Early response to sepsis is characterized by decreased serum T3 and increased rT3 levels. Serum T4 levels decrease within 24–48 hours, and thyroid-stimulating hormone (TSH) levels remain normal, and have no more circadian rhythm. Prolonged sepsis is associated with centrally induced hypothyroidism. In the initial response to sepsis, growth hormone (GH) levels are high with attenuated oscillatory activity and low IGF-1 levels. Later on, GH secretion shows a reduced pulsatile fraction, and correlates with low circulating levels of IGF-1. Exposure to endotoxin caused prompt increase in circulating adrenaline and noradrenalin concentrations. Catecholamines have a very short half-life and are metabolized through captation, enzymatic inactivation, or renal excretion. Plasma catecholamine levels remain elevated in plateau up to a few months after recovery. Insulin levels rapidly increase following LPS as a result of both increased secretion and tissue resistance. The clinical consequences of the stress system activation include behavioral changes, cardiovascular, metabolic, and immune adaptations. The use of exogenous hormones in critical illness has become a standard of care. Hypotension can be corrected by administration of catecholamines, and these drugs are routinely administered in the intensive care unit (ICU). Vasopressin can help improve cardiovascular function in vasodilatory shock. While undoubtedly corticosteroids or insulin prevent critical illness-related morbidity, the survival benefit from treatment with these hormones remains controversial.

Introduction

The critically ill patient has to deal with multiple stressors, including emotional and physical stress, resulting both from an acute aggression such as trauma or infection and from various therapeutic or diagnostic interventions such as surgery, arterial or venous catheterization, laryngeal intubation and mechanical ventilation, and drugs. Of note, critical illness-related stress is sustained at a certain level of intensity for several days with additive and unpredictable surges. Thus, the host response is on one hand reset to counteract a prolonged stress, and on another hand has to remain able to promptly adjust to unpredictable threats. Therefore, the integrity and flexibility of the host response to stressors is essential to survive critical illness.

The "stress system" has two main components: the corticotropin-releasing hormone/vasopressin neurons of the hypothalamus and the locus coeruleus noradrenaline/autonomic neurons of the brainstem [1]. We will summarize recent knowledge on immune regulation of brain activation to generate both neurological and hormonal responses aimed at turning off the immune system when the inflammatory response is no longer needed to fight off, for example, an infectious threat.

Brain Disorders in Critical Illness, ed. Robert D. Stevens, Tarek Sharshar, and E. Wesley Ely. Published by Cambridge University Press. © Cambridge University Press 2013.

Physiological considerations about the neuroendocrine system

Two pathways are used by the organism for inter-organ communication, the central nervous system (CNS) and its peripheral arms and the endocrine system, and these systems cross-talk with a third one, i.e., the immune system [1]. In vertebrates the endocrine organs include anterior and posterior pituitary, ovary and testis, adrenal cortex and medulla, thyroids and parathyroids, islets of Langerhans in the pancreas, and various parts of the intestinal mucosa. The pineal and thymus can also be considered as endocrine organs. In addition, other organs may have some endocrine properties. As examples, the kidney secretes rennin and angiotensin, the heart secretes natriuretic factors. Basically hormones are divided into steroids (cholesterol-derived proteins), peptides, and amines.

There is probably no uniform mechanism for the regulation of hormone activity. For example, parathyroid hormone (PTH or parathormone) release is independent of any nervous stimulation or specific trophic hormone, in contrary to the thyroid, adrenals, and gonads. This review focuses on steroids, catecholamines, and vasopressin. There are two main mechanisms of regulation of endocrine activity: feedback loops and neural control (Figure 19.1). Experiments in which peripheral glands are disconnected from the pituitary showed full cessation of gonad function

whereas the thyroid and adrenal cortex continue to secrete hormones at a lower level depicting their intrinsic activity. Similarly, the anterior pituitary has an intrinsic activity specific to thyroid and adrenal cortex function.

Feedback mechanisms allow circulating hormones to regulate the release of their precursors by the hypothalamus, contributing to a pattern of rhythmic secretion of hormones. The feedback loop also involves central nervous structures such as the hippocampus. This self-balancing system fine tunes the endocrine activity under resting conditions but may be insufficient in the case of enhanced endocrine activity [1]. The hypothalamus plays a key role in regulating the endocrine system. First, it is directly connected to the neurohypophysis and the adrenal medulla. Second, it modulates the anterior pituitary function by releasing, in synchronous pulses (roughly hourly), stimulatory or inhibitory hormones in the hypophysial portal vessels of the pituitary stalk. Stimulatory peptides include corticotropin-releasing hormone (CRH), LH-releasing hormone (LHRH), follicle-stimulating hormone (FSH)-releasing factor (FSHRF), GH-releasing factor (GHRH), prolactin (PRL)-stimulating factor, and thyrotropin-releasing hormone (TRH). Other peptides are inhibiting factors like GH-inhibiting hormone (somatostatin) and PRL-inhibiting hormone. Vasopressin, natriuretic peptides, and catecholamines also influence the pituitary function. The effect of

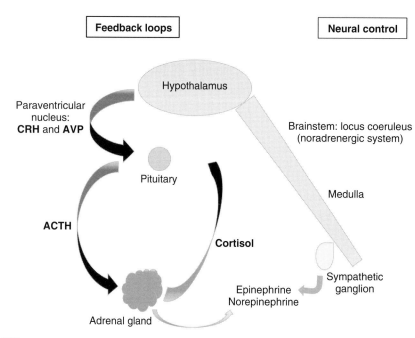

Figure 19.1 Two mechanisms of regulation of endocrine activity. ACTH, adrenocorticotropic hormone; AVP, arginine vasopressin; CRH, corticotropin-releasing hormone.

CRH on ACTH release by the pituitary is permissive and vasopressin acts in synergy with CRH. There are tight interconnections between CRH-synthesizing neurons from the parvocellular nuclei and the locus coeruleus in the brainstem [1]. Thereby, noradrenaline, CRH, and vasopressin can stimulate each other. Through collateral fibers, ultra-short negative feedback loops allow permanent adaptation of the synergy between the two systems. Finally, CRH, vasopressin, and noradrenaline are on the stimulatory control of the serotoninergic, cholinergic, and histaminergic systems and are inhibited by the gamma-aminobutyric acid, benzodiazepine, and opioid systems [1].

Critical illness-related disruption of the neuroendocrine system

The unpredictable nature, duration, and intensity of stressors challenge the host response to critical illness. In a recent work, we showed that in septic rats and in patients with septic shock, ACTH synthesis was decreased, while the expression of its two main regulators CRH and AVP remained roughly unchanged [2]. Acute inflammatory response to LPS include the release of a number of mediators, e.g., tumor necrosis factor alpha (TNFα), interleukin (IL)-1, IL-6, IL-8, nitric oxide, macrophage migration inhibiting factors

(MIF), and high mobility group box (HMGB)-1 [3]. The inflammatory molecules traffic to the brain via multiple routes (Figure 19.2). These mediators reach the hypophysial portal capillaries in the median eminence via the anterior hypophysial arteries. Cytokines can diffuse into the pituitary as these areas are free of the blood–brain barrier [4]. Then, they are carried to the hypothalamus and the brain areas lacking a blood–brain barrier (circumventricular organs), or via specific transport systems [4]. In addition to the blood-borne cytokines, glial cells can produce a number of cytokines such IL-1, IL-2, and IL-6 [5]. Interestingly, i.p. injection of LPS induces IL-1β followed by inducible nitric oxide (NO) synthase (iNOS) mRNA within 2 hours, peaking in 4–6 hours, and then returning to basal values by 24 hours [4]. In this study, IL-1β and iNOS were expressed in the meninges, areas lacking a blood–brain barrier, and also in the parvocellular nuclei and the arcuate nucleus, which contain the hypothalamic-releasing and -inhibiting hormone-producing neurons. Then, a sustained overexpression of NO through iNOS up-regulation prolongs the synthesis of hypothalamic hormones induced by LPS [4]. In addition, cytokines, via activation of GABAergic neurons, block NO-induced LHRH but not FSH release, inhibit GHRH release, and stimulate somatostatin and prolactin release [4].

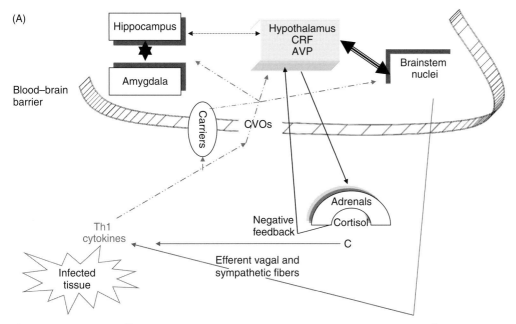

Figure 19.2 Cytokines trafficking to the brain. AVP, arginine vasopressin; CRF, corticotropin-releasing factor; CVOs, circumventricular organs.

(B)

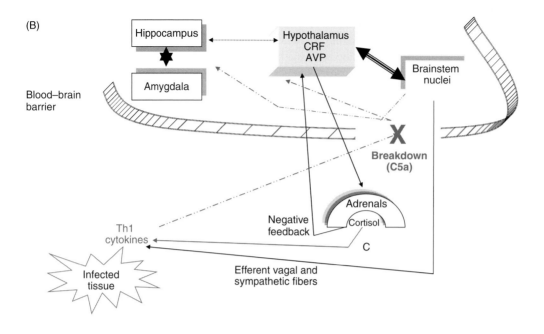

(C)

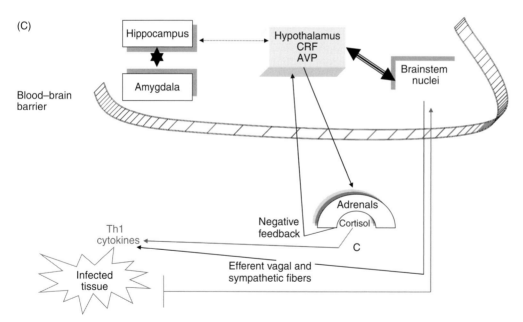

Figure 19.2 (cont.)

Various afferent neurons of the peripheral system sense the threat at the inflammatory sites and stimulate the noradrenergic system and the hypothalamus [1]. Activation of vagal afferent fibers by LPS results in activation of the locus coeruleus, which has neurons with projections that synapse on cholinergic interneurons in the parvocellular nucleus [1]. It has been shown that CRH is released upon acetylcholine stimulation of muscarinic receptor, and that this effect is prevented by non-specific NO antagonists [6].

The efferent vagus nerve controls the systemic inflammatory response by promoting the shift from a T-helper 1 to a T-helper 2 response, an effect mediated by specific nicotinic acetylcholine receptors on immune cell surfaces [7]. This so-called "cholinergic anti-inflammatory reflex" is orchestrated by brain muscarinic networks [8] and requires the integrity of catecholaminergic nerve fibers in the spleen [9].

To mount an appropriate hormonal response, i.e., the general adaptive syndrome, the host recruits additional endocrine cells and up-regulates these cells to release enough hormones. Simultaneously, the feedback loops are inhibited. Then, the net result of the endocrine response is not only increased circulating levels of hormones but also the shift from a rhythmic to a continuous secretion of hormones. In addition, T-helper 1 type cells producing cytokines decrease the clearance of most hormones from the plasma, alter the binding of hormones to their specific transporters or to albumin, and prevent the entrance of hormones into target tissues [1,4]. Tissue utilization of hormones is impaired either as a result of down-regulation of specific receptors or transporters, of transcriptional or post-transcriptional effects [1,4].

Neurohormonal patterns during critical illness

Infection, LPS challenge, major surgery, trauma, or burns elicit very similar patterns of pituitary hormone secretion (Table 19.1). Plasma ACTH and prolactin increase within a few minutes following the insult and is associated with a rapid inhibition of LH and TSH but not FSH secretion. Growth hormone secretion is also stimulated in humans.

Adrenal hormones

Acute stress induces an immediate increase in the amplitude of hypothalamic hormone pulses, mainly CRH and vasopressin, resulting in increased amplitude and frequency of ACTH and cortisol pulses, and the loss of the circadian rhythm [1]. The common feature is characterized by high circulating levels of ACTH and cortisol which remain in plateau as long as the stressful condition is maintained. However, circulating levels of cortisol depend on both synthesis and clearance and do not strictly reflect the HPA axis function. Thus, they vary from < 5 μg/dl to more than 100 μg/dl [10].

Table 19.1 Hormone secretion during critical illness.

Hormones	Main actions
Corticosteroids	Maintenance of vascular tone, of endothelial and vascular permeability Anti-inflammatory and immunosuppressive actions Induce peripheral insulin resistance and free fatty acids and amino-acids release Enhance hepatic gluconeogenesis and glyconeolysis
Vasopressin	Response to stress, memory formation Vasoconstriction, gluconeogenesis, platelet aggregation, release of FVIII and von Willebrand factor ACTH secretion Water reabsorption in the collecting ducts
Thyroid hormones	Increase metabolic rate
Growth hormone	Stimulate the immune system Promote lipolysis, increases protein synthesis, reduces liver uptake of glucose Increase calcium retention and increase bone mineralization
Catecholamines	Modulate vasomotor reactivity, increase systemic vascular resistance, increase the stroke volume Active lipolysis
Insulin	Decrease blood glucose level Decrease gluconeogenesis, proteinolysis, lipolysis Increase fatty acid and glycogen synthesis

Vasopressin

Circulating vasopressin levels are regulated through various stimuli, including changes in blood volume or blood pressure and plasma osmolality, cytokines, and other mediators. In sepsis, vasopressin levels in plasma may follow a biphasic response with initially high concentrations, followed by a decline in concentrations down to the limits of normal range within 72 hours with relative vasopressin insufficiency as a consequence of NO-induced neuronal loss [11]. In a recent work, we showed that about half of patients with septic shock have a blunted vasopressin response to changes in plasma osmolarity [12]. The exact mechanisms underlying the loss of control in vasopressin synthesis remain to be elucidated.

Thyroid hormones

Low T3–T4 syndrome has been described for more than 20 years in fasting conditions and in a wide variety of diseases (e.g., sepsis, surgery, myocardial infarction, transplantation, heart, renal, hepatic failure, cancers, malnutrition, inflammatory diseases) and is also called euthyroid-sick syndrome or non-thyroidal-illness syndrome (NTIS) [13]. In the early phase of stress, there is a decrease in serum triiodothyronine (T3) level, an increase in rT3 level, then serum thyroxine (T4) levels decrease within 24–48 hours, and TSH levels remain within normal range and show no more circadian rhythm. Underlying mechanisms include: (1) decreased conversion of T4 and T3 in extra-thyroid tissues due to inhibition of hepatic 5′-monodeiodination; (2) presence of transport protein inhibitors preventing T4 fixation on the protein; (3) dysfunction of thyrotrophic negative feedback; (4) cytokine (IL-1, IL-6, TNFα, IFNγ)-induced inhibition of the thyrotrophic centers' activity and/or affect the expression of thyroid hormones' nuclear receptors; (5) other inhibitory substances such as dopamine. Prolonged critical illness is associated with centrally induced hypothyroidism as suggested by restoration of T3 and T4 pulses by exogenous TRH infusion.

Growth hormone

The acute phase of critical illness is characterized by high growth hormone levels with attenuated oscillatory activity associated with low levels of insulin-like growth factor (IGF)-1 [14]. Serum concentrations of GH effectors IGF-1 are low during this phase, suggesting resistance to GH as a result of decreased expression of GH receptor. Subsequently, direct lipolysis and anti-insulin effects of GH might be enhanced, liberating metabolic substrates such as free fatty acids and glucose to vital organs, while costly metabolism mediated by IGF-1 is postponed. In prolonged critical illness, the pattern of GH secretion shows a reduced pulsatile fraction that correlated with low circulating levels of IGF-1.

Catecholamines

It is well known that under resting conditions very small amounts of adrenaline and noradrenaline are released from the adrenal medulla (e.g., less than 50 ng/kg/min in the dog). Therefore, removal of the adrenal medulla allows an animal to survive the intervention indefinitely. However, exposure to stressors causes prompt increase in circulating adrenaline and noradrenaline concentrations by 2 to 3 logs, an effect that is prevented by removal of the adrenal medulla. Adrenaline is stored in medulla vesicles. Noradrenaline is present in the subcellular granules of the sympathetic nervous endings. Catecholamines have a very short half-life (10–20 seconds for adrenaline) and are metabolized through captation, enzymatic inactivation (methylation in metadrenaline or normetadrenaline in liver or kidney; oxidative deamination by monoamine oxidase), or renal excretion. The hormonal regulation depends on cortisol, which is necessary for the enzymatic degradation of catecholamine synthesis. The nervous regulation involves cholinergic, preganglionic, parasympathetic pathways via splanchnic nerves. Like cortisol, catecholamine levels in plasma can remain elevated in plateau as long as the stress is maintained, and even up to 3 months after recovery [15].

Insulin

Insulin is involved in glucose metabolism through: (1) mobilization of the store of glucose transport molecules in target cells, such as muscle and fat tissue; (2) activation of hepatic glucokinase gene transcription; (3) activation of glycogen synthetase and inhibition of glycogen phosphorylase [16]. Other actions of insulin include growth stimulation, cellular differentiation, and intra-cellular traffic, increase of lipogenesis, glycogenesis and protein synthesis. These effects result from insulin fixation to a ubiquitous membrane receptor belonging to the tyrosine kinase family, including insulin-like growth factor receptor (IGF-1) and insulin receptor-related receptor (IRR). Insulin levels in plasma are rapidly increased following an acute stress as a result of both increased secretion and tissue resistance. Insulin suppresses and antagonizes the effects of TNF, macrophage migration inhibitory factor (MIF), and superoxide anions, and decreases the synthesis of the acute phase reactants [17]. Moreover, insulin modulates leptin and other adipokines' release from fat cells.

Clinical manifestations of the neuroendocrine response to critical illness

The main objective of the neuroendocrine response to critical illness is to "fight and fly". Then, the immediate manifestations of the activation for the endocrine system, mainly the sympatho-adrenal hormones, include alertness, insomnia, hyperactivity, pupillary dilation, reception of hairs, sweating, salivary secretion, tachycardia, rise in blood pressure with dilation of skeletal muscles' blood vessels and coronary arteries, bronchiolar dilation and polypnea, skin vasoconstriction, mobilization of glucose from liver and hyperglycemia, increased oxygen capacity of the blood via spleen constriction and mobilization of red blood cells, and shortening of coagulation time. However, in practice, fighting is the only option, and the appropriateness of the neuroendocrine activity to the intensity and duration of the stress is the determinant of host survival and recovery. The clinical consequences of the stress system activation roughly include behavioral changes, cardiovascular, metabolic, and immune adaptations (Table 19.2).

Behavior

In animals, infections are associated with anorexia and body weight loss, hypersomnia, psychomotor retardation, fatigue, and impaired cognitive abilities. Similar behavioral changes are consistently reported in humans after cytokine or LPS challenge. The so-called "depression due to a general medical condition" or "sickness behavior" is likely mediated through release of peripheral and brain cytokines, among them IL-1 plays a predominant role [18,19]. Then, when

glucocorticoid and catecholamine responses are insufficient, the critically ill patient will develop brain dysfunction that can result in coma.

Cardiovascular system

The cardiovascular adaptation is mainly driven by the sympatho-adrenal hormones even though thyroid hormones and vasopressin contribute respectively to cardiac adaptation and blood volume and vasomotor tone regulation. Corticosteroids exert important actions on the various elements of the cardiovascular system including the capillaries, the arterioles, and the myocardium. The underlying mechanisms are not fully understood and may involve direct mobilization of intracellular calcium, enzymatic metabolism of adrenaline, increased binding affinity of adrenaline for its receptor or facilitation of the intracellular signalization that follows the coupling of adrenaline to its receptor. Whenever the hypothalamic-pituitary-adrenal axis or the noradrenergic responses are inappropriate, critically ill patients will develop cardiovascular dysfunction. Indeed, septic shock patients with adrenal insufficiency, as defined by a delta cortisol of 9 μg/dl or less, have more pronounced hypotension than those with presumed normal function, and are more likely to develop refractory shock and to die [10]. Adrenal insufficiency is at best recognized at the bedside of critically ill patients by either a low baseline cortisol level (<10 μg/dl) or cortisol increment after

Table 19.2 The clinical consequences of the stress system activation.

Function	Clinical consequence	Metabolic consequence
Behavioral	Anorexia, body weight loss, hypersomnia, psychomotor retardation, fatigue, impaired cognitive abilities, brain dysfunction and coma	Peripheral and brain release of cytokines
Cardiovascular	Loss of cardiovascular adaptation: hypotension, refractory shock	Decrease of the pulsatile activity of the HPA axis Loss of inter-organ communications
Metabolic	Hyperglycemia, insulin resistance, acquisition of superinfection	Cytokine-induced impairment in GLUT-4 metabolism, an imbalance between muscle protein breakdown rate and the rate of muscle protein synthesis
Immune	Increased susceptibility to infection	Suppress T-cell-derived cytokines, and change the Th1/Th2 balance toward excess Th2 cells Up-regulate lymphocyte-derived IL-10 Inhibit the synthesis of many other inflammatory mediators Down-regulate cell surface markers Enhance the occurrence of apoptosis of thymocytes, mature T-lymphocytes, eosinophils, epithelial cells, and precursors of dermal/interstitial dendritic cells, but delay apoptosis of neutrophils Promote locally at the level of inflamed tissues the synthesis of pro-inflammatory mediators

250 μg of corticotropin of < 9 μg/dl [10]. Failure of the noradrenergic system will also result in cardiovascular dysfunction during critical illness. Sepsis is associated with decreased noradrenergic activity that preceded cardiovascular dysfunction [20]. The decrease of the pulsatile activity of the HPA axis and the noradrenergic system result in circulatory and respiratory regulatory functions becoming unable to adjust to stressful conditions, loss in inter-organ communications with multiple organ dysfunction, and death [21]. Finally, inappropriately low vasopressin levels contribute to the vasodilatory shock [22].

Metabolism

The net result from the activation of the endocrine system is hyperglycemia. Tissues that are insulin-dependent cannot uptake glucose which is then available for insulin-independent tissues like the brain or inflammatory cells. The main reason for critical illness-associated insulin resistance is cytokine-induced impairment in GLUT-4 metabolism [23]. Hyperglycemia has been shown to increase mortality in critical illness [24]. The mechanisms underlying glucose toxicity for the cells are still unknown and may include an overloading of the insulin-independent cells such as neurons. Subsequent to low ATP levels in the cells, the excess of intracellular glucose cannot enter the Krebs cycle and results in the generation of free radicals and peroxynitrites which in turn block complex IV of the mitochondria. Then, by killing the mitochondria of insulin-independent cells, hyperglycemia may facilitate acquisition of superinfection, damage the central and peripheral nervous systems, the liver and eventually result in death related to multiple organ dysfunction [23]. Excess in the catabolic hormones, cortisol, adrenaline, and glucagon will also elicit an imbalance between muscle protein breakdown rate and the rate of muscle protein synthesis, resulting in a net catabolism of muscle protein, which may contribute to critical illness-induced muscle weakness and affect long-term prognosis [25].

Immune system

The changes in the immune function again are mainly related to the sympatho-adrenal hormones even though insulin and vasopressin can also influence immunity. Glucocorticoids suppress most, if not all, T-cell derived cytokines, and change the Th1/Th2 balance toward excess Th2 cells [1,10]. They do not affect

IL-10 synthesis by monocytes, and they up-regulate lymphocyte-derived IL-10. They also inhibit the synthesis of many other inflammatory mediators such as cyclooxygenase and inducible NOS, and down-regulate cell surfaces markers such as endotoxin receptor and adhesion molecules. Finally, they enhance the occurrence of apoptosis of thymocytes, mature T-lymphocytes, eosinophils, epithelial cells, and precursors of dermal/interstitial dendritic cells, but delay apoptosis of neutrophils [1,10]. Only Th1 cells expressed beta-2 adrenergic receptors. Activation of these beta-2 receptors inhibits Th1 cell function, thereby catecholamines drive a Th2 shift [26]. They also promote locally at the level of inflamed tissues the synthesis of pro-inflammatory mediators via alpha-adrenergic receptors [27]. Then, the critical illness-associated impaired HPA axis shifts the Th1/Th2 balance to release of pro-inflammatory mediators in the circulation and broadly in body tissues.

Targeting the neuroendocrine response during critical illness

Hormones are routinely used in the management of critically ill patients. The correction of hypotension that is refractory to fluid replacement can almost always be achieved by intravenous administration of catecholamines. Adrenaline and noradrenaline are equipotent in restoring cardiovascular homeostasis during shock [28,29]. Vasopressin may also restore hemodynamic stability in critical illness [29,30]. The current literature suggests that any of dopamine, adrenaline, noradrenaline, or vasopressin can be used for the treatment of shock [29]. Nevertheless, the benefit-to-risk profile may favor the use of noradrenaline in patients with septic shock [31].

Administration of low to moderate doses of corticosteroids may help restore cardiovascular homeostasis in patients with septic shock [32,33] and their immune modulator effects may reverse organ dysfunction [34] and prevent death [32,35]. The use of low to moderate doses of corticosteroids in patients with septic shock continues to be controversial despite two large studies [32,33]. These studies evaluated different populations and came to different conclusions. Similarities between the two studies included steroids' beneficial effects on time to shock reversal, no evidence for increased risk of neuromuscular weakness, and hyperglycemia. Differences between the two studies included entry window (8 vs. 72 hours), duration of hypotension (systolic blood pressure < 90 mmHg for > 1 hour vs. < 1 hour), additional mineralocorticoid treatment (fludrocortisone vs. no fludrocortisone), treatment duration (7 vs. 11 days), weaning (none vs. present), severity of illness (SAPS II scores : 59 vs. 49), proportion of non-responders to corticotropin (77% vs. 47%), differences in steroids' effects according to the response to corticotropin (yes vs. no), increased risk of superinfection (no vs. yes), and whether the study occurred after practice guidelines were published recommending steroids (no vs. yes). Currently, patients with vasopressor-dependent shock should be treated with hydrocortisone [36]. Corticosteroids showed also favorable effects in patients with acute respiratory distress syndrome (ARDS), particularly when treatment was initiated within the first 2 weeks of lung injury [37]. Corticosteroids attenuated systemic and lung inflammation, and restored the hemostatic homeostasis. Subsequently, corticosteroids dramatically reduced the time on a ventilator by almost 1 week, the length of stay in the ICU, and improved survival [37]. Studies have also demonstrated that an impaired HPA axis may account at least partly for prolonged mechanical ventilation in critically ill patients [38]. In that study, patients who failed to be weaned off the ventilator were tested for adrenal function by a standard Synacthen test and non-responders (increment in cortisol of less than 9 µg/dl) were randomized to receive hydrocortisone or its placebo. The authors found that hydrocortisone restored the ability of patients to breathe spontaneously and thus shortened the duration of mechanical ventilation and ICU length of stay. Likewise, impaired HPA axis is a common feature in trauma patients [39,40], and replacement therapy with hydrocortisone improved outcomes of these patients [41].

Recently, intensive treatment with insulin targeting blood glucose levels of 4.4–6 mmol/l was shown to significantly improve morbidity and mortality in both surgical [41] and medical [42] patients. The benefit is mainly observed in the chronic phase of critical illness (after 72 hours) and may be related to protection of cells from glucose toxicity rather than from direct anti-inflammatory effects of insulin. However, two recent multicenter studies did not find any benefit for intensive insulin therapy in critically ill patients [43,44]. One may suggest that the very early increase in blood glucose mainly relates to stress hormones and should not be counteracted, whereas later hyperglycemia relates to cytokine-induced insulin resistance and should be treated. In addition, as compared with the Leuven trials [41,42], subsequent trials failed to achieve normal blood glucose levels and also had much lower daily caloric intake [43,44]. These findings highlighted the need for a better assessment of insulin deregulation in the critically ill to permit an adequate glucose homeostasis.

Other attempts to manipulate the endocrine system during critical illness have included thyroid hormone replacement therapy or growth hormone therapy, and been less successful so far [45,46].

Conclusions

Critical illness is characterized by a disruption in most of the components of the neuroendocrine response. When the balance between the stressors and the sympatho-adrenal response is restored, patients recover from their critical illness with or without sequels. When the intensity or duration of the stress surpasses the counteracting effects of the neuroendocrine system, critical illness progresses with multiple organ failure and eventually death. On the other hand, a too-excessive host response may result in long-term sequelae, including persistent changes in behavior and mood, deregulated metabolic state, and immune dysfunction. Subsequently, patients are exposed to an increased susceptibility to superinfection, risk for chronic muscle fatigue, and posttraumatic stress disorders. Whether the neuroendocrine system can be manipulated to be adjusted to the inflammatory process remains a controversial issue.

References

1. Chrousos GP. The stress response and immune function: clinical implications. The 1999 Novera H. Spector Lecture. *Ann NY Acad Sci* 2000;**917**:38–67.

2. Polito A, Sonneville R, Guidoux C, *et al.* Changes in CRH and ACTH synthesis during experimental and human septic shock. *PLoS One* 2011;**6**(11):e25905.

3. Annane D, Bellissant E, Cavaillon JM. Septic shock. *Lancet* 2005;**365**:63–78.

4. McCann SM, Kimura M, Karanth S, *et al.* The mechanism of action of cytokines to control the release of hypothalamic and pituitary hormones in infection. *Ann NY Acad Sci* 2000;**917**:4–18.

5. Koenig JI. Presence of cytokines in the hypothalamic-pituitary axis. *Prog Neuroendocrino Immunol* 1991;**4**:143–53.

6. Karanth S, Lyson K, McCann SM. Effects of cholinergic agonists and antagonists on interleukin-2-induced

corticotropin-releasing hormone release from the mediobasal hypothalamus. *Neuroimmunomodulation* 1999;**6**:168–74.

7. Wang H, Yu M, Ochani M, *et al.* Nicotinic acetylcholine receptor alpha7 subunit is an essential regulator of inflammation. *Nature* 2003;**421**(6921):384–8.

8. Pavlov VA, Ochani M, Gallowitsch-Puerta M, *et al.* Central muscarinic cholinergic regulation of the systemic inflammatory response during endotoxemia. *Proc Natl Acad Sci USA* 2006;**103**(13):5219–23.

9. Rosas-Ballina M, Ochani M, Parrish WR, *et al.* Splenic nerve is required for cholinergic antiinflammatory pathway control of TNF in endotoxemia. *Proc Natl Acad Sci USA* 2008;**105**(31):11008–13.

10. Annane D. Corticosteroids for severe sepsis: an evidence-based guide for physicians. *Ann Intensive Care* 2011;**1**(1):7.

11. Sharshar T, Gray F, Lorin de la Grandmaison G, *et al.* Apoptosis of neurons in cardiovascular autonomic centres triggered by inducible nitric oxide synthase after death from septic shock. *Lancet* 2003;**362**:1799–805.

12. Siami S, Bailly-Salin J, Polito A, *et al.* Osmoregulation of vasopressin secretion is altered in the postacute phase of septic shock. *Crit Care Med* 2010;**38**(10):1962–9.

13. De Groot LJ. Dangerous dogmas in medicine: the nonthyroidal illness syndrome. *J Clin Endocrinol Metab* 1999;**84**:151–64.

14. Ross R, Miell J, Freeman E, *et al.* Critically ill patients have high basal growth hormone levels with attenuated oscillatory activity associated with low levels of insulin-like growth factor-I. *Clin Endocrinol (Oxf)* 1991;**35**:47–54.

15. Jeschke MG, Gauglitz GG, Kulp GA, *et al.* Long-term persistance of the pathophysiologic response to severe burn injury. *PLoS One* 2011;**6**(7):e21245.

16. Saltiel AR, Kahn CR. Insulin signalling and the regulation of glucose and lipid metabolism. *Nature* 2001;**414**:799–806.

17. Jeschke MG, Boehning DF, Finnerty CC, Herndon DN. Effect of insulin on the inflammatory and acute phase response after burn injury. *Crit Care Med* 2007;**35**(9 Suppl):S519–23.

18. Maier SF, Watkins LR. Cytokines for psychologists: implications of bi-directional immune-to-brain communication for understanding behaviour, mood, and cognition. *Psychol Rev* 1998;**105**:83–107.

19. Dantzer R. Cytokine, sickness behavior, and depression. *Immunol Allergy Clin North Am* 2009;**29**(2):247–64.

20. Annane D, Trabold F, Sharshar T, *et al.* Inappropriate sympathetic activation at onset of septic shock : a spectral analysis approach. *Am J Respir Crit Care Med* 1999;**160**:458–65.

21. Godin PJ, Buchman TG. Uncoupling of biological oscillators: a complementary hypothesis concerning the pathogenesis of multiple organ dysfunction syndrome. *Crit Care Med* 1996;**24**:1107–16.

22. Landry DW, Levin HR, Gallant EM, *et al.* Vasopressin deficiency contributes to the vasodilation of septic shock. *Circulation* 1997;**95**:1122.

23. Minokoshi Y, Kahn CR, Kahn BB. Tissue-specific ablation of the GLUT4 glucose transporter or the insulin receptor challenges assumptions about insulin action and glucose homeostasis. *J Bio Chem* 2003;**278**:33609.60.

24. Van den Berghe G. How does blood glucose control with insulin save lives in intensive care? *J Clin Invest* 2004;**114**:1187.

25. Sharshar T, Bastuji-Garin S, Polito A, *et al.* Hormonal status in protracted critical illness and in-hospital mortality. *Crit Care* 2011;**15**(1):R47.

26. Muthu K, Deng J, Romano F, *et al.* Thermal injury and sepsis modulates beta-adrenergic receptors and cAMP responses in monocyte-committed bone marrow cells. *J Neuroimmunol* 2005;**165**(1–2):129–38.

27. Berczi I, Quintanar-Stephano A, Kovacs K. Neuroimmune regulation in immunocompetence, acute illness, and healing. *Ann N Y Acad Sci* 2009;**1153**:220–39.

28. Annane D, Vignon P, Bollaert PE, *et al.* Norepinephrine plus dobutamine versus epinephrine alone for the management of septic shock. (Abstract). *Intensive Care Med* 2005;**31**:S18.

29. Havel C, Arrich J, Losert H, *et al.* Vasopressors for hypotensive shock. *Cochrane Database Syst Rev* 2011;**5**: CD003709.

30. Russell JA, Walley KR, Singer J, *et al.* Vasopressin versus norepinephrine infusion in patients with septic shock. *N Engl J Med* 2008;**358**(9):877–87.

31. Annane D. Physicians no longer should consider dopamine for septic shock!. *Crit Care Med* 2012;**40**:981.

32. Annane D, Sebille V, Charpentier C, *et al.* Effect of treatment with low doses of hydrocortisone and fludrocortisone on mortality in patients with septic shock. *JAMA* 2002;**288**:862.

33. Sprung CL, Annane D, Keh D, *et al.* Hydrocortisone therapy for patients with septic shock. *N Engl J Med* 2008;**358**:111.

34. Moreno R, Sprung CL, Annane D, *et al.* Time course of organ failure in patients with septic shock treated with hydrocortisone: results of the Corticus study. *Intensive Care Med* 2011;**37**(11):1765–72.

35. Annane D, Bellissant E, Bollaert PE, *et al.* Corticosteroids in the treatment of severe sepsis and septic shock in adults: a systematic review. *JAMA* 2009;**301**(22):2362–75.

36. Dellinger RP, Levy MM, Carlet JM, *et al.* Surviving Sepsis Campaign: international guidelines for management of severe sepsis and septic shock: 2008. *Crit Care Med* 2008;**36**(1):296–327. Erratum in: *Crit Care Med* 2008;36(4):1394–6.

37. Marik PE, Meduri GU, Rocco PR, Annane D. Glucocorticoid treatment in acute lung injury and acute respiratory distress syndrome. *Crit Care Clin* 2011;**27**(3):589–607.

38. Huang CJ, Lin HC. Association between adrenal insufficiency and ventilator weaning. *Am J Respir Crit Care Med* 2006;**173**(3):276–80.

39. Hoen S, Asehnoune K, Brailly-Tabard S, *et al.* Cortisol response to corticotropin stimulation in trauma patients: influence of hemorrhagic shock. *Anesthesiology* 2002;**97**(4):807–13.

40. Roquilly A, Mahe PJ, Seguin P, *et al.* Hydrocortisone therapy for patients with multiple trauma: the randomized controlled HYPOLYTE study. *JAMA* 2011;**305**(12):1201–9.

41. Van den Berghe G, Wouters P, Weekers F, *et al.* Intensive insulin therapy in the critically ill patients. *N Engl J Med* 2001;**345**:1359–67.

42. Van den Berghe G, Wilmer A, Hermans G, *et al.* Intensive insulin therapy in the medical ICU. *N Engl J Med* 2006;**354**:449–61.

43. Brukhorst FM, Engel C, Bloos F, *et al.* Intensive insulin therapy and pentastarch resuscitation in severe sepsis. *N Engl J Med* 2008;**358**:125–39.

44. The NICE-SUGAR Investigators. Intensive versus conventional glucose control in critically ill patients. *N Engl J Med* 2009;**360**:1283–97.

45. Bello G, Paliani G, Annetta MG, Pontecorvi A, Antonelli M. Treating nonthyroidal illness syndrome in the critically ill patient: still a matter of controversy. *Curr Drug Targets* 2009;**10**(8):778–87.

46. Elijah IE, Branski LK, Finnerty CC, Herndon DN. The GH/IGF-1 system in critical illness. *Best Pract Res Clin Endocrinol Metab* 2011;**25**(5):759–67.

Autonomic dysfunction in SIRS and sepsis

Jeremy D. Scheff, Panteleimon D. Mavroudis, Steve E. Calvano,
Stephen F. Lowry, and Ioannis P. Androulakis

SUMMARY

In recent years, much has been learned about the cross-talk between the inflammatory response and the autonomic nervous system. It is also becoming evident that autonomic function may be of importance in inflammatory diseases such as systemic inflammatory response syndrome (SIRS) and sepsis. A common component of the clinical phenotype observed in SIRS and sepsis is a dysregulation of the autonomic nervous system. One of the most promising methods of assessing autonomic dysfunction is by assessing heart rate variability (HRV). Changes in HRV have been correlated with disease state in a number of clinical studies. Another major advantage of this approach is that HRV metrics can be calculated based on ECG data, which is non-invasive and widely available. Through analysis of HRV signals, we can tease out markers of autonomic activity.

Furthermore, a growing body of literature suggests that autonomic dysfunction can be used as a clinical marker for disease severity and that modulation of the autonomic nervous system aimed at restoring normal autonomic function could be a beneficial therapeutic pathway, for instance through vagal stimulation or by drug treatment aimed at restoring robust autonomic function.

In this chapter, we review the current state of mechanistic knowledge concerning autonomic dysfunction in SIRS and sepsis, drawing from experimental models of both systemic inflammation and sepsis. We also highlight recent clinical data illustrating the importance of autonomic dysfunction in the development of and recovery from these diseases. As we continue to increase our understanding of the physiological mechanisms driving autonomic dysfunction in critical illness, new opportunities will likely be revealed in both potential therapeutic targets as well as markers of diagnostic and prognostic value.

Introduction

Systemic inflammatory response syndrome (SIRS) and sepsis impact millions of people in the USA [1]. Although the fatality rate of severe sepsis between 1993 and 2003 has decreased from 46% to 38%, possibly due to more effective treatment, the incidence of sepsis is increasing [2]. Furthermore, despite improvement in clinical outcomes, successful clinical trials of novel drugs are rare and sepsis often resists treatment. The difficulty in developing new and more effective medications for sepsis is due, in part, to our incomplete understanding of the mechanisms driving sepsis, and also of the mechanisms underlying systemic inflammation in general. For instance, it is now well established that autonomic function plays a critical role in the inflammatory response [3], and autonomic dysfunction contributes to the development of sepsis [4]; yet even though metrics of autonomic dysfunction already provide some level of clinical value [5], the biological mechanisms driving autonomic dysfunction are not well defined.

Although sepsis in the past was associated with just an overactivated immune response [6] it is now understood that it is a heterogeneous dynamic syndrome caused by imbalances in the neuroendocrine immune cross-talk [7], as is discussed in Chapter 17, this volume. This realization forces us to look at SIRS and sepsis from a systemic perspective. Additionally, therapies targeting solely the inhibition of pro-inflammatory mediators' surge using antibodies have failed [8,9], revealing the need to take into consideration the multi-compartment nature of this syndrome.

In this chapter, we discuss the current state of mechanistic knowledge concerning autonomic dysfunction in sepsis, drawing from experimental models of both systemic inflammation and sepsis, as well as clinical data illustrating the importance of autonomic

Brain Disorders in Critical Illness, ed. Robert D. Stevens, Tarek Sharshar, and E. Wesley Ely. Published by Cambridge University Press. © Cambridge University Press 2013.

dysfunction in the development of and recovery from sepsis. The growing physiological understanding of autonomic dysfunction will hopefully lead to novel therapeutic targets as well as enhanced clinical diagnosis, prognosis, and stratification.

Autonomic function in inflammation

The autonomic nervous system is commonly divided into two branches, sympathetic and parasympathetic. Although these branches often function antagonistically, under certain circumstances they exhibit complementary behavior [10]; for instance, co-activation of sympathetic and parasympathetic nerves at the sinoatrial region of the heart can produce an increased cardiac output relative to isolated stimulation of either nerve [11]. It is well established that the autonomic nervous system plays a critical role in the progression and resolution of the inflammatory response by communicating through afferent and efferent neural mechanisms with the immune system, which is described in more detail in Chapter 19, this volume. In systemic inflammation, activation of the autonomic nervous system leads to the release of immunomodulatory hormones. Furthermore, it has recently been shown that the activity of the parasympathetic nervous system can more directly modulate the inflammatory response in real time [3]. Much has been learned about neuroimmune cross-talk in inflammation from endotoxemia experiments, both in humans and animals. Endotoxemia is a model of systemic inflammation, a critical component of the early sepsis response. Endotoxemia studies consist of the treatment of subjects with small doses of endotoxin (lipopolysaccharides, LPS). Lipopolysaccharides bind to Toll-like receptor 4 (TLR4) which ultimately leads to the production of inflammatory mediators. This provides a controlled model of TLR4 agonist-induced systemic inflammation which has been used to study how inflammation activates the physiological system (hormonal release, neural activity) as well as how exogenous treatment can modulate inflammation (hormone treatment, vagal stimulation). However, even in this idealized and controlled experimental setting, far from the clinical realities of SIRS and sepsis, the precise relationship between inflammation and the autonomic nervous system is difficult to tease out. Some of this is caused by the convolution of multiple semi-redundant signaling pathways that govern the inflammatory response, but some is also caused by limitations in metrics to assess autonomic activity.

Table 20.1 Metrics of autonomic dysfunction are listed here, along with references of clinical studies showing their application in sepsis. Heart rate variability has been studied most in this context, due to its non-invasive nature and the fact it can be calculated non-invasively from ECG data that are often already recorded for critically ill patients. As discussed in the text, other metrics of autonomic function including microneurography (MSNA) may have future applications in this field, but have not yet been applied in the context of sepsis.

Tools for assessing autonomic function in sepsis	References
Heart rate variability (HRV)	[5, 14, 25–30]
Blood pressure variability (BPV)	[14]
Baroreflex	[15, 17]
Chemoreflex	[15–17]

Assessing autonomic function in inflammation and sepsis

Clinical measurement of autonomic activity is challenging and imprecise, yet there are a variety of techniques that can give some insight into autonomic function, as summarized in Table 20.1. Analysis of heart rate variability (HRV), generally defined as the quantification of some aspect of beat-to-beat variability in heart rate, is commonly used to develop metrics reflecting autonomic activity. As shown in Figure 20.1, the sinoatrial (SA) node, the pacemaker of the heart, is innervated by both sympathetic and parasympathetic branches of the autonomic nervous system. Thus, changes in autonomic outflow provoke changes in the pattern of heartbeats and analysis of HRV allows for the non-invasive assessment of metrics that indirectly reflect cardiac autonomic modulation. Spectral analysis of HRV reveals two distinct frequency bands: low frequency (LF, 0.04–0.15 Hz) and high frequency (HF, 0.15–0.4 Hz) [12]. The spectral power in both frequency bands gives some indication of autonomic activity. The HF band is driven by the respiratory cycle and also responds to vagal signaling. The LF band responds to changes in both sympathetic and vagal activity. Low frequency and HF are often interpreted as reflecting sympathetic and parasympathetic activity, respectively and their ratio is often used to assess autonomic balance. Despite the fact that these metrics are, at best, overlapping and indirect measures of autonomic activity [13], they have still proven to be useful tools in the prognosis and diagnosis of sepsis.

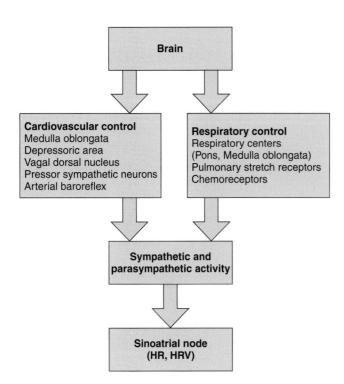

Figure 20.1 Hypothesized signal transduction network linking central autonomic dysfunction with alterations in heartbeat patterns, as suggested in reference [15].

Somewhat similarly to HRV, measuring blood pressure variability (BPV) is another non-invasive technique to assess autonomic function. Blood pressure variability is similar to HRV in that frequency domain peaks occur in similar LF and HF regions with similar mechanistic interpretations [14]. Non-invasive measurements of BPV have shown promise in quantifying autonomic dysfunction in sepsis [14].

Both BPV and HRV reflect, to some extent, baroreflex (blood pressure control) and chemoreflex (breathing pattern regulation) sensitivities as transduced by the autonomic nervous system to LF and HF oscillations, and other methods of estimating baroreflex and chemoreflex sensitivities can be independently used to assess autonomic dysfunction in critical illness [15]. Chemoreflex sensitivity is assessed by acutely altering arterial oxygen pressure and observing how large a change is induced in the heartbeat rhythm, which can be safely performed in critically ill patients [15] and has been shown to correlate with disease severity in patients with multiple organ dysfunction syndrome (MODS) [16]. Baroreflex sensitivity, which can be assessed by injecting phenylephrine and monitoring how much blood pressure increases, has been used as a marker of autonomic dysfunction in MODS patients [17].

Microneurography can assess the autonomic nervous system most directly, such as through muscle sympathetic nerve activity (MSNA), where an electrode tip penetrating peripheral muscle nerve fascicles allows for microneurographic recording [18]. However, microneurography is an invasive procedure; furthermore, it cannot be used to assess autonomic traffic at internal organs of interest, although noradrenaline radiotracer methods can assuage this limitation [19]. While these complications have limited clinical applications relevant to sepsis, a recent study on human endotoxemia did use MSNA assessment in concert with other metrics of autonomic activity to obtain a more comprehensive picture of autonomic dysfunction in endotoxemia [20]. Metrics of autonomic function based on pupillary responses may give insight into sympathetic and parasympathetic activity [21], but experimental support is sparse.

Autonomic dysfunction in sepsis

Sepsis is characterized by the presence of a systemic, whole-body inflammatory state combined with an infection [22]. When the systemic response progresses, patients commonly develop organ dysfunction (e.g., MODS) septic shock, often leading to death [23]. Generally, it is believed that sepsis is driven by inadequate control of inflammatory processes, leading to an imbalanced cytokine response and endothelial dysfunction [24]. Given the importance of appropriate autonomic function as described above, it is not surprising that autonomic dysfunction is an important component in the development and progression of sepsis.

Typically, at the onset of severe sepsis, dysfunction in autonomic output is observed as a component of sepsis-associated encephalopathy, which is more broadly discussed in Chapter 38, this volume. This produces changes in body temperature, hormonal release patterns, HRV, and baroreflex function [4]. Despite challenges in drawing precise mechanistic interpretations of autonomic function from HRV [19], changes in HRV reflecting central autonomic dysregulation have been shown to have prognostic and diagnostic value in sepsis. In general, human studies have convincingly shown that diminished HRV is correlated with disease severity in sepsis [14,25–29]. Particularly in the case of neonatal sepsis, there is a very clear change in HRV patterns prior to the traditional diagnosis of sepsis, which allows the possibility for HRV to inform earlier diagnosis and treatment of neonatal sepsis [30]. A novel monitoring device based on this concept recently went through a large randomized controlled clinical trial which identified decreased mortality when the HRV of infants was monitored [5].

Results from controlled experiments on autonomic-inflammatory links have a general correspondence to what has been observed in sepsis clinically. In both cases, it is clear that there is a relationship between autonomic activity and sepsis/inflammation. Yet also in both cases, precise conclusions are complicated by challenges in accurately measuring and interpreting changes in autonomic activity. Despite these limitations, it is becoming increasingly evident that the dysfunction of autonomic function in sepsis contributes to the overall state of the patient. This is important because it presents an avenue for improved diagnosis and treatment of sepsis. To fully reach this potential, we must explore both the underlying mechanisms driving autonomic dysfunction in addition to higher-level clinical measurables that give insight into autonomic activity.

Mechanisms

There are many steps in signal transduction from the CNS to the heart, and conceptually there are many individual components whose malfunction could, in part, produce the changes in autonomic activity

metrics observed in sepsis. Experimental results suggest several putative mechanisms that may drive autonomic dysfunction in sepsis and SIRS. There is evidence at multiple levels suggesting that autonomic function is diminished and that autonomic-cardiovascular coupling is lost, which may be characteristic of autonomic influences on other systems. Given the immunomodulatory role of autonomic activity in the inflammatory response [3], impaired function of either central (in the brain) or afferent/efferent nerves would produce dysregulated autonomic activity with significant effects on the inflammatory state [15]. In particular, the loss of the anti-inflammatory vagal influence on inflammation would generally result in a heightened local inflammatory response.

Dysregulated neural function can manifest itself in blood pressure (i.e., baroreflex) and respiratory patterns [4], which are proximate drivers of autonomic rhythms in HR. Decreased LF power, traditionally seen as indicative of low sympathetic activity, could be caused by impaired baroreflex sensitivity or by high sympathetic drive saturating the SA node and thus blunting rhythms [14]. Thus, while looking at just an individual component of HRV does not necessarily reveal its mechanistic background, diminished spectral power in the frequency domain of HR in general reflects dysregulation of physiological functions under autonomic control. Furthermore, high sympathetic drive in sepsis may not result in corresponding sympathetic modulation of all peripheral tissues if some component of the efferent signal transduction network is damaged. Impaired cardiovascular sympathetic modulation has been observed in human endotoxemia and sepsis [31].

In addition to efferent neural activity, afferent signaling could also play a role in autonomic dysfunction. Afferent nerves recognize cytokines and other inflammatory mediators, which provokes an autonomic response. In the presence of persistent systemic inflammation, it has been hypothesized that some type of sensory adaptation might inhibit activation of afferent autonomic pathways and thus provoke an insufficient efferent autonomic response [4]. The integrity of autonomic recognition of the inflammatory state may be further complicated by the broad range of molecules at concentrations different from their homeostatic levels during sepsis.

Even if afferent and efferent nerves function correctly, dysregulation of central processing of autonomic signals could still result in overall autonomic dysfunction. A postmortem study found cerebral expression of TNFα and iNOS were elevated in patients with septic shock, as has been observed in endotoxic shock, but only vascular expression of iNOS correlated with autonomic-centre neuronal apoptosis [32]. In this study, despite the significant observed postmortem autonomic neuronal and glial apoptosis, clinical autonomic failure was not detected before death, highlighting the difficulty in assessing autonomic dysfunction with current clinical techniques.

In the absence of neuronal dysregulation as described above, tolerance to efferent autonomic signaling could still produce dysregulated responses to autonomic modulation in sepsis. Catecholamines and glucocorticoids are anti-inflammatory hormones released in sepsis due, at least in part, to autonomic activity. In human endotoxemia experiments, it has been observed that the timing and duration of both epinephrine [33] and cortisol [34] play significant roles in determining the concentration of inflammatory mediators produced in response to LPS. There is evidence that this type of variable sensitivity to anti-inflammatory hormones plays a role in sepsis. In blood sampled from septic patients, stimulation of beta-adrenergic receptors reduced cAMP production [4,35], which is a critical step in signal transduction from circulating epinephrine to the production of anti-inflammatory mediators. Similarly, reduced cortisol responsiveness to corticotropin-releasing hormone (CRH) stimulation was observed in non-survivors of sepsis [4]; however, the interplay between cortisol, autonomic dysfunction, and sepsis is not straightforward, as there are conflicting reports as to whether high or low circulating cortisol levels are correlated with negative outcomes [36]. Desensitization of responses to anti-inflammatory hormones could contribute to further dysregulation of the inflammatory state. Autonomic regulation of the density of cardiac L-type calcium current in myocytes during sepsis may also contribute to changes in heartbeat patterns, as part of a larger remodeling of cardiac autonomic control in sepsis [37]. The importance of responses at the myocytes level in driving changes in HRV is supported by in vitro work showing that rat cardiomyocytes lose beating rate variability in response to endotoxin treatment [38].

These putative mechanisms describing autonomic dysfunction in sepsis are potentially complementary. It is likely that clinically observed changes in metrics of autonomic activity reflect a combination of the factors described here as well as other yet-to-be-discovered mechanisms.

Interpretation of HRV changes in sepsis

Much of the work on assessing autonomic dysfunction in sepsis and SIRS has focused on metrics of HRV. However, conceptually we are still missing a precise interpretation of how autonomic dysregulation is mirrored to decreased HRV and even more to alterations in frequency domain powers of autonomic oscillations [13]. In other words, even though we have some information linking changes in HRV to more fundamental biological processes, we are lacking an overall understanding that would integrate the multi-level experimental findings into one underlying sepsis mechanism. For instance, even in controlled human endotoxemia experiments, the extent of correlation between the inflammatory state (i.e., cytokine levels) and autonomic dysfunction as assessed by HRV is not clear. One study found a weak correlation between various HRV metrics and TNFα [39], yet another found no relationship between HRV and cytokine levels [40], and therapies like exogenous glucocorticoid treatment [41] can alter cytokine responses without a corresponding change in HRV in a dose-dependent manner [42]. These results are not necessarily surprising, as autonomic dysfunction is just one of many physiological changes occurring in inflammation. However, they do suggest that a simple relationship between HRV and inflammatory state is unlikely to be found, particularly in a heterogeneous clinical environment rather than a controlled experimental setting. But even lacking a precise mechanistic interpretation of HRV in inflammation and sepsis, the clinical studies cited earlier show its importance as a prognostic and diagnostic tool.

In an attempt to explain the pathogenesis of multiple organ dysfunction syndrome (MODS), as often occurs in sepsis, it has been hypothesized [43,44] that biological networks are collections of oscillatory systems (organs) that are coupled to one other, and that the maintenance of healthy homeostasis is based both on the integrity of each oscillator and on the coupling between them. This hypothesis predicts that, when interorgan communication is disrupted and organs become isolated, the loss of oscillatory coupling leads to more regular output. This is supported both by a variety of mathematical models [44]

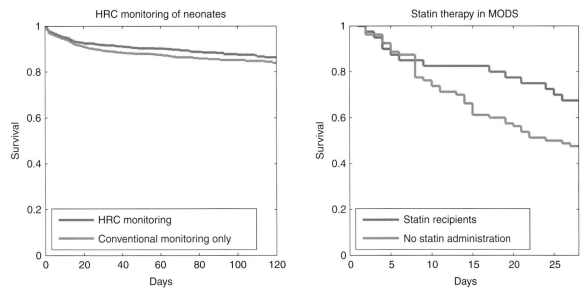

Figure 20.2 Survival curves for two interventions that may be related to autonomic dysfunction. On the left, survival of neonates at risk for sepsis was increased by the presence of a monitor which assesses heart rate characteristics (HRC) [5]. On the right, statin therapy improved outcomes from multiple organ dysfunction syndrome (MODS) [47]. This figure is presented in color in the color plate section.

as well as experimental results. For instance, in response to human endotoxemia, the beats of the heart become more regular while autonomic regulation of HR is diminished [20]. This type of uncoupling of autonomic regulation of the heart has been implicated in pediatric sepsis [45].

A change in autonomic modulation of one tissue does not necessarily imply a similar change has occurred in other tissues. Although much of the results presented here discuss changes in the function of the heart, this is also important in considering the transition to MODS, as centrally impaired neural signaling impacts many target organs. From this perspective, diminished HRV in sepsis and SIRS may not reflect only modulated autonomic activity but the loss of the ability to convey interorgan signals via the autonomic nervous system.

Future outlook

The non-invasive nature of ECG and the relationship between HRV and autonomic dysfunction motivate further applications of HRV towards unraveling the underlying mechanisms of sepsis. Despite limitations in our understanding of the physiological basis of HRV modulation in inflammation, it is clear that variability in HR provides clinically useful information, as exemplified by its recent successful application

towards neonatal sepsis [5]. The present inadequate understanding of sepsis reveals the need for further studies in order to fully comprehend the hierarchy of the intrinsic mechanisms underlying sepsis syndrome, and how these are related to the shift of a beneficial autonomic function into autonomic dysfunction.

Therapies targeted at the restoration of autonomic components of HRV could have beneficial effects in sepsis patients [46]; clinical data supporting this concept are shown in Figure 20.2. For instance, statin therapy has been associated with both the recovery of HRV and reduced mortality [47]. More directly, as detailed in Chapter 22, this volume, vagus nerve stimulation holds promise as a novel treatment of sepsis. Experiments in septic mice have shown that vagus nerve stimulation improves survival [48]. The more we know about the mechanisms of autonomic dysfunction and how they relate to sepsis, the more novel therapies can be designed. But even in the absence of autonomic-based intervention, monitoring the progression of autonomic dysfunction may provide novel metrics to assess the progression of and recovery from disease.

Acknowledgments

JDS, PDM, and IPA acknowledge support from NIH GM082974. JDS, SEC, and SFL are supported, in part, from NIH GM34695.

References

1. Angus DC, Linde-Zwirble WT, Lidicker J, *et al.* Epidemiology of severe sepsis in the United States: analysis of incidence, outcome, and associated costs of care. *Crit Care Med* 2001;**29**(7):1303–10.

2. Dombrovskiy VY, Martin AA, Sunderram J, *et al.* Rapid increase in hospitalization and mortality rates for severe sepsis in the United States: a trend analysis from 1993 to 2003. *Crit Care Med* 2007;**35**(5):1244–50.

3. Tracey KJ. The inflammatory reflex. *Nature* 2002;**420**(6917):853–9.

4. Munford RS, Tracey KJ. Is severe sepsis a neuroendocrine disease? *Mol Med* 2002;**8**(8):437–42.

5. Moorman JR, Carlo WA, Kattwinkel J, *et al.* Mortality reduction by heart rate characteristic monitoring in very low birth weight neonates: a randomized trial. *J Pediatr* 2011;**159**(6):900-6.e1.

6. Bone RC, Balk RA, Cerra FB, *et al.* Definitions for sepsis and organ failure and guidelines for the use of innovative therapies in sepsis. The ACCP/SCCM Consensus Conference Committee. American College of Chest Physicians/Society of Critical Care Medicine. *Chest* 1992;**101**(6):1644–55.

7. Rittirsch D, Flierl MA, Ward PA. Harmful molecular mechanisms in sepsis. *Nat Rev Immunol* 2008;**8**(10):776–87.

8. Fisher CJ Jr, Opal SM, Dhainaut JF, *et al.* Influence of an anti-tumor necrosis factor monoclonal antibody on cytokine levels in patients with sepsis. The CB0006 Sepsis Syndrome Study Group. *Crit Care Med* 1993;**21**(3):318–27.

9. Abraham E, Anzueto A, Gutierrez G, *et al.* Double-blind randomised controlled trial of monoclonal antibody to human tumour necrosis factor in treatment of septic shock. *Lancet* 1998;**351**(9107):929–33.

10. Paton JF, Boscan P, Pickering AE, *et al.* The yin and yang of cardiac autonomic control: vago-sympathetic interactions revisited. *Brain Res Brain Res Rev* 2005;**49**(3):555–65.

11. Koizumi K, Terui N, Kollai M, *et al.* Functional significance of coactivation of vagal and sympathetic cardiac nerves. *Proc Natl Acad Sci USA* 1982;**79**(6):2116–20.

12. Akselrod S, Gordon D, Ubel FA, *et al.* Power spectrum analysis of heart rate fluctuation: a quantitative probe of beat-to-beat cardiovascular control. *Science* 1981;**213**(4504):220–2.

13. Karemaker JM. Autonomic integration: the physiological basis of cardiovascular variability. *J Physiol* 1999;**517**(Pt 2):316.

14. Annane D, Trabold F, Sharshar T, *et al.* Inappropriate sympathetic activation at onset of septic shock: a spectral analysis approach. *Am J Respir Crit Care Med* 1999;**160**(2):458–65.

15. Schmidt HB, Werdan K, Muller-Werdan U. Autonomic dysfunction in the ICU patient. *Curr Opin Crit Care* 2001;**7**(5):314–22.

16. Schmidt H, Muller-Werdan U, Nuding S, *et al.* Impaired chemoreflex sensitivity in adult patients with multiple organ dysfunction syndrome – the potential role of disease severity. *Intensive Care Med* 2004;**30**(4):665–72.

17. Schmidt H, Muller-Werdan U, Hoffmann T, *et al.* Autonomic dysfunction predicts mortality in patients with multiple organ dysfunction syndrome of different age groups. *Crit Care Med* 2005;**33**(9):1994–2002.

18. Mano T, Iwase S, Toma S. Microneurography as a tool in clinical neurophysiology to investigate peripheral neural traffic in humans. *Clin Neurophysiol* 2006;**117**(11):2357–84.

19. Grassi G, Esler M. How to assess sympathetic activity in humans. *J Hypertens* 1999;**17**(6):719–34.

20. Sayk F, Vietheer A, Schaaf B, *et al.* Endotoxemia causes central downregulation of sympathetic vasomotor tone in healthy humans. *Am J Physiol Regul Integr Comp Physiol* 2008;**295**(3):R891–8.

21. Martyn CN, Ewing DJ. Pupil cycle time: a simple way of measuring an autonomic reflex. *J Neurol Neurosurg Psychiatry* 1986;**49**(7):771–4.

22. Hotchkiss RS, Opal S. Immunotherapy for sepsis – a new approach against an ancient foe. *N Engl J Med* 2010;**363**(1):87–9.

23. Akrout N, Sharshar T, Annane D. Mechanisms of brain signaling during sepsis. *Curr Neuropharmacol* 2009;**7**(4):296–301.

24. Bone RC, Grodzin CJ, Balk RA. Sepsis: a new hypothesis for pathogenesis of the disease process. *Chest* 1997;**112**(1):235–43.

25. Barnaby D, Ferrick K, Kaplan DT, *et al.* Heart rate variability in emergency department patients with sepsis. *Acad Emerg Med* 2002;**9**(7):661–70.

26. Garrard CS, Kontoyannis DA, Piepoli M. Spectral analysis of heart rate variability in the sepsis syndrome. *Clin Auton Res* 1993;**3**(1):5–13.

27. Tateishi Y, Oda S, Nakamura M, *et al.* Depressed heart rate variability is associated with high IL-6 blood level and decline in the blood pressure in septic patients. *Shock* 2007;**28**(5):549–53.

28. Piepoli M, Garrard CS, Kontoyannis DA, *et al.* Autonomic control of the heart and peripheral vessels in human septic shock. *Intensive Care Med* 1995;**21**(2):112–19.

29. Korach M, Sharshar T, Jarrin I, *et al.* Cardiac variability in critically ill adults: influence of sepsis. *Crit Care Med* 2001;**29**(7):1380–5.

30. Griffin MP, O'Shea TM, Bissonette EA, *et al.* Abnormal heart rate characteristics preceding neonatal sepsis and sepsis-like illness. *Pediatr Res* 2003;**53**(6):920–6.

31. Annane D, Sebille V, Charpentier C, *et al.* Effect of treatment with low doses of hydrocortisone and fludrocortisone on mortality in patients with septic shock. *JAMA* 2002;**288**(7):862–71.

32. Sharshar T, Gray F, Lorin de la Grandmaison G, *et al.* Apoptosis of neurons in cardiovascular autonomic centres triggered by inducible nitric oxide synthase after death from septic shock. *Lancet* 2003;**362**(9398):1799–805.

33. van der Poll T. Effects of catecholamines on the inflammatory response. *Sepsis* 2001;**4**(2):159–67.

34. Barber AE, Coyle SM, Marano MA, *et al.* Glucocorticoid therapy alters hormonal and cytokine responses to endotoxin in man. *J Immunol* 1993;**150**(5):1999–2006.

35. Bernardin G, Strosberg AD, Bernard A, *et al.* Beta-adrenergic receptor-dependent and -independent stimulation of adenylate cyclase is impaired during severe sepsis in humans. *Intensive Care Med* 1998;**24**(12):1315–22.

36. Annane D, Sebille V, Troche G, *et al.* A 3-level prognostic classification in septic shock based on cortisol levels and cortisol response to corticotropin. *JAMA* 2000;**283**(8):1038–45.

37. Abi-Gerges N, Tavernier B, Mebazaa A, *et al.* Sequential changes in autonomic regulation of cardiac myocytes after in vivo endotoxin injection in rat. *Am J Respir Crit Care Med* 1999;**160**(4):1196–204.

38. Schmidt H, Saworski J, Werdan K, *et al.* Decreased beating rate variability of spontaneously contracting cardiomyocytes after co-incubation with endotoxin. *J Endotoxin Res* 2007;**13**(6):339–42.

39. Jan BU, Coyle SM, Macor MA, *et al.* Relationship of basal heart rate variability to in vivo cytokine responses after endotoxin exposure. *Shock* 2010;**33**(4):363–8.

40. Kox M, Ramakers BP, Pompe JC, *et al.* Interplay between the acute inflammatory response and heart rate variability in healthy human volunteers. *Shock* 2011;**36**(2):115–20.

41. Alvarez SM, Katsamanis Karavidas M, Coyle SM, *et al.* Low-dose steroid alters in vivo endotoxin-induced systemic inflammation but does not influence autonomic dysfunction. *J Endotoxin Res* 2007;**13**(6):358–68.

42. Rassias AJ, Guyre PM, Yeager MP. Hydrocortisone at stress-associated concentrations helps maintain human heart rate variability during subsequent endotoxin challenge. *J Crit Care* 2011;**26**(6):636.e1-5.

43. Godin PJ, Buchman TG. Uncoupling of biological oscillators: a complementary hypothesis concerning the pathogenesis of multiple organ dysfunction syndrome. *Crit Care Med* 1996;**24**(7):1107–16.

44. Pincus SM. Greater signal regularity may indicate increased system isolation. *Math Biosci* 1994;**122**(2):161–81.

45. Ellenby MS, McNames J, Lai S, *et al.* Uncoupling and recoupling of autonomic regulation of the heart beat in pediatric septic shock. *Shock* 2001;**16**(4):274–7.

46. Werdan K, Schmidt H, Ebelt H, *et al.* Impaired regulation of cardiac function in sepsis, SIRS, and MODS. *Can J Physiol Pharmacol* 2009;**87**(4):266–74.

47. Schmidt H, Hennen R, Keller A, *et al.* Association of statin therapy and increased survival in patients with multiple organ dysfunction syndrome. *Intensive Care Med* 2006;**32**(8):1248–51.

48. Huston JM, Gallowitsch-Puerta M, Ochani M, *et al.* Transcutaneous vagus nerve stimulation reduces serum high mobility group box 1 levels and improves survival in murine sepsis. *Crit Care Med* 2007;**35**(12):2762–8.

Sepsis-induced neuronal dysfunction and death

Sadanand M. Gaikwad, Catherine N. Widmann, and Michael T. Heneka

SUMMARY

In the setting of systemic inflammation, the brain mounts a secondary inflammatory response which can lead to severe cell dysfunction and death. This complex response, collectively termed septic encephalopathy (SE), engages different central nervous system (CNS) cell types including microglia, astrocytes, and neurons. Neuronal dysfunction and death may occur during SE as a consequence of exposure to peripherally produced inflammatory molecules or alternatively in response to the local immunological reaction stimulated within the brain itself. Exposure of neuronal structures to inflammatory molecules such as cytokines, complement factors, chemokines, nitrosative or oxidative stress is associated with acute and persisting cognitive disturbances. The brain's reaction to systemic inflammation may depend on the nature or source of infection, but is likely to be shaped by the individual response of the immune system to the inflammatory challenge or by the resistance of the neuronal compartment to such a challenge. Rodent animal models of sepsis have been analyzed for brain dysfunction and neuronal death, however the precise mechanisms and the sequence of events leading to experimental SE remain largely unknown. Studies in animal models but also in human patients are essential to unravel the mechanisms and to develop therapeutic strategies, protecting the brain from either systemic inflammation or its secondary reaction to it. Given the negative influence of SE on the overall outcome or survival of septic patients, brain protection should be a central focus of research in critical care medicine.

Introduction

Despite tremendous advances in medical sciences research, the pathogenesis and long-term effects of sepsis remain poorly understood, posing a major challenge to physicians today. Sepsis is a severe clinical syndrome which is defined as a whole-body systemic inflammatory state, also known as a systemic inflammatory response syndrome (SIRS), and the co-occurrence of a suspected or confirmed infection [1]. In this condition the body's system-wide inflammatory response helps to eliminate pathogens, yet it also increases the permeability of the blood–brain barrier, thereby prolonging and increasing the inflammatory response within the CNS [2]. One consequence of this is septic encephalopathy (SE), also currently known as *sepsis-induced encephalopathy*, *septic encephalitis*, *sepsis-induced delirium*, or *sepsis-associated encephalopathy*. It is a rapid decline in cognitive function usually manifesting itself as delirium or coma. It is reported to occur in 8–70% of septic patients, depending on the criteria used for septic encephalopathy [3,4]. Sepsis and its complications are also the leading causes of mortality in ICUs accounting for 10–50% of deaths [5–7]. Septic encephalopathy has been assumed to be an acute, fairly dispersed and reversible phenomenon in survivors of sepsis. However, recent work indicates it may be linked to cognitive dysfunction and functional impairments persisting for months or years [8,9].

Septic encephalopathy is defined as altered brain functioning associated with the occurrence of pathogens and their toxins in the bloodstream. Many causes of SE have been postulated to date, however no consensus about its etiology is yet in sight. The pathogenesis most likely involves interlinked and dynamic processes: inadequate or disturbed cerebral perfusion, changed CNS or plasma levels of amino acids, systemic metabolic derangement, consequences of multi-organ failure (in more severe cases), complications of medical therapy, and the direct effects of endotoxin or cytokines on the brain. All of these mediators allow the neuronal immune system to respond to

Brain Disorders in Critical Illness, ed. Robert D. Stevens, Tarek Sharshar, and E. Wesley Ely. Published by Cambridge University Press. © Cambridge University Press 2013.

Table 21.1 Summary of mechanisms, clinical outcomes, and cognitive impairment following sepsis.

Sepsis is a leading cause of mortality in intensive care units (ICUs), accounting for 10–50% of deaths.

Recent work indicates that sepsis may be linked to cognitive dysfunction and functional impairments persisting for months and years.

Septic encephalopathy (SE) is a severely rapid global decline in cognitive functions usually manifesting itself as confusion and coma occurring in the majority of severe septic patients.

Pathogenesis of SE most likely involves several interlinked and dynamic processes: disturbed cerebral perfusion, changed central nervous system (CNS) or plasma levels of amino acids, bacterial invasion of the CNS, systemic metabolic derangement, multi-organ failure, complications of medical therapy, and direct effects of endotoxin or cytokines on the brain.

Sepsis raises production of leukocytes which adhere to blood vessels and eventually infiltrate brain.

Brain cytokines and chemokines drive alterations in blood–brain permeability, increasing the influx of inflammatory cells and toxic mediators into the brain and contributing further to brain injury.

Animal models show neurodegeneration in the hippocampal areas CA1, CA2, and prefrontal cortex. Nitric oxide production affects the extent of hippocampal atrophy.

Long-term clinical outcomes in human sepsis patients include higher risk of mortality, lowered quality of life, neurocognitive impairment, limitations in daily functioning, and are linked to greater brain pathology.

To date there is no CNS-specific therapy for patients with sepsis or septic shock and no investigations of neuroprotective substances in patients who have survived severe sepsis.

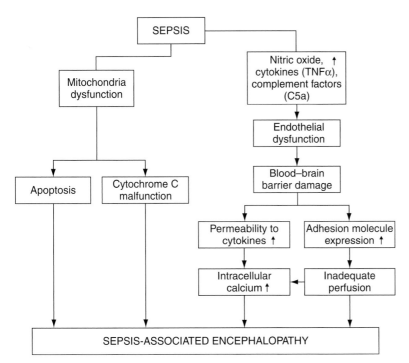

Figure 21.1 The factors implicated in sepsis-associated encephalopathy.

fast-changing circumstances during the course of the systemic inflammatory response. Among the factors implicated in SE are oxidative stress, microglial activation, systemic and local generation of inflammatory cytokines, alterations in cerebral microcirculation, neurotransmitter changes, and organ failure (Figure 21.1) [10,11].

These aspects will be briefly reviewed in the following sections which deal with systemic and cerebral blood flow, animal models of sepsis-induced neuronal death and brain dysfunction, molecular mechanisms involved, and clinical outcomes in human sepsis patients. For a summary of concepts in this chapter, see Table 21.1.

A number of questions still need to be answered regarding SE, e.g., when and how does encephalitis occur during sepsis? Which factors are responsible for triggering neuroprotection and how? How can clinical diagnosis be improved? Is it possible to alter the course and outcome of SE by strengthening anti-inflammatory pathways? Can we prevent potential long-term impairments?

Cerebral blood flow

Among the far-reaching and sustained systemic effects of sepsis is hyperdynamic circulation, which also produces changes in cerebral blood flow implicated in septic encephalopathy. Surprisingly, the effects of endotoxaemia on cerebral blood flow and oxygenation levels are not clear cut, as studies of human and animal models have so far yielded inconsistent results. While some authors have found a significant decrease in cerebral blood flow and cerebral oxygen consumption in septic patients independent of the mean arterial blood pressure, others have found no shift in these parameters in healthy middle-aged volunteers who underwent experimentally induced sepsis [12,13]. Cerebral blood flow can be increased by dobutamine infusions, yet this has not been shown to alter symptoms of septic encephalopathy [14].

Whereas a significant decrease in cerebral blood flow and cerebral oxygenation has been demonstrated in most sepsis animal models, it does not appear to drop low enough to threaten neuronal viability or to directly cause electroencephalogram (EEG) changes. This is reasonable, as cerebral blood flow must drop by more than 33% before anoxic depolarization takes place and must drop by more than 45% before EEG changes become detectable [15]. But even when cerebral blood flow is sufficient to ensure neuronal integrity, slight reductions may still contribute to septic encephalopathy when higher energy demands are made, as in the case of cognitive processing.

Alterations in the blood–brain barrier and brain dysfunction have been found during early stages of sepsis in a rodent model [16]. Unfortunately, there is no clear delineation of the time course of the brain inflammatory response during sepsis and it is not known to what extent this is similar to the systemic response. What is known is that sepsis causes proliferation of leukocytes, which adhere to blood vessels and eventually infiltrate brain. Brain cytokines and chemokines drive alterations in blood–brain barrier permeability that lead to increase influx of inflammatory cells and toxic mediators into the brain, contributing further to brain injury (Figure 21.2).

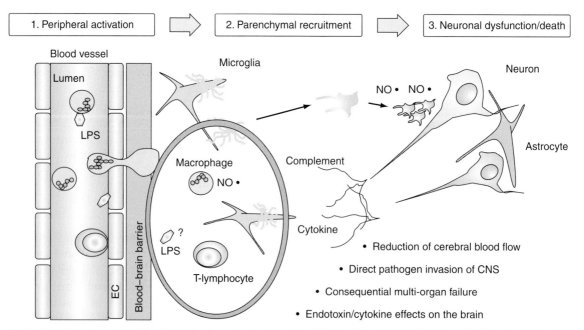

Figure 21.2 Alterations in the blood–brain barrier and brain dysfunction. LPS, lipopolysaccharide; NO, nitric oxide; EC, endothelial cells.

Several innate immune system components, such as complement factors and pro-inflammatory cytokines, may be responsible for altering the permeability of the blood–brain barrier directly via receptor-mediated endocytosis. Inflammatory mediators progress into deeper brain regions and may actively cross the blood–brain barrier via specific carriers [17]. Direct evidence has been found in cerebrovascular endothelial cells via electron microscopy and in electrical resistance [18]. Septic mice lacking the TNF receptor 1 were observed to have less cerebral edema in comparison to control mice [19]. Likewise, neutralizing antibodies with anaphylatoxin C5a has been shown to reduce damage to the blood–brain barrier in a rat model [20]. Hence, blood–brain barrier integrity can be vitiated by interleukin-6 (IL-6), interleukin-1β (IL-1β), and tumor necrosis factor alpha (TNFα), the molecular mechanisms of which will be discussed below.

Animal models of sepsis-induced neuronal death and brain dysfunction

The mechanisms of neuronal death and brain dysfunction have been investigated in animal models over the past two decades. In this section, evidence from animal models about production of cytokines, nitric oxide, slowing of brain activity, and brain metabolism will be summarized.

There are numerous inflammatory signaling cascades associated with the CNS innate immune response during the course of sepsis which lead to brain dysfunction. Expression of inflammation-associated genes such as iNOS, TGF-β, IL-1β, MCP1, and TNFα greatly increases upon microglia activation in the hippocampus and cortex, while the overall number of neuronal cells declines. The aggregation of pro-inflammatory cytokines may merely be a consequence of swelling of the brain [21]. Yet proliferation of IL-1β and TNFα cytokines affects both the function of neurons [22,23] and their survival [24]. Similarly, nitric oxide derived from iNOS can negatively modify or reduce neuronal activity [25], and neuronal viability has been shown to be extremely susceptible to iNOS-dependent nitric oxide (NO) production [26]. Hence, during SE, molecules activate NO and cytokine production intensifies, thereby damaging neuronal integrity and contributing to neurodegeneration.

Slowing electroencephalogram activity and decreased cerebral glucose metabolism confirms diminished neuronal functionality or neuronal cell death. Modeling changes in electroencephalogram activity

during sepsis is important since irregularity of brain activity has been demonstrated to be associated with the diagnosis of SE and the clinical severity [27]. EEG changes in the septic rat brain have not been found to be as prominent as those in human patients [27], yet there is a significant reduction of alpha activity and a concomitant slowing of the overall electroencephalogram [28]. In addition, positron emission tomography (PET) imaging in the preclinical setting or in vivo microPET analysis supports the LPS-induced changes shown in EEG studies. Cerebral glucose uptake decreases drastically after LPS challenge in all cortical areas in the rat brain, allowing inferences to be made about reduction in neuronal activity [29,30].

Among pathogenic mechanisms, circulating bacterial cell wall components initiate a systemic inflammatory response, including leukocyte recruitment, cytokine induction, complement activation, and nitric oxide secretion, consecutively leading to endothelial stimulation and disruption of the blood–brain barrier. Even though there are significant differences between models, these observations each support the theory that exposure of LPS can cause long-term microglia activation and a considerable increase of NOS2, primarily in areas immediately surrounding blood vessels [31]. Neuronal loss in hippocampal subregions and prefrontal cortex and behavioral deficits are long-term consequences found in animal LPS models [32,33]. Neuronal dysfunction or loss has not been linked to any behavioral phenotype (refer to Chapter 11, this volume).

Molecular and neuronal mechanisms

A fundamental aspect of sepsis is the rapid production of cytokines (interleukin-1 (IL-1α and IL-1β), IL-6, and TNFα), chemokines (CXCL1/KC, CXCL9/MIG, CCL2/MIP1, CCL3/MIP-1a), and nitric oxide (NO) derived from iNOS. The neurotoxic effects of these inflammatory mediators are well recognized [34,35]. Cell death within the CNS during sepsis has been described in both rodent models and humans [32,36]. Inflammatory and immune responses evoked in sepsis may cause not only acute brain dysfunction, which occurs in the majority of septic patients [3,4], but possibly also long-term deficits. Nevertheless, only a few sepsis investigations have addressed the underlying biological mechanisms.

Another important aspect of neuroinflammation in SIRS and sepsis is the induction of the inducible isoform of nitric oxide (NO)-producing enzymes (iNOS). Because iNOS is independent of Ca^{2+}, its activity is sustained and can last for days [37], resulting in NO-mediated cell death and tissue damage [38]. iNOS expression in response to sepsis has been detected in peripheral tissue [39], but also in neuronal and glial cells in different animal models of peripheral inflammation [40]. It has been shown that neurons are remarkably sensitive to NO and undergo cell death once exposed to sustained NO generation [26,41]. Slow but prolonged microglial activation has been observed in the innate immune system of wild-type mice, although this effect was not detected in an experiment using mice deficient for NOS2 [31]. A few reports discuss the possibility that the lack of NOS2 in NOS2-deficient mice may protect them from organ failure and septic shock, and decrease levels of cytokine and peripheral toxins [42].

Immune-activated, NOS2-derived nitric oxide accumulation exerts harmful effects on the brain via different mechanisms. Among these are protein nitrosylation, changes in long-term potentiation, and the inhibition of mitochondrial respiration, all of which cause pathological processing in the nerve cell and increases in apoptosis [43–45]. At the neuronal level, synapses are particularly vulnerable in neurodegenerative conditions in general, and this appears to be the case as well in sepsis. A negative impact of NOS2 on proteins responsible for synaptic regulation and subsequent effects on learning and memory have been observed [46]. Specifically, LPS induction has been shown to significantly decrease production of synaptophysin, CaMKII and PSD95 synaptic proteins, which may affect synaptic plasticity and in turn cause memory deficits [47]. Postsynaptic density protein (PSD95) plays a central functional role in the synapse by scaffolding specific large membrane complex receptors such as beta-adrenergic, NMDA, and neuroligin. Severely disturbed spatial memory performance has been found in PSD95 knockout mice [48].

Studies in human sepsis

Among the clinical outcomes briefly reviewed in this section are mortality rates, quality of life, cognitive functioning, activities of daily living, and brain pathologies. Mortality rates, short-term cognitive dysfunction, and quality of life have been well examined in sepsis, yet other long-term outcomes such as cognitive functioning and activities of daily living have so far received limited attention in human research. Generally, total 1-year mortality of sepsis patients after hospital discharge ranges from 25.1% to 71.9%, with older patients dying at significantly higher rates than younger ones [7]. Mortality rates associated with sepsis vary greatly according to severity of disease, country, age, gender, specific clinical setting, and site of organ dysfunction [5,49,50]. Importantly, the occurrence of SE is associated with higher mortality [51].

Among adult survivors of sepsis, quality of life is known to be severely impaired immediately after hospital release [52], and moderately to severely impaired after 6–7 months [53,54]. Less is known about life quality in the very long term, but it is presumed to be equivalent to that of trauma patients or those with chronic diseases such as obstructive pulmonary disease or congestive heart failure [52,55]. It is important to consider the effects of premorbid status, age, severity of disease, comorbidities, and treatment on life quality [56,57]. Psychiatric disease, especially anxiety, depression, and posttraumatic stress disorder, is also known to be elevated in critical illness survivors in general, and is likely the case also in survivors of sepsis.

As mentioned at the outset of this chapter, SE in the acute stage of sepsis has been well documented (see Chapter 11, this volume). Three separate studies using different populations and different methods have demonstrated significant neurocognitive deficits in sepsis survivors years after hospital release [9,58,59], with associated impairments in activities of daily living [9]. Whether acute stage SE or disease severity have a direct association with long-term cognitive or daily functioning is, however, still unconfirmed [8].

Brain pathology in human sepsis patients has suffered from a lack of systematic investigation. Case studies in the acute stage using MRI have reported various brain pathologies including white matter changes and micro abscesses [60,61]. An EEG in the acute stage can reveal sepsis-associated encephalopathy [62]. Postmortem studies of fatal sepsis cases have found diffuse cerebral damage including cerebral infarcts, brain purpura, small white matter hemorrhages, micro abscesses, and a proliferation of astrocytes and microglia in the cerebral cortex [36,63]. One recent study using MRI and EEG to study sepsis survivors revealed hippocampal atrophy with no other structural pathologies and higher resting state delta and theta power in the 6–24 months after ICU stay [59].

Thus, long-term clinical outcomes in human sepsis patients include higher risk of mortality, lowered quality of life, neurocognitive impairment, limitations in daily functioning, and are linked to greater brain pathology. It may be speculated that sepsis survivors are therefore more vulnerable to neurological insults.

Conclusion

This chapter highlights the impact of severe sepsis on brain function and reveals that sepsis can cause persistent learning and memory deficits in mice. It appears that sepsis-induced activation of astrocytes and microglia and subsequent production of NO initiates apoptosis and necrosis of neurons and glial cells. Strategies to modulate sustained microglial activation may represent a valuable therapeutic avenue in patients suffering from severe sepsis. To exclude compensatory responses due to NOS2 deficiency and to test a potential therapeutic benefit, future studies should include treatment protocols with NOS2 selective inhibitors. In particular, inflammatory-induced and nitric oxide-mediated alterations of synapses should be further investigated to unravel the underlying molecular mechanisms, since specific protection of synapses may prove to be beneficial. Studies are needed to evaluate the role of NO in the course of human SE and whether strategies based on selective NO inhibition can be neuroprotective.

References

1. Levy M, Fink M, Marshall J, *et al.* 2001 SCCM/ESICM/ACCP/ATS/SIS International Sepsis Definitions Conference. *Intensive Care Med* 2003;**29**:530–8.

2. Cunningham C. Microglia and neurodegeneration: the role of systemic inflammation. *Glia* 2013;**61**:71–90.

3. Sprung CL, Peduzzi PN, Shatney CH, *et al.* Impact of encephalopathy on mortality in the sepsis syndrome. *Critical Care Med* 1990;**18**:801–6.

4. Young GB, Bolton CF, Austin TW, *et al.* The encephalopathy associated with septic illness. *Clin Invest Med* 1990;**13**:297–304.

5. Vincent JL, Sakr Y, Sprung CL. Sepsis in European intensive care units: results of the SOAP study. *Crit Care Med* 2006;**34**:344–53.

6. Cheng B, Xie G, Yao S. Epidemiology of severe sepsis in critically ill surgical patients in ten university hospitals in China. *Crit Care Med* 2007;**35**:2538–46.

7. Winters BD, Eberlein M, Leung J. Long-term mortality and quality of life in sepsis: a systematic review. *Crit Care Med* 2010;**35**:1276–83.

8. Hopkins RO, Jackson JC. Long-term neurocognitive function after critical illness. *Chest* 2006;**130**:869–78.

9. Iwashyna TJ, Ely EW, Smith DM, Langa KM. Long-term cognitive impairment and functional disability among survivors of severe sepsis. *JAMA* 2010;**304**:1787–94.

10. Wilson JX, Young GB. Progress in clinical neurosciences: sepsis-ssociated encephalopathy: evolving concepts. *Can J Neurol Sci* 2003;**30**:98–105.

11. Teeling JL, Perry VH. Systemic infection and inflammation in acute CNS injury and chronic neurodegeneration: underlying mechanisms. *Neuroscience* 2009;**158**:1062–73.

12. Maekawa T, Fujii Y, Sadamitsu D, *et al.* Cerebral circulation and metabolism in patients with septic encephalopathy. *Am J Emerg Med* 1991;**9**:139–43.

13. Pollard V, Prough DS, Deyo DJ, *et al.* Cerebral blood flow during experimental endotoxemia in volunteers. *Crit Care Med* 1997;**25**:1700–6.

14. Wynn JL, Wong HR. Pathophysiology and treatment of septic shock in neonates. *Clin Perinatol* 2010;**37**:439–79.

15. Hossmann KA. Viability thresholds and the penumbra of focal ischemia. *Ann Neurol* 1994;**36**:557–65.

16. Nishioku T, Dohgu S, Takata F, *et al.* Detachment of brain pericytes from the basal lamina is involved in disruption of the blood–brain barrier caused by lipopolysaccharide-induced sepsis in mice. *Cell Mol Neurobiol* 2009;**29**:309–16.

17. Duchini A, Govindarajan S, Santucci M, Zampi G, Hofman FM. Effects of tumor necrosis factor-alpha and interleukin-6 on fluid-phase permeability and ammonia diffusion in CNS-derived endothelial cells. *J Investig Med* 1996;**44**:474–82.

18. Rettori CA. The mechanism of action of cytokines to control the release of hypothalamic and pituitary hormones in infection. *Ann NY Acad Sci* 2000;**917**:4–18.

19. Alexander JJ, Jacob A, Cunningham P, Hensley L, Quigg RJ. TNF is a key mediator of septic encephalopathy acting through its receptor, TNF receptor-1. *Neurochem Int* 2008;**52**:447–56.

20. Flierl MA, Stahel PF, Rittirsch D, *et al.* Inhibition of complement C5a prevents breakdown of the blood–brain barrier and pituitary dysfunction in experimental sepsis. *Crit Care* 2009;**13**:R12.

21. Semmler A, Hermann S, Mormann F, *et al.* Sepsis causes neuroinflammation and concomitant decrease of cerebral metabolism. *J Neuroinflammation* 2008;**5**:38.

22. Pickering M, Cumiskey D, O'Connor JJ. Actions of TNF-alpha on glutamatergic synaptic transmission in the central nervous system. *Exp Physiol* 2005;**90**:663–70.

23. Kelly A, Lynch A, Vereker E, *et al.* The anti-inflammatory cytokine, interleukin (IL)-10, blocks the inhibitory effect of IL-1 beta on long term potentiation – a role for JNK. *J Biol Chem* 2001;**276**:45564–72.

24. Venters HD, Dantzer R, Kelley KW. A new concept in neurodegeneration: TNF alpha is a silencer of survival signals. *Trends Neurosci* 2000;**23**:175–80.

25. Wang QW, Rowan MJ, Anwyl R. Beta-amyloid-mediated inhibition of NMDA receptor-dependent long-term potentiation induction involves activation of microglia and stimulation of inducible nitric oxide synthase and superoxide. *J Neurosci* 2004;**24**:6049–56.

26. Heneka MT, Loschmann PA, Gleichmann M, *et al.* Induction of nitric oxide synthase and nitric oxide-mediated apoptosis in neuronal PC12 cells after stimulation with tumor necrosis factor-alpha lipopolysaccharide. *J Neurochem* 1998;**71**:88–94.

27. Young GB, Bolton CF, Archibald YM, Austin TW, Wells GA. The electroencephalogram in sepsis-associated encephalopathy. *J Clin Neurophysiol* 1992;**9**:145–52.

28. Lancel M, Mathias S, Schiffelholz T, Behl C, Holsboer F. Soluble tumor necrosis factor receptor (p75) does not attenuate the sleep changes induced by lipopolysaccharide in the rat during the dark period. *Brain Res* 1997;**770**:184–91.

29. Kornblum HI, Araujo DM, Annala AJ, *et al.* In vivo imaging of neuronal activation and plasticity in the rat brain by high resolution positron emission tomography (microPET). *Nat Biotechnol* 2000;**18**:655–60.

30. O'Dwyer MJ, Mankan AK, Stordeur P, O'Connell B, Duggan E, White M. The occurrence of severe sepsis and septic shock are related to distinct patterns of cytokine gene expression. *Shock* 2006;**26**:544–50.

31. Weberpals M, Hermes M, Hermann S, *et al.* NOS2 gene deficiency protects from sepsis-induced long-term cognitive deficits. *J Neurosci* 2009;**29**:14177–84.

32. Semmler A, Okulla T, Sastre M, Dumitrescu-Ozimek L, Heneka MT. Systemic inflammation induces apoptosis with variable vulnerability of different brain regions. *J Chem Neuroanat* 2005;**30**:144–57.

33. Semmler A, Frisch C, Debeir T, *et al.* Long-term cognitive impairment, neuronal loss and reduced cortical cholinergic innervation after recovery from sepsis in a rodent model. *Exp Neurol* 2007;**204**:733–40.

34. Reimann-Philipp U, Ovase R, Weigel PH, Grammas P. Mechanisms of cell death in primary cortical neurons and PC12 cells. *J Neurosci Res* 2001;**64**:654–60.

35. Liu B, Gao HM, Wang JY, *et al.* Role of nitric oxide in inflammation-mediated neurodegeneration. *Ann NY Acad Sci* 2002;**962**:318–31.

36. Sharshar T, Annane D, de la Grandmaison GL, *et al.* The neuropathology of septic shock. *Brain Pathol* 2004;**14**:21–33.

37. Xie Q, Nathan C. The high-output nitric oxide pathway: role and regulation. *J Leuk Biol* 1994;**56**:576–82.

38. Kim PK, Zamora R, Petrosko P, Billiar TR. The regulatory role of nitric oxide in apoptosis. *Int Immunopharmacol* 2001;**1**:1421–41.

39. Thiemermann C. Nitric oxide and septic shock. *Gen Pharmacol* 1997;**29**:159–66.

40. Satta MA, Jacobs RA, Kaltsas GA, Grossman AB. Endotoxin induces interleukin-1beta and nitric oxide synthase MRNA in rat hypothalamus and pituitary. *Neuroendocrinology* 1998;**67**:109–16.

41. Leist M, Volbracht C, Kuhnle S, *et al.* Caspase-mediated apoptosis in neuronal excitotoxicity triggered by nitric oxide. *Mol Med* 1997;**3**:750–64.

42. Wei XQ, Charles IG, Smith A, *et al.* Altered immune-responses in mice lacking inducible nitric-oxide synthase. *Nature* 1995;**375**:408–11.

43. Moncada S, Bolanos JP. Nitric oxide, cell bioenergetics and neurodegeneration. *J Neurochem* 2006;**97**:1676–89.

44. Brown GC. Mechanisms of inflammatory neurodegeneration: iNOS and NADPH oxidase. *Biochem Soc Trans* 2007;**35**:1119–21.

45. Calabrese V, Mancuso C, Calvani M, *et al.* Nitric oxide in the central nervous system: neuroprotection versus neurotoxicity. *Nat Rev Neurosci* 2007;**8**:766–75.

46. Fukunaga K, Miyamoto E. A working model of CaM kinase II activity in hippocampal long-term potentiation and memory. *Neurosci Res* 2000;**38**:3–17.

47. Stagi M, Dittrich PS, Frank N, *et al.* Breakdown of axonal synaptic vesicle precursor transport by microglial nitric oxide. *J Neurosci* 2005;**25**:352–62.

48. Kim EJ, Sheng M. PDZ domain proteins of synapses. *Nat Rev Neurosci* 2004;**5**:771–81.

49. Weycker D, Akhras KS, Edelsberg J, Angus DC, Oster G. Long-term mortality and medical care charges in patients with severe sepsis. *Crit Care Med* 2003;**31**:2316–23.

50. Engel C, Brunkhorst FM, Bone H-G. Epidemiology of sepsis in Germany: results from a national prospective multicenter study. *Intensive Care Med* 2007;**33**:606–18.

51. Eidelman LA, Putterman D, Putterman C, Sprung CL. The spectrum of septic encephalopathy. Definitions, etiologies, and mortalities. *JAMA* 1996;**275**:470–3.

52. Heyland DK, Hopman W, Coo H, Tranmer J, McColl MA. Long-term health-related quality of life in survivors of sepsis. Short Form 36: a valid and reliable measure of health-related quality of life. *Crit Care Med* 2000;**28**:3599–605.

53. Granja C, Dias C, Costa-Pereira A, Sarmento A. Quality of life of survivors from severe sepsis and septic shock may be similar to that of others who survive critical illness. *Crit Care* 2004;**8**:R91–8.

54. Longo CJ, Heyland DK, Fisher HN. A long-term follow-up study investigating health-related quality of life and resource use in survivors of severe sepsis: comparison of recombinant human activated protein C with standard care. *Crit Care* 2007;**11**:R128.

55. Hofhuis JGM, Spronk PE, van Stel HF. The impact of severe sepsis on health-related quality of life: a long-term follow-up study. *Anesth Analg* 2008;**107**:1957–64.

56. Bronner MB, Knoester H, Sol JJ. An explorative study on quality of life and psychological and cognitive function in pediatric survivors of septic shock. *Pediatr Crit Care Med* 2009;**10**:636–42.

57. Clermont G, Angus DC, Linde-Zwirble WT. Does acute organ dysfunction predict patient-centered outcomes? *Chest* 2002;**121**:1963–71.

58. Lazosky A, Young GB, Zirul S, Phillips R. Quality of life after septic illness. *J Crit Care* 2010;**25**:406–12.

59. Semmler A, Widmann CN, Okulla T, *et al.* Persistent cognitive impairment, hippocampal atrophy and EEG changes in sepsis survivors. *J Neurol Neurosurg Psychiatry* 2013;**84**:62–9.

60. Höllinger P, Zürcher R, Schroth G, Mattle HP. Diffusion magnetic resonance imaging findings in cerebritis and brain abscesses in a patient with septic encephalopathy. *J Neurol* 2000;**247**:232–4.

61. Piazza O, Cotena S, De Robertis E, Caranci F, Tufano R. Sepsis associated encephalopathy studied by MRI and cerebral spinal fluid S100B measurement. *Neurochem Res* 2009;**34**:1289–92.

62. Iacobone E, Bailly-Salin J, Polito A, *et al.* Sepsis-associated encephalopathy and its differential diagnosis. *Crit Care Med* 2009;**37**:S331–6.

63. Jackson AC, Gilbert JJ, Young GB, Bolton CF. The encephalopathy of sepsis. *Can J Neurol Sci* 1985;**12**:303–7.

Chapter 22

Neuroimmunomodulation in sepsis

Marion Griton and Jan Pieter Konsman

SUMMARY

Evidence has accumulated over the years indicating that cytokines produced by immune cells can act on the nervous system and that neurotransmitters can modify immune cell functioning. In the present chapter, we will adopt a broad view on neuroimmunomodulation and provide an outline of how immune signals may be channeled to neural circuits that mediate sepsis symptoms and, in turn, modulate immune cell function.

Sepsis is a systemic inflammatory response to infection that can evolve towards severe sepsis and septic shock when hypotension occurs. The systemic inflammatory response in general and fever in particular is often effective against bacterial infection, but involves an increase in energy expenditure and damage to host cells. Activation of primary afferent fibers by prostaglandins, reactive oxygen species, and pro-inflammatory cytokines can mediate rapid immune-to-brain signaling during inflammation. Production of prostaglandins at the blood–brain barrier and the occurrence of pro-inflammatory cytokines in circumventricular organs that lack a blood–brain barrier may be important in immune-to-brain signaling in cases of sepsis with high circulating concentrations of pro-inflammatory cytokines. Neuroanatomical findings indicate that the preoptic area and the paraventricular hypothalamus are part of a neuronal network mediating sympathetic nervous system activation underlying fever and possibly tachycardia during sepsis.

Sympathetic noradrenergic nerve fibers also innervate bone marrow, spleen, thymus, and gut- and bronchus-associated lymphoid tissue where immune cells express beta- and, to a lesser extent, alpha-adrenergic receptors. Noradrenaline release by these fibers may modulate local immune response. In contrast, adrenaline production by the adrenal medulla has the potential to alter immunity systemically. While peritoneal alpha-2-adrenoreceptors may sustain local pro-inflammatory responses, beta-adrenergic receptor activation clearly has anti-inflammatory effects in sepsis models. Stimulation of the vagus nerve also dampens systemic inflammation in sepsis models. This anti-inflammatory effect involves acetylcholine released by vagal terminals in the celiac ganglion as well as acetylcholine produced by splenic T-lymphocytes in response to noradrenaline release by adjacent splenic nerve fibers. Interestingly, the organization of central nervous structures providing input to the spleen and bone marrow through the sympathetic nervous system shows considerable overlap with the pattern of central nervous innervation of brown adipose and cardiac tissue. However, even though the central nervous circuits innervating the spleen and bone marrow and sympathetic- and parasympathetic-mediated modulation of systemic inflammatory responses are known in quite some detail, the brain structures involved in neuroimmunomodulation during sepsis remain to be elucidated.

Introduction

Fever is a core symptom for the diagnosis of sepsis and defined as a regulated rise in body temperature. Since body temperature is controlled by the brain, the occurrence of fever indicates that nervous system functioning is altered during systemic inflammation. Increased heart rate is another symptom of sepsis and a relationship exists between the vagal parameters of heart rate variability and circulating concentrations of pro-inflammatory cytokines in sepsis [1]. These

Brain Disorders in Critical Illness, ed. Robert D. Stevens, Tarek Sharshar, and E. Wesley Ely. Published by Cambridge University Press. © Cambridge University Press 2013.

findings can be interpreted to suggest that the autonomic nervous system influences immune responses during bacterial infection.

Evidence has accumulated over the years indicating that cytokines and other molecules produced by immune cells can act on the nervous system and that neurotransmitters and neuropeptides can modify immune cell functioning. In the present chapter, we will adopt a broad view on neuroimmunomodulation and provide an outline of how immune signals may be channeled to neural circuits that mediate sepsis symptoms and modulate immune cell function.

Inflammation and sepsis

In the clinic a systemic inflammatory response is identified when two of the following are present: temperature over 38 °C or under 36 °C, heart rate over 90 beats per minute, respiratory rate over 20 breaths per minute, and white blood cell count over 12,000/mm^3 or under 4,000/mm^3. Sepsis is a systemic inflammatory response to infection that can evolve towards severe sepsis and septic shock when hypotension occurs. The literature covered in the present chapter will mostly concern rodent models of sepsis and deal with data obtained after peripheral administration of bacterial lipopolysaccharide (LPS) or cecal ligation and puncture.

Tissue macrophages and mast cells express Toll-like receptors (TLR) recognizing bacterial molecular patterns such as LPS and produce pro-inflammatory cytokines that initiate local inflammation by stimulating adhesion molecule expression on endothelial cells and creating chemoattractant gradients for circulating neutrophils. Although mast cells can release proteases with bactericidal activity, neutrophils are true immune effector cells that trap, engulf, and kill pathogens through the production of reactive oxygen species and hypochlorite [2]. Monocytes also emigrate from the bloodstream into infected tissue where they differentiate into macrophages and contribute to the production of reactive oxygen species, but also to subsequent tissue repair by engulfing dead cells and debris [2].

In addition to their localization in the skin, lungs, and intestine where the risk of exposure to environmental microbes is high, macrophages populate the blood-filtering liver and spleen. The spleen is a site of early exposure to circulating bacteria due to specific anatomical characteristics of the marginal zone and the presence of macrophages that, in addition to TLR, express lectins and scavenger receptors recognizing and

clearing encapsulated bacteria. In addition, monocytes and neutrophils are recruited from bone marrow in response to circulating TLR ligands or systemic infection and continuously patrol blood for bacteria [2].

The systemic inflammatory response in general, and fever in particular, is often effective against bacterial infection [3], but involves an increase in energy expenditure and damage to host cells due to production of reactive oxygen and nitrogen species as well as proteases. Inflammatory responses are limited by local production of anti-inflammatory cytokines, such as interleukin-10, but also by pathways involving the nervous system. In the present chapter we will discuss nervous pathways that mediate sepsis symptoms and immunomodulation. Inhibition of innate immune responses by activation of the hypothalamic–pituitary–adrenal axis and endocrine effector mechanisms involving corticoid hormones are discussed in Chapter 20, this volume.

Immune-to-nervous system afferent signaling

The blood–brain and blood–nerve barriers exclude passive entrance of immune cell-derived peptides and proteins into the nervous system except in brain circumventricular organs and at peripheral nerve terminals. In what follows, neural pathways involving activation of peripheral sensory nerves by immune mediators will be distinguished from humoral pathways implicating the bloodstream even though mixed forms of immune-to-nervous system afferent signaling may exist. Additional information on this topic can be found in Chapter 17, this volume.

Neural immune-to-nervous system signaling

Many molecules produced by immune cells in response to detection of bacterial fragments, including complement factors, prostaglandins, leukotrienes, and cytokines, can sensitize or even activate primary afferent nerve fibers. Indeed, intravenous LPS rapidly gives rise to fever through complement factor C5a-stimulated prostaglandin E_2 production in liver macrophages, which, in turn, activates vagal afferents [4]. Alternatively, reactive oxygen species and hypochlorite, which are produced by activated neutrophils, can activate the so-called Transient Receptor Potential Ankyrin 1 channel present on sensory nerve endings [5]. These hydroxyl radicals also play an important role in stimulation of vagal sensory fibers by intravenous bacterial LPS administration [6]. Finally, the pro-inflammatory cytokine interleukin-1ß (IL-1ß) can also directly activate primary afferent nerve fibers in vivo [7,8]. When IL-1ß activates spinal nociceptive primary afferents, it can give rise to pain, while its action on vagal primary afferent fibers mediates behavioral changes [9]. Thus activation of primary afferent fibers by prostaglandins, reactive oxygen species, and pro-inflammatory cytokines can mediate rapid immune-to-brain signaling during inflammation.

Humoral immune-to-nervous system signaling

Brain circumventricular organs are highly vascularized structures that differ from the rest of the brain in that they lack a blood–brain barrier, but contain true macrophages that internalize molecules after their extravasation from the bloodstream [10]. Since these organs express TLR4 and CD14 [11], local macrophages may both neutralize extravasating bacteria and signal the occurrence of systemic infection. Indeed, brain circumventricular organ macrophages express IL-1ß after systemic LPS administration [12]. Moreover, IL-1 action in the brain mediates, at least in part, sustained behavioral changes and neuronal activation in limbic brain structures after peripheral LPS injection [13].

Although the blood–brain barrier prevents pro-inflammatory cytokines from passively entering the brain, they may act on brain endothelial cells and induce the production of prostaglandins and nitric oxide that are capable of diffusing across the blood–brain barrier and activating neurons in the brain parenchyma [14]. Critical testing of this hypothesis by selective knockdown of the signaling IL-1 receptor in endothelial cells abolishes cyclooxygenase-2 expression in brain vascular cells, induction of the cellular activation marker c-Fos in the paraventricular and preoptic hypothalamus, and fever after intravenous administration of IL-1ß [15]. Prostaglandin production at the blood–brain barrier may therefore be important in immune-to-brain signaling in cases of sepsis with high circulating concentrations of pro-inflammatory cytokines.

Nervous-to-immune system efferent signaling

In this section the immunomodulatory effects of mediators released by peripheral nerves and the central nervous innervation of the autonomic nervous system will be discussed. The peripheral nervous system regulates inflammation through the release of neurotransmitters and neuropeptides from autonomic and unmyelinated sensory nerves. Tachykinin neuropeptides released by sensory nerves promote vasodilation, plasma extravasation, and the production of chemotactic and pro-inflammatory cytokines, but also play an important part in organ injury in experimental sepsis models [16,17].

Sympathetic adrenergic immunomodulation during sepsis?

Sympathetic noradrenergic nerve fibers innervate bone marrow, spleen (Figure 22.1), thymus, and gut- and bronchus-associated lymphoid tissue where immune cells express beta- and, to a lesser extent, alpha-adrenergic receptors [18,19]. While noradrenaline release by these fibers may modulate immune response in these organs, adrenaline production by the adrenal medulla has the potential to alter immunity systemically. However, and in spite of the fact that plasma concentrations of catecholamines are increased during clinical and experimental sepsis [20–22], their effects on innate immune responses have not been studied in much detail in vivo.

Alpha-adrenergic receptor-mediated immunomodulation

Naïve immune cells such as peritoneal macrophages from specific pathogen-free rodents have been proposed to express alpha-adrenoreceptors [18]. In these cells, alpha-adrenergic agonists, including noradrenaline, exacerbate LPS-induced pro-inflammatory cytokine production [23]. The gut can be a major source of circulating noradrenaline in sepsis models [22] and alpha-2 adrenergic receptors mediate intestinal and systemic pro-inflammatory cytokine production [24]. It is important to note that immune cells can also produce catecholamines [25]. Stimulation of peritoneal alpha-2-adrenoreceptors by gut-derived or locally produced noradrenaline may thus sustain local pro-inflammatory responses.

Beta-adrenergic receptor-mediated immunomodulation

Electrical stimulation of sympathetic nerve fibers innervating bone marrow induces release of mature neutrophils and egress of hematopoietic stem cells

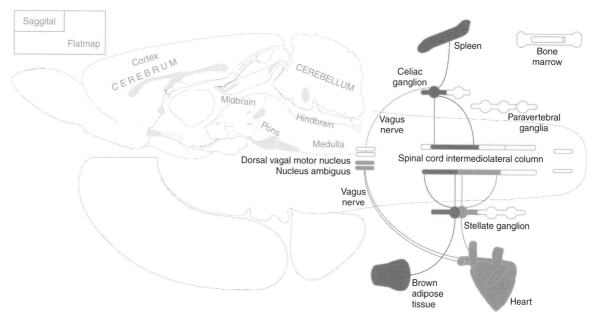

Figure 22.1 Schematic representation of sympathetic and parasympathetic innervation of brown adipose tissue, heart, spleen, and bone marrow in relation to the spinal cord and caudal medulla of the central nervous system. After injection of an attenuated form of the neurotropic pseudorabies herpes virus into the thermogenic brown adipose tissue or heart of rodents, infection occurs in the stellate sympathetic ganglia and in thoracic preganglionic sympathetic neurons of the spinal intermediolateral cell column. Injection of attenuated neurotropic pseudorabies herpes virus into spleen or femoral bone marrow results in infection of neurons in the celiac or prevertebral sympathetic ganglia and in preganglionic sympathetic neurons of the thoracic and lumbar intermediolateral cell column. The presence of viral particles in the vagal preganglionic neurons in the medullar nucleus ambiguus and dorsal motor nucleus of the vagus occurs only after injection of pseudorabies virus into the heart. The flatmap drawing of the central nervous system and the sagittal view on the brain are reproduced with permission from Swanson's *Brain Maps: Structure of the Rat Brain* [53].

[26], but its physiological relevance remains to be established. Administration of low doses of adrenaline in healthy humans and animals is well known to induce leukocytosis, that is a white blood cell count above the normal range, due to increases in T-effector and cytotoxic natural killer cells as well as pro-inflammatory monocytes [27,28]. However, adrenaline infusion exacerbates the experimental sepsis-induced decrease in circulating monocytes through action on beta-adrenergic receptors [29]. In addition, adrenaline attenuates tumor necrosis factor alpha (TNFα) production after LPS administration in rodents through action on beta-adrenergic receptors [30]. In human volunteers, adrenaline infusion also reduces plasma concentrations of pro-inflammatory cytokines and increases that of the anti-inflammatory cytokine interleukin-10 in response to LPS [31,32]. Overall, these findings indicate an anti-inflammatory role for catecholamine action on beta-adrenergic receptors in sepsis models.

Cardiac, renal, lung, and gastrointestinal dysfunction during severe sepsis may be related to sympathetic overstimulation [33]. However, the non-selective beta-blocker propranolol increases experimental sepsis-induced mortality [34]. In a similar vein, administration of a beta-2-adrenoreceptor antagonist increases renal infection-induced mortality and TNFα production and decreases creatinine as well as bacterial LPS clearance [35]. In contrast, selective beta-1-adrenoreceptor antagonists improve survival, attenuate cardiac dysfunction, decrease gut and pulmonary injury, and reduce TNFα production as well as bacterial translocation in experimental sepsis models [36–38]. Although the beta-1-adrenoreceptor is found in cardiac, pulmonary, and renal tissue, its expression in immune cells has not yet been established. The mechanisms through which beta-1-adrenoreceptor antagonists improve attenuate pro-inflammatory cytokine production during experimental sepsis remain therefore unknown.

Vagal cholinergic immunomodulation during sepsis?

Bone marrow, spleen, and thymus are devoid of parasympathetic nerve fibers [19] (Figure 22.1).

However, electrical stimulation of the vagus nerve can attenuate pro-inflammatory cytokine production in experimental sepsis through nicotinic cholinergic alpha-7 receptors [39]. The finding that a selective alpha-7 agonist attenuates LPS-induced cytokine production in blood from sepsis patients [39] suggests that acetylcholine released by vagal terminals can directly act on adjacent immune cells. However, vagal terminals also surround cells in the celiac, superior mesenteric and suprarenal ganglia where cholinergic alpha-7 receptors play a role in neurotransmission (Figure 22.1). Interestingly, both splenectomy and splenic neurectomy abolish the inhibitory effect of vagus nerve stimulation and cholinergic agonists on pro-inflammatory cytokine production in sepsis models [39]. Moreover, vagus nerve stimulation increases splenic noradrenaline via the cholinergic alpha-7 receptor and the splenic nerve. Finally, splenic nerve stimulation mimics vagal and cholinergic induction of noradrenaline release as well as their anti-inflammatory effects, even in alpha-7-deficient mice [39]. These findings support the idea that parasympathetic–sympathetic cross-talk mediates the anti-inflammatory effects of vagus nerve stimulation (Figure 22.1).

Even though electrical stimulation of the vagus nerve increases spleen acetylcholine concentrations, nerve fibers in the spleen do not contain acetylcholine-synthesizing enzymes [39]. Instead, spleen T-lymphocytes release acetylcholine in response to noradrenaline and mediate the suppression of bacterial LPS-induced circulating TNFα by vagus nerve stimulation [39]. Altogether, the literature indicates that the anti-inflammatory effect of vagal stimulation involves acetylcholine released by vagal terminals in the celiac ganglion as well as acetylcholine produced by splenic T-lymphocytes in response to noradrenaline release by adjacent splenic nerve fibers.

Central nervous circuits relevant to sepsis and immunomodulation

Considering the sepsis symptoms fever, tachycardia, changes in white blood cell counts, and hypotension as well as the anti-inflammatory pathways involving the autonomic nervous system, it is of interest to identify the nervous circuits that regulate autonomic activity in thermogenic brown fat, heart, adrenal, bone marrow, and spleen. Injection of an attenuated neurotropic herpes virus in a peripheral organ can reveal a

neuronal network relevant to its function. Indeed, such a virus will first infect neurons of nervous ganglia, then invade preganglionic neurons innervating the first order neurons, and finally neurons in the brain that send projections to the preganglionic neurons. After injection of an attenuated form of the neurotropic pseudorabies herpes virus into the thermogenic brown adipose tissue or heart of rodents, infection occurs in thoracic sympathetic ganglia, preganglionic sympathetic neurons of the spinal cord (Figure 22.1), ventrolateral, ventromedial and caudal dorsomedian medulla, raphe nucleus, and locus coeruleus. In the forebrain, the paraventricular, dorsomedial and lateral hypothalamus, ventral bed nucleus of the stria terminalis, central amygdala, and preoptic area contain viral particles, indicating that they are part of the neuronal networks innervating brown adipose tissue and the heart [40–42] (Figure 22.2).

Injection of a non-infectious retrograde neuronal tracer into the thoracic spinal sympathetic intermediolateral cell column followed by peripheral bacterial LPS injection results in neurons containing both the cellular activation marker c-Fos and the retrograde tracer in the paraventricular hypothalamus and the rostral ventrolateral medulla [43]. In turn, injection of a similar tracer into the paraventricular hypothalamus and subsequent peripheral administration of bacterial LPS leads to c-Fos-tracer double-labeled neurons in the preoptic area, bed nucleus of the stria terminalis, and medullar nucleus of the solitary tract [44]. Finally, lesion and inactivation studies suggest that the preoptic area and paraventricular hypothalamus are involved in bacterial LPS-induced fever [45–47]. Overall these findings indicate that the preoptic area and the paraventricular hypothalamus are part of a neuronal network mediating sympathetic activation underlying fever during sepsis. Central nervous circuits involving preoptic nuclei probably also play a role in sepsis-associated tachycardia and hypotension. Indeed, inactivation of the anterior preoptic hypothalamic area prevents early hypotension after intravenous administration of bacterial LPS in rats and attenuates secondary hypotension [48].

The organization of central nervous structures providing input to the spleen and bone marrow through the sympathetic nervous system shows considerable overlap with the pattern of central nervous innervation of brown adipose and cardiac tissue [49,50] (Figure 22.3). Fore- and hindbrain structures may thus influence immune cell activation and

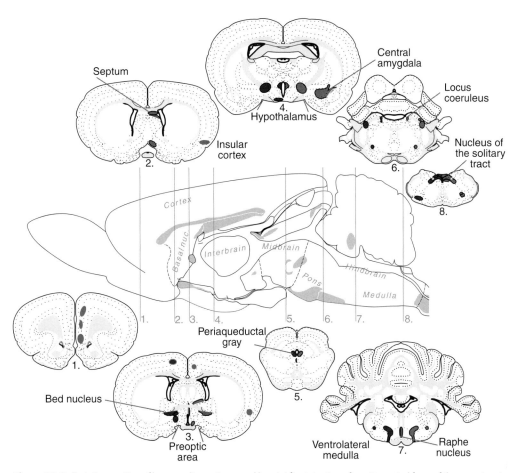

Figure 22.2 Brain innervation of brown adipose tissue and heart. After injection of an attenuated form of the neurotropic pseudorabies herpes virus into the thermogenic brown adipose tissue or heart of rodents, infection occurs in neurons of the ventrolateral and ventromedial medulla, the nucleus of the solitary tract, the caudal raphe, and locus coeruleus. In the pons the periaqueductal gray is consistently labeled after pseudorabies injection into the brown adipose tissue or heart. In the forebrain, the paraventricular, dorsomedial and lateral hypothalamus, central amygdala, the ventral bed nucleus of the stria terminalis, and different parts of the medial preoptic area contain viral particles indicating that they are part of the neuronal networks innervating brown adipose tissue and the heart [40–42]. The presence of viral particles in the vagal preganglionic neurons in the medullar nucleus ambiguus and dorsal motor nucleus of the vagus occurs only after injection of pseudorabies virus into the heart, which is in accordance with the lack of parasympathetic innervation of brown adipose tissue. Drawings of coronal brain sections and the sagittal view on the brain are reproduced with permission from Swanson's *Brain Maps: Structure of the Rat Brain* [53].

traffic. Adrenaline has anti-inflammatory effects (see above) and injection of attenuated pseudorabies virus into the adrenal results in labeling of preganglionic sympathetic neurons of the thoracic spinal cord, but also in the ventromedial and rostral ventrolateral medulla, the caudal raphe nuclei, and the periaqueductal gray as well as in the paraventricular and lateral hypothalamus. Interestingly, injection of different forms of attenuated pseudorabies in the adrenal and the stellate ganglion that contains the cell bodies of the sympathetic neurons to the heart and brown adipose tissue results in double-labeled neurons in the rostroventrolateral medulla, caudal raphe nuclei, periaqueductal gray and in the paraventricular hypothalamus [51]. It may, therefore, well be that medullar and hypothalamic "command" neurons control sympathetic outflow to immune organs relevant to changes in circulating leukocytes and subsequent anti-inflammatory effects during sepsis. These different "command" neurons may, in turn, be under the influence of neurons in the lateral hypothalamus, preoptic area, bed nucleus of the stria terminalis, amygdala, lateral septum, and infralimbic and insular cortices that are labeled after pseudorabies virus injections into the adrenal, stellate, or celiac ganglion [52].

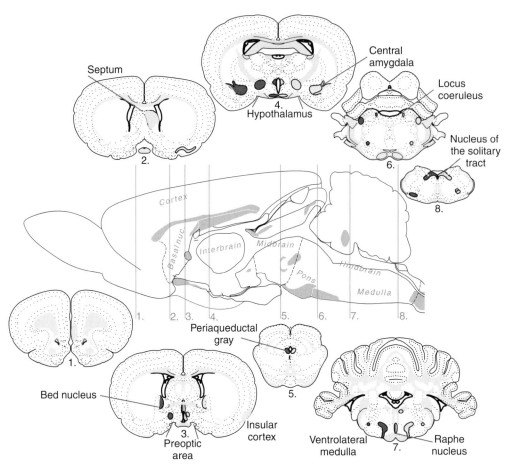

Figure 22.3 Brain innervation of spleen and bone marrow.Injection of attenuated neurotropic pseudorabies herpes virus into spleen or femoral bone marrow results in infection of neurons in the nucleus of the solitary tract, ventrolateral medulla and rostral ventromedial medulla; the raphe nuclei and locus coeruleus consistently contain viral particles as does the pontine periaqueductal gray. In the forebrain viral particles are found in the paraventricular, lateral and dorsomedial hypothalamus, medial preoptic area, bed nucleus of the stria terminalis and central amygdala and to a lesser extent in the lateral preoptic area and the arcuate hypothalamus [49, 50]. Drawings of coronal brain sections and the sagittal view of the brain are reproduced with permission from Swanson's *Brain Maps: Structure of the Rat Brain* [53].

Neuroimmune circuits in sepsis

After the discussion of the immune-to-nervous system afferent and the nervous-to-immune system efferent signaling pathways, a tentative outline of the neuroimmune circuits mediating sepsis symptoms and modulating systemic inflammation will now be presented.

Neuroimmune circuits mediating sepsis symptoms

The role of subdiaphragmatic sensory fibers in the rapid detection of circulating bacterial fragments is illustrated by the finding that vagotomy or perivagal lidocaine application attenuates early fever and hypotension after intravenous administration of bacterial LPS [4,48]. The nucleus of the solitary tract, in which vagal sensory fibers terminate, sends noradrenergic projections to the preoptic area, an important structure in the regulation of brown adipose tissue and cardiovascular output. Intrapreoptic infusion of alpha-adrenergic receptor antagonists attenuates the first two peaks of fever and hypotension after intravenous LPS administration [4,48]. These studies indicate that a vagal-brainstem-noradrenaline-preoptic area circuit mediates early LPS-induced hypotension and fever.

Preoptic noradrenaline-induced increased body temperature depends in part on the prostaglandin-synthesizing enzyme cyclooxygenase-2 [4]. Moreover, intrapreoptic infusion of an alpha-2 adrenergic receptor antagonist reduces the second fever peak and lowers prostaglandin E_2 concentrations after intravenous LPS-administration in a cyclooxygenase-2-dependent way [4]. As mentioned above, preventing circulating IL-1ß action on endothelial cells attenuates cyclooxygenase-2 induction in the brain and fever [15]. Vagal and humoral immune-to-nervous system signaling pathways may thus converge in the preoptic area to activate nervous circuits that give rise to increased heat production in the brown adipose tissue during sepsis.

Anti-inflammatory neuroimmune circuits in sepsis

Based on the central nervous system innervation of immune organs and pharmacological intervention studies, a tentative framework of neuroimmunomodulation in sepsis will now be outlined. Intracerebroventricular administration of the anti-inflammatory drug CNI-1493 inhibits peripheral LPS-induced TNFα production at > 10,000-fold lower concentrations then when given peripherally and in a vagus-dependent manner [39]. Interestingly, CNI-1493 interacts with the muscarinic type 1 receptor and intracerebroventricular, but not peripheral, administration of an agonist of these receptors also inhibits peripheral LPS-induced rises in circulating TNFα [39]. These findings suggest that brain acetylcholine can act on muscarinic receptors to activate the vagus nerve, which, in turn, exerts a peripheral anti-inflammatory effect through nicotinic receptors [39].

Since lateral hypothalamic muscarinic receptors can modulate vagal regulation of visceral functions [39], it is conceivable that they also play a role in adjusting the vagal anti-inflammatory pathway. The lateral preoptic area and lateral hypothalamus contain acetylcholinergic neurons and are part of the central nervous circuits innervating the spleen [49]. Acetylcholinergic neurons in the lateral preoptic area and lateral hypothalamus may therefore play a role in inhibiting splenic pro-inflammatory cytokine production during sepsis via the vagus and splenic nerves.

Although the discussion on the potential central nervous circuits modulating peripheral nervous system-mediated anti-inflammatory mechanisms during sepsis has been limited to classical neuronal circuits, brain cytokine and prostaglandin production may also play a role in neuroimmunomodulation. As indicated above, peripheral administration of bacterial LPS results in IL-1ß production in brain circumventricular organs and in prostaglandin synthesis at the blood–brain barrier. Although it is unknown

if endogenous brain IL-1ß and prostaglandins play a role in neuroimmunomodulation during sepsis, intracerebroventricular administration of IL-1ß or prostaglandin E_2 reduces bacterial LPS-induced production of IL-1ß by spleen macrophages in part through the sympathetic splenic nerve [19].

Conclusions and outstanding questions

It is now well established that immune-to-nervous system signaling during sepsis plays an important role in activation of the preoptic area that, in turn, gives rise to fever through activation of the sympathetic nerves in brown adipose tissue. In addition, the preoptic area also mediates early hypotension in sepsis, which was often thought to result from peripheral inflammation-associated loss of function. Although the central nervous circuits innervating the spleen and bone marrow and sympathetic- and parasympathetic-mediated modulation of systemic inflammatory responses are known in quite some detail, the brain structures involved in neuroimmunomodulation during sepsis remain to be elucidated. In addition, the kinetics of pure sympathetic- versus mixed vagal-sympathetic-mediated anti-inflammatory responses needs to be established during sepsis. Finally, the possibility that noradrenaline action on peritoneal alpha-2-adrenoreceptors sustains local pro-inflammatory responses while adrenaline action on beta-adrenoreceptors exerts systemic anti-inflammatory effects requires further study.

References

1. Jan BU, Coyle SM, Macor MA, *et al.* Relationship of basal heart rate variability to in vivo cytokine responses after endotoxin exposure. *Shock* 2010;**33**(4):363–8.

2. Galli SJ, Borregaard N, Wynn TA. Phenotypic and functional plasticity of cells of innate immunity: macrophages, mast cells and neutrophils. *Nat Immunol* **12**(11):1035–44.

3. Launey Y, Nesseler N, Malledant Y, *et al.* Clinical review: fever in septic ICU patients – friend or foe? *Crit Care* 2011;**15**(3):222.

4. Blatteis CM. The onset of fever: new insights into its mechanism. *Prog Brain Res* 2007;**162**:3–14.

5. Bessac BF, Jordt SE. Breathtaking TRP channels: TRPA1 and TRPV1 in airway chemosensation and reflex control. *Physiology (Bethesda)* 2008;**23**:360–70.

6. Lai CJ, Ruan T, Kou YR. The involvement of hydroxyl radical and cyclooxygenase metabolites in the activation of lung vagal sensory receptors by circulatory endotoxin in rats. *J Appl Physiol* 2005;**98**(2):620–8.

7. Niijima A. The afferent discharges from sensors for interleukin 1 beta in the hepatoportal system in the anesthetized rat. *J Auton Nerv Syst* 1996;**61**(3):287–91.

8. Binshtok AM, Wang H, Zimmermann K, *et al.* Nociceptors are interleukin-1beta sensors. *J Neurosci* 2008;**28**(52):14062–73.

9. Konsman JP, Luheshi GN, Bluthe RM, *et al.* The vagus nerve mediates behavioural depression, but not fever, in response to peripheral immune signals; a functional anatomical analysis. *Eur J Neurosci* 2000;**12**(12):4434–46.

10. Willis CL, Garwood CJ, Ray DE. A size selective vascular barrier in the rat area postrema formed by perivascular macrophages and the extracellular matrix. *Neuroscience* 2007;**150**(2):498–509.

11. Laflamme N, Rivest S. Toll-like receptor 4: the missing link of the cerebral innate immune response triggered by circulating gram-negative bacterial cell wall components. *FASEB J* 2001;**15**(1):155–63.

12. Konsman JP, Kelley K, Dantzer R. Temporal and spatial relationships between lipopolysaccharide-induced expression of Fos, interleukin-1beta and inducible nitric oxide synthase in rat brain. *Neuroscience* 1999;**89**(2):535–48.

13. Konsman JP, Veeneman J, Combe C, *et al.* Central nervous action of interleukin-1 mediates activation of limbic structures and behavioural depression in response to peripheral administration of bacterial lipopolysaccharide. *Eur J Neurosci* 2008;**28**(12):2499–510.

14. Konsman JP, Vigues S, Mackerlova L, *et al.* Rat brain vascular distribution of interleukin-1 type-1 receptor immunoreactivity: relationship to patterns of inducible cyclooxygenase expression by peripheral inflammatory stimuli. *J Comp Neurol* 2004;**472**(1):113–29.

15. Ching S, Zhang H, Belevych N, *et al.* Endothelial-specific knockdown of interleukin-1 (IL-1) type 1 receptor differentially alters CNS responses to IL-1 depending on its route of administration. *J Neurosci* 2007;**27**(39):10476–86.

16. Ng SW, Zhang H, Hegde A, *et al.* Role of preprotachykinin-A gene products on multiple organ injury in LPS-induced endotoxemia. *J Leukoc Biol* 2008;**83**(2):288–95.

17. Hegde A, Tamizhselvi R, Manikandan J, *et al.* Substance P in polymicrobial sepsis: molecular fingerprint of lung injury in preprotachykinin-A-/- mice. *Mol Med* 2010;**16**(5–6):188–98.

18. Elenkov IJ, Wilder RL, Chrousos GP, *et al.* The sympathetic nerve – an integrative interface between two supersystems: the brain and the immune system. *Pharmacol Rev* 2000;**52**(4):595–638.

19. Nance DM, Sanders VM. Autonomic innervation and regulation of the immune system (1987–2007). *Brain Behav Immun* 2007;**21**(6):736–45.

20. Maddens M, Sowers J. Catecholamines in critical care. *Crit Care Clin* 1987;**3**(4):871–82.

21. Hahn PY, Wang P, Tait SM, *et al.* Sustained elevation in circulating catecholamine levels during polymicrobial sepsis. *Shock* 1995;**4**(4):269–73.

22. Yang S, Koo DJ, Zhou M, *et al.* Gut-derived norepinephrine plays a critical role in producing hepatocellular dysfunction during early sepsis. *Am J Physiol Gastrointest Liver Physiol* 2000;**279**(6): G1274–81.

23. Spengler RN, Allen RM, Remick DG, *et al.* Stimulation of alpha-adrenergic receptor augments the production of macrophage-derived tumor necrosis factor. *J Immunol* 1990;**145**(5):1430–4.

24. Zhang F, Wu R, Qiang X, *et al.* Antagonism of alpha2A-adrenoceptor: a novel approach to inhibit inflammatory responses in sepsis. *J Mol Med (Berl)* 2010;**88**(3):289–96.

25. Flierl MA, Rittirsch D, Huber-Lang M, *et al.* Catecholamines-crafty weapons in the inflammatory arsenal of immune/inflammatory cells or opening pandora's box? *Mol Med* 2008;**14**(3–4):195–204.

26. DePace DM, Webber RH. Electrostimulation and morphologic study of the nerves to the bone marrow of the albino rat. *Acta Anat (Basel)* 1975;**93**(1):1–18.

27. Benschop RJ, Rodriguez-Feuerhahn M, Schedlowski M. Catecholamine-induced leukocytosis: early observations, current research, and future directions. *Brain Behav Immun* 1996;**10**(2):77–91.

28. Dimitrov S, Lange T, Born J. Selective mobilization of cytotoxic leukocytes by epinephrine. *J Immunol* 2010;**184**(1):503–11.

29. Oberbeck R, Schmitz D, Wilsenack K, *et al.* Adrenergic modulation of survival and cellular immune functions during polymicrobial sepsis. *Neuroimmunomodulation* 2004;**11**(4):214–23.

30. Monastra G, Secchi EF. Beta-adrenergic receptors mediate in vivo the adrenaline inhibition of lipopolysaccharide-induced tumor necrosis factor release. *Immunol Lett* 1993;**38**(2):127–30.

31. van der Poll T, Coyle SM, Barbosa K, *et al.* Epinephrine inhibits tumor necrosis factor-alpha and potentiates interleukin 10 production during human endotoxemia. *J Clin Invest* 1996;**97**(3):713–19.

32. Jan BU, Coyle SM, Oikawa LO, *et al.* Influence of acute epinephrine infusion on endotoxin-induced

parameters of heart rate variability: a randomized controlled trial. *Ann Surg* 2009;**249**(5):750–6.

33. Dunser MW, Hasibeder WR. Sympathetic overstimulation during critical illness: adverse effects of adrenergic stress. *J Intensive Care Med* 2009;**24**(5):293–316.

34. Schmitz D, Wilsenack K, Lendemanns S, *et al.* Beta-adrenergic blockade during systemic inflammation: impact on cellular immune functions and survival in a murine model of sepsis. *Resuscitation* 2007;**72**(2):286–94.

35. Nakamura A, Niimi R, Yanagawa Y. Renal beta2-adrenoceptor blockade worsens the outcome of an induced *Escherichia coli* renal infection. *J Nephrol* 2010;**23**(3):341–9.

36. Suzuki T, Morisaki H, Serita R, *et al.* Infusion of the beta-adrenergic blocker esmolol attenuates myocardial dysfunction in septic rats. *Crit Care Med* 2005;**33**(10):2294–301.

37. Hagiwara S, Iwasaka H, Maeda H, *et al.* Landiolol, an ultrashort-acting beta1-adrenoceptor antagonist, has protective effects in an LPS-induced systemic inflammation model. *Shock.* 2009;**31**(5):515–20.

38. Mori K, Morisaki H, Yajima S, *et al.* Beta-1 blocker improves survival of septic rats through preservation of gut barrier function. *Intensive Care Med* 2011;**37**(11):1849–56.

39. Huston JM, Tracey KJ. The pulse of inflammation: heart rate variability, the cholinergic anti-inflammatory pathway and implications for therapy. *J Intern Med* 2011;**269**(1):45–53.

40. Standish A, Enquist LW, Escardo JA, *et al.* Central neuronal circuit innervating the rat heart defined by transneuronal transport of pseudorabies virus. *J Neurosci* 1995;**15**(3 Pt 1):1998–2012.

41. Ter Horst GJ, Hautvast RW, De Jongste MJ, *et al.* Neuroanatomy of cardiac activity-regulating circuitry: a transneuronal retrograde viral labelling study in the rat. *Eur J Neurosci* 1996;**8**(10):2029–41.

42. Cano G, Passerin AM, Schiltz JC, *et al.* Anatomical substrates for the central control of sympathetic outflow to interscapular adipose tissue during cold exposure. *J Comp Neurol* 2003;**460**(3):303–26.

43. Zhang YH, Lu J, Elmquist JK, *et al.* Lipopolysaccharide activates specific populations of hypothalamic and brainstem neurons that project to the spinal cord. *J Neurosci* 2000;**20**(17):6578–86.

44. Elmquist JK, Saper CB. Activation of neurons projecting to the paraventricular hypothalamic nucleus by intravenous lipopolysaccharide. *J Comp Neurol* 1996;**374**(3):315–31.

45. Horn T, Wilkinson MF, Landgraf R, *et al.* Reduced febrile responses to pyrogens after lesions of the hypothalamic paraventricular nucleus. *Am J Physiol* 1994;**267**(1 Pt 2):R323–8.

46. Caldwell FT, Graves DB, Wallace BH. Studies on the mechanism of fever after intravenous administration of endotoxin. *J Trauma* 1998;**44**(2):304–12.

47. Lu J, Zhang YH, Chou TC, *et al.* Contrasting effects of ibotenate lesions of the paraventricular nucleus and subparaventricular zone on sleep-wake cycle and temperature regulation. *J Neurosci* 2001;**21**(13):4864–74.

48. Yilmaz MS, Millington WR, Feleder C. The preoptic anterior hypothalamic area mediates initiation of the hypotensive response induced by LPS in male rats. *Shock* 2008;**29**(2):232–7.

49. Cano G, Sved AF, Rinaman L, *et al.* Characterization of the central nervous system innervation of the rat spleen using viral transneuronal tracing. *J Comp Neurol* 2001;**439**(1):1–18.

50. Denes A, Boldogkoi Z, Uhereczky G, *et al.* Central autonomic control of the bone marrow: multisynaptic tract tracing by recombinant pseudorabies virus. *Neuroscience* 2005;**134**(3):947–63.

51. Jansen AS, Wessendorf MW, Loewy AD. Transneuronal labeling of CNS neuropeptide and monoamine neurons after pseudorabies virus injections into the stellate ganglion. *Brain Res* 1995;**683**(1):1–24.

52. Westerhaus MJ, Loewy AD. Central representation of the sympathetic nervous system in the cerebral cortex. *Brain Res* 2001;**903**(1–2):117–27.

53. Swanson LW. *Brain Maps: Structure of the Rat Brain.* 2nd edn. Amsterdam: Elsevier; 1998.

Chapter

23

Clinical neurological assessment of the critically ill patient

Raoul Sutter, Tarek Sharshar, and Robert D. Stevens

SUMMARY

Neurological assessment of critically ill patients requires physical examination, although sensitivity and specificity of findings may be limited by co-existing cognitive impairment, sedative or paralytic medication, endotracheal intubation, mechanical ventilation, neuromuscular weakness, and injuries or surgery involving extracranial tissues. Neurological signs and syndromes are fundamental indicators of severity of illness and prognosis. Neurological syndromes commonly seen in intensive care unit (ICU) patients include disturbances in consciousness, delirium, seizures, generalized weakness, and focal neurological deficits. Neurological examination in responsive patients should include an assessment of mental status, attention, cranial nerves, motor, and sensory findings. If there is persisting diagnostic uncertainty, additional testing should be performed. Computed tomography of the head should be performed if there is a new onset of seizures, focal neurological deficits, and if there is an unexplained alteration of mental status or loss of consciousness. Brain magnetic resonance imaging has greater sensitivity for hyperacute ischemic stroke, microhemorrhagic lesions, anoxic-ischemic damage, and alterations of the white matter and the brainstem. Electroencephalography is needed if seizures or status epilepticus are suspected as a cause or consequence of acute brain dysfunction. Electromyography, nerve conduction velocities, and, in selected patients, cerebrospinal fluid (CSF) examination should be obtained when neuromuscular weakness is severe or cannot be assessed clinically.

Barriers to neurological assessment in the ICU

Physical examination is the cornerstone in the neurological assessment of critically ill patients,

however, the validity and reliability of this examination is constrained by concurrent cognitive impairment and the effects of sedative or paralytic medication. Endotracheal intubation and mechanical ventilation pose significant obstacles to the assessment of cognitive (and in particular language) disturbances and to the interpretation of pathological breathing patterns. Neuromuscular weakness acquired in the ICU, and injuries or surgery may significantly limit the response to stimulation and the yield of neurological assessment [1]. Notwithstanding these constraints, neurological signs remain valuable indicators of severity of illness and prognosis [2–4].

Neurological syndromes in the ICU

Neurological syndromes commonly encountered in critically ill patients include: disturbances in the level of arousal and in cognition, seizures, generalized weakness, and focal neurological alterations.

Coma

Coma is a life-threatening emergency that requires prompt recognition and intervention [5]. It is caused by damage or impairment of neuronal arousal systems linking the rostral brainstem, diencephalon, basal forebrain, and cerebral cortex [6–8]. Coma is a transitional state, evolving either towards recovery of consciousness, or towards death or a chronic disorder of consciousness such as the vegetative state or the minimally conscious state. The onset of coma can be acute as in the setting of a large cerebral infarction, an extensive hemorrhage, or generalized seizures. A more gradual onset of coma may be encountered in toxic or metabolic derangements or in partial seizures with secondary generalization.

Brain Disorders in Critical Illness, ed. Robert D. Stevens, Tarek Sharshar, and E. Wesley Ely. Published by Cambridge University Press. © Cambridge University Press 2013.

Coma is the most severe manifestation in a spectrum of progressively worsening impairments in arousal that includes somnolence, lethargy, obtundation, and stupor. The comatose patient is unresponsive with eyes closed and a complete loss of postural stability and sleep–wake cycles. There is no arousal upon noxious stimuli but reflexive grimacing and flexion or withdrawal movements of the extremities may be preserved. Decorticate or decerebrate posturing responses may occur due to loss of cortical inhibition of brainstem and spinal motor tracts.

Delirium and agitation

Delirium is synonymous with acute confusional state and acute encephalopathy. It is characterized by a relatively sudden onset of impaired attention, associated with altered level of consciousness, disorganized thinking, and a fluctuating course [9]. Associated signs may include perceptual disturbances, altered sleep–wake cycle, increased or decreased psychomotor activity, and memory impairment. Delirium occurs in up to 80% of critically ill patients and has been linked independently to poor outcome [10,11]. Delirium is associated with a global impairment of brain function such as in toxic-metabolic states or systemic infections although focal lesions of the basal ganglia and right fronto-parietal structures may also increase the risk of delirium.

Psychomotor activity in delirious patients may be increased (hyperactive), decreased (hypoactive), or mixed [12,13]. Most critically ill patients are hypoactive, and thus their delirium appears as "quiet" and may be undetected in the absence of bedside screening tests [14,15]. On the other hand, the hyperactive patient will appear agitated and is virtually never missed.

Agitation is an acute psychomotor behavioral disturbance that consists in heightened arousal and increased motor and vocal activity. Agitation is present in a subset of patients with delirium (hyperactive delirium) but it may also occur independently as a manifestation of, or as a response to, physical and/or psychological stressors in the ICU environment including anxiety, pain, noise, and loss of control.

Seizures and status epilepticus

Seizures have been recognized as a major neurological complication of critical illness [16–18], often occurring in patients without a history of epilepsy.

In addition to focal or generalized convulsive seizures, non-convulsive ictal activity is identified in a significant proportion of critically ill patients, underscoring the need for electroencephalographic (EEG) verification. Large-scale EEG studies demonstrate non-convulsive seizure activity in 8–18% of evaluated patients with impaired consciousness [16,19] and suggest that over 80% of all status epilepticus is non-convulsive [18].

Signs of nonconvulsive seizures include depressed mental status, contralesional eye deviation, lip smacking, twitching movements of eyelids or extremities. The examiner should look for physiological manifestation such as increases in heart rate, blood pressure, and hypoxemia. Routine EEG recordings of 20–60 minutes may overlook intermittent paroxysmal ictal phenomena and underestimate the burden of nonconvulsive seizures and status epilepticus. In a single-center study, continuous video-EEG monitoring of ICU patients identified nonconvulsive status epilepticus in over 50% of performed EEGs [20].

Weakness in the ICU

Weakness in the ICU can be caused by pathologic processes involving the central or peripheral nervous system or the intrinsic musculature (Table 23.1) [1,21]. Arguably, the most dramatic and life-threatening etiology of acute weakness is brainstem infarction due to basilar artery thrombosis. This presents with hemi- or quadraparesis with or without hypesthesia that is often associated with dysarthria, facial weakness, vertigo, nausea, drop attacks, and altered consciousness. Ventral pontine lesions sparing arousal systems may result in a "locked-in" syndrome in which patients are conscious but paralyzed, typically only able to communicate via vertical eye movements [22]. Lesions of the spinal cord may result from traumatic, ischemic, inflammatory, infectious, and neoplastic processes. Spinal cord injury above C4 engenders significant diaphragmatic weakness often requiring prolonged mechanical ventilation [23,24]. Intensive care unit acquired weakness (ICUAW) is present in close to 50% of severely ill patients in the ICU [1] and is independently predictive for short-term mortality [25,26]. The diagnosis of ICUAW should be considered in patients with generalized weakness that is not attributable to a condition acquired independently of the underlying critical illness [21]. Factors associated with ICUAW include systemic inflammation and sepsis [27,28], corticosteroids [28], electrolyte disturbances

Table 23.1 Possible etiologies of acute generalized weakness in the intensive care unit.

Bilateral or paramedian brain or brainstem lesions[a]

Trauma
Infarction
Hemorrhage
Infectious and non-infectious encephalitis
Abscess
Central pontine myelinolysis

Spinal cord disorders

Trauma
Non-traumatic compressive myelopathies
Spinal cord infarction
Immune-mediated myelopathies (transverse myelitis, neuromyelitis optica)
Infective myelopathies (e.g., HIV, West Nile virus)

Anterior horn cell disorders

Motor neuron disease
Poliomyelitis
West Nile virus infection
Hopkins syndrome (acute postasthmatic amyotrophy)

Polyradiculopathies

Carcinomatous
HIV-associated

Peripheral nervous disorders

Guillain–Barré syndrome[b]
Diphtheritic neuropathy
Lymphoma-associated neuropathy
Vasculitic neuropathy
Porphyric neuropathy
Paraneoplastic neuropathy
Critical illness polyneuropathy

Neuromuscular junction disorders

Myasthenia gravis
Lambert–Eaton myasthenic syndrome
Neuromuscular-blocking drugs
Botulism

Muscle disorders

Rhabdomyolysis
Disuse myopathy
Cachexia
Infectious and inflammatory myopathies[c]
Mitochondrial myopathies
Drug-induced and toxic myopathies
Critical illness myopathy
Decompensation of congenital myopathies (e.g., myotonic dystrophy, Duchenne muscular dystrophy, adult onset acid maltase deficiency)

HIV, human immunodeficiency virus.
[a] Upper motor neuron signs (increased tone, hyperreflexia) may be absent in the acute setting; [b] includes acute inflammatory demyelinating polyneuropathy, acute motor axonal neuropathy, acute motor and sensory axonal neuropathy; [c] includes polymyositis, dermatomyositis, pyomyositis.
Reprinted from reference [21], with permission from Wolters Kluwer Health.

and hyperglycemia [29,30], immobility [28], and mechanical ventilation [28].

Neurological examination in the ICU

While a comprehensive neurological examination may not be possible in the ICU, a simplified assessment comprising an evaluation of mental status, cranial nerves, and motor responses and strength can be accomplished reliably and rapidly in virtually all patients.

Mental status

Patients should be carefully inspected for spontaneous body position, motor activity, eye opening, or verbalization. Purposeful movements (e.g., reaching for endotracheal tube) and comfort postures (e.g., crossing of the legs) are suggestive of cortical integration. Paroxysmal rhythmic movements may indicate seizures or status epilepticus. Responses to exteroceptive stimuli of graded intensity should then be observed, starting with visual fixation and pursuit, response to verbal commands, progressing to tactile cues and ending with noxious stimulation.

Mental status is explored by evaluating alertness, orientation, attention, memory, visuospatial functioning, executive and language functions. Orientation is determined with respect to person, place, date, and context. Attention may be tested by asking the patient to spell a five-letter word backwards. Memory is assessed in terms of immediate registration, short-term memory (recalling after an interval), and long-term memory (recollection of a well-known historical event). Visuospatial function can be screened by asking the patient to draw a clock, and language is tested by evaluating fluency, comprehension, naming, repetition, and presence or absence of paraphasia.

The widely implemented Glasgow Coma Scale (GCS) assigns a numerical value to the intensity of stimulation necessary to elicit three clinical indicators of arousal: eye opening, verbalization, and motor responses [31]. The Full Outline of UnResponsiveness (FOUR, Table 23.2) score integrates elements of the GCS with an assessment of brainstem reflexes [32]. In a recent pooled analysis, overall GCS and FOUR scores had similar sensitivity and specificity in predicting coma outcome; very low FOUR scores were more accurate in predicting in-hospital mortality [33].

Language or speech difficulties are categorized as dysarthria or aphasia, i.e., if articulation is "slurred" or if there is inability to understand, find, or say the

Table 23.2 Comparison of the FOUR Score with the Glasgow Coma Scale.

FOUR Score	Glasgow Coma Scale
Eye response	*Eye response*
4 = eyelids open or opened, tracking, or blinking to command	4 = eyes open spontaneously
3 = eyelids open but not tracking	3 = eye opening to verbal command
2 = eyelids closed but open to loud voice	2 = eye opening to pain
I = eyelids closed but open to pain	I = no eye opening
0 = eyelids remain closed with pain	*Motor response*
Motor response	6 = obeys commands
4 = thumbs-up, fist, or peace sign	5 = localizing pain
3 = localizing to pain	4 = withdrawal from pain
2 = flexion response to pain	3 = flexion response to pain
I = extension response to pain	2 = extension response to pain
0 = no response to pain or generalized myoclonus state	I = no motor response
Brainstem reflexes	*Verbal response*
4 = pupil and corneal reflexes present	5 = oriented
3 = one pupil wide and fixed	4 = confused
2 = pupil or corneal reflexes absent	3 = inappropriate words
I = pupil and corneal reflexes absent	2 = incomprehensible sounds
0 = absent pupil, corneal, and cough reflexes	I = no verbal response
Respiration	
4 = not intubated, regular breathing pattern	
3 = not intubated, Cheyn–tokes breathing pattern	
2 = not intubated, irregular breathing	
1 = breathes above ventilator rate	
0 = breathes at ventilator rate or apnea	

FOUR = Full Outline of UnResponsiveness.
Reprinted from reference [32], with permission from John Wiley and Sons.

correct words. Dysarthria is caused by lesions affecting any part of the speech system, including the palate, tongue, lips, or facial muscles and the CNS regions controlling those structures. Aphasias are classified as primarily expressive, receptive, or mixed. In patients with stroke, the distinction is important, as expressive (Broca's) aphasia is suggestive of a lesion in the distribution of the anterior/superior division of the middle cerebral artery (MCA), whereas receptive (Wernicke's) aphasia indicates a lesion in the MCA inferior/posterior division. Table 23.3 gives an overview of different types of aphasia and their clinical and anatomical features.

Apraxia generally refers to the "inability to perform" even though the primary sensory and motor systems are intact. It is usually caused by lesions of the higher-order premotor cortex. Verbal requests (e.g., "stick out your tongue," "show me two fingers") can be provided and if that fails, the patient's ability to mimic should be assessed in order to overcome difficulties due to receptive aphasia.

Cranial nerves

The cranial nerve examination provides critical information on the integrity of the brainstem and its afferent/efferent pathways. In patients with impaired consciousness, a fastidious examination of the eyes is particularly valuable given the proximity of centers governing eye movement, pupillary function, and elements of the ponto-mesencephalic brainstem: arousal system. Pupillary changes are dependent on the level of injury of the brainstem: small reactive pupils in comatose patients with diencephalic lesions; large and fixed pupils in patients with pretectal damage; ipsilateral dilated and fixed pupils in patients with lesions of the oculomotor nerve or nucleus; fixed and mid-positioned pupils in comatose patients with midbrain lesions; and pinpoint pupils can be present in pontine injury. Evaluation of brainstem function (Table 23.4) may help not only to localize focal pathological processes but also aids in prognostication (see below).

Motor examination

Motor activity may be classified as involuntary, reflexive, or purposeful. Involuntary movements are seen in seizures, movement disorders, and in metabolic and toxic derangements. Reflexes are stereotypical involuntary motor responses evoked

Table 23.3 Clinical and anatomical characteristics of different types of aphasia.

	Syndrome	Fluency	Comprehension	Repetition	Localization
	Broca's aphasia	Non-fluent	Intact	Impaired	Inferior frontal lobe
	Wernicke's aphasia	Fluent	Impaired	Impaired	Posterior, superior temporal lobe
	Conduction aphasia	Fluent	Intact	Impaired	Arcuate fasciculus
	Anomic aphasia	Fluent	Intact	Intact	Anterior temporal angular gyrus
	Subcortical aphasia	Non-fluent	Impaired	Intact	Thalamus, internal capsule, and basal ganglia
	Transcortical motor aphasia	Non-fluent	Intact	Intact	Medial frontal lobe, superior to Broca's area
	Transcortical sensory aphasia	Fluent	Impaired	Intact	Angular gyrus
	Mixed transcortical aphasia	Non-fluent	Impaired	Intact	Sum of transcortical motor and transcortical sensory area

Table 23.3 (cont.)

	Syndrome	Fluency	Comprehension	Repetition	Localization
	Global aphasia	Non-fluent	Impaired	Impaired	Sum of Broca's and Wernicke's area

Table 23.4 The assessment of brainstem reflexes.

Reflex	Examination technique	Normal response	Afferent pathway	Brainstem	Efferent pathway
Pupils	Response to light	Direct and consensual pupillary constriction	Retina, optic nerve, chiasm, optic tract	Edinger–Westphal nucleus (midbrain)	Oculomotor nerve, sympathetic fibers
Oculocephalic	Turn head from side to side	Eyes move conjugately in direction opposite to head	Semicircular canals, vestibular nerve	Vestibular nucleus. Medial longitudinal fasciculus. Parapontine reticular formation (pons).	Oculomotor and abducens nerves
Vestibulo-occulocephalic	Irrigate external auditory with cold water	Nystagmus with fast component beating away from stimulus	Semicircular canals, vestibular nerve	Vestibular nucleus. Medial longitudinal fasciculus. Parapontine reticular formation (pons).	Oculomotor and abducens nerves
Corneal reflex	Stimulation of cornea	Eyelid closure	Trigeminal nerve	Trigeminal and facial nuclei (pons)	Facial nerve
Cough reflex	Stimulation of carina	Cough	Glossopharyngeal and vagus nerves	Medullary "cough center"	Glossopharyngeal and vagus nerves
Gag reflex	Stimulation of soft palate	Symmetric elevation of soft palate	Glossopharyngeal and vagus nerves	Medulla	Glossopharyngeal and vagus nerves

Reprinted from reference [5], with permission from Wolters Kluwer Health.

by stimulus. Purposeful movements (e.g., localization) imply some degree of cortical processing of environmental variables. Motor function should be assessed routinely in all extremities for bulk, tone, strength, spontaneous (involuntary) movements, and right to left symmetry. Strength can be graded in conscious patients according to the Medical Research Council (MRC) scale [34]. The unconscious patient should be observed for spontaneous or involuntary limb movements and responses to noxious stimuli. Tendon reflexes allow differentiation between upper motor neuron (hyperreflexia) and lower motor neuron involvement (hypo- or

areflexia) with the exception of patients with acute spinal injury where hypo- or areflexia and flaccidity can precede hyperreflexia in the first days after trauma (i.e., spinal shock).

Sensory examination

An accurate examination of sensory function requires alertness and cooperation. Detailed examination is time consuming and may be challenging in the ICU environment. If the patient is conscious, testing of light touch, temperature, and position sense should be performed. Bilateral simultaneous

Table 23.5 The National Institutes of Health Stroke Scale (NIHSS).

NIHSS	
1a. Level of consciousness	0 = Alert; keenly responsive 1 = Not alert, but arousable by minor stimulation 2 = Not alert; requires repeated stimulation 3 = Unresponsive or responds only with reflex
1b. Level of consciousness – questions: – What is the month? – What is your age?	0 = Both answers correct 1 = Answers one question correctly 2 = Answers two questions correctly
1c. Level of consciousness – commands: – Open and close your eyes. – Grip and release your hand.	0 = Performs both tasks correctly 1 = Performs one task correctly 2 = Performs neither task correctly
2. Best gaze	0 = Normal 1 = Partial gaze palsy 2 = Forced deviation
3. Visual fields	0 = No visual loss 1 = Partial hemianopia 2 = Complete hemianopia 3 = Bilateral hemianopia
4. Facial palsy	0 = Normal symmetric movements 1 = Minor paralysis 2 = Partial paralysis 3 = Complete paralysis of one or both sides
5. Motor arm 5a. Left arm 5b. Right arm	0 = No drift 1 = Drift 2 = Some effort against gravity 3 = No effort against gravity; limb falls 4 = No movement
6. Motor leg 6a. Left leg 6b. Right leg	0 = No drift 1 = Drift 2 = Some effort against gravity 3 = No effort against gravity 4 = No movement
7. Limb ataxia	0 = Absent 1 = Present in one limb 2 = Present in two limbs
8. Sensory	0 = Normal; no sensory loss 1 = Mild to moderate sensory loss 2 = Severe to total sensory loss
9. Language	0 = No aphasia; normal 1 = Mild to moderate aphasia 2 = Severe aphasia 3 = Mute, global aphasia
10. Dysarthria	0 = Normal 1 = Mild to moderate dysarthria 2 = Severe dysarthria

Table 23.5 (cont.)

NIHSS	
11. Extinction and inattention	0 = No abnormality 1 = Visual, tactile, auditory, spatial, or personal inattention 2 = Profound hemi-inattention or extinction
Total score	0–42

Reprinted from Lyden P, Lu M, Jackson C, NINDS tPA Stroke Trial Investigators. Underlying structure of the National Institutes of Health Stroke Scale: results of a factor analysis. *Stroke* 1999;**30**:2347–54, with permission from Wolters Kluwer Health.

stimulation may help identify hemineglect, which is often seen in patients with frontoparietal lesions of the non-dominant hemisphere.

Standardized examination protocol for suspected stroke

The National Institutes of Health Stroke Scale (NIHSS, Table 23.5) provides a quantitative assessment of symptom burden in patients with suspected stroke [35] and has robust prognostic value [36]. The NIHSS is weighted to the lesions in the anterior circulation whereas posterior circulation signs such as vertigo, diplopia, nausea and vomiting, pupillary abnormalities, and nystagmus are overlooked by this scale.

Limits of clinical assessment and the need for further testing

When diagnostic uncertainty persists, clinical neurological examination must be supplemented with additional testing, most notably neuroimaging and neurophysiological examination.

Neuroimaging

Imaging with computed tomography (CT) of the head should be obtained whenever there is a new onset of a focal neurological deficit, seizures, any alteration of mental status or loss of consciousness which is not immediately reversible or clearly explained by medication or an underlying metabolic factor [37]. Head CT should be obtained prior to lumbar puncture to evaluate for anatomical shifts, which might increase the risk of herniation. A CT angiography allows additional assessment of the intra- and extracranial arterial and venous circulation, particularly when there is concern for vascular lesions or stroke. Magnetic resonance imaging (MRI) has greater sensitivity for demyelinating and inflammatory diseases, hyperacute ischemic stroke, microhemorrhagic lesions, anoxic-ischemic damage from cardiac arrest, and most disorders affecting the white matter and the brainstem [38,39].

Electroencephalography

An EEG should be obtained whenever there is a concern for seizures or status epilepticus as an underlying cause or consequence of brain dysfunction. When critically ill patients are monitored with EEG, 8–22% of cases are found to have epileptiform activity, most frequently nonconvulsive in nature [17,19,20]. Populations at risk for nonconvulsive seizures or status epilepticus include patients with encephalopathy following cardiac arrest [40], patients following convulsive status epilepticus [41], subarachnoid hemorrhage [42], intracerebral hemorrhage [43], ischemic stroke [43], traumatic brain injury [44], and metabolic-toxic encephalopathy [16].

Evoked potentials

Somatosensory evoked potential (SSEP) recordings are less influenced by drugs and metabolic derangements than EEG. In patients with anoxic-ischemic encephalopathy following cardiac arrest, absence of the cortical N20 response after median nerve stimulation is a highly specific predictor of outcome [45]. A meta-analysis of eight studies demonstrated a false positive rate of 0.7% for poor outcome when bilateral absence of N20 response was recorded [46]. Recent studies completed in cardiac arrest patients who received therapeutic hypothermia confirm the validity of this predictor variable [47,48].

Electromyography and nerve conduction velocities

When neuromuscular weakness cannot be evaluated clinically or is persistent and severe, electromyography and nerve conduction velocities (EMG/NCV) should be obtained [21]. An EMG/NCV will help differentiate between a primarily axonal (reduced compound muscle action potential amplitude, normal latencies) versus a demyelinating (preserved amplitude, increased latencies) polyneuropathy, a fundamental distinction which can orient diagnosis depending on the associated clinical history, time course, and CSF

findings. In patients who are cooperative and able to voluntarily contract muscles, the EMG pattern will help identify an underlying myopathic disturbance. The use of direct muscle stimulation may help separate a neuropathic from a myopathic condition even in the absence of patient cooperation [49]. Neuromuscular junction diseases such as myasthenia gravis and Lambert–Eaton myasthenic syndrome are suggested by decremental responses to repetitive nerve stimulation [50].

References

1. Stevens RD, Dowdy DW, Michaels RK, *et al.* Neuromuscular dysfunction acquired in critical illness: a systematic review. *Intensive Care Med* 2007;**33**(11):1876–91.

2. Bastos PG, Sun X, Wagner DP, *et al.* Glasgow Coma Scale score in the evaluation of outcome in the intensive care unit: findings from the Acute Physiology and Chronic Health Evaluation III study. *Critical Care Med* 1993;**21**(10):1459–65.

3. Hoesch RE, Lin E, Young M, *et al.* Acute lung injury in critical neurological illness. *Critical Care Med* 2012;**40**(2):587–93.

4. Sharshar T, Porcher R, Siami S, *et al.* Brainstem responses can predict death and delirium in sedated patients in intensive care unit. *Critical Care Med* 2011;**39**(8):1960–7.

5. Stevens RD, Bhardwaj A. Approach to the comatose patient. *Critical Care Med* 2006;**34**(1):31–41.

6. Moruzzi G, Magoun HW. Brain stem reticular formation and activation of the EEG. 1949. *J Neuropsychiatry Clin Neurosci* 1995;**7**(2):251–67.

7. Parvizi J, Damasio AR. Neuroanatomical correlates of brainstem coma. *Brain* 2003;**126**(Pt 7):1524–36.

8. Posner JB, Saper CB, Schiff ND, Plum F editors. Examination of the comatose patient. In *Plum and Posner's Diagnosis of Stupor and Coma*. 4th edn. Oxford University Press; 2007:38–87.

9. American Psychiatric Association. *Diagnostic and Statistical Manual of Mental Disorders, Fourth edition, Text Revision* (DSM–IV–TR). Washington, DC: American Psychiatric Association; 2000.

10. Ely EW, Shintani A, Truman B, *et al.* Delirium as a predictor of mortality in mechanically ventilated patients in the intensive care unit. *JAMA* 2004;**291**(14):1753–62.

11. Girard TD, Jackson JC, Pandharipande PP, *et al.* Delirium as a predictor of long-term cognitive impairment in survivors of critical illness. *Critical Care Med* 2010;**38**(7):1513–20.

12. Meagher DJ, O'Hanlon D, O'Mahony E, *et al.* Relationship between symptoms and motoric subtype of delirium. *J Neuropsychiatry Clin Neurosci* 2000;**12**(1):51–6.

13. Meagher DJ, Moran M, Raju B, *et al.* Motor symptoms in 100 patients with delirium versus control subjects: comparison of subtyping methods. *Psychosomatics* 2008;**49**(4):300–8.

14. Spronk PE, Riekerk B, Hofhuis J, *et al.* Occurrence of delirium is severely underestimated in the ICU during daily care. *Intensive Care Med* 2009;**35**(7):1276–80.

15. Peterson JF, Pun BT, Dittus RS, *et al.* Delirium and its motoric subtypes: a study of 614 critically ill patients. *J Am Geriatr Soc* 2006;**54**(3):479–84.

16. Claassen J, Mayer SA, Kowalski RG, *et al.* Detection of electrographic seizures with continuous EEG monitoring in critically ill patients. *Neurology* 2004;**62**(10):1743–8.

17. Oddo M, Carrera E, Claassen J, *et al.* Continuous electroencephalography in the medical intensive care unit. *Critical Care Med* 2009;**37**(6):2051–6.

18. Rudin D, Grize L, Schindler C, *et al.* High prevalence of nonconvulsive and subtle status epilepticus in an ICU of a tertiary care center: a three-year observational cohort study. *Epilepsy Res* 2011;**96**(1–2): 140–50.

19. Towne AR, Waterhouse EJ, Boggs JG, *et al.* Prevalence of nonconvulsive status epilepticus in comatose patients. *Neurology* 2000;**54**(2):340–5.

20. Sutter R, Fuhr P, Grize L, *et al.* Continuous video-EEG monitoring increases detection rate of nonconvulsive status epilepticus in the ICU. *Epilepsia* 2011;**52** (3):453–7.

21. Stevens RD, Marshall SA, Cornblath DR, *et al.* A framework for diagnosing and classifying intensive care unit-acquired weakness. *Critical Care Med* 2009;**37**(10 Suppl):S299–308.

22. Tatu L, Moulin T, Bogousslavsky J, *et al.* Arterial territories of the human brain: cerebral hemispheres. *Neurology* 1998;**50**(6):1699–708.

23. Branco BC, Plurad D, Green DJ, *et al.* Incidence and clinical predictors for tracheostomy after cervical spinal cord injury: a National Trauma Databank review. *J Trauma* 2011;**70**(1):111–15.

24. Como JJ, Sutton ER, McCunn M, *et al.* Characterizing the need for mechanical ventilation following cervical spinal cord injury with neurologic deficit. *J Trauma* 2005;**59**(4):912–16; discussion 916.

25. Ali NA, O'Brien JM, Jr., Hoffmann SP, *et al.* Acquired weakness, handgrip strength, and mortality in critically ill patients. *Am J Resp Crit Care Med* 2008;**178** (3):261–8.

26. Sharshar T, Bastuji-Garin S, Stevens RD, *et al.* Presence and severity of intensive care unit-acquired paresis at time of awakening are associated with increased intensive care unit and hospital mortality. *Critical Care Med* 2009;**37**(12):3047–53.

27. de Letter MA, Schmitz PI, Visser LH, *et al.* Risk factors for the development of polyneuropathy and myopathy in critically ill patients. *Critical Care Med* 2001;**29**(12):2281–6.

28. De Jonghe B, Sharshar T, Lefaucheur JP, *et al.* Paresis acquired in the intensive care unit: a prospective multicenter study. *JAMA* 2002;**288**(22):2859–67.

29. Witt NJ, Zochodne DW, Bolton CF, *et al.* Peripheral nerve function in sepsis and multiple organ failure. *Chest* 1991;**99**(1):176–84.

30. van den Berghe G, Wouters P, Weekers F, *et al.* Intensive insulin therapy in the critically ill patients. *New Engl J Med* 2001;**345**(19):1359–67.

31. Teasdale G, Jennett B. Assessment of coma and impaired consciousness. A practical scale. *Lancet* 1974;**2**(7872):81–4.

32. Wijdicks EF, Bamlet WR, Maramattom BV, *et al.* Validation of a new coma scale: the FOUR score. *Annals Neurol* 2005;**58**(4):585–93.

33. Wijdicks EF, Rabinstein AA, Bamlet WR, *et al.* FOUR score and Glasgow Coma Scale in predicting outcome of comatose patients: a pooled analysis. *Neurology* 2011;**77**(1):84–5.

34. Kleyweg RP, van der Meche FG, Schmitz PI. Interobserver agreement in the assessment of muscle strength and functional abilities in Guillain-Barre syndrome. *Muscle Nerve* 1991;**14**(11):1103–9.

35. Powers DW. Assessment of the stroke patient using the NIH stroke scale. *Emerg Med Serv* 2001;**30**(6):52–6.

36. Hacke W, Donnan G, Fieschi C, *et al.* Association of outcome with early stroke treatment: pooled analysis of ATLANTIS, ECASS, and NINDS rt-PA stroke trials. *Lancet* 2004;**363**(9411):768–74.

37. Stevens RD, Pustavoitau A, Chalela JA. Brain imaging in intensive care medicine. *Semin Neurol* 2008; **28**(5):631–44.

38. Tshibanda L, Vanhaudenhuyse A, Galanaud D, *et al.* Magnetic resonance spectroscopy and diffusion tensor imaging in coma survivors: promises and pitfalls. *Progr Brain Res* 2009;**177**:215–29.

39. Wijman CAC, Mlynash M, Caulfield AF, *et al.* Prognostic value of brain diffusion-weighted imaging after cardiac arrest. *Annals Neurol* 2009;**65**(4):394–402.

40. Rossetti AO, Urbano LA, Delodder F, *et al.* Prognostic value of continuous EEG monitoring during therapeutic hypothermia after cardiac arrest. *Crit Care* 2010;**14**(5):R173.

41. DeLorenzo RJ, Waterhouse EJ, Towne AR, *et al.* Persistent nonconvulsive status epilepticus after the control of convulsive status epilepticus. *Epilepsia* 1998;**39**(8):833–40.

42. Claassen J, Hirsch LJ, Frontera JA, *et al.* Prognostic significance of continuous EEG monitoring in patients with poor-grade subarachnoid hemorrhage. *Neurocritical Care* 2006;**4**(2):103–12.

43. Balami JS, Buchan AM. Complications of intracerebral haemorrhage. *Lancet Neurol* 2012;**11**(1):101–18.

44. Vespa PM, Nuwer MR, Nenov V, *et al.* Increased incidence and impact of nonconvulsive and convulsive seizures after traumatic brain injury as detected by continuous electroencephalographic monitoring. *J Neurosurg* 1999;**91**(5):750–60.

45. Zandbergen EG, Hijdra A, Koelman JH, *et al.* Prediction of poor outcome within the first 3 days of postanoxic coma. *Neurology* 2006;**66**(1):62–8.

46. Wijdicks EF, Hijdra A, Young GB, *et al.* Practice parameter: prediction of outcome in comatose survivors after cardiopulmonary resuscitation (an evidence-based review): report of the Quality Standards Subcommittee of the American Academy of Neurology. *Neurology* 2006;**67**(2): 203–10.

47. Rossetti AO, Oddo M, Logroscino G, *et al.* Prognostication after cardiac arrest and hypothermia: a prospective study. *Annals Neurol* 2010;**67**(3):301–7.

48. Bouwes A, Binnekade JM, Kuiper MA, *et al.* Prognosis of coma after therapeutic hypothermia: a prospective cohort study. *Annals Neurol* 2012;**71** (2):206–12.

49. Rich MM, Bird SJ, Raps EC, *et al.* Direct muscle stimulation in acute quadriplegic myopathy. *Muscle Nerve* 1997;**20**(6):665–73.

50. Baslo MB, Deymeer F, Serdaroglu P, *et al.* Decrement pattern in Lambert-Eaton myasthenic syndrome is different from myasthenia gravis. *Neuromuscul Disord* 2006; **16**(7):454–8.

Chapter 24

Bedside assessment of delirium in critically ill patients

Alawi Luetz and Claudia D. Spies

SUMMARY

Over 14 years ago, delirium was called the "Cinderella of psychiatry": taken for granted, ignored, and seldom studied [1]. Fortunately, the study of acute brain dysfunction, especially in critically ill patients, has rapidly advanced in the last years. The relative paucity of work performed in this area during the last decade of the twentieth century and the significantly rapid rise in publications since the turn of the century is noteworthy [2].

   Devlin and co-workers showed that the use of a validated delirium assessment tool significantly improves the ability of physicians and nurses to identify delirium in ICU patients [3]. Due to the high prevalence and the significantly worse outcomes associated with the development of intensive care unit (ICU) delirium, national and international clinical practice guidelines recommend routine delirium monitoring with a validated delirium assessment tool [4–6]. This might be the main reason for the increasing number of published studies validating and comparing different delirium scores in different clinical settings.

Diagnostic criteria for delirium

Delirium is among the oldest phenomena known to medicine and is a life-threatening organic brain syndrome, affecting 11–87% of critically ill patients [7]. For decades, the definition and labeling of delirium or delirious states was a semantic muddle. The term delirium as a diagnostic entity did not even appear in the formal nomenclature until 1980 when it achieved recognition in the *Diagnostic and Statistical Manual of Mental Disorders*, Third Revision (DSM–III) and was clearly distinguished from dementia or other delirium-like cognitive disorders that do not refer to

a specific organic factor. In contrast to the DSM–III–(R) definition of delirium that was grounded only on expert opinion and a few case studies, the DSM–IV Work Group on Organic Disorders based their work on new data from two large prospective studies. Both studies recorded the incidence of delirium and the presence and severity of each of the DSM–III–(R) criteria. The data revealed that some of the symptoms were more specific than others in identifying delirium and thus significantly improved the development of the DSM–IV criteria for delirium. The World Health Organization developed its own classification system for delirium. It was first published in 1992 with the tenth edition of the *International Classification of Diseases* (ICD–10). Both classification systems include symptoms that must be present for a definite delirium diagnosis and additional qualifying conditions (Table 24.1). One of the major differences between both definitions of delirium is that the ICD–10 criteria have required symptoms of psychomotor retardation, emotional and sleep-wake-cycle disturbances for the diagnosis of delirium. These additional symptoms are suspected to cause the more restrictive performance of the ICD–10 in detecting delirious patients. In a cross-sectional study Laurila and co-workers evaluated the concordance of different diagnostic criteria for delirium in elderly (> 70 years) geriatric hospital patients. The authors found that the DSM–IV was the most inclusive diagnostic tool: the delirium incidence was 25% compared with 10% with the ICD-10 [8]. More importantly, the group of patients with a DSM–IV defined delirium had 1-year and 2-year mortality rates that were comparable to the mortality rates of patients with an ICD–10 defined delirium. Compared with the ICD–10 criteria, these results indicate not only a higher sensitivity for the less restrictive diagnostic tool (DSM–IV) but also a good specificity

Brain Disorders in Critical Illness, ed. Robert D. Stevens, Tarek Sharshar, and E. Wesley Ely. Published by Cambridge University Press. © Cambridge University Press 2013.

Table 24.1 Criteria for delirium diagnosis according to DSM–IV and ICD–10.

Criterion / Disturbance	DSM-IV		ICD-10		Criterion / Disturbance
Consciousness	A	✓	✓	A	Consciousness
Attention		✓	✓		Attention
Memory	B	①	①	B	Memory
Orientation		①	①		Orientation
Speech/Language		①	①		Comprehension
Perceptual disturbance		①	①		Perceptual disturbance
Acute onset	C	✓	①		Hallucination
Fluctuates over the day		✓	❶	C	Hypo-/Hyperactivity
Cause*	D	✓	❶		Speech/Language
Reaction time			❶		Reaction time
Sleep-wake cycle			✓	D	Sleep-wake cycle
Emotional disturbance			✓	E	Emotional disturbance
Comprehension					Acute onset
Hypo-/Hyperactivity					Fluctuates over the day
Hallucination					Cause*

For definite diagnosis, symptoms must be present in this area — ✓ For definite diagnosis, symptom must be present

Symptoms are not defined according to DSM-IV — ① At least one of these symptoms must be present

Additional qualifying conditions according to ICD-10 — ❶ At least one of these symptoms must be present

*General medical condition, substance intoxication, medication use, withdrawal syndrome, more than one etiology, others.

for diagnosing delirium in acutely ill patients. Moreover, the prognostic significance of subsyndromal states of delirium (SSD), especially in critically ill patients, warrants the use of a less restrictive diagnostic tool.

Most study designs validating delirium assessment tools rely on a psychiatrist using the DSM–IV criteria as the "gold standard." However the DSM–IV criteria for diagnosing delirium were not primarily developed to assess ICU delirium, especially in sedated and ventilated patients. Although psychiatrists have formal training to assess disturbance of consciousness and change in cognition, they are often not familiar with patients in the ICU setting receiving analgesia and sedation, being mechanically ventilated, or having critical illness polyneuropathy or critical illness myopathy. Intensivists have more experience assessing the fluctuation of symptoms and evaluating the history, physical examination, or laboratory findings. Clinicians and researchers should use any "gold standard" for delirium by combining the experience from psychiatrists and intensivists. At the patients' bedside, this interdisciplinary team will probably fare better than the sum of its parts. This should be considered, particularly in validation studies of specific delirium assessment tools.

Cultural adaptation and translation of diagnostic screening tools – implications for the use of delirium assessment tools

As a result of the increasing internationalization of clinical trials, the need to translate and adapt Patient Reported Outcome (PRO) instruments for use in countries other than that of the source language has grown rapidly. In 1999 the International Society for PharmacoEconomics and Outcomes Research (ISPOR) established a Translation and Cultural Adaptation (TCA) group to develop guidelines and standards for the translation and cultural adaptation of patient-reported outcome measures. The core of the ISPOR Principles of Good Practice (PGP) is the outline of a structured translation and cultural adaptation

Table 24.2 Steps of the translation and cultural adaptation process.

Step	Key components	Risks of not doing this
Preparation	Obtain permission to use instrument Invite instrument developer	Being prosecuted Misinterpretation of items and concepts
Forward translation	Development of at least two independent *forward translations*	Translation that is too much of one person's own style of writing
Reconciliation	. . . into a *single* forward translation	Biased translation
Back translation	. . . of the reconciled forward translation into the source language The translator should be a native speaker or an accredited interpreter	Biased translation
Back translation review	. . . against the source language	Overlooking mistranslations
Harmonization	. . . of all new translations with each other and the source version The backward translation should also be approved by the original author of the instrument	Overlooking mistranslations and conceptual differences
Cognitive debriefing	. . . of the new translation with: nurses, physicians, and researchers who use the instrument at the patient's bedside; healthy respondents	Missing or inaccurate data resulting Misunderstanding of items
Review and finalization	Cognitive debriefing results are reviewed and the translation finalized	Translation may include words or phrases that are not familiar to healthy respondents (*or the testers*)
Proofreading	. . . of the finalized translation	A final translation that contains spelling, grammatical, and/or other errors
Final report	. . . is written on the development of the translation	Translations of measures that may not be used because of inadequate reporting of methods used in development
Publication	. . . of the finalized translation	– Translations of measures that may not be used because of inadequate reporting of methods used in development – Multiple translation processes of the same instrument in the same language Lack of transparency
Free access	Make the translated instrument available for free to all researchers and practitioners	Multiple translation processes of the same instrument in the same language Insufficient quantity of independent studies conducted with the specific instrument
Validation	. . . of the translated instrument (e.g., against a "gold standard")	Translated instruments with insufficient validity or reliability

process. This process consists of 10 major steps (Table 24.2). Before finalization, the new translation should undergo a cognitive debriefing to avoid misunderstandings of the test items. Usually the newly translated measure should be tested on a group of 5–8 native speakers who adequately represent the target population. However, a potentially delirious ICU patient may not understand the question of a test item due to delirium and not because of an inadequate translation. Therefore a modified cognitive debriefing process would be more appropriate: in this case, ICU nurses and physicians have to evaluate all test items and instructions with respect to intelligibility and language [9]. Finally, to prove that the new translation is sufficient for clinical purposes, this assessment tool should undergo a validation against a "gold standard" (e.g., DSM–IV). If a standardized validation of the new translation reveals insufficient sensitivity or specificity compared with the validation of the instrument in the source language, the new translation should be re-evaluated. In addition, to increase transparency, new translations, including the methodology and results of the cognitive debriefing, should be published in a local journal. Several research groups and the international societies make efforts to increase attention on ICU delirium by developing websites that offer important information, including training materials and translations of different assessment tools. New translations of delirium scores should be available for free to all researchers and practitioners through these websites.

An article by Wild and colleagues addresses the issue of how to approach the problem of creating an instrument in the same language for use in different target countries [10]. The *country-specific approach* would result in different versions of a translation for each major country. The *universal approach* aims to reach a compromise in order to achieve a translation understood by all. If a translation in the target language already exists, it is possible to adopt this language version for use in new countries or populations. Both the universal and the adaptation approach result in one single version. However, each of the mentioned approaches requires a separate debriefing process for each country that should be published anyway.

Validated scores for the detection of delirium in critically ill patients

Delirium assessment tools have advantages over clinical observations in terms of objectivity, standardization, and the availability of normative data. While a number of valid and reliable tools are available to identify delirium in non-ICU populations, a number of unique characteristics in the critically ill restrict the use of these instruments. In particular, the inability of intubated patients to participate in the components of the scales that require verbal responses and the inability of ICU patients to communicate due to the administration of sedative agents, must be considered. The core symptoms of delirium and the specific characteristics of the critically ill help define the qualities of a delirium assessment tool that should be used in this population: (a) an instrument that evaluates unconditional symptoms of delirium (according to DSM–IV or ICD–10 criteria); (b) has proven sufficient validity and reliability in ICU populations; (c) can be completed quickly and easily in clinical routine; and (d) does not require the presence of a psychiatrist. By the end of 2011 we identified eight delirium scores, validated in ICU patients (Table 24.3).

The Cognitive Test for Delirium (CTD) was the first score specifically developed for use in the critically ill. In 1997 an "abbreviated CTD" (CTD-A) was developed when the assessment of only two content areas was found to maintain good reliability [11]. However, both validation studies did not use the ICD–10 or DSM–IV criteria for delirium. More importantly, the number of patients evaluated within these studies is relatively small. The Confusion Assessment Method for the ICU (CAM-ICU) is the most thoroughly investigated delirium score in the critically ill.

The CAM considers three of the four key features of delirium, i.e., both an acute onset of mental status changes or a fluctuating course and inattention, and either disorganized thinking or an altered level of consciousness. In order to be able to assess delirium in mechanically ventilated ICU patients, Ely and co-workers replaced the Mini Mental State Examination (MMSE) with an Attention Screening Examination (ASE) (Chart 1 – CAM-ICU) [12]. Most CAM-ICU validation studies used the DSM–IV criteria as the reference standard, performed the ratings with the help of blinded testers, and included patients with mechanical ventilation. Except for one, all validation studies revealed sufficient sensitivity, specificity, and reliability for the CAM-ICU in detecting delirious patients [12]. Van Eijk and colleagues investigated in a multicenter study the diagnostic value of the CAM-ICU when used in daily practice. Daily bedside nurse assessments of patients were compared with a "gold standard" defined as contemporaneous assessments by teams of three delirium "experts" (psychiatrists, geriatricians, and neurologists) who used cognitive examinations, inspection of medical files, and the DSM–IV criteria for delirium. In contrast to the results of the other validation studies, the sensitivity of the CAM-ICU for diagnosing delirium was quite poor at 47% [13]. The bedside nurses assessed all patients using the CAM-ICU within 3 hours of the expert assessment, without extra training for this study. While centers that always used the CAM-ICU performed better than those that did not, none were close to the sensitivities reported in the research setting. The study was limited by a lack of detail regarding how the bedside nurses actually went about performing the CAM-ICU. One of the reasons for the low sensitivity in this study might be that the quality of training and resources provided for training and implementation of the CAM-ICU were not sufficient.

Table 24.3 Assessment tools for the detection of ICU delirium: methodological characteristics and results of validation studies in the critically ill.

Score/Reference	Pub. (n)	ICD-10	DSM-IV	pros.	blind.	MV	P/A (n)	Sen.	Spe.	Rel.
CAM-ICU	6									
[7]		Ø	✓	✓	✓	✓	(P) 38 (A) 293	95%	89%	0.79
[12]		Ø	✓	✓	✓	✓	(P) 111 (A) 471	93%	98%	0.96
[41]		Ø	✓	✓	✓	✓	(P) 102	91%	98%	0.91
[18]		Ø	✓	✓	✓	✓	(P) 151 (A) 559	79%	97%	0.89
[42]		Ø	✓	✓	✓	✓	(P) 54	88%	92%	0.96
[43]		Ø	✓	✓	✓	?	(P) 181	47%	98%	0.63
ICDSC	3									
[14]		? Psychiatrist	✓	✓	?		(P) 93	99%	64%	0.71
[16]		Ø	✓	✓	✓	✓	(P) 135	43%	94%	Ø
[15]		✓	Ø	✓	✓	Ø	(P) 59	75% 91%[1]	74% 62%[1]	0.75
DDS	2									
[17]		Ø	Ø	✓	Ø	✓	(P) 1073 (A) 3588	69%	75%	0.66
[18]		Ø	✓	✓	✓	✓	(P) 152 (A) 547	25% 79%[2]	89% 81%[2]	0.79
NEECHAM	2									
[20]		Ø	Ø	✓	?	Ø	(P) 19	Ø	Ø	0.81
[21]		Ø	✓	✓	✓	✓	(P) 105 (A) 253	97%	83%	0.60

Table 24.3 (cont.)

Score/Reference	Pub. (n)	ICD–10	DSM–IV	pros.	blind.	MV	P/A (n)	Sen.	Spe.	Rel.
MDAS	1									
[23]		✔	∅	✔	✔	?	(P) 25	100%	95%	0.89
Nu-DESC	1									
[18]		∅	✔	✔	✔	✔	(P) 154 (A) 547	82%	83%	0.68
CTD	1									
[44]		∅	∅	✔	?	?	(P) 22	100%	95%	0.87
CTD-A	1									
[11]		∅	∅	✔	✔	?	(P) 19	95%	99%	0.91

Studies comparing different assessment tools for ICU delirium without using any declared reference standard are not included in this table. Pub. (n), number of published validation studies; pros., prospective; blind., ratings with different instruments were performed independently (blinded testers); MV, patients with mechanical ventilation included; P/A (n), number of included patients (P) and included assessment (A) in data analysis; Sen., sensitivity; Spe., specificity; Rel., reliability; 1 validity using a different cut-off (≥ 3); 2, validity using a different cut-off (>3); ✔, applies; ∅, does not apply; ?, not stated/not calculated.
CAM-ICU, Confusion Assessment Method for the ICU; ICDSC, Intensive Care Delirium Screening Checklist; DDS, Delirium Detection Score; MDAS, Memorial Delirium Assessment Scale; Nu-DESC, Nursing Delirium Screening Scale; CTD, Cognitive Test for Delirium; CTD-A, Abbreviated Cognitive Test for Delirium.

The result of this study is especially important because it emphasizes that reports of high implementation rates for a target instrument do not prove good quality of care. It is rather a question of how an implementation process is organized and monitored.

The Intensive Care Delirium Screening Checklist (ICDSC) consists of 8 items based on unconditional and conditional DSM–IV criteria, but also includes symptoms mentioned in the ICD–10 classification and earlier versions of the DSM (Chart 2 – ICDSC). During the evaluation process, 1 point is given towards each domain that is present, with a score of 4 or higher out of 8 denoting the presence of delirium. The initial validation of the ICDSC revealed good values for sensitivity and specificity in detecting delirium in ICU patients [14]. A study by Georges and co-workers showed that dropping the cut-off for delirium diagnosis from 4 to 3 may lead to a significant higher sensitivity of the ICDSC at almost consistent specificity [15]. A prospective study that compared the CAM-ICU and the ICDSC with a "gold standard" (DSM–IV) revealed a significant higher sensitivity (64%) for the CAM-ICU compared with the ICDSC (43%) [16]. However, all studies comparing both assessment tools reported a *very good agreement* (Cohen's kappa ≥ 0.80) of delirium diagnosing in the critically ill.

The Delirium Detection Score is an 8-item scale modified from the validated Clinical Withdrawal Assessment for Alcohol revised scale (CIWA-Ar), and was initially developed for measuring severity of delirium in ICU patients (Chart 3 – DDS). The first study validated the DDS against the Sedation Agitation Scale (SAS) and demonstrated good validity and reliability for the detection of delirium [17]. However, the DDS was still lacking validation against the DSM–IV criteria for delirium. In 2010, the DDS was validated against the DSM–IV criteria and showed insufficient sensitivity. In order for the DDS to achieve an adequate sensitivity, the cut-off for the DDS was determined with receiver operating characteristic (ROC) analysis to be > 3 [18].

Nurses provide around-the-clock observation and, therefore, play a crucial role in delirium detection. Before the development of the Nursing Delirium Screening Scale (Nu-DESC), the Confusion Rating Scale (CRS) was the only brief nursing delirium-screening instrument. The CRS was not based on DSM–IV criteria and especially overlooked patients in the hypoactive state of delirium. Therefore, Gaudreau and colleagues added a fifth item to the CRS, evaluating unusual psychomotor retardation (Chart 4 – Nu-DESC). The Nu-DESC was initially validated in the oncology inpatient setting and revealed good validity when compared with DSM–IV criteria for delirium. The validation process in the ICU proved similar results with a sensitivity of 82% and a specificity of 83% compared with DSM–IV criteria for delirium [19].

Two studies adopted the NEECHAM confusion scale for use in the ICU. This 9-item scale is separated into three subscales: (a) process information, (b) behavior, and (c) physical conditions. The information-processing domain is given a greater weighting than either behavior or physiological condition, with a lower score reflecting a greater likelihood for the presence of delirium. A score of 19 or more points out of 30 indicates delirium (Chart 5 – NEECHAM). In a small pilot study of 19 patients, the NEECHAM scores and the results of DSM–III ratings showed good correlation [20]. A larger validation study against the DSM–IV criteria for delirium exhibited a high sensitivity and specificity and strong nursing interrater reliability. The *processing subscale* (e.g., attention, command, orientation) had the highest correlation (Cronbach alpha 0.95) [21].

The Memorial Delirium Assessment Scale (MDAS) is a 10-item clinician-rated scale (possible range 0–30) that was initially designed to measure severity of delirium in medically ill patients (Chart 6 – MDAS).

The first validation of the MDAS by Breitbart and co-workers in a group of 33 mixed cancer and AIDS patients established a diagnostic cut-off to be 13 [22]. One single study evaluated the MDAS in the critical care setting. One hundred and twenty patients were evaluated with MDAS score. However, only 25 of these patients were evaluated for delirium by the consultant psychiatrist according to the ICD–10 criteria. The cut-off for the MDAS was determined with ROC analysis to be ≥ 10 [23].

Educational interventions, including the use of a validated delirium assessment instrument, achieved a seven-fold increase in the number of nurses who used the tool (12% vs. 82%) and who used it correctly (8% vs. 62%) [24]. The physicians' ability to accurately detect delirium in ICU patients improved significantly after use of a validated delirium score. Additionally, delirium-specific multidisciplinary education and nurse-led intervention programs in non-ICU settings have resulted in a decrease in the duration and severity of delirium without advising on any specific pharmacotherapy [25].

Choosing among already validated delirium scores especially depends on the appropriateness for the research question or the specific clinical setting. In contrast to a binary delirium score (delirium: yes/no), a graded diagnostic scale (e.g., the ICDSC, DDS, or MDAS), allows calculating the severity of different delirium symptoms. Using these kinds of instruments may have two major advantages: (a) symptom-guided (pharmaco-) therapy or better dose finding; and (b) the detection of patients who are at risk for developing "full-blown" delirium (pre-delirious state). Contrarily, some studies reported that examiners felt unsure about judging the state of the patient correctly when performing the Nu-DESC or the DDS, whereas when performing the CAM-ICU, they felt more confident due to the simplicity and clarity of the task. The delirium diagnosis of graded scales is based on more subjective judgment regarding the presence or absence of specific symptoms. However, no matter which of the validated scores will be used, the intervention of delirium monitoring will emphasize and raise awareness of the ICU staff to delirium symptoms that probably results in improved treatment of these patients.

Subsyndromal delirium and conceptual differences between delirium scores

The phenomenon of a pre- or a subsyndromal delirious state in patients has been discussed for almost three decades. Subsyndromal delirium (SSD) was first described by Lipowski [26], who defined this type of confusional state by the presence of any core delirium symptom or severity scores on rating scales that are below the diagnostic threshold. Official diagnostic criteria for SSD are lacking up to now. DSM–IV recognizes subclinical presentations of delirium but does not distinguish between presentations that precede or follow delirium and presentations that never progress to delirium. However, this clinical syndrome has been extensively described in the geriatric literature. In a prospective study done by Cole and co-workers, 75% of the older (> 65 years) medical inpatients were diagnosed SSD positive [27]. Eight weeks after the SSD diagnosis, 48% of these patients still suffered from SSD. Patients who did not recover from SSD had a significant cognitive decline even 12 months after the

initial diagnosis compared with patients without SSD. In addition, the authors could show that SSD in the elderly falls on a continuum between no symptoms and DSM-defined delirium. The reported prevalence rates of SSD in ICU patients range from 30–50%. Ouimet and colleagues, who evaluated 600 patients with the ICDSC, showed for the first time that SSD is an outcome-relevant clinical syndrome in the critically ill [28]. Since the hazard ratio for mortality was not statistically significant when controlling for potential confounders, the associations (for SSD vs. no delirium) remained significant for ICU length of stay, hospital length of stay, and status following discharge from hospital. We were able to show similar results, by defining SSD with a Nu-DESC >1, which was an independent risk factor for not being discharged to home (defined as death during hospital stay or referral to other hospitals) [18]. These data increase the evidence that delirium, even in the critically ill, is a continuous rather than a categorical syndrome, from no delirium through subsyndromal delirium to clinical delirium, and one that is associated with adverse outcome. Furthermore, these results raised the question whether an assessment tool with a continuous instead of a categorical (or dichotomous) characterization of delirium would be more useful in clinical routine. Several studies demonstrated that the duration of ICU delirium is associated with mortality up to 1 year after ICU admission, even after adjusting for important potential confounders. Pisani and colleagues could show that each day of delirium in the ICU increases the hazard of mortality by 10% [29]. In addition, the results of a study by Heymann and co-workers revealed that patients whose delirium treatment was initiated within 24 h (immediate therapy) after delirium diagnosis had a significantly reduced mortality rate compared with patients with a delayed therapy (> 24 h) [30]. Therefore, it might be outcome-relevant to detect patients who are in a pre-delirious stage, because these patients will probably have a reduced duration of delirium or will even not develop "full-blown" delirium due to earlier treatment. Using a test detecting SSD may be especially useful in settings in which the caregiver–patient relationship is high and from which patients are discharged to settings with lower staffing levels. Except for the CAM-ICU, all validated delirium scores have an ordinal scale for grading severity of delirium symptoms. However, only the ICDSC and the Nu-DESC are explicitly validated for the measurement of SSD in the critically ill (Table 24.4).

Table 24.4 Characteristics of different validated assessment tools for ICU delirium.

Score	Items (n)	Binary	Numeric	Range per Item	Score	Validated for ICU-SSD
CAM-ICU	4	✔	∅	∅	∅	∅
ICDSC	8	✔	✔	0–1	0–8	✔
DDS	8	✔	✔	0,1,4,7	0–56	∅
NEECHAM	9	✔	✔	◆	0–30	∅
MDAS	10	✔	✔	0–3	0–30	∅
Nu-DESC	5	✔	✔	0–2	0–10	✔
CTD	5	✔	✔	0–6	0–30	∅
CTD-A	2	✔	✔	◆	0–24	∅

Studies that did not include a reference rater within the validation process are not mentioned in this table with regards to the detection of ICU-SSD. Binary, binary result diagnoses delirium; Numeric, numeric result diagnoses delirium (defined cut-off); Item, numeric range of each item; Score, numeric range of the score; ◆, items are not counted equally for the test; ✔, applies; ∅, does not apply.
CAM-ICU, Confusion Assessment Method for the ICU; ICDSC, Intensive Care Delirium Screening Checklist; DDS, Delirium Detection Score; MDAS, Memorial Delirium Assessment Scale; Nu-DESC, Nursing Delirium Screening Scale; CTD, Cognitive Test for Delirium; CTD-A, Abbreviated Cognitive Test for Delirium.

The ICDSC as well as the DDS, the NEECHAM, and the MDAS have at least 8 items; the DDS has the largest numeric range from 0 to 56 points. Validated scales that include a variety of different delirium symptoms with a large numeric range may have the potential to guide and monitor pharmacological treatment.

Agitation and pain assessment in the critically ill

In a cross-sectional analytic survey, patients considered pain as the most important physical stressor in the ICU [31]. In particular procedural pain is managed for less than 25% of the patients adequately [32]. Although implementation rates of routine pain assessment up to 80% are reported, the use of appropriate and validated scores for pain measurement is even lower [33]. Chanques and colleagues could show that validity and feasibility of pain assessments varies significantly between different self-report scales; the administrator of the Numeric Rating Scale (NRS) must be sure to provide a scale that is clearly readable [34]. The Behavioral Pain Scale (BPS) is validated for pain assessment in mechanically ventilated ICU patients. However, because the BPS seems to underestimate higher intensity pain, a self-report with the NRS should always be the preferred choice of assessment tool. Unfortunately, using self-report scales is not always possible in non-intubated patients with altered neurological status or delirium. Even if the patient is answering, you cannot be sure that he understands the scale. For these kinds of scenarios the BPS was adapted and validated for non-intubated patients (BPS-NI) [35].

Having pain in the ICU is a significant risk factor for developing delirium [36]. Patients can even show symptoms of delirium-like agitation (hyperactive or mixed delirium), tachycardia or hypertension, due to persistent pain. In a randomized controlled trial among patients with severe dementia, the intervention group, who received individual treatment of pain, had significantly reduced agitation levels compared with the control group [37]. Even though in this study, groups did not differ significantly for activities of daily living or cognition, agitation among non-delirious, critically ill patients is associated with a higher risk of mortality [38]. Therefore, delirium management must include a routine pain assessment with a valid scale. If a patient is scored as delirious, other factors like severe pain (BPS > 5 or NRS > 4) should be excluded or treated if necessary, before starting any pharmacological treatment with antipsychotics. Pain and delirium management are both substantial parts of an evidence-based, multifactorial approach in treating the critically ill.

Implementation of routine delirium screening in the ICU and consequences for the patients' outcome

The availability of a valid assessment instrument is the key component of any systematic strategy to manage delirium in the ICU.

It is likely due to the high prevalence and worse outcome associated with the development of ICU delirium that published articles in this field increased significantly (increase of 5.17 per year) compared to the relative paucity of work in the last decade (increase of 0.87 per year) [2]. Moreover, an increasing number of clinical studies are including delirium as a primary or secondary endpoint. However, national and international surveys could demonstrate a significant discordance between the perceived importance of delirium in the ICU and the practices of delirium monitoring and treatment, with a lack especially regarding the implementation of valid assessment tools. A survey (2006/2007) distributed to 1384 ICU practitioners in North America revealed that more than half (59%) screened for delirium but only 20% of the respondents (n = 258) used a valid delirium assessment tool [39]. A recent European survey revealed a slight increase of the implementation rate of routine delirium monitoring in ICU patients with a specific assessment tool (44%) [33]. These studies show the right trend of increasing awareness to use validated delirium scores in the clinical routine. With the rising use of these instruments more studies will hopefully use delirium as an endpoint in their future clinical trials. Specifically, with regards to the high risk for long-term cognitive impairment after delirium, this endpoint may be more predictive than e.g., ICU length of stay in describing patients' outcome.

The implementation of a valid delirium assessment tool in daily practice significantly increases the detection rate of delirium and the number of patients that receive treatment with haloperidol, even though, after implementation of the CAM-ICU, the individual cumulative doses and the duration of administered haloperidol decreases significantly.

Although intervention programs have been shown to reduce length of hospitalization and mortality when performed in patients outside the ICU [25], there is currently a deficit of evidence demonstrating that a systematic assessment of delirium in ICU patients improves outcome. This probably is due to the fact that numerous prospective intervention and observational studies did not include monitoring and concepts with individual treatment goals for analgesia and sedation. Data regarding the assessment and the management of sedation and analgesia in the ICU reveal that a large proportion of patients are not assessed while receiving treatment for sedation or for analgesia. In a study among 1,360 ICU patients, specific instruments for measuring both sedation and pain in the same patient were used only for 28% of patients [32]. Over 40% of the assessed patients were in a deep state of sedation. Midazolam, which was the most commonly used agent for sedation in this study (70%), was the most consistent and significant predictor of transitioning into delirium. Implementing delirium monitoring in this kind of setting without changing analgesia and sedation practices will probably not result in any significant outcome improvement for the patient. Skrobik and colleagues evaluated the impact of a combined approach including protocolized analgesia, sedation, and delirium management on patient outcome. This combination of protocol implementation significantly reduced the rate of medication-induced coma, sedation levels, the prevalence of delirium and SSD, the duration of mechanical ventilation, ICU, and hospital length of stay. In addition, the percent of patients able to go home increased. These results underline that preventing delirium requires the implementation of a core model of care that combines evidence-based practices: **A**wakening and **B**reathing Coordination, attention to the **C**hoice of Sedation, **D**elirium monitoring, and **E**arly mobility and exercise (ABCDE) [40].

According to the increasing evidence towards integrating a multidisciplinary approach to the management of the critically ill, we developed the following algorithm: all patients receive delirium monitoring with a valid and reliable delirium score for the ICU every 8 hours. If the patient is scored delirium-positive, a symptom-oriented therapy should be initiated. If the patient is not delirious, scoring should be repeated after 8 hours. When delirium scoring cannot be performed and/or RASS < −2 or > +2, the sedation goal should be re-evaluated and/or the sedation level should be adjusted to the target RASS. More importantly, a symptom-oriented pharmacotherapy should only be initiated after exclusion of an insufficient or inadequate sedation and/or analgesia for this patient. If symptoms of delirium persist, pharmacotherapy

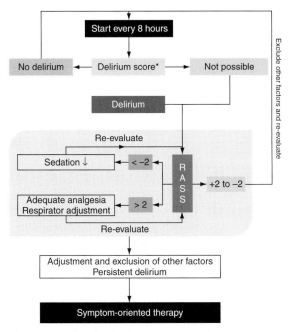

Figure 24.1 Algorithm for the management of intensive care unit (ICU) delirium. Delirium score refers to a valid and reliable score for the ICU, e.g., CAM-ICU, ICDSC, Nu-DESC etc. See text for details. RASS, Richmond Agitation–Sedation Scale.

should be started within the first 24 hours after the first diagnosis of delirium [30]. In cases of agitation, pain management and ventilator settings should be checked and optimized. In some circumstances, delirium monitoring may not be possible despite a RASS of ≥ −2; in that case, staff members should exclude other confounders, such as deaf-muteness or the patient not being familiar with the official language. The suggestion to screen for delirium every 8 hours is due to the fluctuating nature of delirium symptoms over the period of 1 day (Figure 24.1).

References

1. Lipowski ZJ. Delirium, clouding of consciousness and confusion. *J Nerv Ment Dis* 1967;**145**:227–55.

2. Morandi A, Pandharipande P, Trabucchi M, *et al.* Understanding international differences in terminology for delirium and other types of acute brain dysfunction in critically ill patients. *Intensive Care Med* 2008;**34**:1907–15.

3. Devlin JW, Fong JJ, Schumaker G, *et al.* Use of a validated delirium assessment tool improves the ability of physicians to identify delirium in medical intensive care unit patients. *Crit Care Med* 2007;**35**:2721–4.

4. Jacobi J, Fraser GL, Coursin DB, *et al.* Clinical practice guidelines for the sustained use of sedatives and analgesics in the critically ill adult. *Crit Care Med* 2002;**30**:119–41.

5. Martin J, Heymann A, Bäsell K, *et al.* Evidence and consensus-based German guidelines for the management of analgesia, sedation and delirium in intensive care – short version. *Ger Med Sci* 2010;**8**: Doc02.

6. Young J, Murthy L, Westby M, *et al.* Diagnosis, prevention, and management of delirium: summary of NICE guidance. *Br Med J* 2010;**341**:c3704.

7. Ely EW, Inouye SK, Bernard GR, *et al.* Delirium in mechanically ventilated patients: validity and reliability of the confusion assessment method for the intensive care unit (CAM-ICU). *JAMA* 2001;**286**:2703–10.

8. Laurila JV, Pitkala KH, Strandberg TE, *et al.* The impact of different diagnostic criteria on prevalence rates for delirium. *Dement Geriatr Cogn Disord* 2003;**16**:156–62.

9. Luetz A, Radtke FM, Franck M, *et al.* [The nursing delirium screening scale (NU-DESC)]. *Anasthesiol Intensivmed Notfallmed Schmerzther* 2008;**43**:98–102.

10. Wild D, Grove A, Martin M, *et al.* Principles of good practice for the translation and cultural adaptation process for patient-reported outcomes (PRO) measures: report of the ISPOR Task Force for Translation and Cultural Adaptation. *Value Health* 2005;**8**:94–104.

11. Hart RP, Best AM, Sessler CN, *et al.* Abbreviated cognitive test for delirium. *J Psychosom Res* 1997;**43**:417–23.

12. Ely EW, Margolin R, Francis J, *et al.* Evaluation of delirium in critically ill patients: validation of the confusion assessment method for the intensive care unit (CAM-ICU). *Crit Care Med* 2001;**29**:1370–9.

13. van Eijk MM, Slooter AJ. Duration of ICU delirium, severity of the underlying disease, and mortality. *Am J Respir Crit Care Med* 2010;**181**:419–20.

14. Bergeron N, Dubois MJ, Dumont M, *et al.* Intensive care delirium screening checklist: evaluation of a new screening tool. *Intensive Care Med* 2001;**27**:859–64.

15. George C, Nair JS, Ebenezer JA, *et al.* Validation of the Intensive Care Delirium Screening Checklist in nonintubated intensive care unit patients in a resource-poor medical intensive care setting in South India. *J Crit Care* 2011;**26**:138–43.

16. van Eijk MM, van Marum RJ, Klijn IA, *et al.* Comparison of delirium assessment tools in a mixed intensive care unit. *Crit Care Med* 2009;**37**:1881–5.

17. Otter H, Martin J, Bäsell K, *et al.* Validity and reliability of the DDS for severity of delirium in the ICU. *Neurocrit Care* 2005;**2**:150–8.

18. Luetz A, Heymann A, Radtke FM, *et al.* Different assessment tools for intensive care unit delirium: which score to use? *Crit Care Med* 2010;**38**:409–18.

19. Gaudreau JD, Gagnon P, Harel F, *et al.* Fast, systematic, and continuous delirium assessment in hospitalized patients: the nursing delirium screening scale. *J Pain Symptom Manage* 2005;**29**:368–75.

20. Csokasy J. Assessment of acute confusion: use of the NEECHAM confusion scale. *Appl Nurs Res* 1999;**12**:51–5.

21. Immers HE, Schuurmans MJ, van de Bijl JJ. Recognition of delirium in ICU patients: a diagnostic study of the NEECHAM confusion scale in ICU patients. *BMC Nurs* 2005;**4**:7.

22. Breitbart W, Rosenfeld B, Roth A, *et al.* The Memorial Delirium Assessment Scale. *J Pain Symptom Manage* 1997;**13**:128–37.

23. Shyamsundar G, Raghuthaman G, Rajkumar AP, *et al.* Validation of Memorial Delirium Assessment Scale. *J Crit Care* 2009;**24**:530–4.

24. Devlin JW, Marquis F, Riker RR, *et al.* Combined didactic and scenario-based education improves the ability of intensive care unit staff to recognize delirium at the bedside. *Crit Care* 2008;**12**:R19.

25. Lundström M, Edlund A, Karlsson S, *et al.* A multifactorial intervention program reduces the duration of delirium, length of hospitalization, and mortality in delirious patients. *J Am Geriatr Soc* 2005;**53**:622–8.

26. Lipowski ZJ. Transient cognitive disorders (delirium, acute confusional states) in the elderly. *Am J Psychiatry* 1983;**140**:1426–36.

27. Cole MG, McCusker J, Ciampi A, Belzile E. The 6- and 12-month outcomes of older medical inpatients who recover from subsyndromal delirium. *J Am Geriatr Soc* 2008;**56**:2093–9.

28. Ouimet S, Riker R, Bergeron N, *et al.* Subsyndromal delirium in the ICU: evidence for a disease spectrum. *Intensive Care Med* 2007;**33**:1007–13.

29. Pisani MA, Kong SY, Kasl SV, *et al.* Days of delirium are associated with 1-year mortality in an older intensive care unit population. *Am J Respir Crit Care Med* 2009;**180**:1092–7.

30. Heymann A, Radtke F, Schiemann A, *et al.* Delayed treatment of delirium increases mortality rate in intensive care unit patients. *J Int Med Res* 2010;**38**:1584–95.

31. Novaes MA, Aronovich A, Ferraz MB, *et al.* Stressors in ICU: patients' evaluation. *Intensive Care Med* 1997;**23**:1282–5.

32. Payen JF, Chanques G, Mantz J, *et al.* Current practices in sedation and analgesia for mechanically ventilated critically ill patients: a prospective multicenter patient-based study. *Anesthesiology* 2007;**106**:687–95.

33. Luetz A, Balzer F, Radtke F, *et al.* International multicenter study one day prevalence observational study for delirium on ICU (IMPROVE-ICU). *Intensive Care Med* 2011;**37**:254.

34. Chanques G, Viel E, Constantin JM, *et al.* The measurement of pain in intensive care unit: comparison of 5 self-report intensity scales. *Pain* 2010;**151**:711–21.

35. Chanques G, Payen JF, Mercier G, *et al.* Assessing pain in non-intubated critically ill patients unable to self report: an adaptation of the behavioral pain scale. *Intensive Care Med* 2009;**35**:2060–7.

36. Ouimet S, Kavanagh BP, Gottfried SB, *et al.* Incidence, risk factors and consequences of ICU delirium. *Intensive Care Med* 2007;**33**:66–73.

37. Husebo BS, Ballard C, Sandvik R, *et al.* Efficacy of treating pain to reduce behavioural disturbances in residents of nursing homes with dementia: cluster randomised clinical trial. *Br Med J* 2011;**343**:d4065.

38. Marquis F, Ouimet S, Riker R, *et al.* Individual delirium symptoms: do they matter? *Crit Care Med* 2007;**35**:2533–7.

39. Patel RP, Gambrell M, Speroff T, *et al.* Delirium and sedation in the intensive care unit: survey of behaviors and attitudes of 1384 healthcare professionals. *Crit Care Med* 2009;**37**:825–32.

40. Vasilevskis EE, Pandharipande PP, Girard TD, *et al.* A screening, prevention, and restoration model for saving the injured brain in intensive care unit survivors. *Crit Care Med* 2010;**38**:S683–91.

41. Lin SM, Liu CY, Wang CH, *et al.* The impact of delirium on the survival of mechanically ventilated patients. *Crit Care Med* 2004;**32**:2254–9.

42. Guenther U, Popp J, Koecher L, *et al.* Validity and reliability of the CAM-ICU flowsheet to diagnose delirium in surgical ICU patients. *J Crit Care* 2010;**25**:144–51.

43. van Eijk MM, van den Boogaard M, van Marum RJ, *et al.* Routine use of the Confusion Assessment Method for the Intensive Care Unit: a multicenter study. *Am J Respir Crit Care Med* 2011;**184**:340–4.

44. Hart RP, Levenson JL, Sessler CN, *et al.* Validation of a cognitive test for delirium in medical ICU patients. *Psychosomatics* 1996;**37**:533–46.

Chapter 25

Electroencephalography and evoked potentials in critically ill patients

Matthew A. Koenig and Peter W. Kaplan

SUMMARY

Electrophysiological testing of the central nervous system (CNS) remains an important diagnostic tool in critically ill patients. Rather than producing static images of the brain and spinal cord, somatosensory evoked potentials (SSEP) and electroencephalography (EEG) measure electrical surrogates of neurological function in real time. An electroencephalogram continuously measures and displays voltage differences between pairs of scalp electrodes, while SSEP measures evoked conduction of an electrical stimulus along the sensory pathway. In critically ill patients with limited neurological exams and inability to safely transport for radiographic studies, SSEP and EEG can provide an important window into brain function. In addition, real-time measurement of changes in brain electrical activity can allow continuous monitoring for response to therapeutic interventions, secondary injury, and state-dependent changes. The primary indications for EEG and SSEP in critically ill patients are: monitoring for seizure activity in high-risk populations, differentiation between metabolic encephalopathy and non-convulsive status epilepticus (NCSE) as a cause of altered mental status, monitoring of anesthetic depth, prognostication after global brain injuries, and determination of brain death. Continuous monitoring of EEG allows rapid, remote detection of clinically silent seizure activity, which has been demonstrated to occur frequently in patients with severe traumatic brain injury, global anoxic injury, and unexplained coma. For therapeutic interventions for intracranial hypertension or refractory status epilepticus, continuous EEG monitoring is also important for defining therapeutic targets such as seizure suppression and burst-suppression. The SSEP has become an important adjunctive prognostic tool, especially in comatose survivors of cardiac arrest. In this population, bilateral absence of cortical potentials has nearly 100% specificity for poor outcomes. The intensive care unit (ICU) provides a number of challenges to acquisition and interpretation of electrophysiological signals. In particular, differentiation between non-convulsive seizures, metabolic encephalopathy patterns, and injury patterns in patients with diffuse brain injuries can be especially difficult to distinguish from one another. The ICU also provides an abundance of sources of electrical interference which can produce artifacts.

Introduction

Electrophysiological testing of the CNS provides a window into the otherwise black box of the human brain during critical illness. Although advanced imaging with CT angiography and MRI have largely supplanted electrophysiological testing for diagnosing structural brain lesions, these methods still carry some advantages for specific disease states. For unstable patients with critical illness, electrophysiological testing can be performed at the bedside without having to transport the patient to a testing facility. The signal can also be analyzed and interpreted remotely from the ICU. Rather than producing static images of brain structure, electrophysiological testing allows for real-time and continuous assessment of brain function. Changes in brain signal can be measured over time as a means of gauging response to therapeutic interventions, recovery of brain function, or progression of brain injury.

Electrophysiological testing can also provide an objective measure of brain reactivity to the outside world – an indirect measure of consciousness. As a tool to measure brain function, electrophysiological testing is best viewed as a complementary method to imaging, laboratory testing, and bedside clinical assessment. As reviewed in this chapter, electrophysiological testing

Brain Disorders in Critical Illness, ed. Robert D. Stevens, Tarek Sharshar, and E. Wesley Ely. Published by Cambridge University Press. © Cambridge University Press 2013.

in critical illness falls into five main categories – monitoring for seizure activity in high-risk populations, differentiation between metabolic encephalopathy and NCSE as a cause of altered mental status, monitoring of anesthetic depth, prognostication after global brain injury, and determination of brain death [1]. This chapter is meant to be a practical review of each of these categories, focusing entirely on electroencephalography and somatosensory evoked potentials. Although additional electrophysiological testing has been studied using brainstem auditory evoked potentials and cognitive event-related potentials, these topics are beyond the scope of this chapter.

Electroencephalography is the mainstay of electrophysiological testing of the brain, especially for seizure detection, monitoring depth of anesthesia, and diagnosing metabolic encephalopathy. Standard EEG employs a series of surface electrodes cemented to the scalp or needle electrodes inserted subcutaneously. For deeper detection and localization of small seizure foci, depth electrodes can also be placed into the brain or subdural grid electrodes placed directly over the surface of the brain. For routine use in critically ill patients, invasive electrode placement is rarely required. An EEG detects the difference in voltage between sequential pairs of electrodes placed in standard positions along the scalp or between these electrodes and a common reference electrode. Electrical signal is then recorded and displayed in real time, allowing subjective assessment of amplitude, frequency, reactivity, and organization of electrical activity of the brain, as well as detection of abnormal patterns of electrical activity such as triphasic waves, epileptiform discharges, and seizures [2]. In a normal, awake patient, the background rhythm is usually highly organized with a prominent posterior basic rhythm. The normal alpha rhythm in adults usually lies between 8.5 and 12 Hz (see Figure 25.1). With increasing degrees of encephalopathy, the background rhythm becomes less sustained, more disorganized, of higher amplitude with lower frequency. The EEG signal should also be analyzed for side to side differences, e.g., disorganization and slowing on one side can indicate focal brain injury. In encephalopathic patients, it is also important to look for signs of reactivity to the environment. When the eyes are opened, the posterior basic rhythm often suppresses – becoming of lower amplitude and higher frequency. When the eyes are closed again, the posterior basic rhythm should become more prominent. A noxious stimulus should also produce lower amplitude, higher frequency brain activity. The ability of the brain to

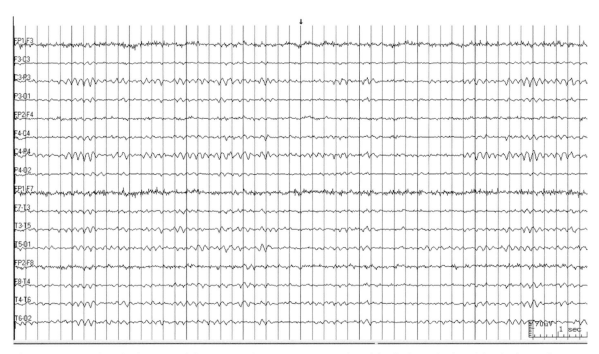

Figure 25.1 Normal awake electroencephalogram (EEG) showing a posterior waking alpha rhythm with relatively less background evident over the frontal regions.

respond to outside stimuli is seen as a surrogate for consciousness. Finally, the pattern of EEG activity should be analyzed over time, looking for spontaneous EEG changes, periodic electrical activity and discharges, and epileptiform discharges. Differentiation between seizure activity and frequent periodic waves is discussed in greater detail below.

The SSEP is similar to EEG in that it measures cortical activity via surface electrodes placed on the scalp or subcutaneous needle electrodes. The SSEP assesses the brain's response to a sensory stimulus via an electrical impulse generated along the median nerve at the wrist. That stimulus then travels along the nerve, through the brachial plexus, up the spinothalamic tract of the spinal cord, through the brainstem, and into the thalamus where it is relayed to the primary sensory cortex. This electrical signal can be detected at various points along the sensory pathways using surface electrodes placed at Erb's Point, over the brachial plexus, along the spinal cord, and on the contralateral scalp. The Erb's Point potential is a quality control measure to determine whether the initial stimulus was of high enough voltage to be transmitted into the central nervous system, that the peripheral nerve conduction is intact, and the velocity of conduction along the peripheral nerve is normal. This measurement is especially important in patients being treated with induced hypothermia, which slows or blocks peripheral nerve conduction, and those with systemic trauma that can cause nerve root avulsion. In normal humans, the latency of conduction is about 16 ms to the brainstem, 18 ms to the thalamus, and 20 ms to the primary sensory cortex. By convention, electrical signal directed upwards from the baseline is referred to as a negative deflection (abbreviated N) and signal below the baseline is called a positive deflection (abbreviated P). Using this naming convention, the cortical signal is termed N20, denoting a negative deflection occurring at about 20 ms after stimulation. In awake patients, after the N20, there is usually a series of negative and positive deflections (P25, N35, and N70) that reflect intra cortical and cortico-thalamo-cortical secondary processing of the stimulus (see Figure 25.2). As with EEG reactivity, this "higher" level processing – referred to as middle or longer latency potentials – may be an indirect measure of the brain's conscious response to stimulation. In patients with greater degrees of encephalopathy (for example, after cardiac arrest), these middle latency potentials are delayed or lost. In progressive brain injury, the primary cortical responses (N20) may also be lost, with signal truncating at the thalamus, brainstem, or spinal cord. The SSEP is commonly used for intraoperative monitoring to provide an early warning

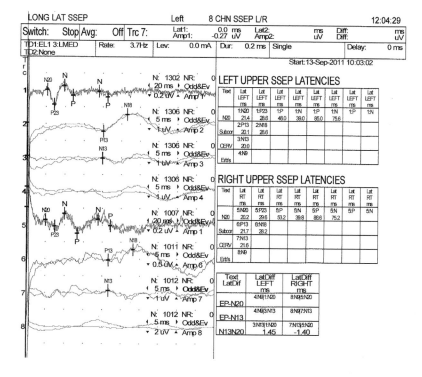

Figure 25.2 This somatosensory evoked potential (SSEP) shows long latency responses in channels 1 and 4 after the N20. Earlier peaks for the N13, P13. N18 are seen in channels 2, 3, 4 and 6, 7, 8. Please note that the timescale for these channels is different, and is at 20 ms/cm vs. 5 ms/cm in the other channels. Channels 1 and 4 show cortical N20 responses, while channels 2 and 5 show subcortical N18 responses. The long latency channels (1 and 4) also reveal responses at about 35 ms – the N35 (labeled as the N after N20) and an N70 (labeled as the second N after N20). These are better developed on the right (in channel 4 of channels 4 through 8). N70s are reported to represent evidence of cognitive processing, and when present after cardiac arrest and anoxia, indicate a favorable prognosis.

system for inadvertent nervous tissue injury during surgery. Although continuous SSEP has been used in an analogous fashion in the ICU, its primary use at this point is for prognostication after global brain injury [2].

Monitoring for electrographic seizures

The primary use for EEG monitoring – either routine studies or continuous monitoring – in the ICU is to detect clinically occult seizure activity. For critically ill patients with unexplained encephalopathy or coma, in particular, EEG monitoring is frequently undertaken to evaluate for NCSE. Convulsive seizures are generally clinically apparent, except if the patient is being treated with a paralytic agent to facilitate ventilatory support or suppress shivering during induced hypothermia. Non-convulsive status epilepticus, on the other hand, may produce subtle clinical signs such as unexplained tachycardia, exaggerated hippus, gaze deviation or spontaneous nystagmus, tachypnea, abnormal posturing, or bruxism [1]. These signs may also be present in a variety of brain injuries, therefore requiring EEG to exclude seizure activity. If EEG is recorded to evaluate a specific movement – for example, extensor posturing and gaze deviation – a routine, 20-minute study may be sufficient to capture several of these movements and definitively exclude seizure activity. If, instead, EEG recording is undertaken to exclude clinically occult seizures as a cause of persistent encephalopathy, longer recordings (24–72 hours) may need to be undertaken [3]. The presence of clinically apparent convulsive seizures, however, does not exclude subsequent non-convulsive seizures as a cause of failure to recover post-ictally. In other words, just because the initial seizure was convulsive, the absence of ongoing convulsive movements does not prove that the patient is not having seizures, or is not in status epilepticus. In a study of patients who did not awaken shortly after a convulsive seizure, EEG monitoring detected subsequent non-convulsive seizures in 48% and ongoing NCSE in 14% [1].

Distinguishing electrographic seizures in NCSE from other periodic EEG patterns – such as periodic epileptiform discharges (PEDs), bilateral periodic epileptiform discharges (BiPEDs), and triphasic waves (TWs) – can be very challenging. This is especially true in patients with underlying brain injuries and/or severe metabolic derangements, in whom periodic EEG patterns are common [4]. The injured brain may not be able to mount well-organized, 3 Hz

generalized spike-wave complexes like the uninjured, epileptic brain. In some cases, rhythmic slowing, burst-suppression patterns, and generalized, rhythmic delta activity may represent seizures. In other words, determining which EEG patterns *cause* brain injury and which are a *marker* of existing brain injury is difficult. For this reason, criteria have been proposed for defining electrographic seizures in NCSE. These criteria require at least one of three primary criteria: (1) repetitive generalized or focal spikes, sharp waves, spike-and-wave, or sharp-and-slow complexes at ≥ 3 Hz; (2) repetitive generalized or focal spikes, sharp waves, spike-and-wave, or sharp-and-slow complexes at a frequency of < 3 Hz and the secondary criterion; or (3) sequential rhythmic, periodic, or quasi-periodic waves ≥ 1 Hz and unequivocal evolution in frequency (incrementing and decrementing over time), morphology, or location and the secondary criterion. The secondary criterion is clinical improvement or emergence of normal, organized background EEG activity in response to benzodiazepine or other anticonvulsant drug administration [5].

The incidence of NCSE differs depending on the population of patients being studied. This can be largely divided into those with known epilepsy or admission for a primary brain injury and those being treated for a systemic critical illness – such as multi-organ failure or sepsis – who secondarily develop unexplained encephalopathy, coma, or NCSE. In a general ICU population with coma and no overt signs of seizure activity, a 30-minute EEG recording captured epileptiform discharges in 5% of patients and electrographic seizure activity in an additional 8% of patients [6]. More prolonged EEG monitoring yields a higher incidence of electrographic seizures, however. In one large, single institution study of ICU patients referred for continuous EEG monitoring, 19% of patients were found to have electrographic seizures, 92% of which were not accompanied by convulsions [3]. Patients at highest risk for seizures were those in coma, under age 18 years, or with known epilepsy or previously documented convulsive seizures during the hospitalization. In 88% of patients with electrographic seizures, ≤ 24 hours of EEG monitoring was sufficient to identify seizure activity. However, 48–72 hours of EEG monitoring was necessary to identify the remaining 12%. Delayed detection of seizures was more common in comatose patients (20%) compared with non-comatose patients (5%) [3]. These data must be interpreted with caution, however, because the denominator reflects patients for whom EEG monitoring was requested – in whom seizures were presumably suspected – rather than all-comers with encephalopathy associated with critical illness. In larger studies of EEG recordings in a general ICU population, the incidence of electrographic seizure activity has been reported at only 0.8% [5]. In patients admitted to the ICU for primary brain injuries, the incidence of electrographic seizure activity may be higher. Among high-grade subarachnoid hemorrhage patients, the incidence of electrographic seizures on continuous EEG monitoring is as high as 19%, most of which is NCSE [1]. In spontaneous intracerebral hemorrhage and traumatic brain injury (TBI), ~20% of patients who underwent continuous EEG monitoring had electrographic seizures [1]. Some examples of EEGs showing NCSE are given in Figures 25.3–25.6.

Evaluation for metabolic encephalopathy

Hepatic encephalopathy is the best characterized metabolic derangement that produces altered mentation along with a characteristic pattern of EEG activity. In actuality, metabolic derangements sufficient to produce severe encephalopathy, coma, and EEG dysfunction can be produced by a variety of conditions, including uremic kidney failure, hypo- or hyperglycemia, electrolyte derangements like hyponatremia and hypocalcemia, sepsis, and sedative drug intoxication [1]. Progressive metabolic encephalopathy is associated with a characteristic evolution of EEG activity. Focusing on liver failure, subclinical encephalopathy may be associated with higher amplitude frontal beta activity – also seen after administration of benzodiazepines and barbiturates. As liver function worsens, there is progressive slowing and increasing disorganization of background EEG, with an initial increase followed by a decrease in EEG amplitude [7]. Encephalopathy is associated with the emergence of triphasic waves, which are bilaterally synchronous bursts of complexes with three phases: an initial negative deflection, followed by a positive deflection, then another negative deflection (Figure 25.6). The duration of triphasic complexes is between 300–600 ms. Triphasic waves typically have a characteristic frontal predominance and an anterior-posterior (A-P) lag, in which the complexes occur slightly later in more posterior electrodes [8]. As hepatic encephalopathy worsens, resulting in diffuse cerebral edema and elevated intracranial pressure, triphasic waves may be replaced by generalized, low-voltage slowing, followed by a discontinuous pattern (burst-suppression), followed by electrical silence [7]. Although initially

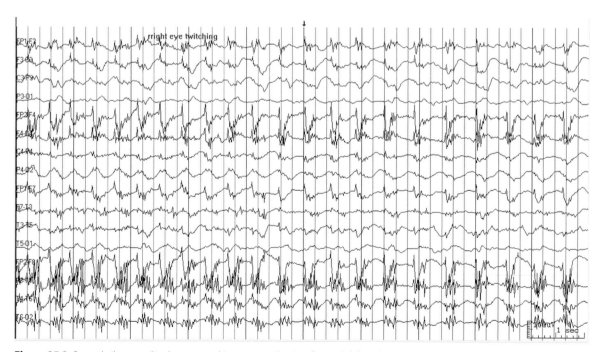

Figure 25.3 Secondarily generalized non-convulsive status epilepticus from a left frontal origin.

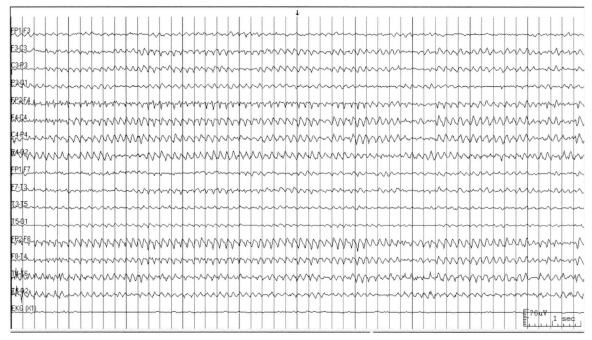

Figure 25.4 The beginning of high frequency buildup of right frontal 9 Hz rhythmic activity initiating right frontal NCSE in the form of cyclic seizures without return to baseline.

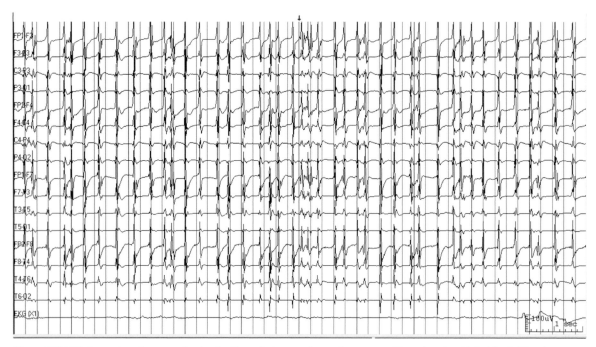

Figure 25.5 Waxing and waning generalized epileptiform discharges after cardiac arrest and hypothermia with facial twitching that lie along the ictal-interictal continuum. The relatively high frequency and evolution would lean towards electrographic status.

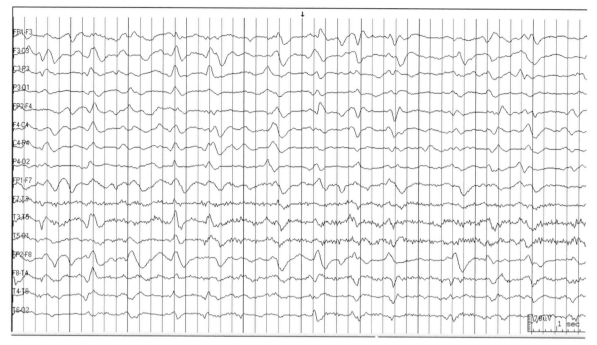

Figure 25.6 Triphasic waves with a metabolic encephalopathy. Note maximum in the fronto-central region. This case shows anterior–posterior phase lag of the triphasic waves.

characterized in hepatic encephalopathy, triphasic waves can also be encountered in other causes of metabolic encephalopathy.

Electroencephalographic monitoring in patients with suspected hepatic encephalopathy can be important to establish the clinical diagnosis of metabolic encephalopathy, exclude alternative causes like NCSE, monitor for worsening encephalopathy, and monitor for response to therapeutic interventions. In a patient with clinically suspected hepatic encephalopathy, the presence of classic triphasic waves can be strong evidence that liver failure is the cause of the patient's altered mentation. As alluded to above, TWs share many features of epileptiform discharges – including high amplitude activity that stands out from the baseline, a combination of sharply contoured components and slow waves, and a clinical background of altered mentation (Figure 25.6). In the right clinical context, triphasic waves may be difficult to distinguish from NCSE in the severely injured brain – i.e., end-stage status epilepticus or global anoxic brain injury, although TWs usually increase with noxious stimulation, while NCSE usually does not. In one study, TWs had slower frequency (< 2 Hz), greater A-P lag,

greater frontal predominance, a higher incidence of background slowing, and were more likely to increase in frequency in response to noxious stimulation. NCSE, on the other hand, had more frequent complexes (> 2 Hz), a higher incidence of polyspikes in addition to the classic triphasic pattern, and did not change in response to noxious stimulation [8]. Both EEG patterns may suppress after administration of benzodiazepines, which is why it is important to determine whether there is clinical improvement or return of normal EEG patterns before interpreting suppression of periodic complexes as evidence of NCSE. Even after TW regression from benzodiazepines, TWs may emerge on noxious stimulation. Complicating matters, metabolic derangements – including hepatic encephalopathy – are a significant risk factor for the development of NCSE. Metabolic encephalopathy and NCSE may also co-exist in the same patient. In one series, 21% of patients with a primary diagnosis of toxic-metabolic encephalopathy had electrographic seizures on continuous EEG monitoring. Conversely, 5–25% of patients with non-convulsive seizures had metabolic derangements as the most likely etiology of seizure activity [1].

Titration of anesthetic medications

The bispectral index (BIS) is a quantitative EEG measure sensitive to slowing and burst-suppression induced by anesthetic agents that is frequently used for intra-operative monitoring of sedation levels. Although EEG is not routinely used to monitor sedation in the ICU – in part because underlying brain abnormalities in critical illness contribute to EEG slowing and discontinuity – it is frequently used as a real-time monitor of anesthetic depth in specific cases [2]. Patients treated with pharmacological coma induced by anesthetic agents – typically, propofol and/or barbiturates – to suppress brain metabolism for treatment of refractory intracranial hypertension and refractory status epilepticus are routinely monitored with continuous EEG. In both of these disease states, the target for anesthetic infusion is to induce EEG burst-suppression (Figure 25.7). Burst-suppression is characterized by alternating periods of generalized electrical silence interrupted by generalized bursts of chaotic, sharply contoured wave forms of variable duration. Physiologically, burst-suppression is believed to be an intrinsic – possibly thalamic – rhythm that emerges with cortical suppression by anesthetic agents or global brain injury (as seen in comatose survivors of cardiac arrest). For metabolic suppression in intracranial

hypertension, anesthetic agents are typically titrated to maintain an initial target of 2–5 bursts per minute [9]. Practically speaking – depending on the duration of bursts – this is equivalent to 1 burst per screen of EEG signal using a standard 10-second epoch display. If ICP remains uncontrolled, deeper sedation may be employed. Because burst-suppression is usually a generalized phenomenon, a limited montage of electrodes may be sufficient to monitor depth of sedation for treatment of ICP crisis. The BIS monitor itself may be used in this scenario, titrating to a BIS of 6–15, while displaying the single-channel EEG signal on the bedside monitor to verify burst-suppression is present [9].

Titration of pharmacological coma for suppression of refractory status epilepticus can be more challenging and typically requires continuous monitoring of a full montage of EEG electrodes [2]. Close monitoring is necessary to confirm that breakthrough electrographic seizures do not occur. In some cases, epileptiform discharges characteristic of the patient's seizures may be admixed within the EEG bursts and subsequently persist into the suppression periods. The presence of breakthrough seizure activity is a risk factor for seizure recurrence after pharmacological coma is withdrawn [10]. In practice, most clinicians advocate for titration of anesthetic medications to

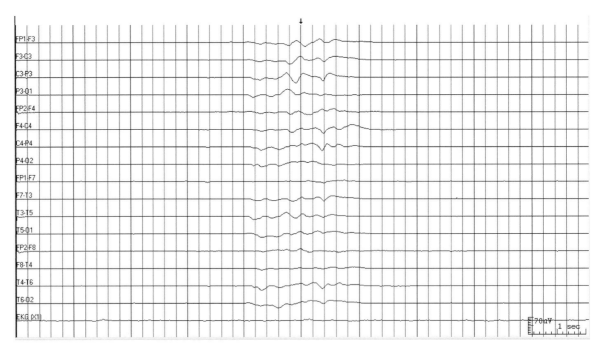

Figure 25.7 Burst-suppression pattern from anesthetic suppression in a patient with status epilepticus. Note 2-s polymorphic burst in the middle of the 10-second epoch. Background during suppression, here, is <5 uV.

induce burst-suppression of similar depth to that described above. Burst-suppression ensures an absence of breakthrough seizures and is more easily recognized by trained clinical staff than simple seizure suppression [10]. Prolonged use of anesthetic medications, however, is associated with high mortality and multiple systemic side effects, including immune suppression, deep venous thrombosis, ileus, and distributive shock [1]. For this reason, other clinicians advocate titration of anesthetic agents just to suppress electrographic seizures rather than to an arbitrary burst-suppression goal [10]. A recent small series found that mortality, seizure control, and outcomes were similar whether refractory status epilepticus patients were treated with pharmacological coma to produce burst-suppression or simple seizure suppression [11]. Although the optimal treatment target has not been defined, both therapeutic goals require continuous EEG monitoring during the entire period of pharmacological coma and anesthetic withdrawal [2].

Prognostication in comatose survivors of cardiac arrest

In addition to monitoring for seizure activity and providing a therapeutic target, electrophysiological recordings of the brain are also undertaken to determine the extent of brain injuries and help prognosticate. The EEG and SSEP have both been extensively studied as prognostic markers among initially comatose survivors of cardiac arrest. An EEG after cardiac arrest is given in Figure 25.5. Among cardiac arrest survivors who have successful return of spontaneous circulation, the majority are initially comatose. Induced moderate hypothermia for 24 hours has been demonstrated to improve neurological outcomes after out-of-hospital cardiac arrest due to ventricular tachycardia or ventricular fibrillation [12]. Induced hypothermia typically requires deep sedation with or without neuromuscular blockade to suppress shivering. During this period of induced hypothermia, the prognosis for neurological recovery remains unclear, but after the end of 24 hours of hypothermia, and on return to normal body temperature, the EEG and SSEP findings are valid. The sobering statistics are that < 10% of patients who are resuscitated from cardiac arrest leave the hospital alive and neurologically intact [12]. In many cases, patients survive cardiac arrest but remain in a persistent vegetative or minimally conscious state.

The American Academy of Neurology (AAN) recently reviewed the strength of evidence for reputed prognostic markers of brain recovery after cardiac arrest. They found strong evidence for the use of SSEP and weaker evidence for EEG as a specific marker of poor outcome (death or persistent vegetative state) after resuscitation from cardiac arrest [12]. A SSEP should be performed 1–3 days after resuscitation, because evoked potentials typically evolve during the first 24 hours. Studies performed too early in the recovery period may result in a falsely pessimistic prognosis. After 24 hours without hypothermia, the persistent bilateral absence of cortical N20 potentials on median nerve SSEP studies has nearly 100% specificity for poor outcome in comatose cardiac arrest survivors with a false positive rate of 0.7% (range 0–3.7%) [12]. Because hypothermia slows peripheral conduction of electrical stimuli, SSEP performed during the hypothermia must be interpreted with caution. Although some authors have assessed the prognostic value of the presence of normal N20 potentials and the presence of middle latency potentials for determining which patients will have good neurological recovery, no reliably specific marker has been identified at this point. Unfortunately, about 50% of patients with preserved N20 potentials still go on to have poor neurological outcomes. The AAN consensus statement relied entirely on prognostic studies performed prior to the widespread use of therapeutic hypothermia. Subsequently, a few small series have determined that the bilateral absence of N20 potentials remains a highly specific marker of poor outcome whether or not patients are treated with hypothermia, as long as the studies are done after rewarming [13].

The EEG has also been extensively studied as a prognostic marker after cardiac arrest, but the ability to perform meta-analyses on the resulting data has been confounded by the variety of grading schemes used in individual studies. Most studies describe a series of malignant EEG patterns after cardiac arrest, including generalized EEG suppression (Figure 25.8), burst-suppression, alpha- or theta-coma (Figure 25.9), and NCSE patterns (Figures 25.2, 25.3, and 25.4) [12]. Alpha- and theta-coma refer to patterns of unwavering, generalized alpha (8–12 Hz) (Figure 25.9) or theta (4–7 Hz) activity that is present in all leads and has no variability in response to external stimulation. As with SSEP, EEG patterns evolve during the first 24 hours of recovery from cardiac arrest. If EEG is performed early enough, most patients progress from electrocerebral

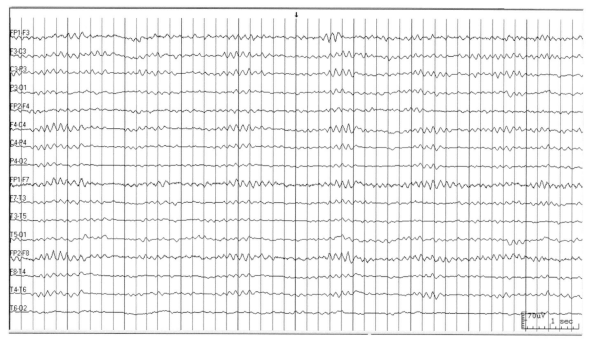

Figure 25.8 This recording shows diffuse 9–10 Hz activity, better seen in the anterior head regions in a comatose patient after cardiac arrest. Such an electroencephalographic (EEG) tracing is referred to as an *alpha-coma* pattern.

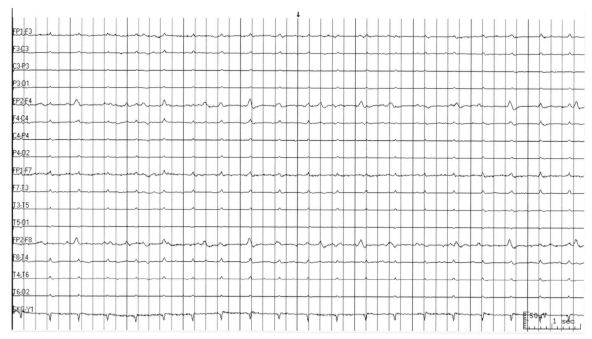

Figure 25.9 Electrocerebral inactivity after cardiac arrest. Electrocardiogram (ECG) and ballisto-cardiographic artifact can be seen, temporally marked by the bottom ECG channel.

silence through a period of burst-suppression prior to regaining continuous, reactive EEG patterns. To a much greater extent than SSEP, EEG is also heavily influenced by use of sedative agents during induction of hypothermia. For these reasons, use of EEG for prognostic purposes should be delayed at least 24 hours until the patient is at normal body temperature. In the AAN consensus statement, the malignant patterns of EEG activity were strongly associated with poor outcomes after cardiac arrest, but they had an unacceptably high false positive rate of 3% (range 0.9–11%) and were not included in the final prognostic algorithm [12]. Like SSEP, EEG is more accurate at determining poor prognosis rather than good prognosis for recovery. In a recent small series of cardiac arrest survivors treated with hypothermia, however, the presence of subjectively determined EEG reactivity was noted in 19/19 survivors – 14 of whom went on to have favorable neurological outcomes – and only 3/15 non-survivors [14]. In addition to prognostication, EEG monitoring is also undertaken to diagnose NCSE after cardiac arrest. Continuous EEG monitoring is especially important in patients being treated with induced hypothermia who require continuous neuromuscular blockade to suppress shivering because of its potential to mask convulsive seizures. In addition, postanoxic myoclonic jerks – a marker of severe brain injury – may be difficult to distinguish from seizures. When continuous EEG monitoring was undertaken in cardiac arrest survivors being treated with hypothermia, NCSE was identified in 12% of patients, the majority of which began within 12 hours of resuscitation [15]. The significance of NCSE is unclear, however, because the prognosis for survival and recovery remains poor whether or not seizures are aggressively treated [15].

Prognostication in severe traumatic brain injury

Although EEG is not well validated as a prognostic tool in severe traumatic brain injury, SSEP has been extensively studied in this population. Similar to data in cardiac arrest survivors, bilateral absence of cortical N20 potentials in comatose TBI patients has been reported to have nearly 100% specificity for poor outcomes (death or persistent vegetative state) at 6 months [16]. On the other hand, presence of N20 potentials alone has poor specificity for good neurological outcomes [16]. In a recent meta-analysis, as a

single prognostic marker of both good and bad outcomes, SSEP performed better than pupillary light reflexes, Glasgow Coma Scale (GCS), CT findings, and EEG [17]. The authors again found nearly 100% specificity for poor outcomes when N20 potentials were bilaterally absent, but significantly lower specificity for good outcomes when cortical potentials were present. In reality, however, SSEP is rarely used as the only prognostic measure and other indicators – like GCS – had better sensitivity and specificity for good outcomes than SSEP [17]. In order to improve the prognostic accuracy of SSEP, some groups have looked beyond simple presence or absence of N20 potentials. In one grading system, N20 is graded as present, absent, or abnormal. Abnormal potentials are graded when the N20 amplitude is asymmetric, the conduction latency is delayed, or the N20 itself is absent but middle latency potentials are present [18]. Although somewhat subjective, use of this grading scale seems to improve the prognostic accuracy for functional outcome at 1 year in a single-center prospective study of serial SSEP performed 1, 3, and 7 days after severe TBI [18]. In this study, normal N20 potentials by the third day and improvement of initially abnormal N20 potentials had the strongest correlation with good functional outcomes at 1 year [18].

Prognostication in neonatal hypoxic-ischemic encephalopathy

Use of electrophysiological tools to prognosticate in neonatal hypoxic-ischemic encephalopathy is not analogous to prognostication after adult cardiac arrest. In particular, the neonatal peripheral nervous system is not developed enough to produce reliable SSEP signal. Normal EEG patterns in neonates – particularly in premature neonates – differ markedly from adult patterns, because the CNS is poorly myelinated (Figure 25.10). For this reason, EEG interpretation in neonates is much more subjective than in older children and adults. Nevertheless, in addition to the clinical exam, continuous EEG monitoring has become a common practice during treatment of neonatal hypoxic-ischemic encephalopathy, both to exclude seizure activity and determine prognosis. Induced moderate hypothermia for 72 hours has been recently shown to improve outcomes and reduce mortality after moderate to severe hypoxic-ischemic neonatal encephalopathy. There is emerging interest to use EEG markers of disease severity to triage

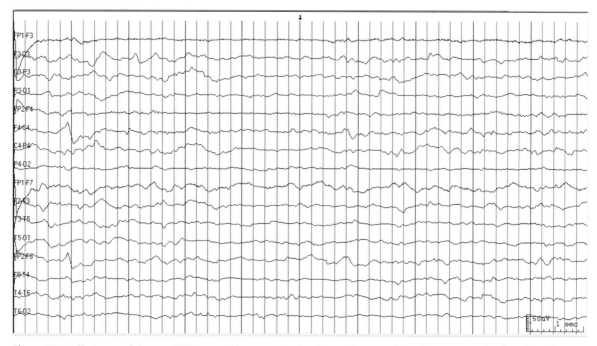

Figure 25.10 Electroencephalogram (EEG) in normal term neonate showing continuous activity with some encoches frontales at the end of the first second of recording, a normal finding in this age group.

neonates to either receive or not receive treatment with hypothermia [19]. These efforts – along with efforts to perform meta-analyses to determine the prognostic accuracy of EEG in neonatal hypoxic-ischemic encephalopathy – have been complicated by the subjective nature of EEG interpretation in this population and the huge variety of proposed criteria that have been published. A recent review found a total of 16 different EEG-based prognostic criteria in neonates [19]. The differences in criteria, EEG timing and technique, and outcome measures rendered it impossible to compare the prognostic accuracy across studies. Common elements to most EEG criteria include: voltage, continuity, frequency, symmetry (see Figure 25.11), presence of normal sleep–wake architecture, and presence of seizures. Most studies defined generalized EEG suppression and burst-suppression patterns as the worst grade and found a strong correlation between the presence of these patterns and poor neurological outcomes. Likewise, normal EEG patterns were strongly correlated with good outcomes. The abnormal and moderately abnormal EEG patterns in the middle – where most patients lie – had very low prognostic consistency between studies, however [19]. Part of the inconsistency in results probably relates to differences in the timing of EEG studies. In one study,

a "moderately abnormal" EEG pattern 6 hours after injury was associated with normal outcome in 100% of neonates, but the same pattern was associated with normal outcomes 43% of the time when recorded 12 hours after injury, 33% at 24 hours, and 0% at 48 hours [19]. Although EEG monitoring is likely to remain an important component of bedside neurological testing in neonatal hypoxic-ischemic encephalopathy, prospective studies using a validated, uniform classification scheme will need to be performed before EEG can be considered a reliable prognostic test.

Determination of brain death

Although state laws and institutional policies differ, a recent consensus statement by the AAN reaffirmed that the gold standard for brain death determination continues to be based on bedside examination by an expert physician [20]. In some cases, however, complete neurological examination cannot be undertaken in a manner that satisfies all of the clinical criteria for brain death. This situation most frequently arises in determination of brain death after severe facial trauma – which may result in inability to examine the eyes for movement or pupillary light responses – or cervical spinal cord trauma – where movement of

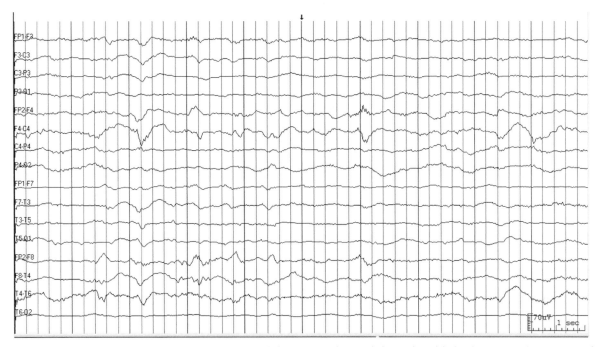

Figure 25.11 Premature infant about 37 weeks. Electroencephalogram (EEG) shows right hemisphere delta brush patterns with suppression of these premature patterns over the left fronto-temporal region.

the extremities cannot be accurately assessed – or severe lung injury that precludes apnea testing. In these situations, additional confirmatory testing is required for declaration of brain death. Alternative methods include nuclear medicine blood flow studies, angiography, and electrophysiological testing with EEG and SSEP. Radiographic studies have a distinct advantage over electrophysiological tests because they are not influenced by severe metabolic derangements or residual sedative medication effects. In unstable patients who cannot be safely transported for radiographic studies, however, bedside electrophysiological testing has an important role in supplementing the clinical exam to confirm brain death. Acceptable electrophysiological signs of brain death include electrocerebral silence on a 30-minute EEG study (Figure 25.6) with appropriate sensitivity settings and absent brainstem, thalamic, or cortical potentials on SSEP [20].

Physiological underpinnings of EEG phenomena

Given the decades of experience with surface EEG recordings, local field potentials, and electrocorticography, surprisingly little is understood about the physiological and neurochemical mechanisms that produce various electrical patterns. Neural electrical activity – whether measured from large populations of neuron volume conducted to the scalp or from invasive local recordings of small populations of neurons – is best regarded as an epiphenomenon of large-scale cell surface receptor activity associated with neuronal depolarization and repolarization. A full review of the physiological underpinnings of electrical phenomena recording during various states of consciousness is beyond the scope of this chapter. In a very elementary sense, however, conscious arousal is associated with amplitude suppression, desynchronization, and increased frequency of basic EEG rhythms. This desynchronization is caused by widespread cortical activation through several redundant pathways. Glutaminergic ascending pathways in the brainstem project through the medial midbrain into divergent pathways through the thalamus and basal forebrain [21]. Activation of non-specific thalamo-cortical projections results in faster cortical rhythms, desynchronization of surface rhythms, and suppression of EEG amplitude [21]. Similarly, these EEG patterns can also be produced by widespread cortical projections from histaminergic, orexinergic, and cholinergic populations in the posterior hypothalamus and basal forebrain [22].

253

Drowsiness and lethargy – either as a prelude to normal sleep or induced by sedative medications or metabolic encephalopathy – results in diminished cortical activation which produces EEG slowing, increased amplitude, synchronous patterns, and lower EEG entropy. These mechanisms account for the loss of arousal patterns and emergence of EEG slowing with increasing degrees of encephalopathy [23]. The physiological and chemical underpinnings of TWs and PED patterns are not well understood.

In terms of specific EEG patterns during encephalopathy, probably the best understood pattern at this point is EEG burst-suppression. Burst-suppression can be observed in a variety of clinical settings, including general anesthesia induced by a variety of agents, deep hypothermia, and global anoxic-ischemic injury caused by cardiac arrest. Burst-suppression is also frequently observed during electrocorticography brain mapping during cortical tumor resections after a region of cortex is undercut, leading to speculation that burst-suppression represents an intrinsic cortical rhythm that emerges when cortex is structurally or functionally deafferented from thalamic inputs [24]. This theory was partially supported by evidence from anesthetic-induced burst-suppression in cats, during which intracellular recordings from thalamic and cortical neurons showed different intrinsic firing patterns [25]. During periods of EEG suppression, cortical neurons showed an almost uniform absence of depolarizations while many thalamic neurons continued to depolarize at a typical intrinsic rhythm [25]. During EEG bursts, intracellular recordings of virtually all cortical neurons demonstrated phasic depolarizations, sometimes leading to action potentials [25]. More recent experiments suggest, however, that bursting events may be triggered by hypersensitivity to subcortical stimuli [26]. In this framework, cortical hyperexcitability results from a reduction of GABA-mediated inhibitory inputs [26]. In this hyperexcitable state, subcortical stimuli set off a series of action potentials in nearly all cortical neurons, producing EEG bursts [26]. The bursting process is limited by depletion of cortical extracellular calcium, leading to failure of synaptic transmission [26]. During the periods of suppression, extracellular calcium levels are restored by neuronal ion pumps and cortical hyperexcitability returns [26]. In this model, the periodicity of bursts and relative duration of bursts and suppressions are determined by the degree of extracellular calcium depletion and the ability of cortical neurons to restore normal gradients, which explains the higher suppression-to-burst ratio with higher degrees of cortical injury [26].

Pitfalls of electrophysiological recordings in the ICU

There are a number of challenges to the recording of electrophysiological tests in the busy electrical environment of the ICU. One of the overarching considerations is the competition for access to the patient who is in need of frequent if not almost constant nursing or medical attention. These demands arise as a function of the underlying medical issues that have resulted in ICU admission. Additionally, the patient may be called away for a CT or an MRI when the electrophysiology technologists have arrived to do the study.

Once access has been gained, there may be physical restrictions for access to the parts of the body to be studied, for example areas of the scalp in the case of neurosurgical and burns patients, or limbs after surgical interventions. The skull or scalp may be open, or covered in bandages. There is clearly a need for sterility, particularly when there are open wounds or burns. With the increasing use of more prolonged monitoring with continuous ICU-EEG, there may be challenges in completing the patient-recording device–interpretation–feedback to physician circuit because of the lack of availability of technicians and study interpreters around the clock. Often ICU personnel, nurses, or intensivists occupy some of these roles during off-hours, such as the re-application of electrodes by nurses or the provisional survey of the EEG data by neurointensivists. Off-site interpretation of cEEG is increasing.

Even with optimal institution of recording devices and techniques, electrodes are subject to a number of environmental artifacts that impede interpretation by introducing electrical noise to the electrode, its wire, an electrode box, or anywhere along this conduit to the amplifiers. Ambient static electricity is generated erratically from a number of sources including clothing and moving machinery that have static charge aligned along their surface. The patient may move, introducing movement-electrode artifact, and sweat can alter the electrolyte contact, producing low-frequency changes. More frequent is the contraction of muscle that produces high-frequency "needle" shaped bursts of beta frequency. For these, the classic appearance of areas more richly endowed with muscle such as the temporal and frontal regions, can alert the interpreter to "account" for these findings as being non-cerebral, and if necessary, use a high-frequency filter moved down to 35 or even 15 Hz in the post-acquisition interpretation of the EEG. More generous and wide-open filtering should be in place during the actual data acquisition and recording. Occipital muscle artifact can sometimes be decreased by positioning a folded or rolled-up towel beneath the neck to enable the patient to relax the neck muscles. When specific recordings are required for subclinical seizure activity or to determine electrocerebral inactivity in support of brain death, paralysis may be warranted to remove all muscle activity contaminants. This procedure must be coordinated with the agreement of the ICU physicians.

A regular, metronomic artifact appearing in one or many leads can be due to a number of causes. Intravenous drip artifact is one, but an often over-looked source of misinterpretation of spikes is artifact from the cardiac beat. Respirators also introduce regular, broad (low-frequency) delta activity every several seconds, but this can be monitored by placing an extra derivation specifically around the respirator tubing which will then signal the specific source of this interference. Somewhat unavoidable is the contamination with 60 Hz artifact from the wiring and sockets as well as machinery which carries current to the ICU. This is often eliminated by the use of a 60 Hz notch filter.

There are fewer artifacts that specifically affect event-related recordings for short-latency evoked potentials. Visual evoked potentials are rarely used in the ICU and, at present, auditory evoked potentials are less used in studies of brain death. They are used without much artifactual interference, in evaluation of brainstem structural abnormalities. The signal averaging eliminates most of the ambient electrical noise, although the automatic artifact rejection may result in a more prolonged acquisition time. More problems occur with long-latency event related potentials, whether auditory or somatosensory, and North American clinicians have less experience in the use of somatosensory N40s and N70s (Figure 25.2), mismatched negativity, and cognitive P300s.

Conclusion

Electrophysiological recordings have become a mainstay of bedside neurological monitoring for encephalopathic or comatose patients in the ICU. Advantages of EEG and SSEP include ready availability, real-time display at the bedside, remote access for interpretation, and continuous measurement of brain function and physiology rather than just a snapshot of brain structure. Widespread use of electrophysiological monitoring of the brain during critical illness has been hampered by the need for expert interpretation of signal that may be subjective or prone to artifacts. This operator-dependence and labor intensiveness limits the utility of these techniques. The holy grail of electrophysiological neuromonitoring remains the ability to design software that identifies and removes artifacts in real time and processes signal into a simplified display or numerical value that can be reliably interpreted by bedside providers with limited training. Advances in quantitative EEG and SSEP have occurred over the last decade, especially in proprietary EEG measures of entropy, automated spike detection, and real-time amplitude-integrated EEG. As clinical trials are undertaken to validate these new technologies and recognition of the frequency of NCSE in critical illness increases, the use of electrophysiological neuromonitoring is likely to continue to increase in the ICU.

References

1. Friedman D, Claasen J, Hirsch LJ. Continuous electroencephalogram monitoring in the intensive care unit. *Anesth Analg* 2009;**109**:506–23.

2. Guérit JM, Amantini A, Amodio P, *et al.* Consensus on the use of neurophysiological tests in the intensive care unit: electroencephalogram, evoked potentials, and electroneuromyography. *Clin Neurophysiol* 2009;**39**:71–83.

3. Claasen J, Mayer SA, Kowalski RG, *et al.* Detection of electrographic seizures with continuous EEG monitoring in critically ill patients. *Neurology* 2004;**62**:1743–8.

4. Bauer G, Trinka E. Nonconvulsive status epilepticus and coma. *Epilepsia* 2010;**51**:177–90.

5. Seidel S, Aull-Watschinger S, Pataraia E. The yield of routine electroencephalography in the detection of incidental nonconvulsive status epilepticus – a prospective study. *Clin Neurophysiol* 2012;**123**(3):459–62.

6. Towne AR, Waterhouse EJ, Boggs JG, *et al.* Prevalence of nonconvulsive status epilepticus in comatose patients. *Neurology* 2000;**54**:340–5.

7. Guerit JM, Amantini A, Fischer C, *et al.* Neurophysiological investigations of hepatic encephalopathy: ISHEN practice guidelines. *Liver Int* 2009;**29**:789–96.

8. Boulanger JM, Deacon C, Lécuyer D, *et al.* Triphasic waves versus nonconvulsive status epilepticus: EEG distinction. *Can J Neurol Sci* 2006;**33**:175–80.

9. Cottenceau V, Petit L, Masson F, *et al.* The use of bispectral index to monitor barbiturate coma in severely brain-injured patients with refractory intracranial hypertension. *Anesth Analg* 2008;**107**:1676–82.

10. Jordan KG, Hirsch LJ. In nonconvulsive status epilepticus, treat to burst-suppression: pro and con. *Epilepsia* 2006;**47**(Suppl 1):41–5.

11. Rossetti AO, Logroscino G, Bromfield EB. Refractory status epilepticus: effect of treatment aggressiveness on prognosis. *Arch Neurol* 2005;**62**:1698–702.

12. Wijdicks EFM, Hijdra A, Young GB, *et al.* Practice parameter: prediction of outcome in comatose survivors after cardiopulmonary resuscitation (an evidence-based review): report of the Quality Standards Subcommittee of the American Academy of Neurology. *Neurology* 2006;**67**:203–10.

13. Oddo M, Rossetti AO. Predicting neurological outcome after cardiac arrest. *Curr Opinion Crit Care* 2011;**17**:254–9.

14. Rossetti AO, Urbano LA, Delodder F, *et al.* Prognostic value of continuous EEG monitoring during therapeutic hypothermia after cardiac arrest. *Crit Care* 2010;**14**:173–81.

15. Rittenberger JC, Popescu A, Brenner RP, *et al.* Frequency and timing of nonconvulsive status epilepticus in comatose post-cardiac arrest subjects treated with hypothermia. *Neurocrit Care* 2012;**16**(1):114–22.

16. Lew HL, Dikmen S, Slimp J, *et al.* Use of somatosensory evoked potentials and cognitive event related potentials in predicting outcomes of patients with severe traumatic brain injury. *Am J Phys Med Rehabil* 2003;**82**:53–61.

17. Carter BG, Butt W. Are somatosensory evoked potentials the best predictor of outcome after severe brain injury: a systematic review. *Intensive Care Med* 2005;**31**:765–75.

18. Houlden DA, Taylor AB, Feinstein A, *et al.* Early somatosensory evoked potential grades in comatose traumatic brain injury patients predict cognitive and functional outcome. *Crit Care Med* 2010;**38**:167–74.

19. Walsh BH, Murray DM, Boylan GB. The use of conventional EEG for the assessment of hypoxic ischaemic encephalopathy in the newborn: a review. *Clin Neurophysiol* 2011;**122**:1284–94.

20. Wijdicks EFM, Varelas PN, Gronseth GS, *et al.* Evidence-based guideline update: determining brain death in adults. *Neurology* 2010;**74**:1911–18.

21. Jones BE. Arousal systems. *Front Biosci* 2003;**8**:438–51.

22. Jones BE. Activity, modulation and role of basal forebrain cholinergic neurons innervating the cerebral cortex. *Prog Brain Res* 2004;**145**:157–69.

23. Kaplan PW. The EEG in metabolic encephalopathy and coma. *J Clin Neurophysiol* 2004;**21**:307–18.

24. Niedermeyer E, Sherman DL, Geocadin RJ, *et al.* The burst-suppression electroencephalogram. *Clin Electroencephalogr* 1999;**30**:99–105.

25. Steriade M, Amzica F, Contreras D. Cortical and thalamic cellular correlates of electroencephalographic burst-suppression. *Electroencephalogr Clin Neurophysiol* 1994;**90**:1–16.

26. Amzica F. Basic physiology of burst-suppression. *Epilepsia* 2009;**50**(Suppl 12):38–9.

Chapter 26

Neuroimaging of delirium

Karen J. Ferguson and Alasdair M. J. MacLullich

SUMMARY

Neuroimaging is routinely used in the investigation of delirium in clinical practice as a means of detecting primary central nervous system causes, for example, stroke and tumors. Yet there are very few studies which can inform the clinician which patients should undergo imaging. Neuroimaging has also been used in a small number of studies as a research tool to help improve understanding of the predisposing factors, acute mechanisms, and consequences of delirium. Currently there are fewer than 20 studies which have explicitly sought to study delirium with neuroimaging. This lack likely reflects the practical and ethical challenges involved in imaging in patients with active delirium. Additionally, to measure change resulting from delirium, or to assess putative neuroimaging predictors of delirium, longitudinal studies incorporating analysis of pre-delirium abnormalities are required. Such studies are costly and challenging and to date have involved recruiting patients undergoing high-risk elective surgery. The currently available research literature has yielded a mixed set of results. Although there are no truly definitive studies, it appears that vascular pathology, as indicated by lacunar infarcts and other white matter lesions, is the finding most consistently found in delirium. This pathology may be important through its role in disrupting fronto-subcortical attentional networks. Some structural studies also suggest an association between various markers of cerebral atrophy and delirium, but no specific brain regions have reliably been implicated. Functional neuroimaging studies of delirium have shown some abnormalities, but the evidence base is not large enough to draw conclusions on which brain areas or systems may be involved. The wider neuroimaging literature provides an extensive array of promising avenues for delirium research. Multiple parameters indicating the volume, integrity, and biochemistry of gray and white matter are now available. There is also scope for more studies on the effective use of neuroimaging in investigating delirium in the clinical setting. This is important in terms of rational use of resources – an important issue given that one in eight hospital inpatients develop delirium, and many undergo neuroimaging as part of their diagnostic work-up. There may also be value in evaluating the clinical value of certain more advanced techniques, such as diffusion tensor imaging, in determining acute causes of delirium. In summary, the field of the neuroimaging of delirium is at a very early stage, but the existing evidence base provides useful early indications of the large potential of neuroimaging to improve our understanding of delirium and also to care for patients more effectively.

Introduction

Delirium is a disorder of the central nervous system (CNS) which can result from primary CNS pathology but which more commonly arises from non-CNS illness or trauma, or as a side effect of drugs. Its pathophysiology remains mysterious. Neuroimaging is routinely used in the investigation of delirium in clinical practice as a means of detecting primary CNS causes of delirium. Such causes include stroke, hemorrhage, and tumors. However, the evidence base informing decisions on which patients might benefit from neuroimaging in delirium is very slight. Studies examining other important questions, such as structural features predicting higher risk of delirium, perfusion changes during delirium, and so on, are also scarce. In a systematic review from 2008, only 12 papers were identified and just seven of these focused on evaluating brain changes predisposing to or resulting from episodes of delirium [1]. Since that review

Brain Disorders in Critical Illness, ed. Robert D. Stevens, Tarek Sharshar, and E. Wesley Ely. Published by Cambridge University Press. © Cambridge University Press 2013.

was published few further substantial studies have emerged. To date, fewer than 400 patients with delirium have been scanned in the entire research literature on delirium and neuroimaging. The contrast with the size of the neuroimaging evidence base in other CNS disorders is striking. Why are there so few imaging studies? The reasons are uncertain but likely reflect the generally low levels of research on delirium, the multifactorial and complex nature of delirium, the practical challenges of performing neuroimaging in patients with active delirium, and the cost of the techniques.

The small evidence base precludes firm conclusions which can be applied to clinical practice or even research studies. However, the existing literature does provide some interesting leads for future research directions. Moreover, there is relevant literature in which patients diagnosed with metabolic or septic encephalopathy, or other conditions essentially falling under the delirium umbrella, can inform thinking about the implications of neuroimaging findings for better understanding of the nature of delirium as well as informing clinical practice in individual cases.

In this chapter we will start by discussing the potential utility as well as the challenges involved in using neuroimaging in delirium research. We then provide an outline of the current research literature, focusing mainly on studies which have explicitly involved patients with *Diagnostic and Statistical Manual of Mental Disorders* (DSM)-or *International Statistical Classification of Diseases and Related Health Problems* (ICD)-defined delirium, but also including relevant studies of patients with labels suggestive of delirium of various etiologies, such as "encephalopathy." As part of the literature review, summaries of each technique are provided. We then go on to discuss the use of neuroimaging in clinical practice.

Neuroimaging of delirium: research

Overview: the potential utility of neuroimaging in delirium research

Neuroimaging has multiple possible functions as a research tool in delirium. These can be categorized as follows: (a) prediction of risk of delirium; (b) the consequences of delirium; (c) the acute causes of current delirium; and (d) the functional and molecular changes associated with current delirium. Prediction of delirium risk using neuroimaging parameters generally requires recruitment of patients awaiting high-risk elective surgery, such as coronary artery bypass grafting or complex vascular surgery. An important caveat here is that selecting patients undergoing a particular type of surgery may give higher weight to risk factors in that population and thus any findings may not be applicable to the general population. For example, patients undergoing coronary bypass surgery may develop delirium with a relatively high frequency, but studying these patients may over-emphasize the importance of vascular disease in delirium pathogenesis. Outwith the high-risk elective surgery experimental design, a large enough cohort study of patients at high risk of delirium from any cause is also possible in principle, though there are no such studies in the literature at present. Prediction of delirium using neuroimaging features could theoretically enhance current models of delirium prediction which are based on clinical variables such as age, cognitive function, and comorbidities. This potential clinical role for neuroimaging would, however, depend on the feasibility of the type of imaging and the analysis method. Widespread *clinical* use of complex MRI modalities along with time-consuming analysis does not appear likely, though it might be possible in high-risk elective surgery as mentioned above. Prediction of clinical risk using simple computed tomography (CT)-based measures is more realistic. Pre-delirium measurement of neuroimaging variables also has the potential to add to our knowledge of the mechanisms of delirium. Although it is known that prior cognitive impairment, particularly dementia, is a strong risk factor for delirium, it is unclear if certain patterns of brain atrophy or other specific regional or neurochemical abnormalities detectable by neuroimaging confer increased risk, or if the general degree of atrophy or white matter changes are more important. Advanced MRI modalities may be used in this context to identify not only the anatomical circuits but also the pathogenic pathways involved in delirium.

Long-term effects of delirium on cognition, for example in conferring an increased risk of dementia [2], are established, but the brain pre- to post-delirium changes corresponding to these behavioral deficits have not been documented. Imaging may also be used here as a means of tracking chronic and progressive effects on brain pathology. Studies of this type would essentially be extensions of studies in those involving prediction. That is, baseline, pre-delirium imaging would be required, followed by at least one additional scan allowing assessment of any changes.

Longitudinal studies of this type are common in dementia research and multiple methods for assessment of change are available. The potential for neuroimaging to inform this crucial area of delirium research is vast, but studies with sufficient power to give definitive results would be large and expensive. This is because even high-risk elective surgery will yield a relatively small proportion of patients with delirium, and the drop-out rate in patients developing delirium will likely be relatively higher because of higher risks of death, complications (including persistent delirium), and prolonged debility. Moreover, the highest-risk patients tend to be frail and are less likely to be recruited into studies requiring multiple hospital visits for imaging and other assessments.

Structural neuroimaging is commonly employed in clinical practice to detect potential acute causes of delirium. However the evidence base evaluating the indications for such imaging is very small. In the research literature, the role of neuroimaging in understanding the neural substrates of delirium with (presumed) non-CNS precipitants of delirium is presently mainly concerned with functional imaging, for example, single photon emission computed tomography (SPECT). Naturally, imaging of patients with delirium for research purposes is highly challenging both ethically and practically. However, imaging is a standard tool of investigation with other severe, acute CNS disorders, demonstrating that research in such vulnerable patients is possible with appropriate safeguards.

Pathophysiology and consequences of delirium: what is known? What can be exploited in imaging?

The pathophysiology of delirium remains poorly understood. However, several predisposing factors have been identified, including some that are well characterized using neuroimaging in general, such as age, cognitive impairment and pre-existing dementia. In addition, delirium shares risk factors and neuropsychological features with other neuropsychiatric conditions that are the subject of extensive study and characterization. Thus, brain pathology associated with these conditions may also be risk factors for delirium, and therefore the same techniques used to study these syndromes could be useful in advancing knowledge of delirium

pathophysiology. Indeed, the application of imaging in some neuropsychiatric disorders such as leukoencephalopathies, Wernicke's encephalopathy (WE) and acute hepatic encephalopathy (AHE) has enhanced understanding of neurobiological correlates of acute cognitive disturbances. Although imaging features in these "encephalopathies" may be to some extent etiology-specific, there may also be some overlap between these syndromes and other delirium groups. In addition, because some encephalopathies have known precipitants, the pathways leading from systemic illness to quantifiable imaging changes are better characterized and may facilitate the application and interpretation of imaging in delirium with less well-defined origins.

Anatomical pathways important in attention

Attentional deficits are the key neuropsychological feature of delirium (see Chapter 8, this volume). Studies in other conditions with significant attentional deficits indicate that integrity of fronto-striatal-pallido-thalamic loops is essential for normal attentional functioning (Figure 26.1). This is in contrast with many other brain systems, which can be damaged without notable effects on attention. Fronto-striatal-pallido-thalamic loops provide constant sampling and interpretation of environmental stimuli and subsequent response adjustment to ensure the behavioral response to the surroundings is appropriate. This set of processes includes distinguishing salient from non-salient or background stimuli and inhibition of behavioral responses to cues lacking salience. Failure of these processes is one plausible route to the attentional deficits observed in delirium.

In most cases of delirium in clinical practice it is difficult to attribute the syndrome to a discrete lesion. Yet the principle that interruption of fronto-striatal-pallido-thalamic loops could cause delirium is supported by many case reports and case series describing delirium-like neuropsychiatric symptoms following hemorrhages and infarcts in the subcortical gray matter (notably the caudate nucleus, particularly on the right) and thalamus (especially the medial nuclei). As well as confusion and altered level of consciousness, symptoms have included persecutory delusions and impaired recognition. In the dorsal caudate nuclei symptoms tended towards apathy, anhedonia, lack of motivation, and goal-directed behavior, as well as attentional deficits including sustaining and focusing attention and impairments in orientation. Ventral lesions were associated with disinhibition,

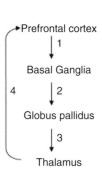

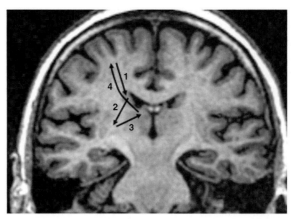

Prefrontal cortex

Basal Ganglia

Globus pallidus

Thalamus

Figure 26.1 Basic frontostriatal pathway. These loops are central to attention and executive function.

inappropriate behavior, and euphoria [3]. However, it is likely that many of these symptoms are due in part to more global processes caused by inflammation and cytokine production resulting from an intracranial hemorrhage. Indeed, symptoms were more pronounced in the acute phase after hemorrhage and in patients in whom bleeding into the ventricle had occurred [4]. Yet in studies where the patients received follow-up cognitive testing, the deficits persisted. This suggests that strategic lesions may play a particularly important role, especially where the delirium is not resolving with management of potential systemic precipitants. Taken together, these findings allow us to propose the related hypotheses that: (a) subcortical lesions are a key specific risk factor for delirium, and (b) acute damage to the basal ganglia may also be a specific cause of delirium.

The putative involvement of frontostriatal circuits in delirium has implications for the application of imaging, because imaging can detect focal or distributed lesions affecting these circuits. Subcortical gray and white matter is particularly vulnerable to age-related brain changes. A significant factor is that these structures receive their blood supply via penetrating lenticulostriate vessels that are prone to micro-angiopathy [5] and subcortical regions are susceptible to hypoperfusion [6] leading to the formation of enlarged perivascular spaces and lacunes or silent brain infarcts (Figure 26.2). These lesions are readily detectable by neuroimaging. Frontostriatal circuits may also be susceptible to the formation of periventricular white matter lesions (Figure 26.3) because of co-location with tracts to the caudate nucleus from the frontal cortex and also from the thalamus back to frontal areas. In vascular dementia some authors have hypothesized that cognitive deficits arising

from frontostriatal disconnection and caudate volumes are associated with higher lesion load [7]. Therefore, focusing on lesions potentially affecting frontostriatal circuits may shed light on the causes of delirium in research settings, or even in particular clinical cases, especially where the delirium is prolonged.

Glial cells

Microglial activation and resulting cytokine production is a key area in delirium pathophysiology research, emanating mainly by Cunningham's prion-based model of delirium in dementia [8–10], but also receiving preliminary support from recent clinical experiments [11]. This is important because imaging research in general has focused mainly on neuronal changes. Yet there is now increasing recognition of a glial contribution to changes in imaging parameters, particularly in associations of some metabolites detectable by proton magnetic resonance spectroscopy (^{1}H-MRS) with inflammation and glial proliferation through tissue biopsies [12,13]. Postmortem studies have shown that microangiopathy and white matter lesions, putative risk factors for delirium and detectable using MRI, are associated with glial activation [14,15]. There is also speculation on the contribution of astrocyte reactivity to changes in diffusion imaging given that hypertrophic astrocytes have greatly enlarged watery cytoplasm and are key in osmoregulation. In addition astrocytes are closely associated with capillaries, and their role in controlling cerebral blood flow [16] has implications for interpreting signals derived from hemodynamic imaging methods.

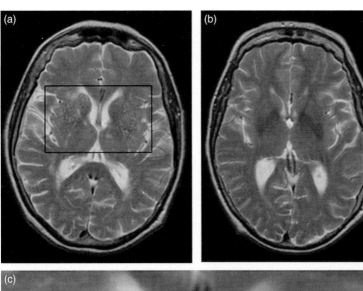

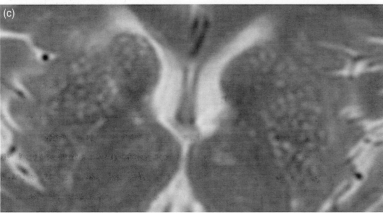

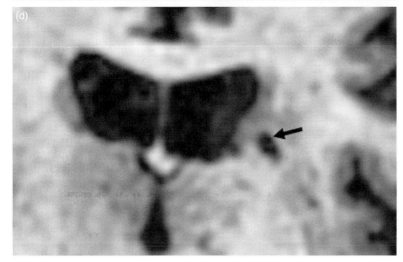

Figure 26.2 Examples of subcortical age-related changes on MRI. Brain from a cognitively normal older individual with a high prevalence of enlarged perivascular spaces (EPVS; (a) and enlarged, (c)) compared with a subject of similar age without EPVS (b). A small lacune or "silent cerebral infarct" in the left internal capsule and caudate nucleus of a cognitively normal older person (d).

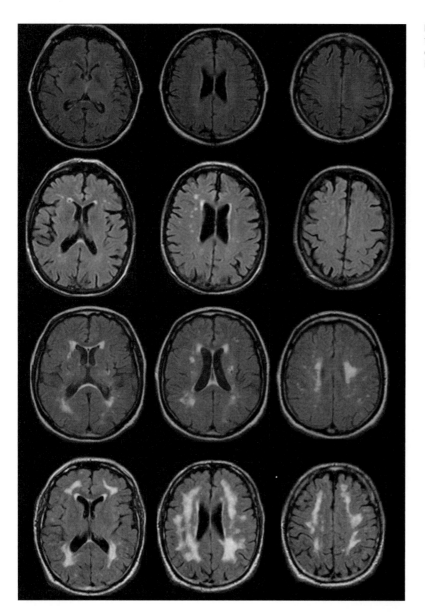

Figure 26.3 Axial FLAIR images showing the range of white matter lesion load observed in cognitively intact elderly individuals.

Astroglial swelling is of particular interest in AHE because brain uptake of ammonia increases following hyperammonemia. Clearance of ammonia leads to accumulation of glutamine within astrocytes, causing extracellular water to enter the astrocytes and making them expand. Concentrations of other osmolytes such as myo-inositol are decreased in compensation. These changes may be functionally important, because astrocytic swelling can lead to neuronal dysfunction through adverse changes in the diffusion and regulation of neurotransmitters [17]. In addition, elevated S100-β, produced (in the CNS) almost exclusively by astrocytes, is higher in plasma in patients with delirium [18]. Therefore, it is possible that glial cells may play a larger role in delirium in general than previously thought, and future imaging studies, particularly ¹H-MRS and positron emission tomography (PET), may provide a means of advancing understanding of this line of enquiry [19].

Neurotransmitters

Delirium resulting from anticholinergic and antipsychotic drug treatment (see Chapter 29, this volume) underpins the hypothesis that cholinergic :

dopaminergic imbalance is key in the emergence of cognitive deficits associated with delirium. In non-drug-induced delirium, neurotransmission may be directly by stress, glial uptake, and cytokine release. Extracellular neurotransmitter levels may also be affected indirectly by vasogenic edema [20]. Positron emission tomography has long been used as an imaging tool for investigating dopamine receptor binding, transport, and turnover. Observations that changes in dopamine transmission detected using PET are associated with attentional deficits in Alzheimer's disease [21] and are susceptible to stress [22,23] make this a useful candidate method in future delirium investigation.

More recently, radioligands have been developed for PET investigation of cholinergic binding and turnover. These have demonstrated reduced acetylcholinesterase activity in Alzheimer's disease and in patients with mild cognitive impairment who later developed Alzheimer's disease [24]. Reduced acetylcholinesterase activity is also associated with increased periventricular white matter lesion severity [25], a possible risk factor for delirium [1], and poorer performance in tasks of reaction time in healthy people and verbal memory, non-verbal memory [24], and attention in Alzheimer's disease [26].

Hemodynamics

Changes in cerebral autoregulation may be a precipitant in delirium onset. Autoregulation is disrupted during surgery [27] and in other pathological states, notably sepsis, in which autoregulation was found to be impaired in patients with delirium compared with non-delirious patients [28].

Chronic impairments in autoregulation are well-studied and may be relevant in the prediction of delirium. PET imaging using ^{15}O shows a decline in cerebral blood flow (CBF), cerebral metabolic rate in oxygen (CMRO$_2$), and cerebral blood volume (CBV) with age, predominantly in frontal regions with increased cerebral oxygen extraction fraction (OEF) [29,30]. Although the relationship between CBF and CMRO$_2$ was preserved, as was the CBF/CBV ratio, increased OEF indicated impaired coupling between oxygen demand and delivery suggestive of inactivation [31]. The neurobiological basis of these changes is not clear, although decline in capillary and synaptic density with age may be a factor. In addition, damage to vessels from atherosclerosis, a known risk factor for delirium, may reduce autoregulatory capacity [32]. It

could be argued that patients with baseline deficits in cerebral circulation may be more susceptible to the effects of further impairments in autoregulation resulting from illness or surgery. Indeed lower baseline CBF is associated with cognitive decline 3 years later in hypertension [33] and faster progression to Alzheimer's disease from mild cognitive impairment [34], suggesting that impaired autoregulation may be a marker for acceleration of cognitive decline. Cerebral hypoperfusion due to extracorporeal circulation in coronary artery bypass graft (CABG) surgery was demonstrated by magnetic resonance perfusion (MR) imaging and associated postoperative cognitive dysfunction in the acute phase following surgery, and also by SPECT 6 months after surgery when CBF remained lower than baseline in some patients [35].

Magnetic resonance perfusion imaging indicates that cerebral blood flow is reduced in patients with higher white matter lesion severity [36] and also in normal-appearing white matter in people with white matter lesions, suggesting that reductions in perfusion precede and may be pathogenic in lesion development [37]. These findings are notable in the light of the apparent association between atherosclerosis and delirium risk.

Long-term cognitive impairment

One emerging area of interest in delirium research is the impact on long-term cognitive performance. It is now known that not only does delirium accelerate cognitive decline in dementia [38] but it is itself a risk for onset of dementia [2]. Moreover, duration of delirium in ICU patients predicts cognitive impairment 1 year after discharge [39]. In healthy aging, decline in cognitive performance is predicted by white matter changes [40,41] and gray matter atrophy [42,43]. One recent imaging study in ICU patients found that delirium severity and duration was associated with reduced white matter integrity at discharge and this predicted poorer cognition 3 months later [44].

Neuroimaging studies of delirium

In this section we summarize the literature on imaging in delirium, extending to the wider literature on encephalopathies where this is informative. A recent systematic review [1] provides more detail on much of the delirium-specific neuroimaging literature. Table 26.1 provides a summary of the literature.

Table 26.1 Neuroimaging studies of delirium: a summary of the literature.

Study/provenance	Design/setting	Imaging modality	Causes of delirium	Mean age of cases (years)	Cases [n (male/female)]	Controls [n (male/female)]	Main positive findings in delirious patients	p
[66] Finland	Case–control; psychiatric hospital (cases), neurological outpatient clinic (controls)	CT	Stroke (22%) Metabolic (13%) Infection (13%) Medications (9%) Epileptic fit (9%) Life change in dementia (9%) Intracranial space-occupying lesion (9%) Carcinoma (6%) Myocardial infarction or insufficiency (4%) Functional psychosis (4%) Trauma (3%)	73.5	69 (29/40)	31 (13/18)	Higher frontal horn index Higher cella media index Greater width of third ventricle Greater width of sylvian fissure Greater mean of the largest cortical sulci Larger proportion of focal abnormalities (e.g., infarcts), especially on the right side Differences between hyperactive, hypoactive, and mixed delirium in: Frontal horn index Width of third ventricle	<.001 <.001 <.001 <.01 .04 <.001 .01 .03
[67] United States	Cohort; psychiatric hospital	MRI	Antidepressant	72.4	5 (2/3)	55 (?)	All cases had basal ganglia lesions plus white matter hyperintensities and either cortical atrophy or ventricular enlargement	<.001[a] .01[a]
[50] United States	Cohort; psychiatric hospital	MRI	ECT	76.1	10 (3/7)	77 (25/52)	Increased incidence of: Basal ganglia lesions Periventricular hyperintensity Deep white matter hyperintensity	 <.01 .02 .02
[51] United States	Case series; psychiatric hospital	CT/MRI	ECT	73.3	6 (3/3)	0	All cases had basal ganglia lesions and white matter hyperintensities	NA
[68] United States	Case–control; psychiatric hospital	CT/MRI	ECT in stroke patients	68.4	4 (2/2)	10 (3/7)	Stroke involved caudate nucleus in 100% of delirious patients vs. 30% of non-delirious patients	.07[a]
[69] Australia	Case series; general hospital	CT	Stroke	72.2	5 (4/1)	0	All cases had right hemisphere subcortical infarcts	NA

Study	Design; setting	Imaging	Cause (%)	Age	n (m/f)	Sample	Findings	p
[70] Japan	Cohort; emergency admissions unit	CT/MRI	Trauma (29%), Cerebrovascular (18%), Acute abdomen (16%), Burn (8%), Circulatory failure (5%), Respiratory failure (3%), Poisoning (3%), Gastrointestinal bleed (3%)	54.9	38 (29/9)	197 (?)	No significant differences in pathological findings on scans	.71[a]
[71] France	Cohort; stroke unit	CT/MRI	Stroke	78 (median)	51 (26/25)	153 (71/82)	Greater cerebral atrophy score; Greater white matter lesion burden	<.01; .05
[64] Japan	Case series; intensive care unit	Xenon CT	Trauma (50%), Acute pancreatitis (30%), Perforated peptic ulcer (10%), Peritonitis carcinomatosa (10%)	47.5	10 (9/1) (all paired "before-and-after" scans)	0	Global reduction in cerebral blood flow; Reduction in regional blood flow in all studied areas: right and left frontal, temporal and occipital lobes, and caudate head, thalamus, and lenticular nucleus	<.01; All <.05
[72] Portugal	Cohort; stroke unit	CT/MRI	Stroke	63.0	19 (7/12)	189 (113/76)	Higher proportion of hemispheric strokes relative to brainstem/cerebellar strokes	.02
[73] United States	Case–control; general hospital	CT	Hypoxia/diffuse cerebral ischemia (25%), Systemic disease (50%), Drug intoxication or withdrawal (15%)	Not stated	20 (?)	50 (?) (total sample 32/38)	No significant differences in intercaudate ratio or periventricular white matter disease	.99[b]; .66[b]
[38] United States	Case–control; general hospital	SPECT	Multifactorial: Medications (77%), Pre-existing cognitive impairment (59%), Infection (50%), Dehydration (36%), Metabolic (36%), Hypoxia (14%), Immobility (11%)	82.1	22 (7/15) (6 paired "before-and-after" scans)	11 (?)	Decreased frontal, parietal, and occipital blood flow (qualitative data); Decreased regional blood flow ratios in the pons, left inferior frontal lobe, right temporal lobe, and right occipital lobe; Paired scan results: Right parietal hypoperfusion (n = 2), Left parietal hyperperfusion (n = 1), Normal (n = 3)	NA; <.01; <.001; <.001; NA

Table 26.1 (cont.)

Study/provenance	Design/setting	Imaging modality	Causes of delirium	Mean age of cases (years)	Cases [n (male/female)]	Controls [n (male/female)]	Main positive findings in delirious patients	p
[59] Japan	Cohort; cardiothoracic unit	MRI/DTI	Cardiac surgery (scheduled)	73.1	19 (13/6)	97 (65/32)	Preoperative reduction in FA values in thalamus, corpus callosum, and deep white matter bilaterally in delirium cases	<.01
[74] South Korea	Case-control; general hospital	fMRI	Cancer (21%) Spinal stenosis (16%) Femur fracture (11%) Pneumonia (11%) Other (47%)	73.6	20 (12/8) during delirium 13 following resolution of delirium (10/3)	22 (13/9)	Positive correlation between posterior cingulate cortex and left dorsolateral prefrontal cortex during delirium and lost after resolution and negatively correlated bilaterally in controls	All <.05
							Functional connectivity strength between precuneus and posterior cingulate negatively correlated with delirium severity and duration	<.05
							Functional connectivity strengths between the intralaminar thalamic nuclei and caudate nucleus and all other subcortical regions were reduced during delirium	All <.05
							Functional connectivity strengths between the intralaminar thalamic nuclei and mesencephalic and ventral tegmental area were restored after resolution of delirium	<.05
[47] United States	Cohort; intensive care unit	MRI	Sepsis/ARDS (30%) Hepatobiliary/pancreatic surgery (21%) CHF/MI/cardiogenic shock (13%) Acute respiratory distress syndrome without infection (9%) COPD/asthma (6%) Vascular surgery (4%) Other (17%)	58 (median of entire cohort)	33 (?) All with paired scans at discharge and 3-month follow-up	14(?)	Duration of delirium associated with increased ventricle-to-brain ratio at discharge and 3 months after discharge	<.05
							Duration of delirium associated with smaller superior frontal lobe and hippocampal volumes at discharge	<.05
							Duration of delirium associated with smaller superior frontal lobe and hippocampal volumes at 3 months post discharge	<.05

[44] United States	Cohort; intensive care unit	MRI DTI	Sepsis/ARDS (30%) Hepatobiliary/pancreatic surgery (23%) CHF/MI/cardiogenic shock (13%) COPD/asthma (9%) Acute respiratory distress syndrome without infection (6%) Other (17%)	58 (median of entire cohort)	33 (?) All with paired scans at discharge and 3-month follow-up	14(?)	Reduced white matter integrity (FA) in genu, body and splenium of corpus callosum, anterior limb of internal capsule at discharge and 3 months after discharge in 3 vs. 0 days of delirium	All <.05
							Lower FA in anterior limb of internal capsule correlated with attention scores at 3 months after discharge	<.01
							Lower FA in genu of corpus callosum correlated with attention scores at 12 months after discharge	p=.05

(?) Data not present in published article.
^{a} p values not included in the original manuscript but derived from published data using Fisher's Exact Test.
^{b} p values not included in the original manuscript but derived from published data using unpaired t test for delirium versus control subjects with depression.
MRI, magnetic resonance imaging; ECT, electroconvulsive therapy; CT, computed tomography; SPECT, single photon emission computed tomography; DTI, diffusion tensor imaging; fMRI, functional magnetic resonance imaging; ARDS, acute respiratory distress syndrome; CHF, congestive heart failure; COPD, chronic obstructive pulmonary disease; MI, myocardial infarction; FA, fractional anisotropy

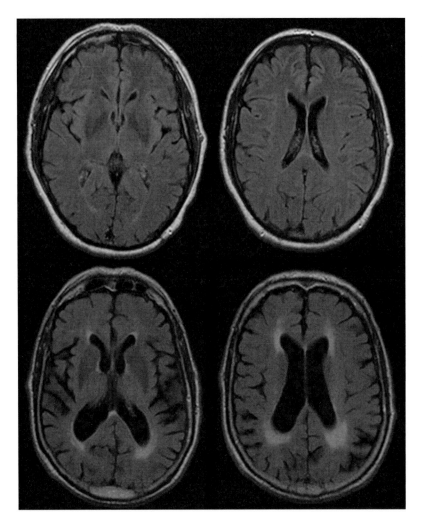

Figure 26.4 Axial FLAIR images in two cognitively intact elderly individuals showing no atrophy (above) and greatly enlarged ventricles and sulci (below). Age-related atrophy is highly variable even in "healthy" subjects. Ventricular enlargement is often accompanied by an increased prevalence of white matter lesions (hyperintense areas adjacent to lateral ventricles in lower case).

Structural changes

Structural changes are those observable on CT and standard structural MR sequences such as T1- and T2-weighted, fluid attenuated inversion recovery (FLAIR) and gradient echo. They reflect differences in volume and also abnormalities in signal in white or gray matter, with or without loss of volume.

Volume and anatomical changes

Methods of assessment include rating of atrophy using qualitative scales and global or regional brain volume measurements. Despite the subjective nature of qualitative scales, experienced neuroradiologists achieve high levels of reliability, especially when using anchored ordinal scales. Qualitative assessment can be more informative than quantitative methods because

volumes, even if corrected for intracranial capacity, reflect longstanding individual differences as well as pathological changes [45]. Several studies in the delirium field have used qualitative assessment rather than volumetric quantification. To date, global changes such as generalized brain atrophy and ventricular enlargement on MRI (Figure 26.4) have been found to be associated with post-ECT delirium in depressed older patients and also in ICU patients. Post-stroke hypoactive delirium is also associated with higher cerebral atrophy scores on the initial CT scan [1].

Simple quantitative methods, such as linear width measurement of ventricles and sulcal fissures, or volumetric methods may be more sensitive in detecting small differences between individuals than qualitative scales, and are less time consuming than formal measurements of volume. However, manual or semi-automated methods combining manual tracing and automatic edge-detection are increasingly allowing reliable measurement of the whole brain, ventricles, and discrete regions such as the subcortical gray matter and hippocampus. High-resolution T1-weighted sequences provide good contrast between gray and white matter and cerebrospinal fluid for this purpose. These are time consuming but provide quantifiable results while maintaining control in adjusting for individual morphological differences. Fully automated methods enable parcellation with good reliability but are often based on atlases derived from young individuals and may not perform as well in a cohort of older subjects. In addition, there is little allowance for morphological variation, although performance is improved by using an age- or cohort-appropriate atlas based on a greater number of subjects [46].

In ICU patients, the duration of delirium has been associated with ventricle-to-brain volume ratio and also with reduced hippocampal volumes and superior frontal lobe volumes measured at discharge. This relationship was still evident at 3 months post-discharge for ventricle-to-brain ratio and superior frontal lobe [47]. Whole brain and regional volume changes have also been reported in a number of conditions in which there is acute deterioration in mental status such as AHE, WE, and sepsis. For example, reduced brain volume in MRI scans prior to liver transplant predicted postoperative AHE. Additionally in WE MRI commonly shows several characteristic lesions, notably mammillary bodies, medial thalamic, hippocampal and cerebellar atrophy [48].

More sophisticated techniques may be more sensitive and particularly useful in longitudinal studies where the effect size may be smaller than the error in more conventional volumetric methods. Co-registration and subtraction of longitudinal scans in AHE have shown small increases in whole brain volume suggestive of low-grade edema and associated with poorer cognition, while decreases in volume were associated with resolution of cognitive function and a better outcome [49]. These studies indicate that different etiologies of delirium may affect the brain in different ways, and that, for example, reductions in brain volume may not always be pathological.

In addition to volume changes, other structural differences have been associated with delirium. In psychogeriatric patients, some imaging studies and case reports have reported that ECT-induced delirium is associated with basal ganglia lacunes [50,51].

Lacunes are cerebrospinal fluid (CSF)-filled 3 mm to 15–20 mm cavities, often clinically silent, in the basal ganglia or white matter. They increase in prevalence with age. Their pathogenesis is unknown but they are thought to result from infarcts. Risk factors include hypertension, diabetes, and alcohol consumption and although these lesions are sometimes "silent" in that they do not cause focal motor or sensory signs, they may indicate subcortical vulnerability. This limited evidence further supports the proposal that basal ganglia lesions are particularly important in delirium.

Intensity changes

White matter lesions

The term white matter lesion (WML) usually refers to hyperintensities observed on T2-weighted and FLAIR images surrounding the anterior and posterior horns of the lateral ventricles, and more focal lesions in the deep white matter becoming confluent with increasing severity of WML load. White matter lesions increase in frequency and severity with age and are progressive, though deep WML are less likely to progress than periventricular lesions [52]. Histologically, age-related WML are characterized by tissue rarefaction with demyelination, astrocytic hypertrophy, increased microglial activation, and loss of ependymal integrity [53]. White matter lesions occur frequently in the "watershed" areas where territories of different cerebral arteries meet. The etiology of WMLs is unclear, but they have been linked with hypoperfusion, and leakage of CSF from the ventricles.

As with brain atrophy, WML loads have commonly been assessed using qualitative scales. However, in contrast with qualitative ratings of the degree of atrophy, inter-rater reliabilities can be low. Selection of the appropriate rating scales used for research is crucial. For example, the simplest scales give the best reliability but lack resolution and high ceiling effects may be found when using scales developed in populations with high lesion loads. Recently, several quantitative methods for measuring WML volume have been developed. These may prove useful in longitudinal studies assessing the consequences of delirium.

Some studies have examined WMLs and delirium [1]. Higher pre-existing WML load was reported to be associated with both post-electroconvulsive therapy and hypoactive post-stroke delirium [50,51]. White matter lesions were observed on MRI in patients with

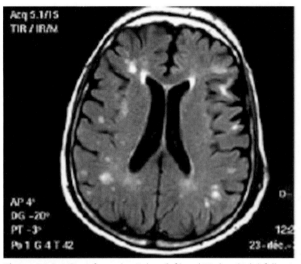 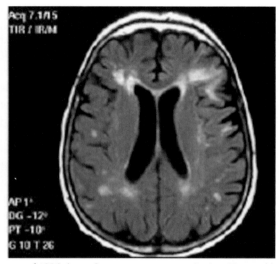

Figure 26.5 MRI performed at 3 days (left) and 30 days (right) following onset of ARDS due to Streptococcus pneumoniae in a 79-year-old woman showing progression of white matter hyperintensities. Reproduced with permission from Sharshar *et al., Intensive Care Med* 2007;**33**:798–806.

delirium in the ICU, with more severe lesions exhibited by older patients [54].

Importantly, hyperintensity in the white matter is non-specific and as well as chronic changes, acute signal abnormalities may occur due to diverse acute illnesses causing vasogenic edema, demyelination, gliosis, and inflammation. It is significant that an imaging study in patients with sepsis showed progression of white matter lesions over the space of a few weeks (Figure 26.5) [55]. These findings have implications for understanding how delirium, particularly in severely unwell patients, may result in chronic cognitive decline. Acute changes are difficult to distinguish from pre-existing lesions with conventional imaging but in contrast to age-related WML, some of these abnormalities may resolve with successful treatment. For example, patients with AHE were found to have multiple focal subcortical white matter lesions that were reduced in size and number on recovery of cognition. This may represent an improvement in brain water balance.

Gray matter

Some of the encephalopathies exhibit increased signal in gray matter; this is thought to be a consequence of edema. These signal changes are not uniformly distributed. Interestingly, in the light of putative fronto-striatal circuitry involvement, many of the gray matter changes affect basal ganglia and medial thalamic nuclei. Sepsis has been associated with significant hyperintensity with FLAIR in basal ganglia and

thalamus: in a case study of a post-renal transplant patient admitted to ICU following a urinary tract infection (UTI), an MRI scan showed pronounced hyperintensity mainly in the basal ganglia and thalamus. Subsequent postmortem after death 13 days after admission showed infarction of the basal ganglia with inflammation, some small focal cortical infarcts, and thalamic edema. Pathological and behavioral changes were attributed to the occlusion of small vessels due to exaggerated inflammatory response [56].

Wernicke's encephalopathy is characterized by abnormal MRI signal in mesencephalic structures such as the medial thalamus, mammillary bodies, tegmentum, periaqueductal region, and tectal plate [57]. One study has suggested that structural MRI scans may be useful in confirming the diagnosis of WE from asymptomatic alcoholics and healthy controls, with increased medial thalamic and periaqueductal T2 signal the best distinguishing features. However, diagnosis of WE could not be eliminated by the absence of these features [58].

Basal ganglia hyperintensities have also been observed on T1 scans in AHE. This is restricted to the globus pallidus and is associated with the regionally specific deposition of manganese, which as a paramagnetic substance alters the behavior of nearby protons, resulting in signal change.

Tissue integrity

Although WML are associated with loss of tissue integrity, they are non-specific. More advanced

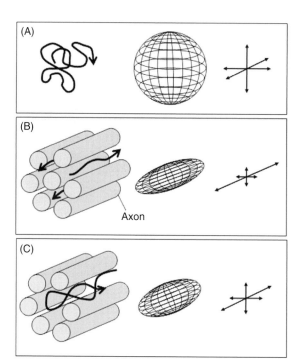

Figure 26.6 Diffusion imaging: The first column shows the trajectory of water diffusion, and the second, the diffusion ellipsoid. In the third column, the longest axis represents the orientation of major water diffusion. (A) Unrestricted, the direction of water diffusion is the same in all directions therefore fractional anisotropy (FA) is equal to 0. (B) When restricted by cellular boundaries, for example in white matter, the direction of water diffusion is dependent on the tissue structure. FA is high in white matter because water preferentially diffuses along white matter tracts rather than between axons and is therefore highly directional. (C) Loss of white matter integrity results in less restriction in water movement, therefore increased diffusion and reduced FA compared to intact tissue.

modalities of MR provide more information concerning microstructural changes. The two main methods used for this purpose are diffusion tensor imaging (DTI) and magnetization transfer ratio (MTR) imaging.

Diffusion tensor imaging

Increases in signal intensity in white and gray matter are commonly due to increased water content and loss of tissue integrity. Diffusion-weighted MR allows specific measurement of water diffusion within brain tissue. Water will diffuse freely in all directions (isotropic) where there are no barriers to diffusion, but with increasing structural order and compaction of tissue, diffusion becomes more directionally dependent or anisotropic (Figure 26.6). This is particularly true in intact white matter where the preferred direction of water diffusion is parallel to the course of the

fiber tracts (Figure 26.7). However, white matter rarefaction or edema results in fewer cellular barriers and therefore more diffusion with a reduction in directional preference. Thus diffusion imaging detects subtle changes in white matter integrity, and is more sensitive than conventional MR imaging and CT. Indeed, changes can be observed in normal-appearing white matter before white matter lesions are apparent in MR imaging. Diffusion tensor imaging provides information on the direction as well as the magnitude of water diffusion allowing fiber pathways to be tracked and differences in connectivity measured.

One study of imaging and cardiac bypass surgery with standardized delirium assessments found that lower fractional anisotropy predicted delirium following surgery [59]. This suggests that reduced white matter integrity is a risk for delirium, complementing the findings of studies which showed that white matter lesions appear to be associated with the risk of delirium. Another study found an association with lower fractional anisotropy (FA) in the corpus callosum and internal capsule measured at discharge from the ICU and delirium duration while in hospital [44]. As these subjects were relatively young, it is likely that the observed DTI changes were due to their critical illness rather than age-related white matter deterioration.

Surgery is a major precipitating factor in delirium. Proposed mechanisms include microembolism, hypotension causing hypoperfusion, adverse reaction to anesthetics, and general factors such as systemic stress responses. In one study using diffusion-weighted imaging [60], seven out of eight patients with post-cardiac surgery encephalopathy showed multiple small lesions, suggesting embolic infarcts throughout the anterior and posterior circulations. Clustering in the region of watershed territories was observed, indicating that smaller vessels were most vulnerable, as expected. Importantly, the lesions were more numerous than observed on conventional MRI, indicating a promising role for this imaging modality in understanding more subtle changes in tissue integrity.

Magnetization transfer ratio

Magnetization transfer ratio imaging enables measurement of free water by determining the transfer of magnetization from protons in water molecules with restricted movement because of binding to macromolecules to those that are able to move freely. Changes in macromolecule density results in reduced ability for

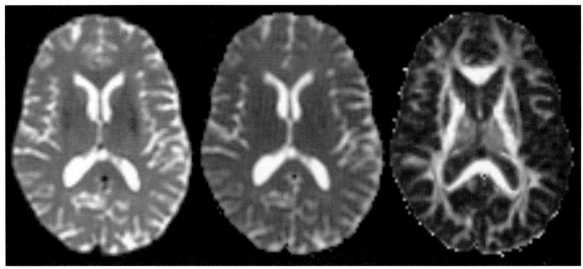

Figure 26.7 Diffusion imaging: The same axial slice showing T2-weighting (left), mean diffusivity (middle), and fractional anisotropy (FA, right). White matter tracts are hyperintense on FA maps due to the highly directional diffusion of water along axons.

magnetization transfer to occur and reduced MTR values. Evidence of low-grade edema is a consistent finding across modalities in MRI of AHE. Magnetization transfer ratio decreases in AHE indicating increased brain water support these findings. Magnetization transfer ratio decreases in globus pallidus and parietal gray matter differentiate cirrhotic patients with AHE from non-AHE cirrhosis whereas changes in other regions were associated with cirrhosis but not AHE.

Biochemistry

Proton magnetic resonance spectroscopy

Levels of metabolites containing protons that resonate close to the frequency of water can be measured using proton magnetic resonance spectroscopy (^{1}H-MRS). In the brain, the most abundant and detectable metabolite measured by ^{1}H-MRS is N-acetylaspartate (NAA) which is specific to neurons, considered to be a marker of neuronal integrity, and is reduced in regions where there is neuronal damage, for example in demyelination, but also where there is increased glial density due to cell proliferation. Another readily detectable chemical is creatine (Cr), which is involved in energy metabolism. High Cr levels may indicate increased cellularity and macrophage infiltration and are found in several neurological illnesses involving inflammation. The choline (Cho) peak represents mainly choline-containing compounds required for phospholipid

membrane synthesis. Increased Cho is thought to indicate higher membrane turnover. Glial cells demonstrate a concentration of Cho that is 2–3 times higher than neurons and increased Cho has been shown to correspond to glial proliferation. However, high Cho levels may also be caused by membrane breakdown resulting in more unbound choline-containing molecules. In addition, there are smaller peaks for myo-inositol (mI) which is involved in osmoregulation, a primary function of astrocytes. Myo-inositol is expressed in astrocytes and mI levels may be a reflection of astrocytic activation and cellular density and also of changes in osmoregulation.

Glycine, glutamate, and GABA are present with overlapping peaks and in low concentrations making their quantification difficult. Lactate, an end-product of anerobic glycolysis, is not detectable in normal brain tissue. It is usually observed in damaged tissue after stroke but positive lactate findings have been observed in a small proportion of healthy older people and in some asymptomatic white matter lesions indicating that lactate production may also occur in "healthy" brain aging.

Proton magnetic resonance spectroscopy following CABG surgery shows decreased NAA/Cr ratios 3 days after surgery compared with baseline levels that correlated with poorer postoperative cognitive performance [61]. Proton magnetic resonance spectroscopy has been used in several studies of AHE. Changes in ^{1}H-MRS are well characterized in this condition; patients exhibit reduced Cho and mI and increased glutamate/glycine [62]. Metabolite changes are associated with the severity of AHE although they are also observed in patients without neuropsychological impairment.

In addition to imaging patients with AHE, hyperammonemia can be induced in patients with cirrhosis by systemic administration of amino acids. Subsequent ^{1}H-MRS enables evaluation of the effects on the brain of hyperammonemia demonstrating how systemic metabolic changes can lead to effects in the brain measurable by imaging. Currently there are no published studies examining MRS in formally defined delirium. The above suggests however that this technique offers considerable potential in understanding the acute changes associated with delirium in patients who are able to tolerate the procedure.

Hemodynamic imaging

Imaging allowing measurement of changes in blood flow, concentrations of various metabolites, and so on, offers substantial promise in determining the processes occurring during acute delirium. Methods using radioligands may have limited application in longitudinal evaluation of delirium due to radioactivity exposure although some of these methods (particularly in CT perfusion) have shown sensitivity in demonstrating changes associated with delirium that resolve in association with functional recovery.

Several small studies have shown CT perfusion methods to be sensitive to changes during delirium that resolve in association with functional recovery. Single photon emission computed tomography allows measurement of regional cerebral blood flow (rCBF) using gamma-emitting radioisotopes injected intravenously. A preliminary SPECT study in six older medical patients showed hypoperfusion predominantly in the frontal and parietal regions with reversal in three of these individuals after resolution of the delirium [63].

Xenon-enhanced computed tomography enables visualization of rCBF using inhaled stable xenon gas which enters the bloodstream and acts as a contrast agent due to its high atomic number. One such study during delirium in ten ICU patients indicated hypoperfusion in all cortical and subcortical regions resolving after recovery from delirium with changes predominantly in the frontal and parietal cortex [64].

Position emission tomography has found reduced oxygen consumption and cerebral blood flow in cirrhotic patients with AHE compared with those with cirrhosis but without AHE and healthy controls. Both CBF and oxygen consumption were negatively correlated with plasma ammonia providing a link between systemic metabolic and neurological changes [65]. There are currently no published studies of PET involving patients with formally diagnosed delirium.

Neuroimaging of delirium in clinical practice

Neuroimaging is used on a very wide scale in clinical practice in the work-up for delirium. There are no published studies indicating the extent of the use of neuroimaging in this clinical context. However, in our own experience, at least one third of older emergency medical patients presenting acutely with formally diagnosed delirium, or indeed changes in mental status labelled as "acute confusion," "encephalopathy," and so on, undergo CT or MRI scanning. Given the very high rates of delirium in general hospital care, this represents a substantial burden on staff time, scanning resources, and associated costs, adds to the number of moves that a vulnerable patient endures, and in the case of CT scanning, the release of radiation. It is surprising that given the extent of these costs, there is little study of the benefits of neuroimaging in delirium, coupled with analysis of the optimal timing and which modalities are best used.

The current paucity of the science means that expert consensus coupled with clinical judgment is the main source of guidance on which patients with delirium should undergo neuroimaging. The 2006 British Geriatrics Society guidelines on delirium suggest that scanning is indicated in patients with delirium who have new focal neurological signs, signs of raised intracranial pressure, or who have recently had a fall or head injury. It is our practice also to request a CT scan in patients with delirium persisting for several days in whom optimal medical management has failed to improve the patient's condition. This is because not all intracranial causes of delirium cause focal neurological signs; for example, small infarcts in areas of the brain not directly involved in motor or sensory functioning, or subdural hemorrhages. Naturally, imaging followed by lumbar puncture is also essential in patients with subarachnoid hemorrhage, or suspected CNS infections, though in the latter case CT scanning will tend only to show gross abnormalities such as cerebral abscesses.

The role of MRI as a second-line investigation in delirium in clinical practice has not been subjected to systematic study. In our experience it has an important place in the investigation of persistent delirium, usually after CT scanning has been done and has either revealed a suspicious lesion or has been negative. A MRI scan may reveal strategic infarcts or small tumors which have not been detected by CT. Mostly, these findings will not change the clinical management in terms of intervention, but they can give crucial prognostic information. Clearly, additional research on the value and indications for CT and MRI in delirium is essential given the billions of dollars a year spent yearly on these investigations.

Conclusions

Neuroimaging of patients with delirium with the aim of excluding structural intracranial pathology is a routine part of clinical practice. Yet the research base informing this is very small. Neuroimaging has been used in delirium research as a means of better understanding the CNS-specific risk factors for delirium, and also, in a handful of patients, what the functional and molecular changes occurring during acute delirium might be. Currently the application of neuroimaging to the understanding of the fundamentals of delirium has been remarkably limited in the face of the enormous burden of the condition along with the potential that neuroimaging has to add knowledge. With the continuing expansion of interest in delirium in both clinical practice and research it may be that delirium researchers find ways of overcoming the practical, ethical, and other barriers of using neuroimaging to shed light on this important yet neglected condition.

References

1. Soiza RL, Sharma V, Ferguson K, *et al.* Neuroimaging findings in delirium: a systematic review. *J Psychosom Res* 2008;**65**:239–48.

2. Davis DH, Muniz Terrera G, Keage H, *et al.* Delirium is a strong risk factor for dementia in the oldest-old: a population-based cohort study. *Brain* 2012;**135**:2809–16.

3. Benke T, Delazer M, Bartha L, Auer A. Basal ganglia lesions and the theory of fronto-subcortical loops: neuropsychological findings in two patients with left caudate lesions. *Neurocase* 2003;**9**:70–85.

4. Caplan LR, Schmahmann JD, Kase CS, *et al.* Caudate infarcts. *Arch Neurol* 1990;**47**:133–43.

5. Seo SW, Kang CK, Kim SH, *et al.* Measurements of lenticulostriate arteries using 7T MRI: new imaging markers for subcortical vascular dementia. *J Neurol Sci* 2012;**322**:200–5.

6. Payabvash S, Souza LC, Wang Y, *et al.* Regional ischemic vulnerability of the brain to hypoperfusion: the need for location specific computed tomography perfusion thresholds in acute stroke patients. *Stroke* 2011;**42**:1255–60.

7. Looi JC, Tatham V, Kumar R, *et al.* Caudate nucleus volumes in stroke and vascular dementia. *Psychiatry Res* 2009;**174**:67–75.

8. Cunningham C, Wilcockson DC, Campion S, Lunnon K, Perry VH. Central and systemic endotoxin challenges exacerbate the local inflammatory response and increase neuronal death during chronic neurodegeneration. *J Neurosci* 2005;**25**:9275–84.

9. Cunningham C, Campion S, Lunnon K, *et al.* Systemic inflammation induces acute behavioral and cognitive changes and accelerates neurodegenerative disease. *Biol Psychiatry* 2009;**65**:304–12.

10. Cunningham C, MacLullich AM. At the extreme end of the psychoneuroimmunological spectrum: delirium as a maladaptive sickness behaviour response. *Brain Behav Immun* 2013;**28**:1–13.

11. MacLullich AM, Edelshain BT, Hall RJ, *et al.* Cerebrospinal fluid interleukin-8 levels are higher in people with hip fracture with perioperative delirium than in controls. *J Am Geriatr Soc* 2011;**59**:1151–3.

12. Bitsch A, Bruhn H, Vougioukas V, *et al.* Inflammatory CNS demyelination: histopathologic correlation with in vivo quantitative proton MR spectroscopy. *AJNR Am J Neuroradiol* 1999;**20**:1619–27.

13. Petroff OA, Graham GD, Blamire AM, *et al.* Spectroscopic imaging of stroke in humans: histopathology correlates of spectral changes. *Neurology* 1992;**42**:1349–54.

14. Simpson JE, Ince PG, Higham CE, *et al.* Microglial activation in white matter lesions and nonlesional white matter of ageing brains. *Neuropathol Appl Neurobiol* 2007;**33**:670–83.

15. Jalal FY, Yang Y, Thompson J, Lopez AC, Rosenberg GA. Myelin loss associated with neuroinflammation in hypertensive rats. *Stroke* 2012;**43**:1115–22.

16. Mulligan SJ, MacVicar BA. Calcium transients in astrocyte endfeet cause cerebrovascular constrictions. *Nature* 2004;**431**:195–9.

17. Häussinger D, Schliess F, Kircheis G. Pathogenesis of hepatic encephalopathy. *J Gastroenterol Hepatol* 2002;**17**:S256–9.

18. van Munster BC, Korevaar JC, Korse CM, *et al.* Serum S100B in elderly patients with and without delirium. *Int J Geriatr Psychiatry* 2010;**25**:234–9.

19. Okello A, Edison P, Archer HA, *et al.* Microglial activation and amyloid deposition in mild cognitive impairment: a PET study. *Neurology* 2009;**72**:56–62.

20. Tourdias T, Mori N, Dragonu I, *et al.* Differential aquaporin 4 expression during edema build-up and resolution phases of brain inflammation. *J Neuroinflammation* 2011;**8**:143.

21. Reeves S, Mehta M, Howard R, Grasby P, Brown R. The dopaminergic basis of cognitive and motor performance in Alzheimer's disease. *Neurobiol Dis* 2010;**37**:477–82.

22. Brunelin J, D'amato T, Van Os J, *et al.* Increased left striatal dopamine transmission in unaffected siblings of schizophrenia patients in response to acute metabolic stress. *Psychiatry Res* 2010;**181**:130–5.

23. Lataster J, Collip D, Ceccarini J, *et al.* Psychosocial stress is associated with in vivo dopamine release in human ventromedial prefrontal cortex: a positron emission tomography study using {^{18}F}fallypride. *Neuroimage* 2011;**58**:1081–9.

24. Marcone A, Garibotto V, Moresco RM, *et al.* {11C}-MP4A PET Cholinergic measurements in amnestic mild cognitive impairment, probable Alzheimer's disease, and dementia with Lewy Bodies: a Bayesian method and voxel-based analysis. *J Alzheimers Dis* 2012;**31**:387–99.

25. Bohnen NI, Bogan CW, Müller ML. Frontal and periventricular brain white matter lesions and cortical deafferentation of cholinergic and other neuromodulatory axonal projections. *Eur Neurol J* 2009;**1**:33–50.

26. Kadir A, Almkvist O, Wall A, Långström B, Nordberg A. PET imaging of cortical 11C-nicotine binding correlates with the cognitive function of attention in Alzheimer's disease. *Psychopharmacology (Berl)* 2006;**188**:509–20.

27. Brady K, Joshi B, Zweifel C, *et al.* Real-time continuous monitoring of cerebral blood flow autoregulation using near-infrared spectroscopy in patients undergoing cardiopulmonary bypass. *Stroke* 2010;**41**:1951–6.

28. Pfister D, Siegemund M, Dell-Kuster S, *et al.* Cerebral perfusion in sepsis-associated delirium. *Crit Care* 2008;**12**:R63.

29. Leenders KL, Salmon EP, Tyrrell P, *et al.* The nigrostriatal dopaminergic system assessed in vivo by positron emission tomography in healthy volunteer subjects and patients with Parkinson's disease. *Arch Neurol* 1990;**47**:1290–8.

30. Aanerud J, Borghammer P, Chakravarty MM, *et al.* Brain energy metabolism and blood flow differences in healthy aging. *J Cereb Blood Flow Metab* 2012;**32**:1177–87.

31. Raichle ME, MacLeod AM, Snyder AZ, *et al.* A default mode of brain function. *Proc Natl Acad Sci USA* 2001;**98**:676–82.

32. Kalaria RN. Vascular basis for brain degeneration: faltering controls and risk factors for dementia. *Nutr Rev* 2010;**68**(Suppl 2):S74–87.

33. Kitagawa K, Oku N, Kimura Y, *et al.* Relationship between cerebral blood flow and later cognitive decline in hypertensive patients with cerebral small vessel disease. *Hypertens Res* 2009;**32**:816–20.

34. Hansson O, Buchhave P, Zetterberg H, *et al.* Combined rCBF and CSF biomarkers predict progression from mild cognitive impairment to Alzheimer's disease. *Neurobiol Aging* 2009;**30**:165–73.

35. Chernov VI, Efimova NY, Efimova IY, Akhmedov SD, Lishmanov YB. Short-term and long-term cognitive function and cerebral perfusion in off-pump and on-pump coronary artery bypass patients. *Eur J Cardiothorac Surg* 2006;**29**:74–81.

36. Markus HS, Lythgoe DJ, Ostegaard L, O'Sullivan M, Williams SC. Reduced cerebral blood flow in white matter in ischaemic leukoaraiosis demonstrated using quantitative exogenous contrast based perfusion MRI. *J Neurol Neurosurg Psychiatry* 2000;**69**:48–53.

37. O'Sullivan M, Lythgoe DJ, Pereira AC, *et al.* Patterns of cerebral blood flow reduction in patients with ischemic leukoaraiosis. *Neurology* 2002;**59**:321–6.

38. Fong TG, Jones RN, Shi P, *et al.* Delirium accelerates cognitive decline in Alzheimer disease. *Neurology* 2009;**72**:1570–5.

39. Girard TD, Jackson JC, Pandharipande PP, *et al.* Delirium as a predictor of long-term cognitive impairment in survivors of critical illness. *Crit Care Med* 2010;**38**:1513–20.

40. van der Flier WM, van Straaten EC, Barkhof F, *et al.* Small vessel disease and general cognitive function in nondisabled elderly: the LADIS study. *Stroke* 2005;**36**:2116–20.

41. Verdelho A, Madureira S, Moleiro C, *et al.* White matter changes and diabetes predict cognitive decline in the elderly: the LADIS study. *Neurology* 2010;**75**:160–7.

42. Whitwell JL, Przybelski SA, Weigand SD, *et al.* 3D maps from multiple MRI illustrate changing atrophy patterns as subjects progress from mild cognitive impairment to Alzheimer's disease. *Brain* 2007;**130**:1777–86.

43. Risacher SL, Saykin AJ, West JD, *et al.* Baseline MRI predictors of conversion from MCI to probable AD in the ADNI cohort. *Curr Alzheimer Res* 2009;**6**:347–61.

44. Morandi A, Rogers BP, Gunther ML, *et al.*; VISIONS Investigation, VISualizing Icu SurvivOrs Neuroradiological Sequelae. The relationship between delirium duration, white matter integrity, and cognitive impairment in intensive care unit survivors as determined by diffusion tensor imaging: the VISIONS prospective cohort magnetic resonance imaging study. *Crit Care Med* 2012;**40**:2182–9.

45. Ferguson KJ, Wardlaw JM, MacLullich AM. Quantitative and qualitative measures of hippocampal atrophy are not correlated in healthy older men. *J Neuroimaging* 2010;**20**:157–62.

46. Aribisala BS, Cox SR, Ferguson KJ, *et al.* Assessing the performance of atlas-based prefrontal brain parcellation in an aging cohort. *J Comput Assist Tomogr* 2013;**37**:257–64.

47. Gunther ML, Morandi A, Krauskopf E, *et al.*; VISIONS Investigation, VISualizing Icu SurvivOrs Neuroradiological Sequelae. The association between brain volumes, delirium duration, and cognitive outcomes in intensive care unit survivors: the VISIONS cohort magnetic resonance imaging study. *Crit Care Med* 2012;**40**:2022–32.

48. Sullivan EV, Pfefferbaum A. Neuroimaging of the Wernicke-Korsakoff syndrome. *Alcohol Alcohol* 2009;**44**:155–65.

49. Garcia-Martinez R, Rovira A, Alonso J, *et al.* Hepatic encephalopathy is associated with posttransplant cognitive function and brain volume. *Liver Transpl* 2011;**17**:38–46.

50. Figiel GS, Coffey CE, Djang WT, Hoffman G, Doraiswamy PM. Brain magnetic resonance imaging findings in ECT-induced delirium. *J Neuropsychiatry Clin Neurosci* 1990;**2**:53–8.

51. Figiel GS, Krishnan KR, Doraiswamy PM. Subcortical structural changes in ECT-induced delirium. *J Geriatr Psychiatry Neurol* 1990;**3**:172–6.

52. Prins ND, van Straaten EC, van Dijk EJ, *et al.* Measuring progression of cerebral white matter lesions on MRI: visual rating and volumetrics. *Neurology* 2004;**62**:1533–9.

53. Fazekas F, Kleinert R, Offenbacher H, *et al.* The morphologic correlate of incidental punctate white matter hyperintensities on MR images. *AJNR Am J Neuroradiol* 1991;**12**:915–21.

54. Morandi A, Gunther ML, Vasilevskis EE, *et al.* Neuroimaging in delirious intensive care unit patients:

a preliminary case series report. *Psychiatry (Edgmont)* 2010;**7**:28–33.

55. Sharshar T, Carlier R, Bernard F, *et al.* Brain lesions in septic shock: a magnetic resonance imaging study. *Intensive Care Med* 2007;**33**:798–806.

56. Finelli PF, Uphoff DF. Magnetic resonance imaging abnormalities with septic encephalopathy. *J Neurol Neurosurg Psychiatry* 2004;**75**:1189–91.

57. Cerase A, Rubenni E, Rufa A, *et al.* CT and MRI of Wernicke's encephalopathy. *Radiol Med* 2011;**116**:319–33.

58. Antunez E, Estruch R, Cardenal C, *et al.* Usefulness of CT and MR imaging in the diagnosis of acute Wernicke's encephalopathy. *AJR Am J Roentgenol* 1998;**171**:1131–7.

59. Shioiri A, Kurumaji A, Takeuchi T, *et al.* White matter abnormalities as a risk factor for postoperative delirium revealed by diffusion tensor imaging. *Am J Geriatr Psychiatry* 2010;**18**:743–53.

60. Wityk RJ, Goldsborough MA, Hillis A, *et al.* Diffusion- and perfusion-weighted brain magnetic resonance imaging in patients with neurologic complications after cardiac surgery. *Arch Neurol* 2001;**58**:571–6.

61. Bendszus M, Reents W, Franke D, *et al.* Brain damage after coronary artery bypass grafting. *Arch Neurol* 2002;**59**:1090–5.

62. Naegele T, Grodd W, Viebahn R, *et al.* MR imaging and (1)H spectroscopy of brain metabolites in hepatic encephalopathy: time-course of renormalization after liver transplantation. *Radiology* 2000;**216**:683–91.

63. Fong TG, Bogardus ST Jr, Daftary A, *et al.* Cerebral perfusion changes in older delirious patients using 99mTc HMPAO SPECT. *J Gerontol A Biol Sci Med Sci* 2006;**61**:1294–9.

64. Yokota, H, Ogawa, S, Kurokawa, A, Yamamoto, Y. Regional cerebral blood flow in delirium patients. *Psychiatry Clin Neurosci* 2003;**57**:337–39.

65. Iversen P, Sørensen M, Bak LK, *et al.* Low cerebral oxygen consumption and blood flow in patients with cirrhosis and an acute episode of hepatic encephalopathy. *Gastroenterology* 2009;**136**:863–71.

66. Koponen H, Hurri L, Stenback U, *et al.* Computed-tomography findings in delirium. *J Nerv Ment Dis* 1989;**177**:226–31.

67. Figiel GS, Krishnan KRR, Breitner JC, Nemeroff CB. Radiologic correlates of antidepressant-induced delirium: the possible significance of basal ganglia lesions. *J Neuropsychiatry Clin Neurosci* 1989;**1**:188–90.

68. Martin M, Figiel GS, Mattingly G, Zorumski CF, Jarvis MR. ECT-induced interictal delirium in patients with a

history of a CVA. *J Geriatr Psychiatry Neurol* 1992;**5**:149–155.

69. Nagaratnam N, Nagaratnam P. Subcortical origins of acute confusional states. *Eur J Intern Med* 1995;**6**:55–58.

70. Kishi Y, Iwasaki Y, Takezawa K, Kurosawa H, Endo S. Delirium in critical care unit patients admitted through an emergency room. *Gen Hosp Psychiatry* 1995;**17**:371–9.

71. Henon H, Lebert F, Durieu I, *et al.* Confusional state in stroke – relation to preexisting dementia, patient characteristics, and outcome. *Stroke* 1999;**30**:773–9.

72. Caeiro L, Ferro JM, Albuquerque R, Figueira ML. Delirium in the first days of acute stroke. *J Neurol* 2004;**251**:171–8.

73. Samton JB, Ferrando SJ, Sanelli P, *et al.* The Clock Drawing Test: diagnostic, functional, and neuroimaging correlates in older medically ill adults. *J Neuropsychiatry Clin Neurosci* 2005;**17**:533–40.

74. Choi SH, Lee H, Chung TS, *et al.* Neural network functional connectivity during and after an episode of delirium. *Am J Psychiatry* 2012;**169**:498–507.

Chapter

27

Environmental modification

Yoanna Skrobik

SUMMARY

Critical care units are currently designed to physically accommodate the mechanical and technological support the patients require, and to provide staff with easy and speedy access to patients with open working areas, monitoring devices and their alarms, and a focus on safety aided by technology rather than on a patient-centered reassuring environment. In this chapter, the focus will be this environment in relationship to cognitive well-being and psychological or psychiatric symptom prevention and palliation. Environment can be defined in many ways: physical and structural, in terms of light and sound, in terms of local practice and culture, such as nursing practice regarding restraints and patient visiting policies, and as a consideration of available resources such as physiotherapy. The link between features of the environment as defined above, and the vulnerable critically ill patient's well-being, is reviewed herein.

Introduction

The anxiety, fear, paranoid delusions, and discouragement that characterize many a critically ill patient's experience is viewed by medical caregivers through the narrow prism of the neurological or psychiatric diagnosis. Medical culture [1] necessarily espouses this rigid approach. In settings outside critical care, it is understood that a patient's well-being depends on psychological integrity and on a reassuring physical environment. The foreign, disturbing, and overwhelmingly technological setting of the intensive care unit (ICU) is an antithesis to this patient comfort. Some authors have drawn parallels between the critical care environment and the torture imposed on political prisoners [2], including social isolation, sleep deprivation, and inattention to needs. This wretchedness is

complicated by a complete dependence on machines and personnel. What little autonomy patients retain is seldom fostered or encouraged. The relationship with a significant person in the patient's life, which contributes to healing, or to a more serene journey towards death, is disrupted in many ways, particularly if the patient becomes delirious or comatose, and if, in addition, local rules such as limited visiting hours are imposed. Dimensions such as illness (the patients' perception of the self) and sickness (the social dimension and impact of the disease), both influenced by environment, cause the patient distress. Patient recovery and post-discharge outcomes may be related to these dimensions of illness and sickness; however, our inadequate understanding of these facets as experienced by patients, their caregivers, and loved ones limits an evidence-based approach to holistic care.

The attention of the critical care community has been drawn over recent years to the treatment and the prevention of delirium as well as the study of associated risk factors. Delirium, one of the psychological or psychiatric dimensions of the critical care experience, is believed to be the consequence of many concomitant features; risk models for patients outside the ICU have been constructed, and incorporate predisposing and precipitating factors. Predisposing factors are not modifiable; precipitating factors can be related to the acute illness but also, importantly, to the environment and therefore can, potentially, be changed to benefit the patient. Other psychological and psychiatric disturbances common to the ICU patient such as depression or posttraumatic stress disorder have not been described with such risk model stratification in critical care, probably because of their more recent description.

In this chapter, the focus will be the patient's environment with a specific emphasis on cognitive well-

Brain Disorders in Critical Illness, ed. Robert D. Stevens, Tarek Sharshar, and E. Wesley Ely. Published by
Cambridge University Press. © Cambridge University Press 2013.

being and psychological or psychiatric symptom prevention and palliation. Environment can be defined in many ways: physical and structural, in terms of light and sound, in terms of local practice and culture, such as nursing practice regarding restraints and patient visiting policies, and as a consideration of available resources such as physiotherapy. This chapter is, however, limited by the dearth of information on the topic in the current literature.

Physical environment

Architects interested in hospital and ICU environment design publish reviews that link the physical environment to patient and staff outcomes in four areas: the reduction of staff stress and fatigue, including increased effectiveness in delivering care; improvements in patient safety; the reduction of patient stress and associated improved outcomes; and improvement in overall healthcare quality [3]. Because of this volume's focus on patient neurological and cognitive function, only patient outcome-based environmental elements will be described here, with a focus on noise, light, and sleep. Ergonomics play a key role in ICU functionality but have not been presented from a patient-centered perspective, and are therefore not elaborated upon here.

Florence Nightingale wrote in 1859 that "unnecessary noise, or noise that creates an expectation in the mind, is that which hurts a patient." Critical care environments are notoriously noisy. Sound is usually measured in decibels (dB), and an increase of 10 dB is perceived by the human ear as a sound twice as loud. The World Health Organization recommends that the average background noise in hospitals not exceed 30 A-weighted decibels [dB (A)], with peaks during the night time of less than 40 dB (A). Studies report average noise levels of 60–70 dB (A) in critical care units, with peaks over 90 dB (A) 24 hours a day. The generation of noise is multifactorial, and generally due to behaviour, as loud voices are louder than the telephone or alarms; equipment noise accounts for the greater part of the balance. Nebulizers are recorded at 80 dB (A); hoods used for continuous positive airway pressure reach levels of above 100 dB (A). A table with ICU noise levels placed in the context of familiar sounds illustrates this point (Table 27.1).

Noise in the ICU is considered one of the environmental causes of sleep disruption. Sound pressure levels of below 40 dB (A) are generally required to enable sleep, although the auditory threshold for waking may increase when individuals are continually

Table 27.1 Examples of commonplace noises and their decibel levels.

Type of noise	Sound level [dB(A)]
Jet aircraft taking off at 50 m	120
Loud music in a disco	100
Lawn mower at 1 m	90
Vacuum cleaner at 1 m	70
Average ICU sound level	60–70
Conversation at 50 m	55
Soft whisper in a library	40

exposed to a noisy environment. Patients perceive noise as a common cause of sleep disruption in the ICU and may find it difficult to get to sleep because of the continuous background sound level. It has been suggested that the disruption to sleep caused by noise may become more important as a patient begins to recover from critical illness.

Earplugs have been shown to lessen the sleep deterrent impact of the noise made by mechanical ventilators, monitoring alarms, and other ICU apparatuses in normal subjects [4]. Patients in the ICU could technically benefit from being offered earplugs in the clinical setting with an aim of reducing noise and helping them sleep. However, the experience in my hospital center has been the patients are frightened of what will happen if they cannot hear what is going on around them. Their use has not been validated in a prospective study.

The human sleep–wake cycle is closely linked to the environment; the light–dark cycle is probably its most significant component. Sleep–wake cycles can be altered in the absence of such cycles; in some ICUs, patients are never exposed to any natural light. Light has mostly been used in critical care to re-establish day–night cycle normality, and in an attempt to move away from the technical need to light the environment well to more patient-centered lighting. Morning bright light administration to a small group of post-esophagectomy patients was associated, in a pilot study, with earlier mobility and lower delirium rates [5], and assumed to be attributable to light-triggered improvement in circadian rhythm. Lack of exposure to daylight appears to increase the risk for delirium in the only large ICU study that explicitly included environmental features. Patients with no visible daylight had an OR of 2.39 for delirium in comparison to patients exposed to rooms with windows [6] (Figure 27.1).

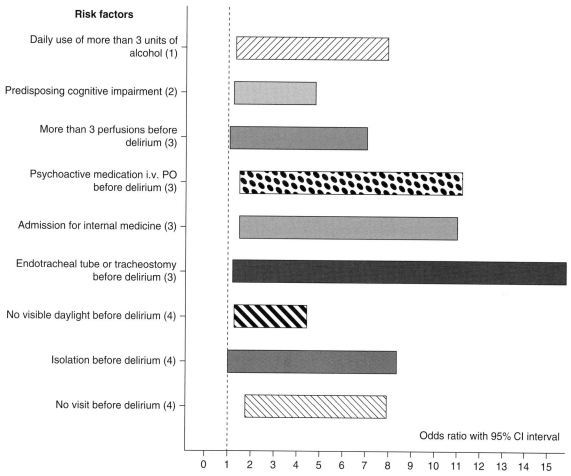

Figure 27.1 Environmental risk factors associated with delirium, among significant associated risks; adapted from [6].

General noise reduction strategies and a pleasant, appropriately lit environment do seem to be beneficial to patients and reduce delirium duration in a single site pre–post study [7], and are very unlikely to do harm. This is tempered by the increase in delirium incidence observed when patients are isolated in infection isolation rooms, even though these are quieter (OR of 2.89). Isolation may account for this risk, since patients with no visitors also appear to have a higher delirium risk (OR 3.73) [6], although whether this is a result of premorbid characteristics or a true ICU experience association is not certain. Some authors have argued that noise reduction, pleasant lighting, and more ergonomic environments are measures that may not only increase patient well-being but staff satisfaction and performance [8], and that improving nursing staffing ratios and promoting a more humane environment is beneficial for caregivers and patients alike. When

environmental factors such as organizational structures and professional sociological processes are correlated with organizational attributes and patient care outcomes, noise levels and lighting, enhancing communication, and eliminating over- and under-stimulation consistently favorably influence the quality of care.

Humane appreciation of visitors' environmental needs may also lessen the patients' distress. Families should be accommodated through the availability of showers, lockers, and internet access.

Nursing practice

Physical restraint

The use of physical restraint in the ICU varies broadly between nations and continents. In the USA, Australia, and mainland Europe, it is conventional practice in the

ICU setting. In the UK, it is rarely used, similarly to Scandinavian countries where 'chemical' restraint is favored [9]. In an observational American study of 40 hospitals in six cities, ICUs accounted for 56% of all restraint days despite having only 16% of all the patient-days [10].

The patient 's psychological experience in response to restraint has been reported to include increased agitation, withdrawal, emotional devastation, fear, and loss of dignity [11]. Adverse physical effects have included all the associated side effects of immobility, impaired circulation, and nerve injury. Although touted as a safety measure, physical restraints are associated with a higher rate of self-extubation [12]. In a recent study by Van Rompaey and colleagues [6], the preventive use of soft wrist restraints to protect the position of catheters, tubes, and drains seemed to be associated with a higher delirium incidence (OR 33.84). In addition to being controversial, the use of restraints has been associated with posttraumatic stress disorder (PTSD) [13] among critically ill patients. Ideally, restraint must not substitute for inadequate human and environmental resources, and should only be used when alternative therapeutic measures have proved ineffective.

Visiting hours and framing families

Visitation policies vary considerably among institutions. In the ICU study with careful documentation of environmental features, patients without visitors were at greater risk of developing delirium (OR 3.73) [6]. Recent literature pointed at the possible beneficial effects of visitors in the ICU. An open visitor policy has not been associated with patient harm. Descriptions by observers, and stories [14] told by individual patients, describe the anguish, fear, and harrowing nature of patient perceptions in a delirious state. Some narratives and recall studies describe the positive impact of reassuring or reality-orienting caregivers within the critical care setting. The added contribution made by visiting family members and loved ones are in keeping with the positive impact of nurse-facilitated family participation in the care of a delirious patient [15].

Nursing culture and symptom management

Critically ill patients are by definition vulnerable and marginalized populations; their nursing services experience needs are seldom acknowledged or integrated into intervention and treatment plans. Framing nursing care around the concept of "Nursing their way not our way" [16] may improve patient comfort and perception of comfort by responding to explicitly expressed patient wishes. Several of these have been raised in studies addressing sources of patient anxiety and discomfort: pain and untreated pain; amnesia as to ICU events and the distress associated with this amnesia (particularly in patients with delirium, who experience amnesia more frequently [17]); and anxiety. Most patients are aware of their surroundings while they are in the ICU; many nursing authors emphasize how important ICU nursing education is to include issues regarding all aspects of patient care, including optimizing their feelings of security, comfort, and self-respect.

Self-reported distress in terms of pain, psychological problems, and frustration as to the ability to communicate are common (44, 60, and 90% respectively) in the critically ill mechanically ventilated patient. Regular assessments of pain are beneficial to patient outcome; they certainly appear to be linked to lower mechanical ventilation time and better wound healing in surgical patients. In addition to moderate to severe pain being common, it is debilitating to ICU survivors. However, pain assessments are not routinely performed despite evidence that pain occurs in patients in whom caregivers do not expect it [18], and is poorly screened for in the critically ill in general. Treating patients for pain and adjusting the medications to their sedation needs appear to be associated with a lower incidence of subsyndromal delirium [19].

The role of psychological distress is not negligible in the perception and experience of delirium. Delirium in the ICU has been described by some authors as a "psychosomatic" problem in the context of stress response syndrome after surgery or as a defense mechanism against death anxiety [20]. Such psychological factors may be resolved more efficiently with the collaboration of psychologists and psychiatrists in the ICU. Psychological support in the ICU to families and to patients appears to lessen burden and improve outcome. Narratives in other psychologically stressed populations, such as combat-zone medical or trauma patients, appear to aid greatly in reducing PTSD and are a useful, cost-effective method to improve outcomes. One study suggests that early and targeted psychological intervention, consisting of five or six face-to-face meetings involving direct ICU patient counseling, stress management, support, and education by a clinical psychologist [21], offers better outcomes from PTSD than standard ICU care.

Public health data of the World Health Organization revealed that smoking is common in 24% of adults in the USA, and 37% in Europe. Nicotine withdrawal may be associated with delirium according to some studies, although the benefit of nicotine patches in patients without myocardial ischemia is not proven for all ICU populations. Delirium tremens is rare, but alcohol consumption has been associated with significantly increased ICU delirium risk in several studies. Careful documentation of alcohol and tobacco consumption by nurses and physicians may aid in identifying high-risk patients.

Prevention

Early physiotherapy and mobilization, when implemented to aid myopathy, significantly reduce delirium rates [22,23] and are an element of "environment" described by others in this book. These results raise the question of whether non-pharmacological interventions, which encourage patients to focus on their autonomy, may prevent or alleviate delirium. Sedatives and analgesics, when carefully titrated and administered according to symptoms, are associated with lower rates of subsyndromal delirium and an increase in the probability of a patient being able to return home. The association of cognitive and psychiatric syndromes with sedative agents and the potential benefits of specific drugs such as dexmedetomidine are discussed elsewhere in this book.

Other environmental resources

Non-medical interventions can be helpful in many psychiatric and psychological disturbances. Outside the ICU, prevention of syndromes such as delirium through the use of interventions such as rehydration, reorientation, and warm milk and massages in the evening can sometimes yield spectacular results [24] and are extremely cost-effective. Interventions such as managing pain and anxiety with music may be beneficial to patients, help, and are extremely unlikely to do harm [25]. A bedside diary may aid the most severely traumatized survivor make sense of his or her experience [26]. Finally, opportunities for ICU survivors to tell their tale in a structured fashion may be therapeutic [27]. The narrative has also been described as a tool for healing in the context of illness in many settings,

and as a crucial instrument in transforming suffering for the individual who is telling the tale. Which type of follow-up care, with narratives or without, would best profit ICU survivors is uncertain [28], although routine screening after ICU discharge and as-needed referral services may be of benefit [29,30].

References

1. Good BJ. How medicine constructs its objects. In *Medicine, Rationality, And Experience: An Anthropological Perspective*. Cambridge: Cambridge University Press; 1994:35–87.

2. Dyer I. Preventing the ITU syndrome, or how not to torture an ITU patient: Part 1. *Intensive Crit Care Nurs* 1995;**11**(3):130–139; Part 2. *Intensive Crit Care Nurs* 1995;11(4):223–232.

3. Ulrich R, Zimring C, Quan X, Joseph A, Choudhary R. *Role of the Physical Environment in the Hospital of the 21st Century*. The Center for Health Design; 2004.

4. Wallace CJ, Robins J, Alvord LS, Walker JM. The effect of earplugs on sleep measures during exposure to simulated intensive care unit noise. *Am J Crit Care* 1999;**8**(4):210–19.

5. Taguchi T, Yano M, Kido Y. Influence of bright light therapy on postoperative patients: a pilot study. *Intensive Crit Care Nurs* 2007;**23**(5):289–97.

6. Van Rompaey B, Elseviers MM, Schuurmans MJ, *et al.* Risk factors for delirium in intensive care patients: a prospective cohort study. *Crit Care* 2009;**13**(3):R77.

7. Zaal IJ, Peelen LM, Spruyt CF, Kesecioglu J, Slooter AJ. Nursing environment and delirium in ICU patients. *Crit Care* 2011;**15**(Suppl 1):P334.

8. Mitchell PH, Armstrong S, Simpson TF, Lentz M. American Association of Critical Care Nurses demonstration project: profile of excellence in critical care nursing. *Heart Lung* 1989;**18**:219–37.

9. Martin B, Mathisen L. Use of physical restraints in adult critical care: a bicultural study. *Am J Crit Care* 2005;**14**(2):133–42.

10. Minnick AF, Mion LC, Johnson ME, *et al.* Prevalence and variation of physical restraint use in acute care settings in the US. *J Nurs Scholar* 2007;**39**:30–7

11. Fletcher K. Use of restraints in the elderly. *AACN Clin Issues* 1996;**7**(4):611–35.

12. Chang LY, Wang KW, Chao YF. Influence of physical restraint on unplanned extubation of adult intensive care patients: a case-control study. *Am J Crit Care* 2008;**17**(5):408–15.

13. Jones C, Bäckman C, Capuzzo M, *et al.* Precipitants of post-traumatic stress disorder following intensive care: a hypothesis generating study of diversity in care. *Intensive Care Med* 2007;**33**(6):978–85.

14. Misak CJ. The critical care experience: a patient's view. *Am J Respir Crit Care Med* 2004;**170**:357–9.

15. Black P, Boore JR, Parahoo K. The effect of nurse-facilitated family participation in the psychological care of the critically ill patient. *J Adv Nurs* 2011;**67**:1091–101.

16. Wilson D, Neville S. Nursing their way not our way: working with vulnerable and marginalised populations. *Contemp Nurse* 2008;**27**(2):165–76.

17. Roberts BL, Rickard CM, Rajbhandari D, Reynolds P. Factual memories of ICU: recall at two years post-discharge and comparison with delirium status during ICU admission – a multicentre cohort study. *J Clin Nurs* 2007;**16**(9):1669–77.

18. Desbiens NA, Wu AW, Alzola C, *et al.* Pain during hospitalization is associated with continued pain six months later in survivors of serious illness. The SUPPORT Investigators. Study to Understand Prognoses and Preferences for Outcomes and Risks of Treatments. *Am J Med* 1997;**102**(3):269–76.

19. Skrobik Y, Ahern S, Leblanc M, *et al.* Protocolized intensive care unit management of analgesia, sedation, and delirium improves analgesia and subsyndromal delirium rates. *Anesth Analg* 2010;**111**:451–63.

20. Reich M, Rohn R, Lefevre D. Surgical intensive care unit (ICU) delirium: a "psychosomatic" problem? *Palliat Support Care* 2010;**8**(2):221–5.

21. Peris A, Bonizzoli M, Iozzelli D, *et al.* Early intra-intensive care unit psychological intervention promotes recovery from post traumatic stress disorders, anxiety and depression symptoms in critically ill patients. *Crit Care* 2011;**15**:R41.

22. Schweickert WD, Pohlman MC, Pohlman AS, *et al.* Early physical and occupational therapy in mechanically ventilated, critically ill patients: a randomized controlled trial. *Lancet* 2009;**373**: 1874–82.

23. Needham DM, Korupolu R, Zanni JM, *et al.* Early physical medicine and rehabilitation for patients with acute respiratory failure: a quality improvement project. *Arch Phys Med Rehabil* 2010;**91**:536–42.

24. Inouye SK, Bogardus ST, Charpentier PA, *et al.* A multicomponent intervention to prevent delirium in hospitalized older patients. *N Engl J Med* 1999;**340**:669–76.

25. Hunter BC, Oliva R, Sahler OJ, *et al.* Music therapy as an adjunctive treatment in the management of stress for patients being weaned from mechanical ventilation. *J Music Ther* 2010;**47**:198–219.

26. Jones C, Bäckman C, Capuzzo M, *et al.* Intensive care diaries reduce new onset post traumatic stress disorder following critical illness: a randomised, controlled trial. *Crit Care* 2010;**14**:R168.

27. Williams SL. How telling stories helps patients to recover psychologically after intensive care. *Nurs Times* 2010;**106**:20–3.

28. Cuthbertson BH, Rattray J, Johnston M, *et al.* A pragmatic randomised, controlled trial of intensive care follow up programmes in improving longer-term outcomes from critical illness. The PRACTICAL study. *BMC Health Serv Res* 2007;**7**:116.

29. Schandl AR, Brattström OR, Svensson-Raskh A, *et al.* Screening and treatment of problems after intensive care: a descriptive study of multidisciplinary follow-up. *Intensive Crit Care Nurs* 2011;**27**:94–101.

30. Pattison NA, Dolan S, Townsend P, Townsend R. After critical care: a study to explore patients' experiences of a follow-up service. *J Clin Nurs* 2007;**16**:2122–31.

Chapter 28

New paradigms in sedation of the critically ill patient

Christopher G. Hughes and Pratik P. Pandharipande

SUMMARY

Critically ill patients are routinely provided medications to treat pain and anxiety, permit invasive procedures, and improve tolerance of mechanical ventilation. Untreated pain and anxiety lead to negative short- and long-term consequences; however, oversedation is common and is also associated with worse clinical outcomes, including delirium. In addition, a wide discrepancy in the approach to sedation of critically ill patients exists secondary to regional preferences, institutional bias, and individual patient and practitioner variability. Practitioners can improve patient outcomes by incorporating analgesia, sedation (arousal), and delirium protocols, targeted arousal levels, daily interruption of sedation, linked spontaneous awakening and breathing trials, and early mobilization of patients into clinical management. Furthermore, altering conventional sedation paradigms by providing necessary analgesia, incorporating propofol or dexmedetomidine to reach arousal targets, and reducing benzodiazepine exposure can further improve outcomes, including time on mechanical ventilation and development of acute brain dysfunction.

General principles of sedation in the intensive care unit

In critically ill patients, pain and anxiety contribute to an already exaggerated sympathetic stress response that includes increased endogenous catecholamine activity, increased oxygen consumption, tachycardia, hypercoagulability, hypermetabolism, and immunosuppression [1]. Furthermore, unrelieved anxiety and agitation can lead to the removal of lifesaving medical devices (e.g., endotracheal tubes, intravascular lines) and may be a significant source of physical and psychological stress during the acute event and months after discharge [e.g., posttraumatic stress disorder (PTSD)] [2]. Analgesia and sedation are thus administered to provide comfort and ensure patient safety; however, oversedation occurs frequently and is associated with longer time on mechanical ventilation and in the ICU, greater need for radiological evaluations of mental status, and higher probability of developing delirium [3–6]. In order to optimize patient care, safety, and comfort while minimizing the negative outcomes associated with psychoactive medications, healthcare professionals must achieve the right balance of analgesic and sedative drug administration.

Hemodynamic instability, drug interactions, altered protein binding, and impaired organ function cause unpredictable pharmacokinetics and pharmacodynamics in ICU patients, thus increasing the difficulty of achieving benefit from analgesic and sedative medications without harm from their associated complications. Drug accumulation from continuous infusions, redistribution, and tachyphylaxis also confound the utilization of sedation, highlighting the importance of techniques to prevent systemic drug accumulation. Thus, in order to develop the best treatment strategy for analgesia and sedation, the specific medical condition necessitating treatment must be recognized. Thereafter, objective routine assessments of pain, arousal, and acute brain dysfunction (e.g., delirium and coma) are necessary to guide the adjustment of goal-directed therapeutic targets that change with the medical condition of the patient [1].

Analgesia

Endotracheal intubation, invasive monitoring, surgical procedures, nursing interventions, and pre-existing diseases are only a few sources of discomfort commonly experienced by ICU patients. Insufficient pain relief can contribute to increased stress response,

Brain Disorders in Critical Illness, ed. Robert D. Stevens, Tarek Sharshar, and E. Wesley Ely. Published by Cambridge University Press. © Cambridge University Press 2013.

deficient sleep, disorientation, anxiety, delirium, and PTSD; however, pain is often undertreated, secondary to concerns about respiratory depression and/or hemodynamic compromise.

Pain assessment

Routine monitoring of pain levels, including intensity, quality, and location, has been associated with lower analgesic and sedative utilization and decreased time on mechanical ventilation and, thus, should be elicited as part of the patient's vital signs [7]. The FACES scale (Figure 28.1) and Behavioral Pain Scale (Table 28.1) are examples of validated tools for assessing pain in ICU patients unable to communicate [8,9].

Analgesic therapy

Systemic analgesics should be administered as part of a goal-directed analgesia and sedation protocol. Systemic therapies include non-steroidal anti-inflammatory

drugs and acetaminophen, but opioids are the most common ICU therapy secondary to their analgesic and sedative properties. The most commonly used opioids in the ICU are morphine, hydromorphone, fentanyl, and remifentanil.

The selection of an opioid has traditionally depended on the pharmacology of the specific opioid and the likely duration of analgesic infusion, for few comparative trials have been performed in ICU patients [1]. In one randomized double-blind study, remifentanil provided better outcomes than morphine with regards to time at optimal arousal level, necessity of supplemental sedation, duration of mechanical ventilation, and extubation time [10]. Fentanyl and remifentanil have displayed equal efficacy in achieving sedation goals with no difference in extubation times [11]. Patients receiving fentanyl required more breakthrough sedatives but experienced less pain after extubation compared with patients receiving remifentanil [11]. Higher cost and reports of withdrawal and hyperalgesia have also limited the utilization of remifentanil for ICU analgesia. In general, fentanyl's rapid onset, short duration of action, relatively short half-life, minimal histamine release, and lack of renal elimination allow easy titration as a continuous infusion and makes it the opioid of choice in hemodynamically unstable patients.

With regards to brain dysfunction outcomes, adequate pain control likely reduces delirium. In a prospective cohort study of hip fracture patients, those who received more than 10 mg of parenteral morphine equivalents per day were less likely to develop delirium than patients who received less analgesic medications [12]. Additionally, studies in trauma and burn patients have reported lower risk of developing delirium in patients receiving morphine and methadone [5,13]. However, meperidine and morphine have also been associated with increased risk for delirium in other studies [14,15]. Thus, it appears that in patients at high risk for pain, providing

Table 28.1 The Behavioral Pain Scale (adapted from [9]).

Item	Description	Score
Facial expression	Relaxed	1
	Partially tightened (e.g., brow lowering)	2
	Fully tightened (e.g., eyelid closing)	3
	Grimacing	4
Upper extremity movement	No movement	1
	Partially bent	2
	Fully bent with finger flexion	3
	Permanently retracted	4
Ventilator compliance	Tolerating movement	1
	Coughing but tolerating ventilation	2
	Fighting ventilator	3
	Unable to control ventilation	4

Wong–Baker FACES pain rating scale

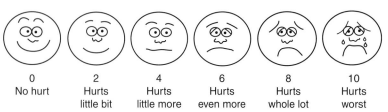

0	2	4	6	8	10
No hurt	Hurts little bit	Hurts little more	Hurts even more	Hurts whole lot	Hurts worst

Figure 28.1 FACES scale. Reproduced with permission from Hicks CL, *et al.* The Faces Pain Scale-Revised: toward a common metric in pediatric pain measurement. *Pain* 2001;**93** (2):173–83.

analgesia with opioids may be protective of acute brain dysfunction, while excessive opioid administration to achieve sedation may be detrimental.

Sedation

Pain, excessive stimulation, dyspnea, delirium, inability to communicate, sleep deprivation, and metabolic disturbances are potential causes of anxiety and agitation commonly seen in critically ill patients. Left untreated, agitation can have substantial physical and psychological consequences in the short and long term, and may become life-threatening if it leads to the removal of lifesaving equipment. However, sedative medications also lead to worse patient outcomes, necessitating methods such as target-based protocols to decrease patients' psychoactive drug exposure while still providing adequate patient comfort and safety.

Arousal assessment

The reliability and validity of arousal scales among adult ICU patients allow these scales to be utilized for goal-directed sedative therapy; however, assessment of arousal is part of the neurological examination of all critically ill patients and should not be exclusively linked to sedative drug administration. The Riker Sedation–Agitation scale (Table 28.2), Ramsay scale, and Richmond Agitation–Sedation scale (RASS) are a few of the commonly utilized scales [16–18]. Importantly, the RASS (Table 28.3) has also been shown to detect variations in the level of consciousness over time or in response to changes in analgesic and sedative drug therapy [18]. Along with level of consciousness, critically ill patients should also be monitored for acute brain dysfunction. Delirium, a common clinical presentation of acute brain dysfunction, is an acute fluctuating change in mental status characterized by inattention, perceptual disturbances, and altered levels of consciousness. Its prevalence and associated morbidity, mortality, and cost mandate delirium monitoring in ICU patients [19,20]. Healthcare personnel can assess for the presence of delirium with the Intensive Care Delirium Screening Checklist and the Confusion Assessment Method for the ICU, which have both been validated in non-verbal patients and are reliable in the hands of bedside critical care nurses [21,22]. Thus, arousal scales provide an assessment of the level of consciousness while the delirium monitoring instruments provide further insight into the "quality" and "content" of that consciousness. Increased adaptation of these assessment tools is necessary to promote the widespread cultural change required to improve the care of our critically ill patients.

Table 28.2 The Riker Sedation–Agitation scale (adapted from [16]).

7	Dangerously agitated	Trying to remove tubes and catheters, thrashing, climbing out of bed, striking at staff
6	Very agitated	Requiring restraints and/or frequent verbal reminders of limits, biting endotracheal tube
5	Agitated	Anxious and/or physically agitated, calms to verbal instructions and support
4	Calm and cooperative	Easily arousable, calm, follows commands with minimal stimulation
3	Sedated	Awakens to verbal or physical stimuli, difficult to arouse, able to follow commands when stimulated
2	Deeply sedated	Arouses to physical stimuli, does not follow commands or communicate
1	Unarousable	Minimal or no response to stimulation, does not follow commands or communicate

Table 28.3 The Richmond Agitation–Sedation scale (adapted from [18]).

+4	Combative	Combative, violent, immediate danger to staff
+3	Very agitated	Pulls or removes tubes or catheters, aggressive
+2	Agitated	Frequent non-purposeful movement, fights ventilator
+1	Restless	Anxious, apprehensive, but movements not aggressive or vigorous
0	Alert and calm	
−1	Drowsy	Not fully alert, but has sustained (>10 s) awakening (eye opening/ contact) to voice
−2	Light sedation	Drowsy, briefly (<10 s) awakens to voice or physical stimulation
−3	Moderate sedation	Movement or eye opening (but no eye contact) to voice
−4	Deep sedation	No response to voice, but movement or eye opening to physical stimulation
−5	Unarousable	No response to voice or physical stimulation

Sedation protocols

The provision of protocol-based, goal-directed therapy reduces sedative administration, decreases patient discomfort, and improves patient outcomes [23,24]. Furthermore, the daily interruption of sedation, as well as linking spontaneous awakening trials to daily spontaneous breathing trials, has been shown to increase time off mechanical ventilation and shorten ICU length of stay [4,25]. By incorporating this linked approach, the Awakening and Breathing Controlled Trial also demonstrated a significant reduction in mortality 12 months after hospitalization [25].

While these studies attest to the fact that deep sedation is not required in the majority of ICU patients and that lighter sedation goals improve outcomes, it is important to note that interrupted sedation methods have not been associated with an increase in long-term neuropsychological outcomes such as PTSD [26,27]. In fact, sedative utilization (in particular lorazepam) has been associated with PTSD, and days of sedation have been positively correlated with symptoms of PTSD and depression [28]. While unpleasant memories of their ICU course may contribute to psychological distress in survivors [29], PTSD is more often related to having delusional and non-factual memories of the ICU stay [30]. Additionally, patients with recall of their ICU stay had less cognitive dysfunction than patients with complete amnesia [31], further emphasizing that deep sedation may have prolonged neuropsychological and cognitive effects.

Sedation management

The specific medical condition (e.g., respiratory failure, septic shock) requiring intensive care treatment must be recognized in order to appropriately manage anxiety and agitation. Furthermore, the optimal target arousal level for the individual patient and medical condition must then be determined to guide therapy. If pain is present, an analgesic should be the initial therapeutic choice. Once analgesic therapy has been initiated, propofol, dexmedetomidine, and benzodiazepines are the drugs most commonly utilized if the target arousal level has not been achieved.

Analgosedation

Analgesia-based sedation has been studied primarily with remifentanil and morphine. Remifentanil sedation led to significantly shorter neurological assessment times and time to extubation in patients with brain injury when compared with propofol or midazolam [32]. Both the duration of mechanical ventilation and duration of weaning were significantly shorter in patients receiving remifentanil than midazolam in another comparative study [33]. A randomized multicenter study examined sedation regimens based on propofol or benzodiazepine (with as-needed opioid) versus analgosedation with remifentanil (with as-needed propofol) and found a shortened duration of mechanical ventilation and ICU length of stay in the analgosedation group [34]. More recently, a single-center randomized controlled study compared the use of an analgesia-based protocol incorporating morphine (intervention group) to sedation with propofol and found that the intervention group had shorter times on mechanical ventilation and in the ICU with no adverse events [35]. While approximately 80% of the patients in the intervention group were managed with morphine alone, the ICU had 1 : 1 nursing ratios and other personnel available to reassure patients, limiting the generalizability of this study to most other ICUs.

Sedative medications

Beyond target-based and goal-directed sedation with daily interruption of sedatives, the choice of sedative also has significant implications on patient outcomes. Diazepam, midazolam, and lorazepam have traditionally been the benzodiazepines (gamma-aminobutyric acid (GABA) agonists) most frequently utilized in the ICU. Currently, use of benzodiazepine sedation in the ICU has been curtailed in favor of other sedation regimens, primarily propofol and dexmedetomidine, secondary to mounting evidence of increased morbidity with benzodiazepine administration. Propofol is a diisopropylphenol anesthetic and a GABA agonist with rapid onset and short duration of action. Its side effects include hypotension due to vasodilation and myocardial depression, respiratory depression, hypertriglyceridemia, and propofol-related infusion syndrome (characterized by severe lactic acidosis and rhabdomyolysis) [36]. Dexmedetomidine is an alpha-2 receptor agonist with a sedation site of action at presynaptic neurons in the locus coeruleus and analgesic site of action in the spinal cord, producing sedation and analgesia without significant respiratory depression [37,38]. Its most common side effects include bradycardia, hypotension, and hypertension (stimulation of post-junctional alpha receptors usually during bolus administration).

Comparative studies of sedative regimens

Compared with individual benzodiazepines in several studies, propofol has been shown to increase duration at target arousal level, reduce mechanical ventilation days, and reduce cost per patient [39,40]. The MENDS and SEDCOM studies compared dexmedetomidine to benzodiazepines (lorazepam and midazolam, respectively) and demonstrated that patients sedated with dexmedetomidine had shorter durations of acute brain dysfunction (delirium and coma) [41,42]. In the SEDCOM study, patients on dexmedetomidine also spent less time on mechanical ventilation and developed less tachycardia, and a post hoc analysis demonstrated a significant per-patient reduction in cost associated with dexmedetomidine. Furthermore, decreased mortality was seen in a subgroup of septic patients sedated with dexmedetomidine during the MENDS trial [43].

The first studies comparing dexmedetomidine with propofol demonstrated similar sedation efficacy and mechanical ventilation weaning times between the two agents [44,45]. In post-surgical patients, dexmedetomidine use resulted in the need for less supplemental analgesics than propofol [44]. Similarly, utilization of beta-blockers, antiemetics, epinephrine, and diuretics were reduced with dexmedetomidine sedation in postoperative patients after cardiac surgery [45]. A subsequent meta-analysis additionally suggested that sedation with dexmedetomidine decreases ICU length of stay [46].

In a recently published multicenter study, dexmedetomidine was compared with midazolam (MIDEX) and propofol (PRODEX) for sedation in patients requiring mechanical ventilation [47]. Time at target arousal level was equivalent between dexmedetomidine and the control groups. Patients in the dexmedetomidine group more often required a rescue drug than those in the propofol group, and discontinuation due to lack of efficacy occurred more often in patients sedated with dexmedetomidine. Dexmedetomidine reduced duration of mechanical ventilation compared with midazolam, and time to extubation was faster in dexmedetomidine than either midazolam or propofol. The dexmedetomidine groups also had less delirium and improved arousability, communication, and patient cooperation. Overall, length of ICU and hospital stay and mortality were similar between groups.

These studies attest to the fact that reducing benzodiazepine exposure by utilizing alternative sedation paradigms (e.g., propofol, dexmedetomidine)

improves patient outcomes, including brain organ dysfunction outcomes. For the treatment of delirium tremens, other withdrawal syndromes, and seizures, however, benzodiazepines remain the drugs of choice. An empiric protocol (Figure 28.2) for the management of analgesia and sedation is provided as a reference, although clinicians are advised to incorporate local culture, patient characteristics, and expert opinion to determine the best protocol for their ICUs.

Pharmacological paralysis

The utilization of neuromuscular blockade in ICU sedation has decreased considerably given the increasing evidence of the harm associated with deep sedation techniques. Pharmacological paralysis remains utilized in patients with postoperative open abdomens and in patients with progressive respiratory failure and high peak inspiratory pressures unresponsive to conventional ventilation. Cisatracurium is the recommended agent for maintenance of paralysis in the critically ill, secondary to its non-steroidal benzyl-isoquinoline structure, Hoffman elimination, independence of hepatic or renal elimination, and lack of histamine release. A recent multicenter randomized controlled trial demonstrated that early utilization of cisatracurium paralysis decreased mechanical ventilation time and mortality in patients with acute respiratory distress syndrome without a witnessed increase in muscle weakness [48]. The results of this study need to be confirmed, and the ramifications with regards to sedation techniques still need to be further evaluated.

Early mobilization

Initiating physical therapy early during a critically ill patient's hospital stay has been proven feasible and safe and has been associated with decreased length of stay both in the ICU and hospital [49]. Combining daily interruption of sedation with physical and occupational therapy has been shown to decrease duration of delirium in the ICU and hospital by almost 50%, and lead to significant improvement in functional status at hospital discharge [50].

Sedation paradigms and brain dysfunction

The temporal association of sedative medications and acute brain dysfunction has been studied in

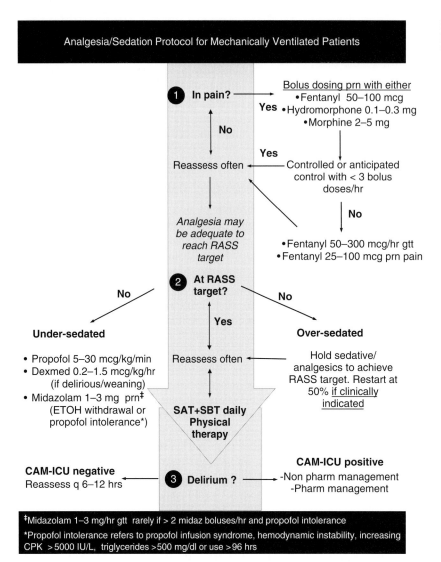

Figure 28.2 Empiric sedation protocol. With permission from http://www.icudelirium.org.

multiple ICU cohorts. In mechanically ventilated medical ICU patients, lorazepam was an independent risk factor for daily development of delirium after adjusting for important covariates such as age, severity of illness, and presence of sepsis [51]. Similar associations between midazolam and acute brain dysfunction outcomes have been found in trauma, burn, and surgical ICU cohorts [5,13]. As noted earlier, data on the effects of opioid analgesics are not consistent. The utilization of dexmedetomidine for sedation, however, has been shown to decrease duration of brain organ dysfunction when compared with benzodiazepine sedation [41,42].

Conclusion

Physicians must strive to balance the necessity and utilization of analgesic and sedative medications with their potential to negatively affect patient outcomes. By incorporating into their practice a systematic management approach that follows the general principles outlined in this chapter, physicians can maximize patient comfort and safety while reducing the likelihood and cost of iatrogenic complications. A liberation and animation strategy of the critically ill patient focusing on the ABCDEs (**A**wakening and **B**reathing **C**oordination, attention to the **C**hoice of Sedation, **D**elirium monitoring, and **E**arly mobility and exercise) [52] is one such organizational framework that can improve patient outcomes.

Acknowledgments

Dr. Hughes is supported by a Foundation for Anesthesia Education and Research Mentored Research Training Grant. Dr. Pandharipande is supported by the VA Clinical Science Research and Development Award (VA Career Development Award).

Conflicts of interest

Dr. Pandharipande has received honoraria from Hospira Inc. and Orion Pharma.

References

1. Jacobi J, Fraser GL, Coursin DB, et al. Clinical practice guidelines for the sustained use of sedatives and analgesics in the critically ill adult. *Crit Care Med* 2002;**30**(1):119–41.

2. Kapfhammer HP, Rothenhausler HB, Krauseneck T, Stoll C, Schelling G. Posttraumatic stress disorder and health-related quality of life in long-term survivors of acute respiratory distress syndrome. *Am J Psychiatry* 2004;**161**(1):45–52.

3. Kollef MH, Levy NT, Ahrens TS, et al. The use of continuous i.v. sedation is associated with prolongation of mechanical ventilation. *Chest* 1998;**114**(2):541–8.

4. Kress JP, Pohlman AS, O'Connor MF, Hall JB. Daily interruption of sedative infusions in critically ill patients undergoing mechanical ventilation. *N Engl J Med* 2000;**342**(20):1471–7.

5. Pandharipande P, Cotton BA, Shintani A, et al. Prevalence and risk factors for development of delirium in surgical and trauma intensive care unit patients. *J Trauma* 2008;**65**(1):34–41.

6. Boogaard M, Pickkers P, Slooter AJ, et al. Development and validation of PRE-DELIRIC (PREdiction of DELIRium in ICu patients) delirium prediction model for intensive care patients: observational multicentre study. *Br Med J* 2012;**344**:e420.

7. Payen JF, Bosson JL, Chanques G, Mantz J, Labarere J. Pain assessment is associated with decreased duration of mechanical ventilation in the intensive care unit: a post hoc analysis of the DOLOREA study. *Anesthesiology* 2009;**111**(6):1308–16.

8. Hicks CL, von Baeyer CL, Spafford PA, van Korlaar, I, Goodenough B. The Faces Pain Scale-Revised: toward a common metric in pediatric pain measurement. *Pain* 2001;**93**(2):173–83.

9. Payen JF, Bru O, Bosson JL, et al. Assessing pain in critically ill sedated patients by using a behavioral pain scale. *Crit Care Med* 2001;**29**(12):2258–63.

10. Dahaba AA, Grabner T, Rehak PH, List WF, Metzler H. Remifentanil versus morphine analgesia and sedation for mechanically ventilated critically ill patients: a randomized double blind study. *Anesthesiology* 2004;**101**(3):640–6.

11. Muellejans B, Lopez A, Cross MH, et al. Remifentanil versus fentanyl for analgesia based sedation to provide patient comfort in the intensive care unit: a randomized, double-blind controlled trial [ISRCTN43755713]. *Crit Care* 2004;**8**(1):R1–R11.

12. Morrison RS, Magaziner J, Gilbert M, et al. Relationship between pain and opioid analgesics on the development of delirium following hip fracture. *J Gerontol A Biol Sci Med Sci* 2003;**58**(1):76–81.

13. Agarwal V, O'Neill PJ, Cotton BA, et al. Prevalence and risk factors for development of delirium in burn intensive care unit patients. *J Burn Care Res* 2010;**31**(5):706–15.

14. Dubois MJ, Bergeron N, Dumont M, Dial S, Skrobik Y. Delirium in an intensive care unit: a study of risk factors. *Intensive Care Med* 2001;**27**(8):1297–304.

15. Marcantonio ER, Goldman L, Orav EJ, Cook EF, Lee TH. The association of intraoperative factors with the development of postoperative delirium. *Am J Med* 1998;**105**(5):380–4.

16. Riker RR, Picard JT, Fraser GL. Prospective evaluation of the Sedation-Agitation Scale for adult critically ill patients. *Crit Care Med* 1999;**27**(7):1325–9.

17. Ramsay MA, Savege TM, Simpson BR, Goodwin R. Controlled sedation with alphaxalone-alphadolone. *Br Med J* 1974;**2**(5920):656–9.

18. Ely EW, Truman B, Shintani A, et al. Monitoring sedation status over time in ICU patients: reliability and validity of the Richmond Agitation-Sedation Scale (RASS). *JAMA* 2003;**289**(22):2983–91.

19. Ely EW, Shintani A, Truman B, et al. Delirium as a predictor of mortality in mechanically ventilated patients in the intensive care unit. *JAMA* 2004;**291**(14):1753–62.

20. Milbrandt EB, Deppen S, Harrison PL, et al. Costs associated with delirium in mechanically ventilated patients. *Crit Care Med* 2004;**32**(4):955–62.

21. Bergeron N, Dubois MJ, Dumont M, Dial S, Skrobik Y. Intensive Care Delirium Screening Checklist: evaluation of a new screening tool. *Intensive Care Med* 2001;**27**(5):859–64.

22. Ely EW, Inouye SK, Bernard GR, et al. Delirium in mechanically ventilated patients: validity and reliability of the confusion assessment method for the intensive care unit (CAM-ICU). *JAMA* 2001;**286**(21):2703–10.

23. Brattebo G, Hofoss D, Flaatten H, *et al.* Effect of a scoring system and protocol for sedation on duration of patients' need for ventilator support in a surgical intensive care unit. *Qual Saf Health Care* 2004;**13**(3):203–5.

24. Brook AD, Ahrens TS, Schaiff R, *et al.* Effect of a nursing-implemented sedation protocol on the duration of mechanical ventilation. *Crit Care Med* 1999;**27**(12):2609–15.

25. Girard TD, Kress JP, Fuchs BD, *et al.* Efficacy and safety of a paired sedation and ventilator weaning protocol for mechanically ventilated patients in intensive care (Awakening and Breathing Controlled trial): a randomised controlled trial. *Lancet* 2008;**371**(9607):126–34.

26. Jackson JC, Girard TD, Gordon SM, *et al.* Long-term cognitive and psychological outcomes in the Awakening and Breathing Controlled Trial. *Am J Respir Crit Care Med* 2010;**182**(2):183–91.

27. Kress JP, Gehlbach B, Lacy M, *et al.* The long-term psychological effects of daily sedative interruption on critically ill patients. *Am J Respir Crit Care Med* 2003;**168**(12):1457–61.

28. Girard TD, Shintani AK, Jackson JC, *et al.* Risk factors for posttraumatic stress disorder symptoms following critical illness requiring mechanical ventilation: a prospective cohort study. *Crit Care* 2007;**11**(1):R28.

29. Rotondi AJ, Chelluri L, Sirio C, *et al.* Patients' recollections of stressful experiences while receiving prolonged mechanical ventilation in an intensive care unit. *Crit Care Med* 2002;**30**(4):746–52.

30. Granja C, Gomes E, Amaro A, *et al.* Understanding posttraumatic stress disorder-related symptoms after critical care: the early illness amnesia hypothesis. *Crit Care Med* 2008;**36**(10):2801–9.

31. Larson MJ, Weaver LK, Hopkins RO. Cognitive sequelae in acute respiratory distress syndrome patients with and without recall of the intensive care unit. *J Int Neuropsychol Soc* 2007;**13**(4):595–605.

32. Karabinis A, Mandragos K, Stergiopoulos S, *et al.* Safety and efficacy of analgesia-based sedation with remifentanil versus standard hypnotic-based regimens in intensive care unit patients with brain injuries: a randomised, controlled trial [ISRCTN50308308]. *Crit Care* 2004;**8**(4):R268–80.

33. Breen D, Karabinis A, Malbrain M, *et al.* Decreased duration of mechanical ventilation when comparing analgesia-based sedation using remifentanil with standard hypnotic-based sedation for up to 10 days in intensive care unit patients: a randomised trial [ISRCTN47583497]. *Crit Care* 2005;**9**(3):R200–10.

34. Rozendaal FW, Spronk PE, Snellen FF, *et al.* Remifentanil-propofol analgo-sedation shortens duration of ventilation and length of ICU stay compared to a conventional regimen: a centre randomised, cross-over, open-label study in the Netherlands. *Intensive Care Med* 2009;**35**(2):291–8.

35. Strom T, Martinussen T, Toft P. A protocol of no sedation for critically ill patients receiving mechanical ventilation: a randomised trial. *Lancet* 2010;**375**(9713):475–80.

36. Barr J. Propofol: a new drug for sedation in the intensive care unit. *Int Anesthesiol Clin* 1995;**33**(1):131–54.

37. Maze M, Scarfini C, Cavaliere F. New agents for sedation in the intensive care unit. *Crit Care Clin* 2001;**17**(4):881–97.

38. Morandi A, Watson PL, Trabucchi M, Ely EW. Advances in sedation for critically ill patients. *Minerva Anestesiol* 2009;**75**(6):385–91.

39. Carson SS, Kress JP, Rodgers JE, *et al.* A randomized trial of intermittent lorazepam versus propofol with daily interruption in mechanically ventilated patients. *Crit Care Med* 2006;**34**(5):1326–32.

40. Barrientos-Vega R, Mar Sanchez-Soria M, Morales-Garcia C, *et al.* Prolonged sedation of critically ill patients with midazolam or propofol: impact on weaning and costs. *Crit Care Med* 1997;**25**(1):33–40.

41. Pandharipande PP, Pun BT, Herr DL, *et al.* Effect of sedation with dexmedetomidine vs lorazepam on acute brain dysfunction in mechanically ventilated patients: the MENDS randomized controlled trial. *JAMA* 2007;**298**(22):2644–53.

42. Riker RR, Shehabi Y, Bokesch PM, *et al.* Dexmedetomidine vs midazolam for sedation of critically ill patients: a randomized trial. *JAMA* 2009;**301**(5):489–99.

43. Pandharipande PP, Sanders RD, Girard TD, *et al.* Effect of dexmedetomidine versus lorazepam on outcome in patients with sepsis: an a priori-designed analysis of the MENDS randomized controlled trial. *Crit Care* 2010;**14**(2):R38.

44. Venn RM, Grounds RM. Comparison between dexmedetomidine and propofol for sedation in the intensive care unit: patient and clinician perceptions. *Br J Anaesth* 2001;**87**(5):684–90.

45. Herr DL, Sum-Ping ST, England M. ICU sedation after coronary artery bypass graft surgery: dexmedetomidine-based versus propofol-based sedation regimens. *J Cardiothorac Vasc Anesth* 2003;**17**(5):576–84.

46. Tan JA, Ho KM. Use of dexmedetomidine as a sedative and analgesic agent in critically ill adult patients: a meta-analysis. *Intensive Care Med* 2010;**36**(6):926–39.

47. Jakob SM, Ruokonen E, Grounds RM, *et al.* Dexmedetomidine vs midazolam or propofol for

sedation during prolonged mechanical ventilation: two randomized controlled trials. *JAMA* 2012;**307**(11):1151–60.

48. Papazian L, Forel JM, Gacouin A, *et al*. Neuromuscular blockers in early acute respiratory distress syndrome. *N Engl J Med* 2010;**363**(12):1107–16.

49. Morris PE, Goad A, Thompson C, *et al*. Early intensive care unit mobility therapy in the treatment of acute respiratory failure. *Crit Care Med* 2008;**36**(8):2238–43.

50. Schweickert WD, Pohlman MC, Pohlman AS, *et al*. Early physical and occupational therapy in

mechanically ventilated, critically ill patients: a randomised controlled trial. *Lancet* 2009;**373**(9678):1874–82.

51. Pandharipande P, Shintani A, Peterson J, *et al*. Lorazepam is an independent risk factor for transitioning to delirium in intensive care unit patients. *Anesthesiology* 2006;**104**(1):21–6.

52. Vasilevskis EE, Pandharipande PP, Girard TD, Ely EW. A screening, prevention, and restoration model for saving the injured brain in intensive care unit survivors. *Crit Care Med* 2010;**38**(10 Suppl):S683–91.

Chapter 29

Pharmacological management of delirium

Dustin M. Hipp and E. Wesley Ely

SUMMARY

Pharmacological management of delirium may be necessary for some critically ill patients after a thorough investigation of underlying causes, modification of potentially reversible risk factors, and utilizing appropriate non-pharmacological strategies such as orientation and early mobilization. Important considerations for pharmacological intervention include discontinuation of potentially deliriogenic medications; the use of analgesics and sedatives associated with decreased duration or less frequency of delirium; and the use of psychoactive agents for treatment of acute delirium. While there is currently no Food and Drug Administration (FDA)-approved medication for the management of delirium, the 2002 Society of Critical Care Medicine clinical practice guidelines recommend haloperidol due to its various delivery routes (intramuscular, intravenous, enteral), its rapid onset of action, and its minimal effects on hemodynamics or respiratory drive. Attention has also been given to the atypical antipsychotics such as quetiapine and ziprasidone, which are viewed by many clinicians as equally efficacious with less risk for extrapyramidal symptoms. Both typical and atypical antipsychotics carry varying risk for cardiac abnormalities (QTc prolongation, torsades de pointes, sudden cardiac death), warranting electrocardiographic monitoring during treatment in the intensive care unit (ICU). While multiple small trials with varying designs support the use of antipsychotics in the treatment of ICU delirium, more robust and prospective randomized controlled trials are needed to solidify the scientific basis for utilization of this drug class. The alpha-2 agonists used for sedation, particularly dexmedetomidine, also demonstrate favorable properties for reducing the likelihood of transition to delirium. Patients receiving dexmedetomidine should be monitored for bradycardia and hypotension. Other agents such as the cholinesterase inhibitors have proven either unhelpful or require further study.

General principles of pharmacological management of delirium

Overarching concepts through which to approach this chapter have to do with the balance between non-pharmacological and pharmacological aspects of delirium management as follows.

The clinician interested in managing delirium must begin by focusing on addressing/treating the recognized underlying disease processes that are leading to the patient's brain dysfunction, then moving to drug removal (not addition), and then modification of environmental factors (hearing and vision aids, removal of restraints and early mobility, and sleep hygiene). At the bedside, we summarize these via the mnemonic Dr. DRE (Diseases, Drug Removal, and Environment). These are covered and operationalized in the evidence-based ABCDEs of ICU Care, which stands for Awakening and Breathing Coordination, attention to the Choice of Sedation, Delirium monitoring, and Early mobility and exercise. When patients remain delirious even after following these precepts, then we focus on pharmacological management with specific agents that are discussed in this chapter.

As described in previous chapters, delirium is a form of acute brain dysfunction characterized by inattention, fluctuating mental status, and altered level of consciousness or disorganized thinking. It is common in the critically ill population, yet under-diagnosed in large part to its variable presentation as hypoactive, hyperactive, and mixed motoric subtypes. Awareness of delirium as a clinically relevant and potentially modifiable entity has increased over the last decade

Brain Disorders in Critical Illness, ed. Robert D. Stevens, Tarek Sharshar, and E. Wesley Ely. Published by Cambridge University Press. © Cambridge University Press 2013.

due to improved methods in screening and assessment for the presence of delirium. These valid and reliable instruments include arousal scales such as the Riker Sedation–Agitation Scale (SAS) and the Richmond Agitation–Sedation Scale (RASS), as well as delirium instruments such as the Confusion Assessment Method for the ICU (CAM-ICU) and the Intensive Care Delirium Screening Checklist (ICDSC). As mentioned in Chapter 24, delirium monitoring should be part of an ICU's screening armamentarium as part of an integrated, evidence-based approach (for example, the "D" for delirium monitoring and management in the ABCDE bundle, see Chapter 28, this volume).

When the critically ill patient develops delirium, a thorough investigation regarding its etiology should first be undertaken. A full neurological exam should be performed, with attention for any localizing signs that would suggest macro-injury such as a stroke. The risk factors for development and causes of delirium are many and have been described in detail previously (acute illness, patient predisposition, environmental or iatrogenic factors). Reversible factors such as introduction of new medications should be considered and, if possible, these contributing agents should be discontinued. Infection, another common and potentially life-threatening cause of delirium in adults, should also be considered, and respective cultures sent and appropriate antibiotics initiated. The key principle (as outlined above) is that delirium management hinges first and foremost on the identification and treatment of the underlying cause (or causes, as in reality delirium in most patients is likely multifactorial), whether it be medications, infection, metabolic causes, or electrolyte disturbances. Next, in conjunction with addressing potentially modifiable contributors to delirium, we must also consider non-pharmacological management of delirium, which includes both modification of environmental factors (Chapter 27, this volume) and initiation of early physical and occupational therapy when appropriate (Chapter 31, this volume).

Nevertheless, despite the recognition of clinical delirium, the modification of reversible risk factors, and the use of non-pharmacological interventions such as reorientation and restoring sleep–wake cycles, delirium may persist for some patients. In these cases, the next appropriate step may be pharmacological intervention. Pharmacological management of delirium in critically ill adults includes three categories of therapeutic strategies:

1. Discontinuation of potentially deliriogenic medications (First, do no harm).
2. Use of analgesics and sedatives associated with less frequency or decreased duration of delirium.
3. Treatment of the clinical symptoms of delirium.

Chapter 28 discussed both the discontinuation of potentially deliriogenic medications (such as lorazepam and midazolam, benzodiazepines commonly used in the ICU) [1,2], as well as the use of sedatives associated with less frequency or decreased duration of delirium (alpha-2 agonists such as dexmedetomidine). Therefore, this chapter will focus on a discussion of the psychoactive medications most commonly used in the ICU, the best available evidence for pharmacological management of delirium with these drug classes (specifically the typical and atypical antipsychotics), and the potential adverse affects associated with these medications.

Once the decision has been made to consider pharmacological intervention, the next step is the choice of psychoactive agent used and the duration of treatment. Given that the psychoactive medications used to treat delirium also carry the risk of adverse effects (for instance, antipsychotics and the risk for extrapyramidal symptoms, EPS), another important principle is that these drugs should be used *at an appropriate dose* and *for the shortest duration possible*, as many of these medications, if their use results in oversedation, may contribute to confusion, further cloud the patient's sensorium, and prolong time on mechanical ventilation. Underutilization of analgesics also may contribute to delirium, as pain that is undertreated has been shown to be a risk factor for delirium. Therefore, targeted sedation, judicious analgesia, and use of delirium assessment tools are all recommended. The use of a validated delirium assessment tool has been shown to result in less exposure to haloperidol [3]. An example delirium treatment protocol that combines the use of an arousal scale, a delirium assessment tool, and non-pharmacological management strategies with pharmacological treatment guidelines is shown in Figure 29.1 and available on the website of the ICU Delirium and Cognitive Impairment Study Group (http://www.icudelirium.org).

Antipsychotics

Currently there are no medications approved by the FDA for the prevention or treatment of delirium. Past versions of the Society of Critical Care Medicine

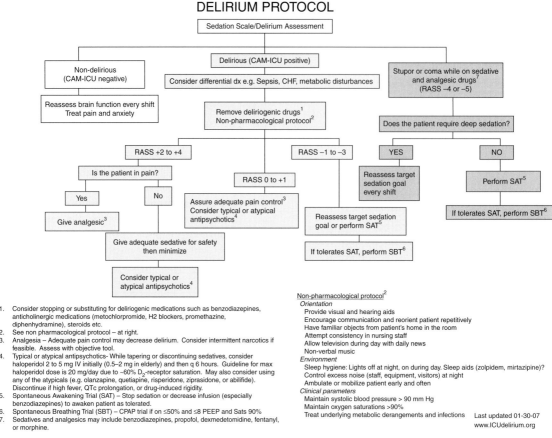

DELIRIUM PROTOCOL

Sedation Scale/Delirium Assessment

Non-delirious (CAM-ICU negative)

Reassess brain function every shift
Treat pain and anxiety

Delirious (CAM-ICU positive)

Consider differential dx e.g. Sepsis, CHF, metabolic disturbances

Remove deliriogenic drugs[1]
Non-pharmacological protocol[2]

RASS +2 to +4

Is the patient in pain?

Yes

No

Give analgesic[3]

RASS 0 to +1

Assure adequate pain control[3]
Consider typical or atypical antipsychotics[4]

Give adequate sedative for safety then minimize

Consider typical or atypical antipsychotics[4]

RASS –1 to –3

Reassess target sedation goal or perform SAT[5]

If tolerates SAT, perform SBT[6]

Stupor or coma while on sedative and analgesic drugs[7]
(RASS –4 or –5)

Does the patient require deep sedation?

YES

Reassess target sedation goal every shift

NO

Perform SAT[5]

If tolerates SAT, perform SBT[6]

1. Consider stopping or substituting for deliriogenic medications such as benzodiazepines, anticholinergic medications (metochlorpromide, H2 blockers, promethazine, diphenhydramine), steroids etc.
2. See non pharmacological protocol – at right.
3. Analgesia – Adequate pain control may decrease delirium. Consider intermittent narcotics if feasible. Assess with objective tool.
4. Typical or atypical antipsychotics- While tapering or discontinuing sedatives, consider haloperidol 2 to 5 mg IV initially (0.5–2 mg in elderly) and then q 6 hours. Guideline for max haloperidol dose is 20 mg/day due to ~60% D_2-receptor saturation. May also consider using any of the atypicals (e.g. olanzapine, quetiapine, risperidone, ziprasidone, or abilifide). Discontinue if high fever, QTc prolongation, or drug-induced rigidity.
5. Spontaneous Awakening Trial (SAT) – Stop sedation or decrease infusion (especially benzodiazepines) to awaken patient as tolerated.
6. Spontaneous Breathing Trial (SBT) – CPAP trial if on ≤50% and ≤8 PEEP and Sats 90%
7. Sedatives and analgesics may include benzodiazepines, propofol, dexmedetomidine, fentanyl, or morphine.

Non-pharmacological protocol[2]
Orientation
Provide visual and hearing aids
Encourage communication and reorient patient repetitively
Have familiar objects from patient's home in the room
Attempt consistency in nursing staff
Allow television during day with daily news
Non-verbal music
Environment
Sleep hygiene: Lights off at night, on during day. Sleep aids (zolpidem, mirtazipine)?
Control excess noise (staff, equipment, visitors) at night
Ambulate or mobilize patient early and often
Clinical parameters
Maintain systolic blood pressure > 90 mm Hg
Maintain oxygen saturations >90%
Treat underlying metabolic derangements and infections   Last updated 01-30-07
www.ICUdelirium.org

Figure 29.1 Example delirium protocol that builds on the Society of Critical Care Medicine guidelines and combines pharmacological and non-pharmacological strategies. This protocol, which is expected to be updated with new evidence and adapted for use by local experts at adopting medical centers, is available online (http://www.icudelirium.org).

clinical practice guidelines for analgesia and sedation supported the use of haloperidol for the treatment of acute delirium [4]. This recommendation was based on Level C support and limited case studies, as no large prospective randomized controlled trial has been undertaken (yet) to show that haloperidol or any other psychoactive medication is both effective and safe for critically ill patients.

Based largely on these SCCM guidelines and anecdotal experience, haloperidol has emerged as the standard pharmacological treatment for delirium in the ICU, used by 75–80% of intensivists, followed by atypical antipsychotics used by 35–40% of intensivists [5–7]. Nevertheless, numerous recent systematic reviews have emphasized the dearth of strong statistical evidence supporting the safety and efficacy of antipsychotics for the treatment of delirium, and the need for larger, well-designed studies in the future [8–12].

Haloperidol

Haloperidol is a butyrophenone-derived typical antipsychotic (or "neuroleptic") that binds with high affinity to D_2 receptors, relatively low affinity to D_1 receptors, and exhibits little adrenergic or muscarinic activity compared with low-potency neuroleptics such as chlorpromazine. Its mechanism of action is dopamine antagonism at cortical D_2 receptors, in the nigrostriatal pathway and basal ganglia, and disinhibition of acetylcholine (resulting in acetylcholine release) [13]. Positron emission tomographic studies have shown that haloperidol induces D_2 receptor occupancy in a therapeutic range (53–72%) even at low daily doses (2–4 mg), suggesting that the adverse effects associated with high doses can be avoided [14]. Haloperidol may have some anti-inflammatory effects that mitigate organ dysfunction in the critically ill patient, though these data are very limited [15,16].

In the critical care setting, haloperidol can be quickly administered either intramuscularly (i.m.) or intravenously (i.v.) with high bioavailability, nearly 100%, and rapid onset of action (3–20 minutes i.v.) [4,17]. Its mean half-life is 21 hours (range 18–54 h). It is rapidly distributed throughout tissues (V_d 9.5–21.7 L/kg) and extensively protein-bound with a free fraction in human plasma 7.5–11.6%. It is extensively oxidized and metabolized by the liver (CYP3A4 and CYP2D6) with ~1% excreted in urine unchanged. Theoretically, haloperidol metabolism can be affected by other medications metabolized via the CYP3A4 pathway, such as phenobarbital, rifampin, quinidine, and carbamazepine. However, these medications are rarely used in the critical care setting and so are unlikely to contribute to problematic drug–drug interactions.

Haloperidol is typically given initially at a dose between 1 and 5 mg i.v. for a rapid response in the acutely delirious patient, followed by maintenance doses every 6–12 hours. The lower dose range of 0.5–2 mg are used for the elderly and the demented, as they are at increased risk for oversedation and cardiac adverse effects (see "Safety profile of antipsychotics"). With the administration of higher doses (> 20 mg daily), the marginal benefit is believed minimal, and the risk for QTc prolongation increases. Haloperidol can also be administered via the oral or enteral route; however, given that oral haloperidol has been associated with unpredictable absorption, more adverse effects (extrapyramidal symptoms [EPS]) [18], and delayed reversal of delirium, this is not usually a preferred delivery route [19].

Initially a drug used to treat schizophrenia, haloperidol gained more acceptance for use in the critical care setting in the mid-1990s when Riker *et al.* showed that continuous infusion of haloperidol could successfully manage agitation, as well as reduce sedative drug requirements and nursing attention [20]. Such large doses with continuous infusion of haloperidol have fallen out of favor over time, as evidence has shown similar therapeutic benefit at lower doses and with less risk for extrapyramidal symptoms and arrhythmias. Milbrandt *et al.* also suggested a survival benefit in a retrospective cohort analysis of 989 patients, which demonstrated that mechanically ventilated patients who received haloperidol had significantly lower hospital mortality compared with those who did not receive haloperidol [15].

Atypical antipsychotics

The atypical antipsychotics have more recently gained attention as a potential alternative to haloperidol for the treatment of acute delirium. The premise is that atypical antipsychotics may be as efficacious as haloperidol and the typical neuroleptics for treating delirium, with less risk for extrapyramidal symptoms [21].

The most commonly studied atypical antipsychotics for the treatment of delirium thus far are olanzapine, ziprasidone, risperidone, and quetiapine. These second-generation antipsychotics are characterized pharmacologically as having reduced affinity for D_2 receptors relative to neuroleptics (hence, less EPS), and a wider variety of reported affinities for serotonin, adrenergic, histaminic, and muscarinic receptors. For instance, ziprasidone is an antagonist at serotonin receptors (5-HT_{1D}, 5-HT_{2A}, 5-HT_{2C}), dopamine receptors (D_2, D_3), and alpha-1 receptors, as well as an agonist at 5-HT_{1A} receptors [22]. Quetiapine has been shown to block serotonin receptors (5-HT_2, 5-HT_6), dopamine receptors (D_1, D_2), alpha-1 and alpha-2 adrenergic receptors, and histaminic (H_1) receptors [22].

Currently, no study has shown an atypical antipsychotic to be superior to haloperidol; however, atypical antipsychotics have been shown to be as efficacious as haloperidol in delirium management [21]. The results of the limited number of randomized controlled trials are described below and summarized in Table 29.1.

In 2003, Skrobik *et al.* randomized 73 medical/surgical ICU patients diagnosed with delirium using the Intensive Care Delirium Screening Checklist (ICDSC) to receive either olanzapine or haloperidol [23]. They concluded that olanzapine was a safe alternative treatment to haloperidol with comparable clinical improvement in delirium and less EPS.

In 2010, two pilot studies were published simultaneously that laid the groundwork for future prospective randomized controlled trials. Devlin *et al.* studied the use of scheduled quetiapine [24] in 36 delirious ICU patients requiring as-needed haloperidol, compared with placebo. Quetiapine was associated with reduced duration of delirium, shorter time to first resolution of delirium, less agitation, and a greater rate of discharge to rehabilitation or home. Patients receiving quetiapine also were noted to require fewer days of as-needed haloperidol. The incidence of QTc prolongation was similar in the two study groups. More somnolence was observed in patients receiving quetiapine, though this was not statistically significant.

Table 29.1 Randomized controlled trials of typical and atypical antipsychotics for treatment of delirium.

Reference	Patients	Starting mean dose	Medication	Delirium assessment tool	Summary
[24]	73 medical-surgical ICU	2.5–5 mg haloperidol qid; 5 mg/daily olanzapine	Haloperidol vs. Olanzapine	ICDSC	Olanzapine is safe alternative to haloperidol, less EPS
[25]	36 ICU patients, ICDSC >/= 4, as-needed haloperidol, tolerating enteral nutrition	50 mg every 12 hours either quetiapine or placebo; as-needed haloperidol 1–10 mg q2h	Quetiapine vs. Placebo	ICDSC	Quetiapine added to as-needed haloperidol led to faster delirium resolution, less haloperidol, less agitation, greater rate of transfer to rehabilitation/home
[26]	101 medical-surgical mechanically ventilated patients	15.0 mg/day haloperidol; 113.3 mg/day ziprasidone	Haloperidol vs. Ziprasidone vs. Placebo	CAM-ICU	Feasibility study, no improvement in number of days alive without delirium/coma, no increased adverse outcomes
[27]	64 medical-surgical ward patients	0.25 mg haloperidol 2–3 times daily; 0.25–0.5 mg/day risperidone; 1.25–7.5 mg/day olanzapine	Haloperidol vs. Risperidone vs. Olanzapine	DRS-R98, MMSE	Significant reduction in delirium scores, improvement in MMSE scores, no difference between groups, similar side effects
[28]	457 patients, >65 years of age, admitted to ICU after non-cardiac surgery	0.5 mg i.v. haloperidol bolus followed by 0.1 mg/h continuous infusion for 12 h	Haloperidol vs. placebo	RASS, CAM-ICU	Lower incidence of delirium, shorter ICU stay for patients receiving short-term, low-dose prophylactic i.v. haloperidol

ICDSC, Intensive Care Delirium Screening Checklist; CAM-ICU, Confusion Assessment Method for the Intensive Care Unit; DRS-R98, Delirium Rating Scale-Revised-98; EPS, extrapyramidal symptoms; MMSE, Mini Mental Status Examination.

The Modifying the INcidence of Delirium (MIND) Trial, published in 2010 [25], studied the feasibility and safety of a randomized controlled trial comparing placebo, haloperidol, and ziprasidone in 101 medical and surgical ICU patients. The primary endpoint measured was number of days patients were alive without coma or delirium (also known as delirium-coma free days). Interestingly, in this pilot feasibility trial, treatment with antipsychotics was not associated with a difference versus placebo in the number of delirium-coma free days. However, the trial was not powered for efficacy and its feasibility reinforced the need for a larger prospective randomized controlled trial to test the hypothesis that antipsychotics improve delirium duration in critically ill patients. Rates of adverse effects such as akathisia and other EPS symptoms were similar among all three groups.

Grover et al. conducted a small single-blind prospective comparative efficacy study of olanzapine and risperidone versus haloperidol in 64 patients [26].

Delirium was assessed using the Delirium Rating Scale-Revised-98 (DRS-R98) and the Mini Mental Status Examination (MMSE). In all three study groups, significant reduction in DRS-R98 scores and improved MMSE scores were noted with treatment, though no significant difference was noted between the groups. They too concluded that risperidone and olanzapine are as efficacious as haloperidol in the treatment of delirium. Lastly, a study by Wang et al. [27] in China of low severity of illness ICU patients showed that *prophylactic* haloperidol might have benefit and complemented a previous prophylaxis trial by Kaalisvaart [28], though this approach too requires further study and application to sicker patient cohorts before being adopted widely.

Other small open-trial and non-randomized studies have been published that consider amisulpride [29], quetiapine [29,30], risperidone [31,32], and aripiprazole [33]; however, it is difficult to compare or generalize the results of these studies based on heterogeneity in study design (retrospective analysis, observational), heterogeneity in patient population studied (non-critically ill, oncology, ICU), small sample size, the use of different atypical antipsychotics with different dosing regimens, and the use of different delirium assessment tools.

Safety profile of antipsychotics

As with all pharmacotherapies, the benefits of treatment should exceed the risks, and this is just as true for the pharmacological management of ICU delirium with haloperidol as well as the atypical antipsychotics. Many of the adverse effects associated with haloperidol have been well established such as EPS (akinesia, dystonia, akathisia, tardive dyskinesia), neuroleptic malignant syndrome, and sedation to some degree. These adverse effects are usually worse with enteral haloperidol therapy and occur less with intravenous haloperidol therapy [34]. The risk for EPS with neuroleptics is generally thought to be greater relative to atypical antipsychotics due to increased D_2 receptor blockade. There are also reports of lower mortality in geriatric patients receiving risperidone and olanzapine versus haloperidol [29], all initially suggesting that the atypical antipsychotics may be safer than haloperidol.

However, both typical and atypical antipsychotics have been associated with other adverse effects such as glucose and cholesterol abnormalities [35], venous thromboembolism [36], and particularly cardiac dysrhythmias. These cardiac complications include QTc prolongation, ventricular tachyarrhythmias such as torsades de pointes, and even sudden cardiac death [37]. Multiple high-profile reports have raised concerns for these cardiac complications, especially in the elderly and the demented receiving both haloperidol and the atypical antipsychotics [38,39]. This risk for QTc prolongation and torsades de pointes has been designated by the FDA as a "cross-class" risk for all antipsychotics; therefore, while some may argue this risk is less with one agent relative to another, it should be considered by the diligent intensivist for all antipsychotics. These reports further underscore the need to conduct placebo-controlled clinical trials that demonstrate not only the efficacy, but also the safety of the antipsychotics for the treatment of ICU delirium.

It is therefore generally recommended that patients have a baseline electrocardiogram to assess the QTc interval prior to treatment. Then, if QTc prolongation is noted upon initiation of treatment with an antipsychotic, then the antipsychotic should be discontinued immediately if at all possible.

Alpha-2 agonists

In the last decade, a number of studies have suggested that the alpha-2 agonists, particularly dexmedetomidine, may be a useful sedative in reducing the risk of transition to delirium. The role of dexmedetomidine in sedation protocols was described in more detail in Chapter 28, this volume. However, a review of the evidence for dexmedetomidine as an effective pharmacotherapy for delirium is warranted. The randomized controlled trials for dexmedetomidine with a summary of relevant delirium data are shown in Table 29.2. Clonidine, also an alpha-2 agonist, is used more frequently in Europe and has also been associated with decreased delirium, particularly in the postoperative setting after cardiac or vascular surgery [40]. However, there are overall limited data on clonidine and delirium, including an occasional case report of clonidine-induced delirium [41], hence this discussion will focus more on dexmedetomidine.

Gregoretti describes the alpha-2 adrenergic receptor, targeted by both clonidine and dexmedetomidine, as "the body's most important presynaptic receptor" [42]. Activation of the alpha-2 receptor is thought to result in decreased sympathetic activity and reduction in norepinephrine release. The highest concentration of alpha-2 receptors are located in the locus coeruleus, which is thought to modulate wakefulness, as well as the intermediolateral cell column and substantia gelatinosa in the spinal column, which are implicated in pain modulation [42]. Dexmedetomidine has significantly greater affinity for the alpha-2 receptor compared with clonidine. It does not depress ventilatory drive and also allows for "cooperative sedation" in which patients can quickly be neurologically assessed. There is also some evidence that dexmedetomidine may be neuroprotective and may mimic physiological sleep better than the GABA-acting sedatives. Although dexmedetomidine has been approved in the USA only for short-term sedation of ICU patients (< 24 h) at a maximal dose of 0.7 µg/kg/h (up to 1.0 µg/kg/h for procedural sedation), several studies demonstrate the safety and efficacy of infusions administered for > 24 h (i.e., MENDS up to 5 days, PRODEX/MIDEX up to 14 days, and SEDCOM up to 28 days) and at higher doses (up to 1.5 µg/kg/h) [43]. In these three trials (MENDS, SEDCOM, and PRODEX/MIDEX), the most reproducible and significant adverse effect associated with dexmedetomidine was bradycardia, which typically resolved without event and infrequently required adjunctive treatment beyond discontinuation of the drug.

Table 29.2 Randomized controlled trials of alpha-2 agonists for sedation and related delirium outcomes.

Study	Patients	Medications	Arousal scale, Delirium assessment tool	Summary
[44], MENDS Trial	106 medical-surgical ICU patients	Dexmedetomidine vs. lorazepam	RASS, CAM-ICU	Dexmedetomidine resulted in significantly more days alive without delirium/coma and coma-free days, not delirium-free days
[45], SEDCOM Trial	375 mechanically ventilated ICU patients	Dexmedetomidine vs. midazolam	RASS, CAM-ICU	Prevalence of delirium in patients receiving dexmedetomidine decreased within 1 day; no difference in percentage of time in target RASS range
[47], DEXCOM Study	306 ICU patients after cardiac surgery	Dexmedetomidine vs. morphine	MAAS, CAM-ICU	Incidence of delirium was similar, duration of delirium shorter in patients receiving dexmedetomidine
[48]	85 medical-surgical patients expecting ICU stays > 48 h and requiring sedation > 24 h	Dexmedetomidine vs. propofol or midazolam	RASS	Dexmedetomidine was comparable to propofol or midazolam for long-term light sedation but not deep sedation
[49], ANIST Trial	30 intubated patients, both brain-injured and non-brain-injured	Dexmedetomidine/ fentanyl vs. propofol/fentanyl	RASS, CAM-ICU, ACE	Statistically significant improved ACE scores for patients receiving dexmedetomidine, patients with brain injury required less sedation, modest bradycardia with dexmedetomidine
[50]	20 mechanically ventilated medical-surgical ICU patients, delirious but ready for extubation	Haloperidol vs. dexmedetomidine	RASS, ICDSC	Dexmedetomidine significantly shortened median time to extubation, decreased ICU length of stay, and reduced by half the proportion of time ongoing propofol sedation was required
[51], MIDEX/ PRODEX Trial	998 mechanically ventilated ICU patients needing light to moderate sedation > 24 h	Midazolam or propofol vs. dexmedetomidine	VAS, RASS, CAM-ICU assessed 48 h after stopping study drugs	Dexmedetomidine not inferior to midazolam or propofol; dexmedetomidine reduced time to extubation, fewer neurocognitive disorders than propofol, similar to midazolam

RASS, Richmond Agitation–Sedation Scale; CAM-ICU, Confusion Assessment Method for the Intensive Care Unit; MAAS, Motor Activity Assessment Scale; ACE, Adapted Cognitive Exam; ICDSC, Intensive Care Delirium Screening Checklist; VAS, Visual Analog Scale.

It is important to state that both the bradycardia and hypotension can be significant enough to warrant discontinuation and use of another sedative. This is particularly true for patients with compromised ventricular function or some degree of heart block at baseline.

The favorable properties of dexmedetomidine demonstrated in the MENDS and SEDCOM trials were described in Chapter 28, this volume [44–46]. MENDS was the first randomized controlled trial to show that acute brain dysfunction (delirium and coma) could be reduced through the choice of sedative. The SEDCOM trial demonstrated that dexmedetomidine could achieve the same targeted sedation as midazolam; even more interesting, the prevalence of delirium in the study

group receiving dexmedetomidine was significantly lower within 1 day compared with those receiving midazolam, and this effect lasted for the entire week of study. Together, these two trials raise the question as to whether this difference in observed acute brain dysfunction is *a result of receiving an alpha-2 agonist*, or rather *the avoidance of a GABA-acting agent*. A follow-up analysis of the SEDCOM trial revealed that the duration of delirium was the strongest independent predictor of death, ventilation time, and ICU stay after adjusting for covariates [46]. The DEXCOM study [47] compared dexmedetomidine to morphine-based pain management and sedation after cardiac surgery. This study found similar incidence of duration between the two groups but reduced duration of delirium in those receiving dexmedetomidine. Ruokonen *et al.* [48] did not directly study delirium but compared dexmedetomidine to standard card (either propofol or midazolam) for patients requiring long-term sedation. The authors found that dexmedetomidine was indeed comparable for maintaining light to moderate sedation (RASS 0 to −3) but not comparable for deep sedation.

In the Acute Neurological ICU Sedation Trial (ANIST), Mirski *et al.* assessed whether sedative regimens utilizing dexmedetomidine compared with propofol resulted in sedation and anxiolysis without compromising arousal or cognition [49]. Patients receiving dexmedetomidine were found to have improved Adapted Cognitive Exam (ACE) scores, relative to patients receiving propofol who scored significantly worse on this cognitive exam. This randomized double-blind, crossover study controlled trial further supports the hypothesis that dexmedetomidine may provide sufficient sedation and anxiolysis while maintaining the patient's mental engagement and arousability. The incidence of delirium, assessed using the CAM-ICU, was found to be minimal and similar in both groups.

In Reade *et al.*, dexmedetomidine was compared with haloperidol in 20 mechanically ventilated patients with agitated delirium that prevented extubation [50]. Use of dexmedetomidine in facilitating extubation was found to significantly shorten median time to extubation, as well as decrease ICU length of stay significantly. For patients who also required ongoing propofol sedation, dexmedetomidine was found to halve the proportion of time propofol was required.

Most recently, Jakob *et al.* published the MIDEX/PRODEX trials, two parallel randomized controlled trials that enrolled nearly 1000 patients in multiple countries [51]. Dexmedetomidine was compared with either midazolam or propofol for mechanically ventilated ICU patients requiring light to moderate long-term sedation. Dexmedetomidine was not inferior to either midazolam or propofol. Use of dexmedetomidine reduced duration of mechanical ventilation compared with midazolam (not propofol). Patients' ability to interact and communicate pain, measured using a visual analog scale (VAS), was significantly improved with dexmedetomidine compared with either drug. Patients receiving dexmedetomidine also experienced fewer neurocognitive disorders, including delirium, in follow-up compared with propofol. Similar to other trials, more bradycardia and hypotension were observed with dexmedetomidine.

In summary, a growing body of evidence suggests that the choice of sedative (the "C" in the ABCDE bundle) is an important consideration when choosing a pharmacological strategy to achieve targeted sedation and analgesia while minimizing risk for developing acute brain dysfunction. The alpha-2 agonists, particularly dexmedetomidine, exhibit many favorable properties for use in light to moderate sedation in mechanically ventilated patients, who are particularly vulnerable to development of ICU delirium. Bradycardia and hypotension can occur not infrequently with administration of dexmedetomidine; however, this generally resolves with discontinuation of dexmedetomidine and replacement with another sedating agent. Further studies are needed to delineate whether this seemingly neuroprotective effect is truly due to the alpha-2 agonist's mechanisms of action, or rather the avoidance of other sedatives that can further contribute to the patient's delirium.

Cholinesterase inhibitors

One of the prevailing hypotheses generated outside the ICU regarding the pathophysiology of delirium remains the cholinergic deficiency theory [13]. According to this theory, delirium is related to a deficiency of acetylcholine and increase in dopamine. Therefore, it was hypothesized that the cholinesterase inhibitors used to treat dementia may in fact improve symptoms of delirium by increasing synaptic acetylcholine levels. Unfortunately this theory at this point is a theoretical construct and has not led to the successful development of new therapies.

In 2010, van Eijk *et al.* [52] evaluated the effect of rivastigmine as an adjunct to usual care with haloperidol in reducing the duration of delirium. This was intended to be a multicenter, double-blind, randomized controlled trial that would enroll over 400 patients. However, after enrollment of just 104 patients, the trial was halted, as the treatment group receiving rivastigmine was noted to have statistically significant higher mortality. In fact, patients receiving rivastigmine experienced increased duration of delirium. Therefore, the cholinesterase inhibitors are not recommended for the treatment of delirium [53]. This example highlights well the need to understand further the pathophysiology of delirium, and the present challenges to drug development specifically for ICU delirium.

Benzodiazepines

The benzodiazepines are among the most commonly used medications in the intensive care setting. However, they are not recommended for the treatment of non-alcoholic ICU delirium [54]. In fact, in one study, lorazepam was found to be an independent risk factor for transition to delirium [1]. Use of benzodiazepines has also been associated with longer duration of a first episode of delirium [55]. Benzodiazepines remain the recommended drugs for the treatment of seizures and delirium tremens in the context of acute alcohol withdrawal.

Conclusions

The identification of safe and efficacious agents to reduce the duration, incidence, and severity of ICU is currently an important priority in critical care research and will remain so given the rapidly aging population and clinical equipoise at this time regarding the best approach to pharmacological management of delirium. Much remains to be discovered, and hopefully improved understanding of the pathophysiological mechanisms of delirium will contribute to new and emerging pharmacological strategies. In the meantime, the best evidence suggests that delirium is best prevented and treated using a combination of both non-pharmacological means (such as spontaneous awakening trials and spontaneous breathing trials) and pharmacological strategies, which include both avoiding medications that may contribute to delirium, as well as the prudent use of medications for the treatment of acute delirium. For each patient, the benefits of using a particular drug class must be carefully weighed against the risks. Currently, the medical evidence supports the use of antipsychotics for ICU delirium. Dexmedetomidine as an alpha-2 agonist may also be an appropriate choice as sedative for many patients in the intensive care setting. The use of benzodiazepines or cholinesterase inhibitors is not currently supported by the literature for treatment of delirium in the critically ill patient.

Acknowledgments

Dr. Ely is supported by the National Institutes of Health grants (AG-027472–01A5 and AG-035117–01A1) and the VA Geriatric Research Education and Clinical Center (GRECC).

Conflicts of interest

Dr. Ely has received grants and honoraria from Hospira, grants from Eli Lilly, and consults for Cumberland and Masimo.

References

1. Pandharipande P, Shintani A, Peterson J, *et al.* Lorazepam is an independent risk factor for transitioning to delirium in intensive care unit patients. *Anesthesiology* 2006;**104**(1):21–6.

2. Pandharipande P, Cotton BA, Shintani A, *et al.* Prevalence and risk factors for development of delirium in surgical and trauma intensive care unit patients. *J Trauma* 2008;**65**:34–41.

3. van den Boogaard M, Pickkers P, van der Hoeven H, *et al.* Implementation of a delirium assessment tool in the ICU can influence haloperidol use. *Crit Care* 2009;**13**(4):R131.

4. Jacobi J, Fraser GL, Coursin DB, *et al.* Clinical practice guidelines for the sustained use of sedatives and analgesics in the critically ill adult. *Crit Care Med* 2002;**30**(1):119–41.

5. Ely EW, Stephens RK, Jackson JC, *et al.* Current opinions regarding the importance, diagnosis, and management of delirium in the intensive care unit: a survey of 912 healthcare professionals. *Crit Care Med* 2004;**32**(1):106–12.

6. Patel RP, Gambrell M, Speroff T, *et al.* Delirium and sedation in the intensive care unit: survey of behaviors and attitudes of 1384 healthcare professionals. *Crit Care Med* 2009;**37**(3):825–32.

7. MacSweeney R, Barber V, Page V, *et al.* A national survey of the management of delirium in UK intensive care units. *QJM* 2010;**103**(4):243–51.

8. Lacasse H, Perreault MM, Williamson DR. Systematic review of antipsychotics for the treatment of hospital-associated delirium in medically or surgically ill patients. *Ann Pharmacother* 2006;**40**(11):1966–73.

9. Seitz DP, Gill SS, van Zyl LT. Antipsychotics in the treatment of delirium: a systematic review. *J Clin Psychiatry* 2007;**68**(1):11–21.

10. Lonergan E, Britton AM, Luxenberg J, Wyller T. Antipsychotics for delirium. *Cochrane Database Syst Rev* 2007;**2**:CD005594.

11. Campbell N, Boustani MA, Ayub A, *et al.* Pharmacological management of delirium in hospitalized adults – a systematic evidence review. *J Gen Intern Med* 2009;**24**(7):848–53.

12. Bledowski J, Trutia A. A review of pharmacologic management and prevention strategies for delirium in the intensive care unit. *Psychosomatics* 2012;**53**(3):203–11.

13. Hshieh TT, Fong TG, Marcantonio ER, Inouye SK. Cholinergic deficiency hypothesis in delirium: a synthesis of current evidence. *J Gerontol A Biol Sci Med Sci* 2008;**63**(7):764–72.

14. Kapur S, Remington G, Jones C, *et al.* High levels of dopamine D2 receptor occupancy with low-dose haloperidol treatment: a PET study. *Am J Psychiatry* 1996;**153**:948–50.

15. Milbrandt EB, Kersten A, Kong L, *et al.* Haloperidol use is associated with lower hospital mortality in mechanically ventilated patients. *Crit Care Med* 2005;**33**(1):226–9.

16. Song C, Lin A, Kenis G, Bosmans E, Maes M. Immunosuppressive effects of clozapine and haloperidol: enhanced production of the interleukin-1 receptor antagonist. *Schizophr Res* 2000;**42**(2):157–64.

17. Kudo S, Ishizaki T. Pharmacokinetics of haloperidol: an update. *Clin Pharmacokinetics* 1999;**37**:435–56.

18. Menza MA, Murray GB, Holmes VF, Rafuls WA. Decreased extrapyramidal symptoms with intravenous haloperidol. *J Clin Psychiatry* 1987;**48**(7)278–80.

19. Wang EHZ, Mabasa VH, Loh GW, Ensom MHH. Haloperidol dosing strategies in the treatment of delirium in the critically ill. *Neurocrit Care* 2012;**16**:170–83.

20. Riker R, Fraser G, Cox P. Continuous infusion of haloperidol controls agitation in critically ill patients. *Crit Care Med* 1994;**22**:433–40.

21. Rea RS, Battistone S, Fong JJ, Devlin JW. Atypical antipsychotics versus haloperidol for treatment of delirium in acutely ill patients. *Pharmacotherapy* 2007;**27**(4):588–94.

22. Morandi A, Gunther ML, Ely EW, Pandharipande P. The pharmacological management of delirium in critical illness. *Curr Drug Ther* 2008;**3**:148–57.

23. Skrobik YK, Bergeron N, Dumont M, Gottfried SB. Olanzapine vs haloperidol: treating delirium in a critical care setting. *Intensive Care Med* 2004;**30**(3):444–9.

24. Devlin JW, Roberts RJ, Fong JJ, *et al.* Efficacy and safety of quetiapine in critically ill patients with delirium: a prospective, multicenter, randomized, double-blind, placebo-controlled pilot study. *Crit Care Med* 2010;**38**(2):419–27.

25. Girard TD, Pandharipande PP, Carson SS, *et al.* Feasibility, efficacy, and safety of antipsychotics for intensive care unit delirium: the MIND randomized, placebo-controlled trial. *Crit Care Med* 2010;**38**(2):428–37.

26. Grover S, Kumar V, Chakrabarti S. Comparative efficacy study of haloperidol, olanzapine and risperidone in delirium. *J Psychosom Res* 2011;**71**(4):277–81.

27. Wang W, Li HL, Wang DX, *et al.* Haloperidol prophylaxis decreases delirium incidence in elderly patients after noncardiac surgery: a randomized controlled trial. *Crit Care Med* 2012;**40**(3):731–9.

28. Kalisvaart KJ, de Jonghe JF, Bogaards MJ, *et al.* Haloperidol prophylaxis for elderly hip-surgery patients at risk for delirium: a randomized placebo-controlled study. *J Am Geriatr Soc* 2005;**53**(10):1658–66.

29. Lee KU, Won WY, Lee HK, *et al.* Amisulpride versus quetiapine for the treatment of delirium: a randomized, open prospective study. *Int Clin Psychopharmacol* 2005;**20**(6):311–14.

30. Pae CU, Lee SJ, Lee CU, Lee C, Paik IH. A pilot trial of quetiapine for the treatment of patients with delirium. *Hum Psychopharmacol* 2004;**19**(2):125–7.

31. Nasrallah HA, White T, Nasrallah AT. Lower mortality in geriatric patients receiving risperidone and olanzapine versus haloperidol: preliminary analysis of retrospective data. *Am J Geriatr Psychiatry* 2004;**12**(4):437–9.

32. Han CS, Kim YK. A double-blind trial of risperidone and haloperidol for the treatment of delirium. *Psychosomatics* 2004;**45**(4):297–301.

33. Boettger S, Friedlander M, Breitbart W, Passik S. Aripiprazole and haloperidol in the treatment of delirium. *Aust N Z J Psychiatry* 2011;**45**(6):477–82.

34. Riker RB, Fraser GL, Richen P. Movement disorders associated with withdrawal from high-dose intravenous haloperidol therapy in delirious ICU patients. *Chest* 1997;**111**:1778–81.

35. Leucht S, Corves C, Arbter D, *et al.* Second-generation versus first-generation antipsychotic drugs for schizophrenia: a meta-analysis. *Lancet* 2009;**373**(9657):31–41.

36. Liperoti R, Pedone C, Lapane KL, *et al.* Venous thromboembolism among elderly patients treated with atypical and conventional antipsychotic agents. *Arch Intern Med* 2005;**165**(22):2677–82.

37. Ray WA, Chung CP, Murray KT, Hall K, Stein CM. Atypical antipsychotic drugs and the risk of sudden cardiac death. *N Engl J Med* 2009;**360**(3):225–35.

38. Wang PS, Schneeweiss S, Avorn J, *et al.* Risk of death in elderly users of conventional vs. atypical antipsychotic medications. *N Engl J Med* 2005;**353**(22):2335–41.

39. Liperoti R, Gambassi G, Lapane KL, *et al.* Conventional and atypical antipsychotics and the risk of hospitalization for ventricular arrhythmias or cardiac arrest. *Arch Intern Med* 2005;**165**(6):696–701.

40. Rubino AS, Onorati F, Caroleo S, *et al.* Impact of clonidine administration on delirium and related respiratory weaning after surgical correction of acute

type-A aortic dissection: results of a pilot study. *Interact Cardiovasc Thorac Surg* 2010;**10**(1):58–62.

41. Delaney J, Spevack D, Doddamani S, Ostfeld R. Clonidine-induced delirium. *Int J Cardiol* 2006;**113**:276–8.

42. Gregoretti C, Moglia B, Pelosi P, Navalesi P. Clonidine in perioperative medicine and intensive care unit: more than an anti-hypertensive drug. *Curr Drug Targets* 2009;**10**:667–86.

43. Guinter JR, Kristeller JL. Prolonged infusions of dexmedetomidine in critically ill patients. *Am J Health-Syst Pharm* 2010;**67**:1246–53.

44. Pandharipande PP, Pun BT, Herr DL, *et al.* Effect of sedation with dexmedetomidine vs lorazepam on acute brain dysfunction in mechanically ventilated patients: the MENDS randomized controlled trial. *JAMA* 2007;**298**(22):2644–53.

45. Riker RR, Shehabi Y, Bokesch PM, *et al.* Dexmedetomidine vs midazolam for sedation of critically ill patients: a randomized trial. *JAMA* 2009;**301**(5):489–99.

46. Shehabi Y, Riker RR, Bokesch PM, *et al.* Delirium duration and mortality in lightly sedated, mechanically ventilated intensive care unit patients. *Crit Care Med* 2010;**38**(12):2311–18.

47. Shehabi Y, Grant P, Wolfenden H, *et al.* Prevalence of delirium with dexmedetomidine compared with morphine based therapy after cardiac surgery: a randomized controlled trial (DEXmedetomidine COmpared to Morphine-DEXCOM Study). *Anesthesiology* 2009;**111**(5)1075–84.

48. Ruokonen E, Parviainen I, Jakob SM, *et al.* Dexmedetomidine versus propofol/midazolam for long-term sedation during mechanical ventilation. *Intensive Care Med* 2009;**35**(2):282–90.

49. Mirski MA, Lewin JJ, III, Ledroux S, *et al.* Cognitive improvement during continuous sedation in critically ill, awake and responsive patients: the Acute Neurological ICU Sedation Trial (ANIST). *Intensive Care Med* 2010;**36**(9):1505–13.

50. Reade MC, O'Sullivan K, Bates S, *et al.* Dexmedetomidine vs. haloperidol in delirious, agitated, intubated patients: a randomised open-label trial. *Crit Care* 2009;**13**(3):R75.

51. Jakob SM, Ruokonen E, Grounds RM, *et al.* Dexmedetomidine vs. midazolam or propofol for sedation during prolonged mechanical ventilation: two randomized controlled trials. *JAMA* 2012;**307**(11) 1151–60.

52. Van Eijk MM, Roes KC, Honing ML, *et al.* Effect of rivastigmine as an adjunct to usual care with haloperidol on duration of delirium and mortality in critically ill patients: a multicentre, double-blind, placebo-controlled randomised trial. *Lancet* 2010;**376**:1829–37.

53. Overshott R, Karim S, Burns A. Cholinesterase inhibitors for delirium. *Cochrane Database Syst Rev* 2008;**1**:CD005317.

54. Lonergan E, Luxenberg J, Areosa Sastre A, Wyller TB. Benzodiazepines for delirium. *Cochrane Database Syst Rev* 2009;**211**:CD006379.

55. Pisani MA, Murphy TE, Araujo KL, *et al.* Benzodiazepine and opioid use and the duration of intensive care unit delirium in an older population. *Crit Care Med* 2009;**37**(1):177–83.

Chapter 30

Pharmacogenomics and cerebral dysfunction

Yoanna Skrobik

SUMMARY

More medications are administered in critical care units than in most hospital wards; intensive care unit (ICU) pharmacy expenditures often approach 20% of a hospital pharmacy's budget. The cost of this level of care is complicated by inadvertent events that increase costs even further. Adverse drug reactions (ADRs) occur in 6.7% of hospitalized patients [1], and are twice as common among the critically ill [2]. Many quality assurance initiatives have been proposed to mitigate other costly pharmacy performance-related issues, such as medication administration errors. In contrast, ADRs require an understanding of pharmacokinetics and pharmacogenomics.

Sedatives and opiate analgesics are routinely administered in severely ill and mechanically ventilated patients, and rank among the top six medication categories responsible for ADRs in critical care [3,4]. The therapeutic efficacy and the toxicity associated with the metabolism or transport of sedative and analgesic medications, on one hand, and neurological findings such as deep sedation or coma, and delirium, are linked. The mechanistic pathway rationale for this association, and clinical examples and data supporting that these interactions occur and are or may be clinically significant, are presented in this chapter.

Introduction

Severe adverse drug events relevant to critical care practitioners were described in 1957 [5] with the rare but dramatic complication of succinylcholine administration to inherited butyrylcholinesterase variant carriers [6]. The 1 in 3,500 affected Whites with a genetically determined single amino acid substitution [7] develop severe complications after the short-term paralytic agent succinylcholine is administered. The following decades have brought better understanding of genetic determinants of drug metabolism; publications addressing pharmacogenomics have increased further since the completion of the human genome project [6] (Figure 30.1). Genetically or metabolically influenced drug–drug interactions, alterations in metabolic pathways, and variable pharmacokinetics are understood and described in many clinical settings. Most of these reports, however, focus on cardiovascular or oncological drugs [8]. Complex drug interactions in other patient populations can lead to dramatic complications such as respiratory failure and coma [9]. This type of complication requires critical care admission, and should be familiar to the intensive care caregiver. In addition, multiple and often interacting drugs are administered in the critical care setting, highlighting the relevance of pharmacology and drug interaction-related clinical effects, such as confusion and coma, to the critical care practitioner.

Many drug interactions and genetic variants affect consciousness and cognition. Caregivers administer sedation to mitigate the patient's perception of the ICU experience; significant proportions of patients respond only to pain or are unresponsive. Patients with acute respiratory distress syndrome, who account for 5% of ICU admissions [10], may require deep sedation because of severe hypoxia. However, coma-like sedation levels occur in 75% of mechanically ventilated patients [11–13]. Sedative metabolism changes associated with age make this deep sedation, which can be considered a pharmacological complication, more likely [14]. Short- or medium-term decreases in consciousness in ICU are associated with increased morbidity, mortality, and expenditure [12,15–17]. Follow-up studies [18] associate decreases in consciousness with increased mortality [15,19], prolonged duration of both ventilation and

Brain Disorders in Critical Illness, ed. Robert D. Stevens, Tarek Sharshar, and E. Wesley Ely. Published by Cambridge University Press. © Cambridge University Press 2013.

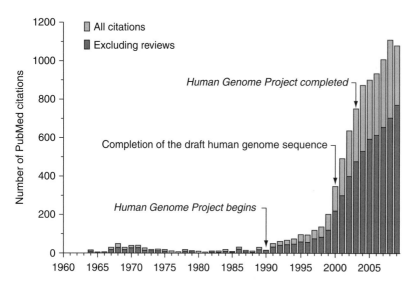

Figure 30.1 The emergence of pharmacogenomics. Number of citations including the terms pharmacogenetics or pharmacogenomics in PubMed are plotted vs. year. A dramatic increase is observed paralleling advances in technology and the completion of the Human Genome Project. Adapted from Meyer [6].

ICU stay [12], neuropsychological dysfunction [20], and functional decline [21–23]. Either interrupting or titrating [24] and minimizing drug administration benefits patients, shortens mechanical ventilation duration, reduces costs [25], and does not worsen psychological stress [26]. Current ICU sedation research and practice recommendations [27] therefore advocate optimizing and individualizing sedation goals. However, careful symptom-driven drug dosing is not always possible. In addition, even with careful protocol-driven sedation and analgesia, iatrogenic coma incidence is reduced only by half [27]. This apparent paradox suggests that ICU patients' pharmacokinetic and pharmacodynamic characteristics differ from those described in patients receiving short-term sedatives and analgesics for general anesthesia or in the procedural context.

Drug-metabolizing enzymes

Cytochrome P450 enzymes

Cytochrome P450s (CYP) are a superfamily of 57 hepatic enzyme coding genes that metabolize many drugs. Cytochrome pathways are responsible for the metabolism of most medications administered in critical care. Enzymes of drug metabolism pathways, including CYP450, are subject to genetic polymorphisms that may alter their metabolic activity. The genetic polymorphism of these enzymes thus plays a significant role in their metabolic activity and should be taken into account when administering these drugs, although there is a dearth of information as to the impact of genetic polymorphisms in critical care. Slow, intermediate, fast and

ultra-fast metabolizers have been described with, in some of the clinical examples described within the chapter below, dramatic clinical consequences. Genetic polymorphisms thus explain some of the drug response variability between individuals. Regulation of CYP activity is primarily transcriptional: nuclear receptors are recognized as key mediators in drug metabolism enzyme modulation. Their ligands are both endogenous and exogenous substances, which may have an agonistic or antagonistic effect on these transcription factors. The protein structure within different cytochromes determines affinity, and therefore specificity, for various substrates. Some substrates modify biotransformation enzyme activity; by increasing or decreasing it, they are classified as inducers or inhibitors. Co-administration of medication, a common occurrence in critical care, whether agonist or antagonist nuclear receptor ligands, can lead to severe toxicity, loss of therapeutic efficacy, or metabolic imbalance. Thus, CYP activity is dependent on both genotype and the environment.

The CYP3A system is the most abundantly expressed; more than 50% of medications in clinical use are isoenzyme CYP3A substrates [28,29]. CYP3A4 and CYP3A5 are its principal isoforms. CYP3A4/5 determines the metabolism of many therapeutic agents, among them midazolam, fentanyl, and antifungal agents such as fluconazole. The concurrent administration of drugs metabolized by this pathway leads to increases in serum drug levels and to potentiated therapeutic effect in studies conducted outside the ICU [30]. Excessive sedation is known to occur when benzodiazepines such as midazolam, triazolam, alprazolam, or diazepam, or non-benzodiazepine sedatives such as zopiclone and buspirone, are administered with CYP3A4 inhibitors [31]. Published expert reviews describe cytochrome P450's importance as a critical determinant of drug clearance, and as involved in the mechanism of numerous clinically relevant drug–drug interactions observed in critically ill patients [32]. However, these biologic and pharmacologic premises are not supported by many clinical descriptions. Indeed, and despite sound rationale that these interactions should and do occur, data are sparse as to what effects occur and the extent to which they are clinically significant.

The few clinical descriptions that drug interactions exist in the ICU and have an impact in day-to-day clinical practice are nevertheless compelling. One example of potentially significant interactions is depicted in Figure 30.2 (prototypical individual patient, unpublished data). Mathematical modeling to project expected fentanyl levels based on administered doses and infusion rates failed to predict the measured fentanyl levels when fluconazole was being co-administered (such as the individual whose values in hours 0–50 are shown in Figure 30.2). The higher fentanyl levels correlated with deep sedation. The effect was no longer present with similar fentanyl doses once fluconazole was discontinued (> 100 hours, Figure 30.2). How constant this effect is across cohorts and with different CYP4503A4 inhibitors is not known.

Computerized cytochromic interaction alerting software exists to identify potential drug interactions in vulnerable populations receiving multiple medications. It has been shown to improve detection and adjustment of medication based on identified interactions in geriatric patients [33]. In 100 elderly patients receiving five or more medications, a total of 238 cytochrome P450 drug–drug interactions were identified, of which over 70% involved CYP3A4. Medication adjustments and follow-up were deemed to be required in over 50% of the patients based on the information provided by the software. Similar smart alert or detection systems have not been tested to date in critically ill adults, or correlated with clinical outcomes.

The CYP3A5 variant is present in 10% or so of the White population [34,35] but in as many as 30% or more African Americans. Such patients metabolize CYP4503A4 pathway drugs more quickly [36]. Midazolam requirements, sedation levels, and serum midazolam measurements were compared in critically ill patients homozygous for this polymorphism, and in critically ill heterozygotes [37]. No significant differences were found. Whether a difference might be detected if CYP3A5 *1/*1, CYP3A5 *1/*3, and CYP3A5 *3/*3 carriers were compared, or how this genetic variant influences fentanyl requirements for adequate analgesia, is currently unknown. Whether competitive inhibition of cytochrome P4503A5 is similar to 3A4 is also unknown; the potential differences have been suggested in a study showing that ketoconazole inhibited CYP3A4 more than it did CYP3A5 for midazolam metabolism [38].

No genetic polymorphism is currently described for CYP3A4. Its activity varies considerably; pro-inflammatory cytokines down-regulate CYP450 enzyme content and activity in the animal model [39].

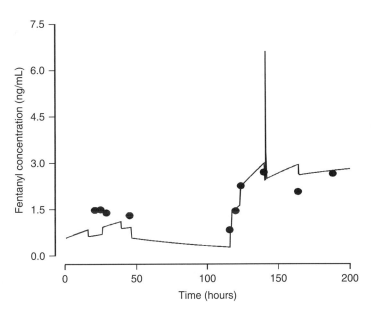

Figure 30.2 Mathematical modeling fit during administration of fluconazole (0–50 hours) vs. after fluconazole cessation in an ICU patient receiving intravenous infusions of fentanyl. The measured fentanyl serum level was nearly the double of the projected level when a medication competing for the same metabolic pathway was given concurrently.

This same effect has been described in humans. Patients requiring critical care after undergoing elective aortic aneurysm repair or major general surgery patients were assessed with carbon-14 [14C] erythromycin breath testing as a surrogate for CYP 3A4 activity; interleukin- 6 (IL-6) was used as a surrogate marker for inflammation. Cytochromic activity initially increased over the 24 hours after the intervention, followed by a marked reduction over 72 hours [40]. Higher levels of IL-6 were associated with significantly lower cytochromic activity. When leukocyte counts and C-reactive protein levels were used as inflammation markers in critically ill children, however, no relationship with midazolam metabolism (inferred on the basis of midazolam requirements rather than levels, and presumed to be CYP3A4 mediated) could be identified [41]. Midazolam clearance was assumed strictly on the basis of midazolam requirements and sedation levels. Sepsis-associated encephalopathy [42,43] may thus be at least in part related to inflammatory mediators and their direct physiological effects. However, if the patient is receiving sedatives or opiates metabolized by the cytochrome 3A4 pathway, drug metabolism and clearance may vary not only because of co-administered drugs but also because of variable levels in inflammatory mediators.

The metabolism of sedatives and opiates by CYP450s

Fentanyl and midazolam are commonly administered in the critical care setting [44] and are extensively metabolized by the same CYP450 isoenzymes, namely, CYP3A4/5 [45,46]. Co-administration of FEN and MDZ, or of either, with other drugs metabolized by the CYP3A4/5 isoenzyme [30] increases serum drug levels by competitive inhibition; metabolism and excretion of these drugs decreases with age [47]. In vitro studies suggest that fentanyl competitively inhibits metabolism of midazolam using a human hepatic microsome and recombinant cytochrome P450 isoforms model. Fentanyl competitively inhibits metabolism of midazolam to l'-OH MDZ by CYP3A4 [48]. Propofol, another commonly used sedative, is metabolized by a different CYP450 (CYP2C19); its presence inhibits 2D6 function [49] and alters 2D6 substrates (such as haloperidol, codeine, oxycodone, and tramadol) and antipsychotic metabolism. However, its impact on CYP4503A4/5 activity is believed to be mediated by metabolic inhibition; fentanyl and midazolam levels are increased through that mechanism [49].

We compared the biological and drug treatment characteristics in 100 patients who developed coma or delirium while receiving sedatives or opiate analgesics in the ICU [37]. Coma was not associated with the fentanyl dose received prior to the occurrence of coma, but was associated with the co-administration of CYP3A inhibitors (r = 0.31, p = 0.005) and with fentanyl plasma levels (3.7 ± 4.7 vs. 2.0 ± 1.8 ng/ml, p = 0.0001), while delirium was not. Similarly, coma was not associated with midazolam doses administered prior to the occurrence of coma, but was associated with midazolam plasma levels (1050 ± 2232 vs. 168 ± 249 ng/ml, p = 0.0001), while delirium was not. These data suggest that iatrogenic coma in the critical care setting is at least partly attributable to cytochromic pathway drug–drug interaction. In addition, the data suggest the mechanistic pathways leading to coma or to delirium may differ, and that cerebral dysfunction may not predictably be a disease spectrum of "brain failure" as has been proposed.

The pharmacokinetics of midazolam (MDZ) are well characterized, and its pharmacodynamics are predictable in healthy adults [50]. Midazolam is exclusively metabolized by CYP3A4 and metabolic clearance in healthy populations is preserved over a relatively narrow range [51,52]. Information on the effect of critical illness, however, on the PK and PD of midazolam is less reported. Midazolam drug levels were sampled daily in nine septic critically ill patients and compared with otherwise stable outpatients receiving midazolam for procedural sedation. Plasma levels, half-life, and terminal half-life varied within a considerably broader range than that reported in the literature to date, and in comparison with normal subjects [53], with very broad intra- and inter-subject variability (Tables 30.1 and 30.2, and Figures 30.3 and 30.4). In addition, terminal half-life, which is determined after drug infusion cessation, was prolonged in all patients, and contrasted with previously published

Table 30.1 Midazolam dosing duration and mean concentration.

	Continuous infusion	Intermittent dosing[*]
Days	8.8	4.8
MDZ	265 ± 177	100 ± 134

[*] Bolus dosing in the same nine critically ill patients administered on an as-needed basis following discontinuation of midazolam infusion; concentrations are expressed in ng/ml, and presented as mean ± SD.

Table 30.2 Pharmacokinetic (Pk) parameters in study participants and healthy controls. Comparison of midazolam clearance and half-life in nine septic ICU patients and four patients receiving MDZ for procedural outpatient interventions.

PK parameter	Study patients		Healthy controls	
	Mean ± SD	Range	Mean ± SD	Range
CL_{ss} (ml/min)	418 ± 324	31–1157	376	267–485
$T_{1/2}$ (h)	16.0 ± 9.6	2.3–34.9	3.2	1.0–4.0

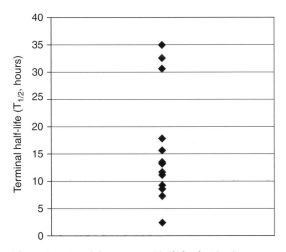

Figure 30.3 Variability in terminal half-life of midazolam among nine septic intensive care unit (ICU) patients.

values in less ill populations. These characteristics are in keeping with description in a pediatric critical care population where lower midazolam elimination was observed in comparison to other studies in pediatric patients [54], and felt to be attributable, among others, to covariates such as renal failure, hepatic failure, and concomitant administration of CYP3A inhibitors.

Disease- and genotype-associated drug metabolism alterations

The vulnerable critically ill metabolize sedatives differently than do healthy elective surgery patients [37,54,55]. This, in addition to drug–drug interactions, can lead to excessive sedation and elevated opiate and benzodiazepine levels [37]. Because renal dysfunction, hepatic abnormalities, and drug–drug interactions are prevalent, particularly in older critically ill patients, analgesic and sedative pharmacokinetics may contribute to alterations in level of consciousness. Poorly defined entities such as septic encephalopathy may at least partly be attributable to inflammatory or other pharmacologically related, and therefore modifiable, effects.

While no CYPP4503A4/5 genotypic variants have been shown to cause a phenotypic change in drug metabolism, various genotypes of the CYP2D6 are associated with clear and clinically significant drug metabolism differences. Twenty percent of drugs are metabolized by cytochrome P4502D6. Approximately 80 allele variations in CYP2D6 have been identified [55]; their impact on clinical outcomes is primarily linked to their effect on metabolism. Individuals with two non-functional alleles at 2D6 are considered poor metabolizers. O-demethylation of codeine by CYP2A6 metabolism accounts for only 10% of the administered codeine's metabolism, but is essential in producing its active metabolite, morphine. The 7–10% of Whites with the poor metabolizer genotype cannot get analgesic effect from codeine because of their inability to produce morphine. Persons with one or two functional alleles are considered extensive metabolizers, and those with duplicate or amplified active CYP2D6 are considered ultra-rapid metabolizers. A minority of North American or European Whites, but more than 25% of Ethiopians, for instance, have genetically determined ultra-rapid metabolism. Ultra-rapid metabolizers produce serum levels of morphine 20–80 fold higher than those produced by extensive metabolizers given the same codeine dose. The 2D6 pathway produces active metabolite but only accounts for a small proportion of drug disposal. N-demethylation of codeine, and its glucoronidation, account for 80% of the remaining metabolism [56]. N-demethylation is CYP3A4 dependent.

The importance of understanding genetic variability, and active metabolite and elimination pathways, was elegantly illustrated in a case report describing an ultra-rapid metabolizer who received a moderate dose

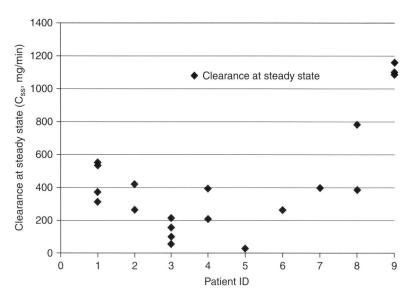

Figure 30.4 Observed intra- and inter-subject variability in MDZ clearance at steady state.

of codeine [9]. In this case, the featured patient received codeine while receiving voriconazole and clarithromycin, two CYP3A4 inhibitors. The patient had concomitant renal failure. He became unconscious and developed hypercarbic respiratory failure, required mechanical ventilation, intensive care admission, and a naloxone infusion. Genotyping and serum drug sampling confirmed very high serum morphine levels, induced by the ultra-rapid metabolizer profile, which were compounded by his inability to clear the morphine or morphine-3-glucorinide and morphine-6-glucorinide, morphine's neurotoxic metabolites, because of the co-administration of CYP3A4 inhibitors and the concomitant renal failure. Since this publication, other cases of respiratory depression and death due to codeine administration in rapid metabolizers have been reported [57].

Whether ultra-rapid CYP2D6 metabolizers are at risk for other forms of toxicity than high serum morphine levels after codeine administration is not clear. One study seeking to link postoperative cognitive dysfunction (POCD) to cytochrome P450 polymorphism by genotyping of 2D6 and 2C19 in 337 patients showed no link between polymorphisms and POCD outcome [58]. The 2D6 ultra-rapid metabolizers had, however, by far the highest incidence of POCD, at 25% on first assessment, and with a two-fold incidence of POCD at both 1-week and 3-month postoperative testing in comparison to all other metabolizer profiles. This difference was not considered statistically significant on multivariate analysis, however, when age and type of surgery were considered.

P-glycoprotein (P-gp)

P-glycoprotein is an efflux transporter with the capacity to extrude intracellular medication to the extracellular matrix; it exists on the apical surface of intestinal epithelial cells, in the biliary tree, in the kidney tubules, and on the blood–brain barrier [59–61]. P-glycoprotein (P-gP) limits xenobiotic absorption and acts as a protector against drug accumulation by promoting urinary and biliary xenobiotic efflux. Cerebral cells are protected by P-gP at the blood–brain barrier (BBB0 level). P-glycoprotein is a key transporter for many therapeutic agents, among them fentanyl [62]. In a pilot cohort of 100 patients receiving fentanyl and midazolam, we measured P-glycoprotein polymorphism to test whether it was associated with the occurrence of delirium or iatrogenic coma and found no correlation [37]. P-glycoprotein inhibitor administration was, however, associated with the number of days patients were deemed delirious (r = 0.32, p = 0.002). Whether this effect had any relationship with cerebral accumulation of fentanyl, midazolam, or their potentially toxic metabolites was not tested, as cerebrospinal fluid was not sampled in that study.

Pharmacokinetic variables

The responses to acute physiological stress, aggressive hemodynamic resuscitation, and organ dysfunction significantly alter drug response in the critically ill and in a critically ill individual over time. One example of this effect is the wide variations in serum albumin attributable to alterations in liver synthesis and dilution. This may affect highly protein-bound drugs such as propofol, midazolam, and fentanyl. When in vitro plasma protein binding and distribution in blood of fentanyl was studied in healthy human volunteers, in plasma, 84.4% of fentanyl was bound [63]. Propofol significantly raises the rate of albumin-unbound free midazolam in an in-vitro albumin model [64]. The effects of acute illness and protein shifts on midazolam and fentanyl bioavailability may thus vary with fluid resuscitation and protein synthesis by the liver.

Inflammation and neurotransmitters

The relationship between sepsis and cerebral dysfunction is explored elsewhere in this book. Several reports suggest a relationship between systemic inflammation and behavioral changes, some of which may be attributable to blood–brain barrier permeability. An increase in plasma levels of pro-inflammatory cytokines has been linked to delirium [65] and depression [66]. IL-1β injected into rat brains causes an increase in blood–brain barrier permeability [67]. IL-8 is a potent neutrophil chemotactic agent; its expression may also act to increase blood–brain barrier dysfunction [68]. IL-6 is able to cause a substantial increase in the permeability of the blood–brain barrier [69]. Chemokines have also been shown to modulate blood–brain barrier permeability [70]. In one small human ICU study, an association was found with IL-8 levels and delirium [71]. Other reports identify variable drug transport across the blood–brain barrier with accumulation of toxic metabolites in the brain. IL-6 influenced morphine metabolite transport across the blood–brain barrier in critically ill patients [72], raising the possibility that it may also modulate the distribution of other drugs.

In a pilot cohort of 100 patients receiving fentanyl and midazolam studied to assess determinants of delirium or iatrogenic coma, delirious patients had higher levels of IL-6 than comatose patients (129.3 vs. 35.0 pg/ml, p = 0.05), suggesting that the inflammatory mediator patterns may differ in various clinical presentations of alterations in consciousness combined with cognitive abnormalities, that some authors have termed "cerebral dysfunction" to describe this spectrum in the critically ill.

The ICU environment is unique in that it contextually associates factors associated with critical illness with some of the mechanisms postulated to cause delirium [73,74]. These include neurotransmitter imbalance, inflammation, blood–brain barrier permeability, as well as abnormal levels of large neutral amino acids. Some amino acid precursors such as tryptophan are believed, in the context of increased plasma concentrations, to influence both neurotransmitter levels and neuroinflammation [75]. Tryptophan competes with tryrosine and leucine for transport across the blood–brain barrier; increased cerebral uptake of tryptophan and phenylalanine leads to elevated levels of neurotransmitters such as serotonin and norepinephrine. Decreased ratio of tryptophan to other large amino acids has been associated with delirium. A recent study investigated the association between plasma kynurenine concentrations and kynurenine/tryptophan ratios, and acute brain dysfunction, defined as the presence of either delirium or coma [76]. Among the 84 patients studied, and after adjusting for age, sedation regimen, and severity of illness, elevated kynurenine and kynurenine/tryptophan ratio were associated with fewer delirium/coma-free days, leading to speculation as to a biochemical mechanistic pathway. There were, however, limitations to the analysis. Assessment of the plasma kynurenine/tryptophan ratio (the most common tool in clinical investigations of tryptophan–kynurenine metabolism) does not distinguish between the activity of two rate-limiting enzymes of kynurenine formation from tryptophan: tryptophan 2,3-dioxygenase (TDO) and indoleamine 2,3 dioxygenase (IDO). Each enzyme activity is enhanced by other factors common in the critically ill: TDO by stress hormones (cortisol) and IDO by pro-inflammatory cytokines (tumor necrosis factor alpha [TNFα] and interferon-gamma) [77]. These enzymatic pathway activities have been studied in depression, and are suspected to play an important role in psychosis and cognition [77]. The rate of kynurenine metabolism, or changes associated with the ability of kynurenine metabolites to penetrate the central nervous system, cannot be differentiated given the challenges of measuring the direct metabolites of kynurenine (e.g., kynurenic acid). In addition, a single plasma kynurenine and tryptophan measurement as described in the study would not capture the association between changes in the kynurenine/tryptophan ratio over time and delirium, coma, or both, or account for the fluctuating nature of both delirium and coma during the ICU stay. Moreover, the validity of combining delirium and coma as a single outcome is the subject of some debate, since no biological rationale supports an association between the kynurenine pathway with unresponsiveness, in addition to recent data suggesting that iatrogenic coma and delirium in the ICU are not mechanistically linked [37].

Conclusion

Some authors deplore the lack of timely transmission of pharmacogenomic interactions into clinical practice [78], and the relative paucity of prospectively validated genetic risk data on the vulnerable and expensive critically ill population [79]. That drug–drug interactions and genomic variations impact on level of consciousness appears clear from data in critically ill adult and pediatric populations to date. Delirium and its association to sedatives and analgesics present several challenges. Screening tool inconsistencies and potential confounding by sedation, in addition to the pharmacological findings described above, make the association between benzodiazepines and delirium less convincing. Overall, drug interactions in the critically ill are probably common and may be harmful; identifying the most significant ones, identifying their clinical impact, and raising the awareness of the critical care community is a scientific and educational challenge.

References

1. Lazarou JPB, Pomeranz BH, Corey PN. Incidence of adverse drug reactions in hospitalized patients: a meta-analysis of prospective studies. *JAMA* 1998;**279**(15):1200–5.

2. Cullen BD, Small SD, Cooper JB, Nemeskal AR, Leape LL. The incident reporting system does not detect adverse drug events: a problem for quality improvement. *Jt Comm J Qual Improv* 1995;**21**(10):541–8.

3. Kopp BJ, Erstad BL, Allen ME, Theodorou AA, Priestley G. Medication errors and adverse drug events in an intensive care unit: direct observation approach for detection. *Critical Care Med* 2006;**34**(2):415–25.

4. Kane-Gill SL, Kirisci L, Verrico MM, Rothschild JM. Analysis of risk factors for adverse drug events in critically ill patients. *Critical Care Med* 2012;**40**(3):823–8.

5. Kalow W. Pharmacogenetics and anesthesia. *Anesthesiology* 1964;**25**:377–87.

6. Meyer UA. Pharmacogenetics – five decades of therapeutic lessons from genetic diversity. *Nat Rev Genet* 2004;**5**(9):669–76.

7. McGuire MC, Noqueira CP, Bartels CF, *et al.* Identification of the structural mutation responsible for the dibucaine-resistant (atypical) variant form of human serum cholinesterase. *Proc Natl Acad Sci USA* 1989;**86**(3):953–7.

8. Empey PE. Genetic predisposition to adverse drug reactions in the intensive care unit. *Crit Care Med* 2010;**38**(6 Suppl):S106–16.

9. Gasche Y, Daali Y, Fathi M, *et al.* Codeine intoxication associated with ultrarapid CYP2D6 metabolism. *N Engl J Med* 2004;**351**:2827–31.

10. Esteban A, Ferguson ND, Meade MO, *et al.* Evolution of mechanical ventilation in response to clinical research. *Am J Resp Crit Care Med* 2008; **177**(2):170–7.

11. Girard TD, Jackson JC, Pandharipande PP, *et al.* Delirium as a predictor of long-term cognitive impairment in survivors of critical illness. *Crit Care Med* 2010;**38**(7):1513–20.

12. Shehabi Y, Bellomo R, Reade MC, *et al.* Early intensive care sedation predicts long-term mortality in ventilated critically ill patients. *Am J Resp Crit Care Med* 2012;**186**(8):724–31.

13. Girard TD, Kress JP, Fuchs BD, *et al.* Efficacy and safety of a paired sedation and ventilator weaning protocol for mechanically ventilated patients in intensive care (Awakening and Breathing Controlled trial): a randomised controlled trial. *Lancet* 2008;**371**(9607):126–34.

14. Hammerlein A, Derendorf H, Lowenthal DT. Pharmacokinetic and pharmacodynamic changes in the elderly. Clinical implications. *Clin Pharmacokinet* 1998;**35**(1):49–64.

15. Ouimet S, Kavanagh BP, Gottfried SB, Skrobik Y. Incidence, risk factors and consequences of ICU delirium. *Intensive Care Med* 2007;**33**(1):66–73.

16. Herridge MS, Tansey CM, Matte A, *et al.* Functional disability 5 years after acute respiratory distress syndrome. *N Engl J Med* 2011;**364**(14):1293–304.

17. Ely EW, Shintani A, Truman B, *et al.* Delirium as a predictor of mortality in mechanically ventilated patients in the intensive care unit. *JAMA* 2004;**291**(14):1753–62.

18. Treggiari MM, Romand JA, Yanez ND, *et al.* Randomized trial of light versus deep sedation on mental health after critical illness. *Crit Care Med* 2009;**37**(9):2527–34.

19. Watson PL, Shintani AK, Tyson R, *et al.* Presence of electroencephalogram burst suppression in sedated, critically ill patients is associated with increased mortality. *Crit Care Med* 2008;**36**(12):3171–7.

20. Granja C, Gomes E, Amaro A, *et al.* Understanding posttraumatic stress disorder-related symptoms after

critical care: the early illness amnesia hypothesis. *Crit Care Med* 2008;**36**(10):2801–9.

21. Samuelson K, Lundberg D, Fridlund B. Memory in relation to depth of sedation in adult mechanically ventilated intensive care patients. *Intensive Care Med* 2006;**32**(5):660–7.

22. Samuelson KA, Lundberg D, Fridlund B. Light vs. heavy sedation during mechanical ventilation after oesophagectomy – a pilot experimental study focusing on memory. *Acta Anaesthesiol Scand* 2008;**52**(8):1116–23.

23. Nelson BJ, Weinert CR, Bury CL, Marinelli WA, Gross CR. Intensive care unit drug use and subsequent quality of life in acute lung injury patients. *Critical Care Med* 2000;**28**(11):3626–30.

24. Mehta S, Burry L, Cook D, *et al.* Daily sedation interruption in mechanically ventilated critically ill patients cared for with a sedation protocol: a randomized controlled trial. *JAMA* 2012;**308**(19):1985–92.

25. Awissi DK, Begin C, Moisan J, Lachaine J, Skrobik Y. I-SAVE study: impact of sedation, analgesia, and delirium protocols evaluated in the intensive care unit: an economic evaluation. *Annals Pharmacother* 2012;**46**(1):21–8.

26. Roberts DJ, Haroon B, Hall RI. Sedation for critically ill or injured adults in the intensive care unit: a shifting paradigm. *Drugs* 2012;**72**(14):1881–916.

27. Barr JM, Fraser GL, Puntillo K, *et al.* Clinical practice guidelines for the management of pain, agitation, and delirium in adult patients in the intensive care unit. *Critical Care Med* 2013;**41**(1):263–306.

28. Skrobik Y, Ahern S, Leblanc M, Marquis F, Awissi DK, Kavanagh BP. Protocolized intensive care unit management of analgesia, sedation, and delirium improves analgesia and subsyndromal delirium rates. *Anesth Analg* 2011;**11**(2):451–63.

29. Rendic S, Di Carlo FJ. Human cytochrome P450 enzymes: a status report summarizing their reactions, substrates, inducers, and inhibitors. *Drug Metab Rev* 1997;**29**(1–2):413–580.

30. Guengerich FP. Cytochrome P-450 3A4: regulation and role in drug metabolism. *Annu Rev Pharmacol Toxicol* 1999;**39**:1–17.

31. Saari TI, Laine K, Neuvonen M, Neuvonen PJ, Olkkola KT. Effect of voriconazole and fluconazole on the pharmacokinetics of intravenous fentanyl. *Eur J Clin Pharmacol* 2008;**64**(1):25–30.

32. Dresser GK, Spence JD, Bailey DG. Pharmacokinetic-pharmacodynamic consequences and clinical relevance of cytochrome P450 3A4 inhibition. *Clin Pharmacokinet* 2000;**38**(1):41–57.

33. Spriet I, Meersseman W, de Hoon J, *et al.* Mini-series: II. Clinical aspects. Clinically relevant CYP450-mediated drug interactions in the ICU. *Intensive Care Med* 2009;**35**(4):603–12.

34. Zakrzewski-Jakubiak H, Doan J, Lamoureux P, *et al.* Detection and prevention of drug–drug interactions in the hospitalized elderly: utility of new cytochrome p450-based software. *Am J Geriatr Pharmacother* 2011;**9**(6):461–70.

35. Kuehl P, Zhang J, Lin Y, *et al.* Sequence diversity in CYP3A promoters and characterization of the genetic basis of polymorphic CYP3A5 expression. *Nat Genet* 2001;**27**(4):383–91.

36. van Schaik RH van der Heiden IP, van den Anker JN, Lindemans J. CYP3A5 variant allele frequencies in Dutch Caucasians. *Clin Chem* 2002;**48**(10):1668–71.

37. Lin YS, Dowling AL, Quigley SD, *et al.* Co-regulation of CYP3A4 and CYP3A5 and contribution to hepatic and intestinal midazolam metabolism. *Mol Pharmacol* 2002;**62**(1):162–72.

38. Skrobik Y, Leger C, Cossette M, Michaud V, Turgeon J. Factors predisposing to coma and delirium: fentanyl and midazolam exposure, CYP3A5, ABCB1 and ABCG2 genetic polymorphisms, and inflammatory factors. *Critical Care Med* 2013;**41**(4):999–1008.

39. Michaud V, Simard C, Turgeon J. Characterization of CYP3A isozymes involved in the metabolism of domperidone: role of cytochrome b(5) and inhibition by ketoconazole. *Drug Metab Lett* 2010;**14**(2):95–103.

40. Haas CE, Kaufman DC, Jones CE, Burstein AH, Reiss W. Cytochrome P450 3A4 activity after surgical stress. *Critical Care Med* 2003;**31**(5):1338–46.

41. Vet NJ, de Hoog M, Tibboel D, de Wildt SN. The effect of critical illness and inflammation on midazolam therapy in children. *Pediatr Crit Care Med* 2012;**13**(1):48–50.

42. Siami S, Annane D, Sharshar T. The encephalopathy in sepsis. *Critical Care Clinics* 2008;**24**(1):67–82.

43. Sharshar T, Polito A, Checinski A, Stevens RD. Septic-associated encephalopathy – everything starts at a microlevel. *Crit Care* 2010;**14**(5):199.

44. Mehta S, Burry L, Fischer S, *et al.* Canadian survey of the use of sedatives, analgesics, and neuromuscular blocking agents in critically ill patients. *Critical Care Med* 2006;**34**(2):374–80.

45. Feierman DE, Lasker JM. Metabolism of fentanyl, a synthetic opioid analgesic, by human liver microsomes. Role of CYP3A4. *Drug Metab Dispos* 1996;**24**(9):932–9.

46. Gorski JC, Hall SD, Jones DR, Van den Branden M, Wrighton SA. Regioselective biotransformation of midazolam by members of the human cytochrome P450 3A (CYP3A) subfamily. *Biochem Pharmacol* 1994;**47**(9):1643–53.

47. Greenblatt DJ, Abernethy DR, Locniskar A, *et al*. Effect of age, gender, and obesity on midazolam kinetics. *Anesthesiology* 1984;**61**(1):27–35.

48. Hamaoka N, Oda Y, Hase I, *et al*. Propofol decreases the clearance of midazolam by inhibiting CYP3A4: an in vivo and in vitro study. *Clin Pharm Ther* 1999;**66**(2):110–17.

49. McKillop D, Wild MJ, Butters CJ, Simcock C. Effects of propofol on human hepatic microsomal cytochrome P450 activities. *Xenobiotica* 1998;**28**(9):845–53.

50. Albrecht S, Ihmsen H, Hering W, *et al*. The effect of age on the pharmacokinetics and pharmacodynamics of midazolam. *Clin Pharm Ther* 1999;**65**(6):630–9.

51. Malacrida R, Fritz ME, Suter PM, Crevoisier C. Pharmacokinetics of midazolam administered by continuous intravenous infusion to intensive care unit patients. *Crit Care Med* 1992;**20**:1123–26.

52. Dresser GK. Coordinate induction of both cytochrome P4503A and MDR1 by St John's wort in healthy subjects. *Clin Pharm Ther* 2003;**73**:41–50.

53. Ovakim D, Bosma KJ, Young GB, *et al*. Effect of critical illness on the pharmacokinetics and dose–response relationship of midazolam. *Crit Care Med* 2012;**16**(Suppl 1):330.

54. de Wildt SN, de Hoog M, Vinks AA, van der Giesen E, van den Anker JN. Population pharmacokinetics and metabolism of midazolam in pediatric intensive care patients. *Crit Care Med* 2003;**31**(7):1952–8.

55. Eichelbaum M, Evert B. Influence of pharmacogenetics on drug disposition and response. *Clin Exp Pharmacol Physiol* 1996;**23**:983–5.

56. Desmeules J, Gascon MP, Dayer P, Magistris M. Impact of environmental and genetic factors on codeine analgesia. *Eur J Clin Pharmacol* 1991;**41**(1):23–6.

57. Ciszkowski C, Madadi P, Phillips MS, Lauwers AE, Koren G. Codeine, ultrarapid-metabolism genotype, and postoperative death. *N Engl J Med* 2009;**361**(8):827–8.

58. Steinmetz J, Jespersgaard C, Dalhoff K, *et al*. Cytochrome P450 polymorphism and postoperative cognitive dysfunction. *Minerva Anestesiol* 2012;**78**(3):303–9.

59. Thiebaut F, Tsuruo T, Hamada H, *et al*. Cellular localization of the multidrug-resistance gene product P-glycoprotein in normal human tissues. *Proc Natl Acad Sci USA* 1987;**84**(21):7735–8.

60. Fromm MF. The influence of MDR1 polymorphisms on P-glycoprotein expression and function in humans. *Adv Drug Deliv Rev* 2002;**54**(10):1295–310.

61. Nakamura Y, Ikeda S, Furukawa T, *et al*. Function of P-glycoprotein expressed in placenta and mole. *Biochem Biophys Res Commun* 1997;**235**(3):849–53.

62. Henthorn TK, Liu Y, Mahapatro M, Ng KY. Active transport of fentanyl by the blood–brain barrier. *J Pharmacol Exp Ther* 1999;**289**(2):1084–9.

63. Meuldermans WE, Hurkmans RM, Heykants JJ. Plasma protein binding and distribution of fentanyl, sufentanil, alfentanil and lofentanil in blood. *Arch Int Pharmacodyn Ther* 1982;**257**(1):4–19.

64. Ohmori J, Maeda S, Higuchi H, *et al*. Propofol increases the rate of albumin-unbound free midazolam in serum albumin solution. *J Anesth* 2011;**25**(4):618–20.

65. de Rooij SE, van Munster BC, Korevaar JC, Levi M. Cytokines and acute phase response in delirium. *J Psychosom Res* 2007;**62**:521–5.

66. Dantzer R, O'Connor JC, Freund GG, Johnson RW, Kelley KW. From inflammation to sickness and depression: when the immune system subjugates the brain. *Nat Rev Neurosci* 2008;**9**:46–56.

67. Saija A, Princi P, Lanza M, *et al*. Systemic cytokine administration can affect blood-brain barrier permeability in the rat. *Life Sci* 1995;**56**:775–84.

68. Scholz M, Cinatl J, Schadel-Hopfner M, Windolf J. Neutrophils and the blood–brain barrier dysfunction after trauma. *Med Res Rev* 2007;**27**:401–16.

69. de Vries HE, Bloom-Roosemalen M, van Oosten M, *et al*. The influence of cytokines on the integrity of the blood–brain barrier in vitro. *J Neuroimmunol* 1996;**64**:37–43.

70. Stamatovic SM, Shakui P, Keep RF, *et al*. Monocyte chemoattractant protein-1 regulation of blood–brain barrier permeability. *J Cereb Blood Flow Metab* 2005;**25**:593–606.

71. van den Boogaard M, Kox M, Quinn KL, *et al*. Biomarkers associated with delirium in critically ill patients and their relation with long-term subjective cognitive dysfunction; indications for different pathways governing delirium in inflamed and noninflamed patients. *Crit Care* 2011;**15**(6):29.

72. Roberts DJ, Goralski KB, Renton KW, *et al*. Effect of acute inflammatory brain injury on accumulation of morphine and morphine 3- and 6-glucuronide in the human brain. *Crit Care Med* 2009;**37**:2767–74.

73. McGrane S, Girard TD, Thompson JL, *et al*. Procalcitonin and C-reactive protein levels at admission as predictors of duration of acute brain dysfunction in critically ill patients. *Crit Care* 2011;**15**(2):R78.

74. Forrest CM, Mackay GM, Oxford L, *et al*. Kynurenine metabolism predicts cognitive function in patients following cardiac bypass and thoracic surgery. *J Neurochem* 2011;**119**(1):136–52.

75. Oxenkrug GF. Interferon-gamma-inducible kynurenines/pteridines inflammation cascade:

implications for aging and aging-associated psychiatric and medical disorders. *J Neural Transm* 2011;**118**:75–85.

76. Adams-Wilson JR, Morandi A, Girard TD, *et al.* The association of the kynurenine pathway of tryptophan metabolism with acute brain dysfunction during critical illness. *Crit Care Med* 2012;**40**(3):835–41.

77. Oxenkrug GF. Tryptophan–kynurenine metabolism as a common mediator of genetic and environmental impacts in major depressive disorder: the serotonin hypothesis revisited 40 years later. *Isr J Psychiatry Relat Sci* 2010;**47**(1):56–63.

78. Manolopoulos VG. Pharmacogenomics and adverse drug reactions in diagnostic and clinical practice. *Clin Chem Lab Med* 2007;**45**(7):801–14.

79. Chiang AP, Butte AJ. Data-driven methods to discover molecular determinants of serious adverse drug events. *Clin Pharmacol Ther* 2009;**85**(3):259–68.

Chapter 31

Early physical and occupational therapy

John P. Kress

SUMMARY

Intensive care unit (ICU) patients who require mechanical ventilation frequently suffer from severe neuromuscular weakness and neurocognitive dysfunction. Prolonged immobility due to illness and sedation contributes to this problem. Aggressive physical and occupational therapy is feasible in such patients. Such therapy can begin extremely early during critical illness, even while patients still require mechanical ventilation. Such unconventional approaches to patient care have been shown to improve functional and neurological outcomes in ICU survivors.

Introduction

Survival after critical illness has improved greatly over the last few decades [1–5]. Accordingly, recovery from previously fatal acute illnesses is now a reality. Traditionally, because respiratory failure requiring endotracheal intubation and mechanical ventilation is a life-threatening condition, the standard care strategy had been to stabilize cardiopulmonary function regardless of the impact on other organ systems. This strategy started with a philosophy of "taking over," whereby full mechanical ventilatory support and stabilization of circulatory insufficiency with intravenous fluids and vasoactive drugs became the norm. However, most sick patients do not respond passively to aggressive interventions such as endotracheal intubation. This "conflict" typically led to a strategy of deep sedation in order to ensure a passive, docile patient. Since most sedative and analgesic drugs were originally studied for use in the operating room, the ICU became a natural extension of the operating room environment. In retrospect, it seems that a short-term goal of ICU survival was the major focus of this approach to care, with relatively little attention given

to longer-term cognitive and neuromuscular function in those who actually did survive their acute illness. However, a number of recent publications have addressed the abundant longer-term issues of ICU survivorship, particularly with regard to those suffering from respiratory failure requiring mechanical ventilation [6–10]. Herridge and colleagues reported 1-year outcomes in patients recovering from acute respiratory distress syndrome (ARDS). One hundred percent of the patients evaluated reported loss of muscle bulk, proximal muscle weakness, and fatigue; half of this relatively young group of patients were unemployed 1 year after their ICU experience [6]. Follow-up studies from these investigators noted similar problems in this cohort of patients at the 2- and 5-year marks for many of these patients with lung injury [7]. The complex syndrome, referred to as "ICU-acquired weakness" (ICUAW), has received a great deal of attention in recent literature. Though a precise pathophysiology of this syndrome has not been identified, the state of prolonged immobility is thought to be a major contributor to the problem. Many ICU patients remain relatively motionless for days to weeks. This state has been referred to as one of suspended animation [11].

In such a state of suspended animation, ICU delirium is extremely common [12]. The short- and long-term effects of ICU delirium are well described. They include increased hospital length of stay, fewer days alive without mechanical ventilation, and a risk of 6-month mortality that is greater than three-fold higher compared with those without ICU delirium. Cognitive impairment is also greater in those with ICU delirium. Ely and colleagues noted that ICU patients with delirium were more than nine times more likely to have cognitive impairment at hospital discharge than those without ICU delirium [13].

Brain Disorders in Critical Illness, ed. Robert D. Stevens, Tarek Sharshar, and E. Wesley Ely. Published by Cambridge University Press. © Cambridge University Press 2013.

Not only the presence, but also the duration of ICU delirium is important. Girard, *et al.* reported that increasing duration of delirium was an independent predictor of worse cognitive performance in ICU survivors evaluated at 3- and 12-month follow-up times [14]. Given the importance of these above-mentioned problems, this chapter will explore the current evidence on the association between early physical and occupational therapy and improved brain function in critically ill patients.

Physical exercise and mental health

The harmful effects of complete bed rest have been recognized for more than 60 years. Asher's description of the perils of bed rest in 1947 in the *British Medical Journal* is actually quite apropos, even today: "... consider the mental changes, the demoralizing effects of staying in bed ... the patient may acquire an exaggerated idea of the seriousness of his illness and think 'Surely, I must be very ill if I am kept in bed'. At a later stage, a dismal lethargy overcomes the victim. He loses the desire to get up and even resents any efforts to extract him from his supine stupor. The end result can be a comatose, vegetable existence in which, like a useless but carefully tended plant, the patient lies permanently in tranquil torpidity" [15]. Clearly, much has been written about brain dysfunction in critical illness, as discussed in other chapters written in this book. The notion that physical and mental function are intimately intertwined has been recognized for centuries. However, the impact of this relationship on management strategies for patients in modern intensive care is a relatively new concept.

Numerous studies outside the intensive care setting have described the importance of physical function on cognition [16–21]. Inouye and colleagues published an important study more than a decade ago describing a strategy to reduce delirium in hospitalized, non-ICU patients [22]. In a trial using an intervention-matched control approach, patients were studied to evaluate an intervention to reduce delirium. Immobility was one of six targeted risk factors for delirium in these patients. The immobility intervention was an early mobilization protocol that involved ambulation or active range-of-motion exercises multiple times per day. The protocol also focused on minimization of immobilizing equipment such as bladder catheters or physical restraints. This mobilization protocol occurred successfully during 84% of patient hospital days. There was a significant

reduction in delirium incidence in these high-risk hospitalized patients (9.9% vs. 15.0%); likewise, the *cumulative* incidence of delirium was lower in the intervention group.

Laurin and colleagues reported a 5-year observational study of more than 9,000 patients [17]. Physical activity was associated with lower risks of cognitive impairment, Alzheimer's disease, and dementia when compared with no exercise. This positive association was greater in those with higher levels of exercise than in those with lesser exercise. Yaffe and colleagues studied almost 6,000 women who were 65 years or older. In a prospective trial spanning 6–8 years, women with greater baseline physical activity level were less likely to experience cognitive decline during the 6–8-year follow-up evaluations [18]. Together, these studies suggest that there is a strong relationship between physical activity and cognitive function. This mind–body relationship clearly suggests an opportunity for interventions to improve brain dysfunction in critical illness.

In the last few years, several investigators have begun reporting specifically on a culture shift in ICU care. The traditional model of deep sedation and prolonged bed rest in mechanically ventilated patients has been challenged with the novel strategy of physical mobilization of ICU patients, even while still undergoing mechanical ventilation. With a culture of ICU care embracing minimization of sedation [2,23–26], intubated patients can be awake and mentally animated [27].

Needham and colleagues reported a before/after quality improvement project seeking to avoid oversedation and reduce delirium in medical ICU patients [28]. The interventions in this project sought to facilitate mobilization in ICU patients, thereby improving functional mobility. The intervention involved a multidisciplinary team in the medical ICU, which included increased staffing, including full-time physical and occupational therapists. There was also a concerted focus on systematically reducing ICU sedation. This "culture change" away from the tradition of deep sedation and bed rest to systematic mobilization throughout the ICU was mandated at a multidisciplinary level. After this quality improvement project, sedative and opiate use decreased, and ICU delirium improved. The investigators noted a greater fraction of patients who were alert (67% vs. 30%) and fewer who were delirious (28% vs. 36%). These changes were associated with patients receiving more rehabilitation treatments and accomplishing a higher level of functional mobility. Intensive care unit length of stay decreased by an average of 2.1

days (95% CI, 0.4–3.8); hospital length of stay decreased by 3.1 days (95% CI, 0.3–5.9).

Schweickert and colleagues performed a prospective randomized blinded trial of very early physical and occupational therapy from the inception of respiratory failure requiring mechanical ventilation [29]. In this trial, mobilization therapy began a median of 1.5 days after endotracheal intubation. Those randomized to the intervention group underwent a progressive physical and occupational therapy regimen focused on mobilization and achievement of occupational tasks (i.e., activities of daily living [ADL]). The standard care control group did not receive mobilization while undergoing mechanical ventilation. Since patients in both groups received daily sedative interruption [23], daily spontaneous breathing trials [30], early enteral nutrition, and tight glucose control [31], the benefits seen were clearly due to early mobilization itself rather than attempts to reduce sedation and/or liberate patients from mechanical ventilation. The primary endpoint of the trial was the return to "functional independence" at hospital discharge – defined as the ability to perform ADLs (bathing, dressing, eating, grooming, transfer from bed to chair, toileting) and walk independently. The intervention led to a 1.7-fold increase in patients who were functionally independent when they left the hospital (59 vs. 35%, p = 0.02). More patients in the early mobilization group went directly home after hospitalization than in the control group (43% vs. 24%, p = 0.06). The early mobilization patients had better maximal walking distances (33.4 vs. 0 meters, p = 0.004), and more ventilator-free days (23.5 vs. 21.1, p = 0.05). As noted in Figure 31.1, the impact of the early mobilization intervention with regard to recovery of functional status was delayed for approximately 2 weeks, a time when most patients were no longer in the ICU. This figure shows that an ICU intervention can have an important impact on patient outcome beyond the time when care is being provided by ICU clinicians.

Interestingly, the intervention of very early mobilization led to a 50% reduction in ICU delirium days (2.0

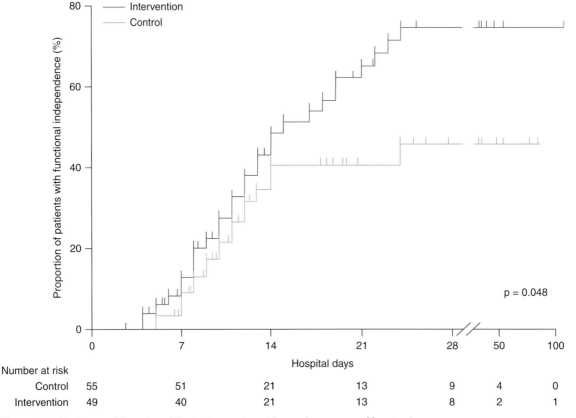

Figure 31.1 The impact of the early mobilization intervention with regard to recovery of functional status.

vs. 4.0 days, p = 0.03). Hospital delirium days were similarly reduced. These findings were noted in spite of the fact that the doses of sedative were not different between the two groups. The findings from this trial strongly suggest the existence of an important mind–body relationship, even in the sickest patients in the ICU. The reasons for the finding of reduced delirium are likely multifactorial. Clearly, maintaining physical coordination requires mental engagement. Patients standing upright with an endotracheal tube in place must be mentally sharp in order to perform such a maneuver. Our anecdotal experiences, both during our early mobilization trial and subsequently during routine patient care, confirm this notion. Our physical and occupational therapists noted repeatedly that the patients who were most alert, physically performed at the highest level. We also noted that many patients actually remembered the intervention of mobilization in the ICU. The intervention was described with words such as "refreshing" and "exhilarating." Several patients stated that they looked forward to the mobilization sessions. One patient actually described ICU mobilization as a needed "break from the monotony of the ICU" – even while intubated! Another possible benefit of ICU mobilization is the potential for restoring the sleep–wake cycle of ICU patients. It is well known that sleep during critical illness is abnormal. Perhaps physical activity during daytime hours improves sleep at night. Certainly, this experience is well known to anyone who engages in regular physical exercise. Obviously, this speculative explanation for the improvements in delirium noted in those who undergo early mobilization requires careful study to confirm its importance.

Conclusions

Intensive care unit survivors recovering from respiratory failure requiring mechanical ventilation often have neuromuscular weakness and functional impairment. A growing body of literature suggests that physical and occupational therapy for mechanically ventilated patients can improve both physical and mental functional status in these survivors. It is clear from recent literature that early mobilization of mechanically ventilated patients is feasible, and that the benefits appear to be substantial. The reductions in ICU delirium recently reported in the literature suggest that early physical and occupational therapy in ICU patients is a potent intervention to combat brain dysfunction in critical illness. More research is needed to determine whether the beneficial effects of early mobilization of delirium translate into improvements in long-term cognitive function. Ongoing attention to the problems associated with deep sedation and prolonged immobility is necessary to ensure improvements in mental and physical animation in this group of high-risk patients.

References

1. The Acute Respiratory Distress Syndrome Network. Ventilation with lower tidal volumes as compared with traditional tidal volumes for acute lung injury and the acute respiratory distress syndrome. *N Engl J Med* 2000;**342**(18):1301–8.

2. Girard TD, Kress JP, Fuchs BD, *et al.* Efficacy and safety of a paired sedation and ventilator weaning protocol for mechanically ventilated patients in intensive care (Awakening and Breathing Controlled trial): a randomised controlled trial. *Lancet* 2008;**371**(9607):126–34.

3. Bernard GR, Vincent JL, Laterre PF, *et al.* Efficacy and safety of recombinant human activated protein C for severe sepsis. *N Engl J Med* 2001;**344**(10):699–709.

4. Brochard L, Mancebo J, Wysocki M, *et al.* Noninvasive ventilation for acute exacerbations of chronic obstructive pulmonary disease. *N Engl J Med* 1995;**333**(13):817–22.

5. Papazian L, Forel JM, Gacouin A, *et al.* Neuromuscular blockers in early acute respiratory distress syndrome. *N Engl J Med* 2010;**363**(12):1107–16.

6. Herridge MS, Cheung AM, Tansey CM, *et al.* One-year outcomes in survivors of the acute respiratory distress syndrome. *N Engl J Med* 2003;**348**(8):683–93.

7. Cheung AM, Tansey CM, Tomlinson G, *et al.* Two-year outcomes, health care use, and costs of survivors of acute respiratory distress syndrome. *Am J Respir Crit Care Med* 2006;**174**(5):538–44.

8. Dowdy DW, Eid MP, Dennison CR, *et al.* Quality of life after acute respiratory distress syndrome: a meta-analysis. *Intensive Care Med* 2006;**32**(8):1115–24.

9. Dowdy DW, Eid MP, Sedrakyan A, *et al.* Quality of life in adult survivors of critical illness: a systematic review of the literature. *Intensive Care Med* 2005;**31**(5):611–20.

10. Herridge MS, Angus DC. Acute lung injury – affecting many lives. *N Engl J Med* 2005;**353**(16):1736–8.

11. Schweickert WD, Kress JP. Implementing early mobilization interventions in mechanically ventilated patients in the ICU. *Chest* 2011;**140**(6):1612–17.

12. Vasilevskis EE, Ely EW, Speroff T, *et al.* Reducing iatrogenic risks: ICU-acquired delirium and weakness – crossing the quality chasm. *Chest* 2010;**138**(5):1224–33.

13. Ely EW, Shintani A, Truman B, *et al.* Delirium as a predictor of mortality in mechanically ventilated patients in the intensive care unit. *JAMA* 2004;**291**(14):1753–62.

14. Girard TD, Jackson JC, Pandharipande PP, *et al.* Delirium as a predictor of long-term cognitive impairment in survivors of critical illness. *Crit Care Med* 2010;**38**(7):1513–20.

15. Asher RA. The dangers of going to bed. *Br Med J* 1947;**2**(4536):967.

16. Kramer AF, Colcombe SJ, McAuley E, Scalf PE, Erickson KI. Fitness, aging and neurocognitive function. *Neurobiol Aging* 2005;**26**(Suppl 1):124–7.

17. Laurin D, Verreault R, Lindsay J, MacPherson K, Rockwood K. Physical activity and risk of cognitive impairment and dementia in elderly persons. *Arch Neurology* 2001;**58**(3):498–504.

18. Yaffe K, Barnes D, Nevitt M, Lui LY, Covinsky K. A prospective study of physical activity and cognitive decline in elderly women: women who walk. *Arch Int Med* 2001;**161**(14):1703–8.

19. Barnes DE, Blackwell T, Stone KL, *et al.* Cognition in older women: the importance of daytime movement. *J Am Geriatrics Soc* 2008;**56**(9):1658–64.

20. Barnes DE, Cauley JA, Lui LY, *et al.* Women who maintain optimal cognitive function into old age. *J Am Geriatrics Soc* 2007;**55**(2):259–64.

21. Colcombe S, Kramer AF. Fitness effects on the cognitive function of older adults: a meta-analytic study. *Psychol Sci* 2003;**14**(2):125–30.

22. Inouye SK, Bogardus ST, Jr., Charpentier PA, *et al.* A multicomponent intervention to prevent delirium in hospitalized older patients. *N Engl J Med* 1999;**340**(9):669–76.

23. Kress JP, Pohlman AS, O'Connor MF, Hall JB. Daily interruption of sedative infusions in critically ill patients undergoing mechanical ventilation. *N Engl J Med* 2000;**342**(20):1471–7.

24. Brook AD, Ahrens TS, Schaiff R, *et al.* Effect of a nursing-implemented sedation protocol on the duration of mechanical ventilation. *Crit Care Med* 1999;**27**(12):2609–15.

25. Strom T, Martinussen T, Toft P. A protocol of no sedation for critically ill patients receiving mechanical ventilation: a randomised trial. *Lancet* 2010;**375**(9713):475–80.

26. De Jonghe B, Bastuji-Garin S, Fangio P, *et al.* Sedation algorithm in critically ill patients without acute brain injury. *Crit Care Med* 2005;**33**(1):120–7.

27. Petty TL. Suspended life or extending death? *Chest* 1998;**114**(2):360–1.

28. Needham DM, Korupolu R, Zanni JM, *et al.* Early physical medicine and rehabilitation for patients with acute respiratory failure: a quality improvement project. *Arch Phys Med Rehabil* 2010;**91**(4):536–42.

29. Schweickert WD, Pohlman MC, Pohlman AS, *et al.* Early physical and occupational therapy in mechanically ventilated, critically ill patients: a randomised controlled trial. *Lancet* 2009;**373**(9678):1874–82.

30. Ely EW, Baker AM, Dunagan DP, *et al.* Effect on the duration of mechanical ventilation of identifying patients capable of breathing spontaneously. *N Engl J Med* 1996;**335**(25):1864–9.

31. van den Berghe G, Wouters P, Weekers F, *et al.* Intensive insulin therapy in the critically ill patients. *N Engl J Med* 2001;**345**(19):1359–67.

Probing consciousness in non-communicating patients

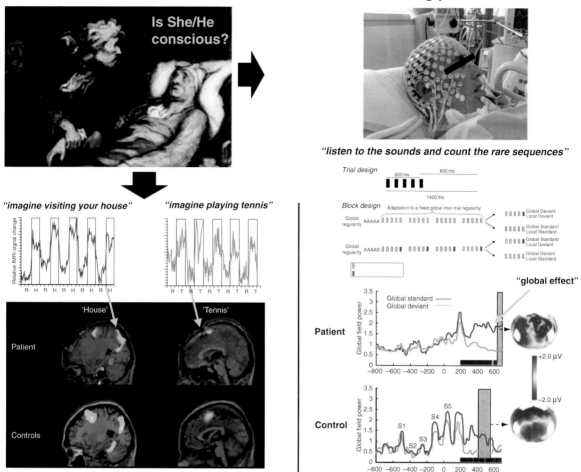

Figure 7.1 Two recent illustrations of active paradigms using functional brain imaging (EEG and fMRI) to probe consciousness in non-communicating patients. The mental navigation and mental motor imagery tasks designed by the group of Owen (left) allow the detection of sustained fMRI BOLD activations in cortical networks specific to each of these two mental imagery tasks [32]. The global regularity auditory task designed by the group of Naccache [42] allows the detection of late and sustained P3-like EEG responses when patients detect the occurrence of global regularity violations. In these two paradigms, the presence of a significant effect is highly suggestive of conscious processing.

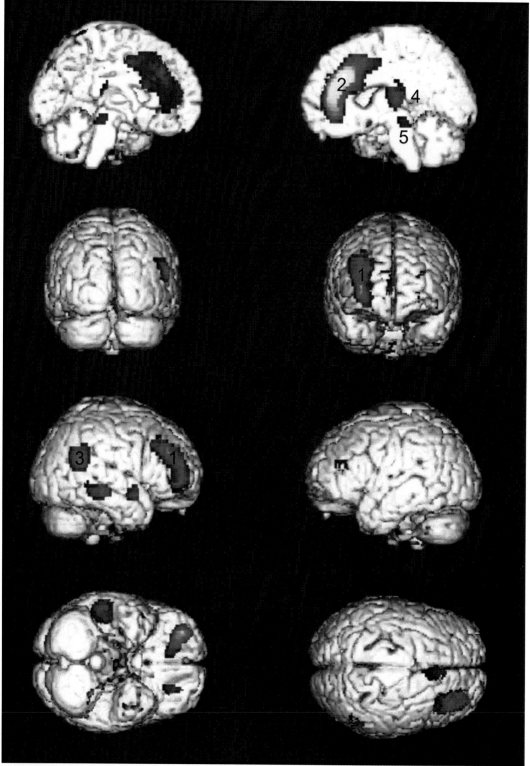

Figure 8.1 Positron emission tomography activations for a task of sustained attention with visual stimuli. The predominantly right hemisphere network encompasses the dorsolateral prefrontal cortex (1), the anterior cingulate gyrus (2), the inferior parietal cortex (3), the thalamus (4) and the ponto-mesencephalic tegmentum, possibly involving the locus coeruleus (5). From Sturm, W. (2009). Aufmerksamkeitsstörungen. In Sturm W, Herrmann M, Münte TF. (Hrsg.): *Lehrbuch der Klinischen Neuropsychologie*. 2. Aufl. (421–443). Heidelberg: Spektrum. Reprinted with the authors' permission.

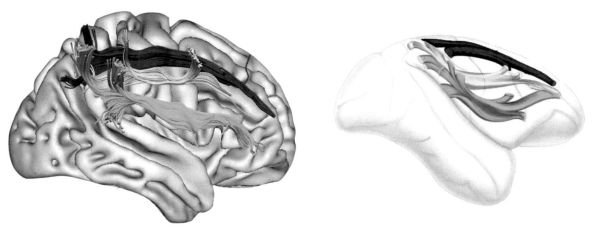

Figure 8.3 The three branches of the superior longitudinal fasciculus in a human brain (left) and a monkey brain (right). Modified from [25] with the author's permission.

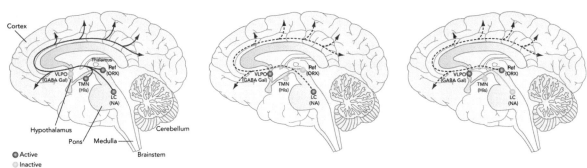

Figure 9.1 Brainstem and hypothalamic nuclei mediate the hypnotic effects of GABAergic anesthetics but do not affect noradrenergic signaling. Active nuclei are depicted in red and inactive nuclei are depicted in blue. (a) In the awake state, certain "awake-active" neural nuclei, including the noradrenergic (NA) locus coeruleus (LC), the orexinergic (ORX) perifornical nucleus (Pef), and the histaminergic (His) tuberomamillary nucleus (TMN) provide excitatory input to the corticothalamic network. When awake a "sleep-active" nucleus, the venterolateral preoptic nucleus (VLPO) is silent. During sleep the VLPO is active and the LC, Pef, and TMN are inactive. (b) During GABAergic hypnosis, potentiated inhibitory actions of the VLPO reduce neural activity in both the Pef and TMN but allow activity to proceed unimpeded in the LC (resulting in intact noradrenergic signaling; active signaling shown with a dotted red line). Reproduced with permission from *Intensetimes.*

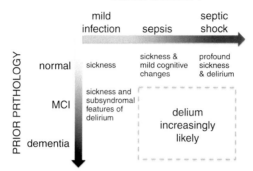

Figure 11.2 A schematic prediction for how severity of insult and prior pathology interact to increase the likelihood of delirium during sepsis. While mild infection is likely to induce only symptoms of sickness behavior in individuals who have no pathology at baseline, similar insults may produce subsyndromal delirium in individuals with mild cognitive impairment at baseline, and may produce florid delirium in those with existing dementia. Thus, as severity of sepsis and severity of underlying pathology increase, so increases the probability of delirium. MCI, mild cognitive impairment.

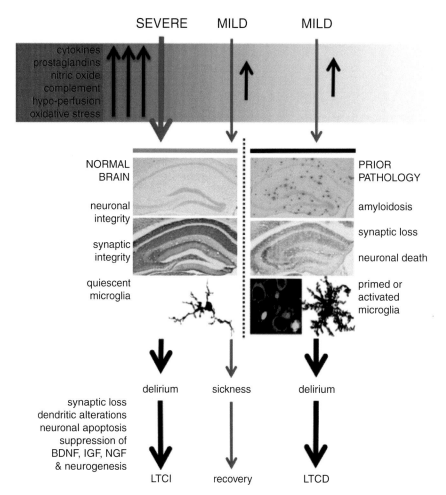

INSULT SEVERITY

SEVERE   MILD   MILD

cytokines
prostaglandins
nitric oxide
complement
hypo-perfusion
oxidative stress

NORMAL
BRAIN

neuronal
integrity

synaptic
integrity

quiescent
microglia

PRIOR
PATHOLOGY

amyloidosis

synaptic loss

neuronal death

primed or
activated
microglia

synaptic loss
dendritic alterations
neuronal apoptosis
suppression of
BDNF, IGF, NGF
& neurogenesis

delirium   sickness   delirium

LTCI   recovery   LTCD

Figure 11.3 Possible routes to delirium and long-term cognitive impairment resulting from infection. The concentrations of cytokines, prostaglandins, nitric oxide, complement factors, and the degree of hypoperfusion and oxidative stress increase as a function of the severity of sepsis (↑↑↑ versus ↑). This will influence the severity of the cognitive symptoms. Compared with the normal brain, the aged or neurodegenerative brain may show increased amyloid pathology, decreased presynaptic terminal density, and increased numbers of dying neurons and primed microglia. Systemic inflammatory mediators and tissue perfusion will have fundamentally different consequences in the brain, depending on the pathological state of that brain at baseline. Mild insults may produce nothing more than reversible sickness symptoms in the normal brain. However, even moderate inflammation may have effects on synaptic function, dendritic structure, growth factor synthesis and maturation, and indeed on neurogenesis. The impacts of these changes will be considerable in a brain that is functioning with limited cognitive reserve. Furthermore, in those with overt pathology, microglia may be primed to produce exaggerated CNS inflammatory responses, effectively amplifying the severity of the systemic insult. Interleukin-1β, TNFα, prostaglandin E2, and nitric oxide have been directly implicated in the cognitive deficits in animal models. In addition to acute cognitive changes, more severe inflammatory responses are likely to induce neuronal damage and death. In pathologically normal patients who experience severe sepsis this is likely to lead to *de novo* inflammatory damage and long-term cognitive impairment (LTCI). For those with existing progressive disease, these patients are likely to suffer accelerated long-term cognitive decline (LTCD). BDNF, brain-derived neurotrophic factor; IGF, insulin-like growth factor; NGF, nerve growth factor.

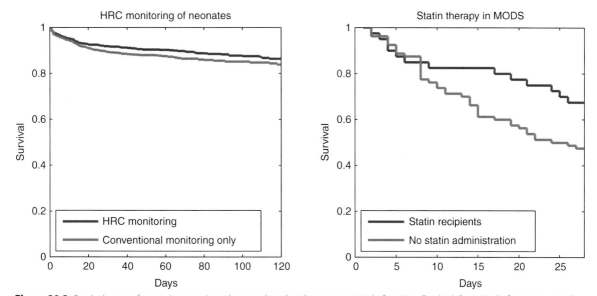

Figure 20.2 Survival curves for two interventions that may be related to autonomic dysfunction. On the left, survival of neonates at risk for sepsis was increased by the presence of a monitor which assesses heart rate characteristics (HRC) [5]. On the right, statin therapy improved outcomes from multiple organ dysfunction syndrome (MODS) [47].

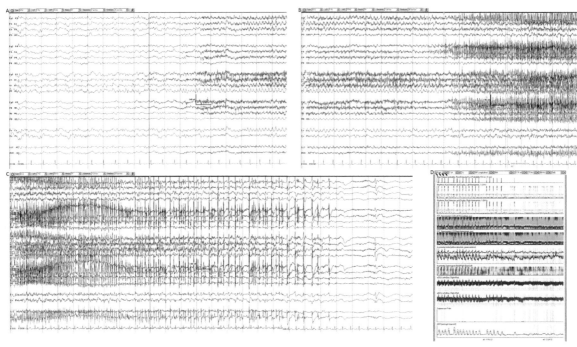

Figure 39.1 Convulsive status epilepticus in a patient with epilepsy. A woman in her 40s with a history of static encephalopathy and epilepsy who presented with hyponatremia and subtherapeutic anticonvulsant levels. Continuous electroencephalography (cEEG) demonstrated left temporal 1–2Hz quasi-periodic sharp waves (not clearly seen here) with (A) gradual evolution to 4–5Hz sharply contoured ictal theta. (B, C) Seizures lasted 50–80 seconds and manifest as behavioral arrest followed by tonic right arm movement, leftward head deviation, and rightward eye deviation. (D) On quantitative EEG, there was a clear cyclic component with seizures occurring at regular intervals every 5–20 minutes. From the top to the bottom, rows on this quantitative EEG montage include: seizure probability, rhythmic run detection on left and right, color spectrogram on left and right, relative and absolute asymmetry indices, asymmetry spectrogram, amplitude integrated EEG on left and right, suppression ratio, and alpha/delta ratio on left and right. Four typical seizures on the quantitative montage are indicated by arrows.

Chapter 32

Rehabilitation after critical illness

Richard D. Griffiths and Christina Jones

SUMMARY

To aid recovery from the legacy of brain dysfunction described in earlier chapters requires an appreciation of the factors that impact physically, psychologically, emotionally, and socially on their pathway back to health. A focus, for instance, solely on the important rehabilitation of cognitive function would ignore the myriad of factors that also impinge on recovery. The key lesson over the last 25 years supported by the testimony of patients and their carers is that a "total rehabilitation" approach is needed that incorporates consideration of mind and body, starts early as an integral part of ICU care, involves physical and psychological care, and ideally should manage the relative or carer in this process. As brain dysfunction is so frequent yet diverse this chapter aims to give a general practical perspective on a comprehensive approach to the rehabilitation of the critically ill from the joint experiences of a general intensive care physician and a nurse specialist rather than an expert discussion of specific cognitive rehabilitation.

Identification

A "total rehabilitation" approach incorporates consideration of mind and body, starts early as an integral part of ICU care and involves physical and psychological care and ideally should manage the relative or carer in this process [1]. Because planning for rehabilitation starts within the ICU it is necessary to have processes in place that can identify those most at risk where help and support may benefit their recovery. Prolonged critical illness, major systemic sepsis, severe pulmonary dysfunction, profound weakness, coma, and confusion are not difficult to recognize. Similarly are those patients that have required prolonged and heavy use of sedative drugs and those where early physiotherapy and mobilization have proved impractical and their illness has been characterized by immobility.

It is equally important to appreciate that the majority of ICU patients, especially those only having a brief stay in the ICU, are likely to need little or no additional support to recover. However awareness and a clinical screening process within the ICU that identifies those with persistent delirium, drug dependency or drug withdrawal issues or history of anxiety or prior psychiatric illness and those lacking family or social support can be helpful.

In the patient who is no longer delirious the recognition of mild cognitive impairment clinically is difficult within the ICU without formal testing and does not lend itself readily to routine screening, though a short adapted cognitive examination for use in the ICU has been developed [2]. This is an area of keen research and the reader is referred to Chapter 2, this volume for a more detailed expert discussion of this important consequence of severe illness.

The clinical recognition of depression and anxiety within the ICU can only be made reliably once voice is returned and impossible unless delirium excluded. However it is not difficult to recognize stress in their relatives and this indicates whether they are coping or not with what can be their most devastating life experience. This can manifest in many patterns including avoidance, withdrawal and depression, sleep disturbance, or overt anxiety and anger [3].

In the UK, for instance, it is recommended that a clinical risk assessment and screening process should be maintained during an ICU stay and be formalized on leaving the ICU to plan for the immediately apparent problems (e.g., weakness) and start screening for possible psychological issues, such as acute anxiety states [4].

Brain Disorders in Critical Illness, ed. Robert D. Stevens, Tarek Sharshar, and E. Wesley Ely. Published by Cambridge University Press. © Cambridge University Press 2013.

Prevention

Prevention is, of course, preferable and the importance of instituting measures within the ICU that can have profound effects on long-term recovery cannot be underestimated. Sadly the immediacy of the acute critical illness and its complex management has clouded the perspective of critical care practitioners and marginalized any attention to factors that impinge on long-term well-being. The earlier chapters emphasize new sedation paradigms, drug avoidance, and reduced sedation, waking and weaning protocols and early mobilization and delirium management. Added to this we should include vigorous drug review and protocols for the management of drug weaning in certain situations (e.g., after extensive benzodiazepine use).

Perhaps forgotten in prevention is the need to anticipate rehabilitation and prepare the ground to which the patient will return. This means early handling of a relative's stress and the delivery of coping support to bring them into a "culture of rehabilitation therapy" in anticipation of the recovery period. The experienced ICU nurse both recognizes and can deliver valued coping support for the immediate problems [5,6] but to fully help relatives they must also extend it to the promotion of a rehabilitation culture.

The family need to understand and even, where appropriate, assist with physical, psychological, and emotional support at all stages of recovery. Even while the patient may be ventilated and unaware the relatives' or carers' involvement with a patient diary record may itself be of benefit as a measure of participation, but they help also to deliver a tool that can be used later (see below).

Management within and after ICU

The avoidance of immobility by an active program of mobilization within and after ICU is a fundamental culture change that has occurred over the last 25 years. The concept that a critically ill patient was ventilated, paralyzed, and sedated and therefore immobilized until they left ICU to then recover with "bed rest" has fortunately been dismissed with our better understanding of the harmful consequences of immobility and the benefits of maintaining activity. In the past this legacy of profound weakness and debility was not seen by ICU practitioners unless it impacted on weaning from the ventilator, but rather was left to ill-informed general ward staff and distressed relatives to cope with. With no appreciation

of its severity or the timescales of recovery patient and family have unrealistic expectations and disappointment ensues. Our understanding of intensive care unit acquired weakness (ICUAW) [7] has matured with the recognition of how muscle wasting can be ameliorated by passive [8] and active movement [9] and that preservation of neuromuscular activity and mobility has wider benefits on metabolism, immune function, and cognitive function. For a more detailed expert discussion of the influence of early mobilization on functional status the reader is referred to Chapter 4, this volume.

The early and active physiotherapy that is started within the ICU needs to continue as the patient leaves and this culture of therapy must transfer and be seen as important to subsequent carers and relatives over the whole course of their recovery. Experience suggests, and in keeping with our understanding of the severity of muscle wasting and how patients recover, a simple aide-memoire to give patients *and* relatives a perspective on the timescale of physical recovery is for a young patient for each day in the ICU they need 1 week of recovery and for the older patient this is 2 weeks for every day spent ill in the ICU.

Memory and amnesia: why it matters?

Effective amnesia for an unpleasant event is appropriate for elective surgery where the recipient has a desire to be pain free, not distressed, and holds an understanding of why and the duration it is necessary. Therefore this short-term amnesia has no major consequence. Transferred into intensive care the elective operation that is anticipated to require only a day longer is also unlikely to be an issue. However for the majority of emergency ICU patients, in particular the sicker and longer-stay patients, memory disturbance and amnesia present a serious and underappreciated problem. Unlike the less ill trauma patients, it is not unusual for the ventilated major trauma patients to have no recall of their accident; and, similarly many severe sepsis patients also lose any recall of how they were admitted to hospital. The impact of brain dysfunction during intensive care treatment means that the intensive care experience is a mixture of amnesia or profound distortion in time, place, and content. There are even some patients who despite having apparently been awake and aware while in the ICU in the later stages subsequently fail to maintain any memory of intensive care. We have had patients vigorously deny being in intensive care despite the assertion of their relatives. Any significant periods of amnesia has consequences later and are associated with an impact on well-being during recovery [10]. The most direct consequence of simple amnesia is the loss of the patient's own autobiography to place the changes that have occurred to them (e.g., wasting and weakness) into context and allow them to have an understanding of why it has happened and how they will recover [11]. In its simplest form this lack of understanding can be addressed by information and timescale discussion but needs to be repeated because it is often not retained initially.

There has been much debate over the years regarding the impact of the memory and experiences on ICU and their impact on subsequent recovery. Because of acute brain dysfunction, most commonly manifesting as delirium [12], it is apparent that patient memories are highly abnormal, and apart from amnesia for the real early ICU events, for some patients their ICU experience is dominated by frank delusions and later by highly distorted interpretations of events. It had been assumed that unpleasant real ICU experiences might trigger acute stress reactions and lead onto posttraumatic stress disorder (PTSD), however research suggested that frightening delusional experiences, particularly associated with early amnesia were a stronger predictor of PTSD and the relationship with real ICU experiences was not primarily responsible [13]. Initial retrospective studies had implicated unpleasant ICU experiences as a factor [14] but subsequent prospective studies confirmed that the strongest association with the development of PTSD was the suffering of frightening delusional experiences [15] followed as a risk factor by heavy sedation use, which others have also noted [16]. This important manifestation of delirium and acute brain dysfunction results in an incidence of new PTSD in about 10% of patients who stay more than a few days. For all patients delusional experiences are vivid and strongly retained in memory over real events. For some the delusions are not troubling, however for others they are life threatening in nature and where amnesic may be the only memory retained of the critical illness. This patient-specific impact on long-term well-being even at 5 years has been shown to be dependent on the experience or not of delusional or distorted memories within ICU [17].

Principles of care

As the patient progresses through intensive care, the hospital ward, and home a patient-specific program that focuses on their personal needs and goals should be established and should incorporate review processes to recognize any evolving need. At its simplest level the "culture of rehabilitation therapy" needs to be continued using a combination of information, setting realistic goals and timescales, positive reinforcement, normalizing issues of distress, and supporting effective coping mechanisms and encouraging physical rehabilitation. This is encapsulated in recent UK guidance from the National Institute of Health and Clinical Excellence [4].

Beyond this an initial watch and wait approach is advocated for psychological issues using review and screening to identify those not coping (e.g., screening for acute anxiety/PTSD symptoms [18]). It is important not to over-medicalize and to allow patients to regain control. For a more detailed expert discussion of psychiatric disorders following critical illnesses the reader is referred to Chapter 3, this volume.

Because of memory disturbance one must be prepared to repeat what is said often. For practical purposes it is better to assume memory is impaired initially in most patients and that memory processing and decision making is poor or abnormal in many patients. This cognitive impairment is often poorly recognized [19]. This impacts directly on how information is given, patients' decisions made and how patient autonomy is protected.

It is neither sensible nor realistic to specifically separate physical from psychological rehabilitation since there is a close social and psychological impact from participating in physical programs and vice versa. Significant psychological morbidity may confound participation in physical activity and where sleep is affected may also add to fatigue. Evidence on the importance of physical activity on brain function goes further as an authoritative review [20] suggests that across many age ranges exercise has a beneficial effect on many aspects of cognitive function, and even has a greater and a more generalizable effect than specific cognitive training programs [21].

The right time and tempo of rehabilitation is patient specific and as explained earlier starts within the ICU. However it is important not to confuse rehabilitation with "post ICU follow-up." The latter is an inclusive, cross-sectional observational process of all

Table 32.1 Differences between intensive care unit (ICU) follow-up and rehabilitation.

ICU follow-up	ICU rehabilitation
For the benefit of future patients	Primarily for individual patient benefit
Rarely involves families	Involves family and carers
Starts after ICU	Starts early within ICU
Inclusive and general	Highly selective and specific
Screens to include	Screens to filter out and exclude
Assessment of complications	Assessment for risk avoidance
Generally pathology independent	Highly pathology dictated
Cross-sectional and serial	Step-wise longitudinally
Set time points, patient independent	Patient dictated, no set time points
No therapy role, primarily observational	Involves specific therapies as required

patients at specific times to describe incidence of patient problems and predominantly involves outpatient clinics a few months after ICU discharge (see Table 32.1 outlining the differences). Rehabilitation after intensive care however is a patient-specific therapy process delivered only if and when needed irrespective of place or timing using a variety of inpatient and outpatient services (Table 32.2). Post-ICU clinics serve an important role in the initial stages of developing services, monitoring progress and for research observation but probably play a modest role in any established therapy pathway and should not be considered the mainstay of any ICU rehabilitation program as the therapy benefit of "ICU follow-up" based around a clinic at 3 months involving many short-stay patients cannot be measured [22].

For these reasons we considered that a patient-centered self-help program run by a rehabilitation coordinator would provide support to rehabilitation that allowed the patient and importantly the relatives together to engage with their recovery as the patients move through hospital to home.

Table 32.2 Components of rehabilitation after critical illness care in an intensive care unit (ICU).

Identification	
	Clinical risk assessment during ICU and on discharge Exclude the many low risk able to cope (e.g., short stay, less ill)
Prevention	
Patient	Early mobilization, active measures to limit sedation use, waking and weaning Delirium and confusion management Drug avoidance and weaning Orientation, visual, and hearing support Reassurance that the "hard work" of physical therapy pays off "Bed rest" is harmful
Family/relative	Emphasize a culture of rehabilitation therapy (exercise as treatment) Encourage involvement with a diary Family coping support and timescales Stress and anxiety management
After ICU	Identify any specific issues and select most appropriate support Involve the relatives/family Positive re-enforcement, repetition Timescales (months not days) and realistic daily/weekly goal setting Memory management, normalizing, and advice Foster normal coping and screen for psychological distress Watch and wait where necessary but act on indications Patient and family use of diary record Continue generic mobilization therapy Self-guided multimodal programs (several weeks to months) Specific guided physical training programs Take measures to identify risks of rare complications

Specific approaches and evidence

A patient-centered and self-guided rehabilitation multimodal physical, psychological, and social program in the form of a manual such as the "ICU Recovery Manual," combining information on recovery from critical illness, weekly exercise diaries, and self-directed exercise programs has been shown in longer-stay patients (median ICU stay 14 days) to aid physical recovery [23]. The design is based on educational principles and allows patients to tailor the program to their individual needs with the information available to share with their family. This gives the control of their recovery back to the patient and their family. However, such a program only had a short-term impact at 8 weeks on psychological recovery, which was not sustained to the end of the study at 6 months possibly because it did not manage the delusional experiences of some patients which we addressed later in the "diary study" (see below).

Outpatient-based rehabilitation programs, which are in the same model as pulmonary rehabilitation programs, are feasible. One program, predominantly but not uniquely with a more physical focus designed at the Manchester Royal Infirmary (UK) follows early ICU mobilization and intensive inpatient exercise physiotherapy with 2 hours of supervised outpatient exercise and education sessions each week and two unsupervised home exercise sessions each week for 6 weeks. The exercise sessions comprise ten 1-minute stations in a gym of various combinations of exercise involving all major muscle groups repeated once for a total exercise time of 20 minutes with effort targeted to moderate or somewhat severe breathlessness combined with periods of recovery. Heart rate and oxygen saturation are monitored and patients stratified for high- or low-risk heart rate reserve. A group exercise session teaches additional home exercise which they are encouraged to repeat 2–3 times during the following week. Assessments were undertaken at 1 week before the start of the program and 1 week after completion. The distance patients walked in 6 minutes improved by 160 meters ($p < 0.001$), and there were significant improvements in anxiety ($p = 0.001$) and depression ($p = 0.001$) scores [24].

Outpatient clinics have adapted from their follow-up role to become a clinical monitoring and feedback stage in any program, a helpful closure for some and an important contact for patients who were recruited into research. Some clinics are multidisciplinary and

able to address several management issues in one visit but since the best time for particular therapies is patient specific this is not always convenient. In our experience the most important role of any outpatient clinic visit involves the patient and relative (who must always attend) in reconciliation about what has happened and their fears, and to ensure they are in dialog together and have the same understanding on the timescales of recovery. This becomes less important when patients have followed a detailed program and used the ICU diary together.

Proving the efficacy of a rehabilitation therapy is very challenging in such a heterogeneous post-ICU patient population with diverse pathologies, ages, and expected timescales of recovery and where the benefit of the intervention may have only a modest additive effect to normal recovery and where the tempo of recovery may be widely different from patient to patient. There are some studies started later following an ICU stay that have been unable to demonstrate a benefit and involve the recruitment of many short-stay patients (median ICU stay only 2.9 days) whose reversible recovery may be independent of any measure within this period [22], or similarly where the therapy is started only later after leaving hospital when at home but also in relatively shorter-stay patients (median 6 days) [25]. Other models of multi-component rehabilitation that consider functional aspects and include goal management cognitive training [26] are being piloted but their effectiveness is not yet established [27].

All rehabilitation programs, however, will be challenged if the lack of autographical memory for the period of critical illness is not addressed. Coupled with the presence of frightening delusional memories, it can make it difficult for patients to make sense of what has happened to them when they were at their sickest. The use of an ICU diary is becoming increasingly popular across Scandinavia and the UK. The diary is a daily account of the stay in ICU, written in everyday language by the ICU staff, with the relatives contributing where they feel able to. They are encouraged to not only write about what is happening in the ICU but also about what the patient may be missing at home. The text is complemented with appropriate photographs at points of change in the patients' treatment or condition. These should be of good enough quality to allow the patient to recognize themselves. Once the patient is ready to read the diary and look at the photographs an ICU nurse should guide them through this to ensure that they completely understand what has been written and the content of the pictures [28]. The diary allows the patient to fill in the gaps in their memory and helps put any delusional memories into context [29–31]. Two recent randomized controlled trials have also demonstrated that the provision of an ICU diary can have an impact on anxiety and depression [32], and in the larger multicenter study has been shown to significantly reduce the incidence on new-onset PTSD [33]. In addition the patient receiving an ICU diary may reduce the level of PTSD-related symptoms in their family members [34] which is important since PTSD is recognized to occur also in family members [35,36].

Specific additional psychological support and practical observations

Early psychological distress in the first month following critical illness may resolve spontaneously without any intervention. However high levels of early anxiety, depression, or posttraumatic stress symptoms may not resolve without formal therapy. The key is to recognize those patients and/or families who are not coping with their symptoms and then offer appropriate and timely help without interfering unnecessarily [37]. Counseling/therapy services following critical illness for some may be needed for severe anxiety, depression, and PTSD and is effective in helping both patients and their relatives get back to normal functioning [38]. Therapies such as cognitive behavioral therapy (CBT) and eye movement desensitization and reprocessing (EDMR) have been shown to be effective in the treatment of significant psychological distress. Cognitive behavioral therapy uses a goal-oriented, systematic procedure to change the individuals' feelings and thoughts about their present difficulties [39], while EMDR was developed initially to resolve traumatic disorders [40] caused by exposure to distressing events such as rape. When a traumatic experience occurs the individuals' normal coping mechanisms may be overwhelmed and the memories inadequately processed. Eye movement desensitization and reprocessing has as its goal the processing of these distressing memories allowing individuals to develop more adaptive coping mechanisms.

Addressing major psychological morbidities such as PTSD is important as a specific treatment for instance, a recent study of treatment of PTSD symptoms showed significant improvements in cognitive

deficits such as executive function [41]. Following on from this study a randomized controlled trial of therapy targeting resilience resource (e.g., positive emotional engagement and social connectedness) to PTSD also showed broader benefits, both alleviating anxiety and depressive symptoms and improving emotional and cognitive function [42]. Importantly, as has been shown in studies on war veterans, improvement in cognitive function may come from addressing the functional psychological disturbance.

Over 25 years of working with patients and their families they have reported to the authors various tricks to help them cope with memory problems and other issues. One patient who had a large number of hospital appointments, which she tended to forget or muddle, got into the habit of sticking the appointment cards onto the front of the fridge in date order and on making her breakfast coffee would check if she had an appointment that day. Some patients who had never kept a diary before their critical illness got into the habit of routinely filling their diary with anything they needed to remember, including lists of questions that they needed to ask their doctor. The recent ploy used by UK hospitals, to improve outpatient attendance, of sending a text to the patient the day before is helpful but has to be done consistently as they do become reliant on them. Recently one patient missed a physiotherapy appointment because they normally sent him a text and it was forgotten, and he then decided he had confused the date.

Conclusion

It is important not to mistake follow-up with rehabilitation. The former is the observation of patients to inform future care and by definition occurs after the event, while the latter is an early active process to avoid anticipated problems. It is a mistake to assume all patients are the same and follow a similar pathway and need all aspects of rehabilitation. While patients may share some similar features there is no single "post-ICU syndrome" but a myriad of pathologies, ages, and problems which mean that patient support and trajectories may be very different [43]. Also, another mistake is to assume *all* patients need rehabilitation when there are many short-stay patients who have well-developed coping mechanisms, family support, and personal motivation that comfortably exceed any external provision.

The cardinal mistake is not listening to your patients. Preformed questionnaires used in "follow-up" assume that problems are understood and much may be missed. Our experience suggests that the greatest contribution to improve rehabilitation care and understanding the unexpected (for instance, the impact of delusions) has come through a frequent enquiring dialog with patients and relatives. The development of rehabilitation of the critically ill requires a caring attitude and an early "culture of rehabilitation therapy" combined with an open-minded diagnostic problem-solving approach.

References

1. Griffiths RD, Jones C. Seven lessons from 20 years of follow up of intensive care unit survivors. *Curr Opin Crit Care* 2007;**13**:508–13.

2. Lewin JJ III, LeDroux SN, Shermock KM, *et al*. Validity and reliability of The John Hopkins Adapted Cognitive Exam for critically ill patients. *Crit Care Med* 2012;**40**(1):139–44.

3. Davidson J, Jones C, Bienvenu OJ. Family response to critical illness: postintensive care syndrome – family. *Crit Care Med* 2012;**40**(2):618–24.

4. National Institute for Health and Clinical Excellence. *Rehabilitation after Critical Illness: NICE Clinical Guideline 83*. London: NICE; 2009. http://www.nice.org.uk/CG83.

5. Jones C, Hussey R, Griffiths RD. Social support in the intensive care unit. *Br J Intensive Care* 1991;**1**:66–9.

6. Jones C, Griffiths RD. Social support and anxiety levels in relatives of critically ill patients. *Br J Intensive Care* 1995;**5**:44–7.

7. Griffiths RD, Hall J. Intensive care unit-acquired weakness. *Crit Care Med* 2010;**38**(3):779–87.

8. Griffiths RD, Palmer TEA, Helliwell T, Maclennan P, Macmillan RR. Effect of passive stretching on the wasting of muscle in the critically-ill. *Nutrition* 1995;**11**:428–32.

9. Burtin C, Clerckx B, Robbeets C, *et al*. Early exercise in critically ill patients enhances short-term functional recovery. *Crit Care Med* 2009;**37**:2499–505.

10. Granja C, Lopes A, Moreira S, *et al*. Patients' recollections of experiences in the intensive care unit may affect their quality of life. *Critical Care* 2005;**9**: R96–109.

11. Griffiths RD, Jones C. Filling the intensive care memory gap? *Intensive Care Med* 2001;**27**:344–6.

12. Ely EW, Gautam S, Margolin R, *et al*. The impact of delirium in the intensive care unit on hospital length of stay. *Intensive Care Med* 2001;**27**:1892–900.

13. Jones C, Griffiths RD, Humphris G. Acute post traumatic stress disorder: a new theory for its development after intensive care. *Critical Care Med* 2001;**29**:573–80.

14. Schelling G, Stoll C, Haller M, *et al*. Health-related quality of life and posttraumatic stress disorder in survivors of the acute respiratory distress syndrome. *Crit Care Med* 1998;**26**(4):651–9.

15. Jones C, Bäckman C, Capuzzo M, *et al*. Precipitants of post traumatic stress disorder following intensive care: a hypothesis generating study of diversity in care. *Intensive Care Med* 2007;**33**:978–85.

16. Girard TD, Shintani AK, Jackson JC, *et al*. Risk factors for post-traumatic stress disorder symptoms following critical illness requiring mechanical ventilation: a prospective cohort study. *Crit Care* 2007;**11**(1):R28.

17. Ringdal M, Plos K, Örtenwall P, Bergbom I. Memories and health-related quality of life after intensive care: a follow-up study. *Critical Care Med* 2010;**38**(1):38–44.

18. Twigg E, Humphris G, Jones C, Bramwell R, Griffiths RD. Use of a screening questionnaire for post-traumatic stress disorder (PTSD) on a sample of UK ICU patients. *Acta Anaesthesiol Scand* 2008;**52**(2):202–8.

19. Jones C, Griffiths RD, Slater T, Benjamin KS, Wilson S. Significant cognitive dysfunction in non-delirious patients identified during and persisting following critical illness. *Intensive Care Med* 2006;**32**(6):923–6.

20. Hillman CH, Rickson KI, Kramer AF. Be smart, exercise your heart: exercise effect on brain and cognition. *Nature Reviews Neurosci* 2008;**9**(1):58–65.

21. Smith GE, Housen P, Yaffe K, *et al*. A cognitive training programme based on principles of brain plasticity. *J Am Geriatr Soc* 2009;**57**(4):594–603.

22. Cuthbertson BH, Rattray J, Campbell MK, *et al*. The PRaCTICaL study of nurse led, intensive care follow-up programmes for improving long term outcomes from critical illness: a pragmatic randomised controlled trial. *Br Med J* 2009;**339**:b3723–31.

23. Jones C, Skirrow P, Griffiths RD, *et al*. Rehabilitation after critical illness: a randomised, controlled trial. *Crit Care Med* 2003;**31**(10):2456–61.

24. McWilliams DJ, Atkinson D, Carter A, *et al*. Feasibility and impact of a structured, exercise-based rehabilitation programme for intensive care survivors. *Physiother Theory Pract* 2009;**25**(8):566–71.

25. Elliott D, McKinley S, Alison J, *et al*. Health-related quality of life and physical recovery after a critical illness: a multi-centre randomised controlled trial of a home-based physical rehabilitation program. *Crit Care* 2011;**15**:R142–52.

26. van Hooren SAH, Valentijn SAM, Bosma H, *et al*. Effect of a structured course involving goal management training in older adults: a randomized controlled trial. *Patient Educ Couns* 2007;**65**:205–13.

27. Jackson JC, Ely EW, Morey MC, et al. Cognitive and physical rehabilitation of ICU survivors: results of the RETURN randomized, controlled pilot investigation. Crit Care Med 2012;40(4):1088–97.

28. Bäckman CG, Jones C. Implementing a diary programme in your ICU. ICU Management 2011;11(3):10–16.

29. Bäckman CG, Walther SM. Use of a personal diary written on the ICU during critical illness. Intensive Care Med 2001;27:426–9.

30. Bergbom I, Svensson C, Berggren E, Kamsula M. Patients' and relatives' opinions and feelings about diaries kept by nurses in an intensive care unit: pilot study. Intensive Crit Care Nurs 1999;15(4):185–91.

31. Egerod I, Christensen D, Schwartz-Nielson KH, Ågård AS. Constructing the illness narrative: a grounded theory exploring patients' and relatives' use of intensive care diaries. Crit Care Med 2011;39(8):1922–8.

32. Knowles RE, Tarrier N. Evaluation of the effect of prospective patient diaries on emotional well-being in intensive care unit survivors: a randomized controlled trial Crit Care Med 2009;37(1):184–91.

33. Jones C, Bäckman C, Capuzzo M, et al. Intensive Care diaries reduce new onset PTSD following critical illness: a randomised, controlled trial. Crit Care 2010;14:R168–78.

34. Jones C, Bäckman C, Griffiths RD. Intensive Care diaries reduce PTSD-related symptom levels in relatives following critical illness: a pilot study. Am J Critical Care 2012;21(3):172–6.

35. Jones C, Skirrow P, Griffiths RD, et al. Post-traumatic stress disorder-related symptoms in relatives of patients following intensive care. Intensive Care Med 2004;30 (3):456–60.

36. Azoulay E, Pochard F, Kentish-Barnes N, et al. Risk of post-traumatic stress symptoms in family members of intensive care unit patients. Am J Respir Crit Care Med 2005;171(9):987–94.

37. Jones C, Griffiths RD. Patient and caregiver counseling after the intensive care unit: what are the needs and how should they be met? Curr Opin Crit Care 2007;13:503–7.

38. Jones C, Hall S, Jackson S. Benchmarking a nurse-led ICU counseling initiative. Nursing Times 2008;104(38):32–4.

39. Foa E, Rothbaum B, Furr J. Augmenting exposure therapy with other CBT procedures. Psychiatr Annals 2011;33(1):47–56.

40. Shapiro F. EMDR as an Integrative Psychotherapy Approach: Experts of Diverse Orientations Explore the Paradigm Prism. Washington, DC: American Psychological Association; 2002, pp. 3–26.

41. Walter KH, Palmieri PA, Gunstad J. More than symptom reduction: changes in executive function over the course of PTSD treatment. J Traumatic Stress 2010;23(2):292–5.

42. Kent M, Daavis MC, Stark SL, Stewart LA. A resilience-oriented treatment for posttraumatic stress disorder: results of a preliminary randomized clinical trial. J Traumatic Stress 2011;24(5):591–5.

43. Griffiths RD. Rehabilitating the critically ill: a cultural shift in intensive care unit care. Crit Care Med 2012;40(2):681–2.

Chapter

33

Drug-induced encephalopathy

Bruno Mégarbane

SUMMARY

Intoxications represent a frequent cause of patient admission to the emergency department and intensive care unit (ICU). Drug-induced encephalopathy and coma require rapid management as they may result in life-threatening conditions. Several other neurological features related to drugs are also possible, including seizures, involuntary movements, sensory impairments, and disturbances in brainstem functions. Diagnosis is first based on determination of medical history and detailed clinical examination focusing on the identification of toxidromes. Vital signs, body temperature, respiratory pattern, pupil abnormalities, odor of breath, and clothing represent useful parameters for the clinical orientation. When collecting a patient's different neurological features, recognition of one toxidrome helps the physician in charge to assess a toxicological etiology to the patient's encephalopathy and suspect a family of involved toxicants. The main toxidromes involving the central nervous system (CNS) to be known by an intensivist include lethargic, opioid, anticholinergic, cholinergic, adrenergic, and serotonin syndromes.

The clinical approach allows not only obtaining a toxicological diagnosis but also ruling out any other non-toxicological hypothesis. Administration of supportive treatments and emergent antidotes are based on this detailed clinical examination. Pharmacodynamic tests using specific antidotes like naloxone for opioids or flumazenil for benzodiazepines and analogs complete the physical examination. The Glasgow Coma Scale is largely used to indicate intubation of poisoned patients, although the decision to intubate should also take into account ventilation impairment, the risk of aspiration, the severity of encephalopathy, and the elimination kinetics of the involved toxicant. Electrocardiogram (ECG) and routine laboratory tests are mandatory to assess the final diagnosis, while brain imaging and electroencephalography (EEG) can be useful in certain situations. Finally, toxicological analysis using specific and sensitive assays is required for a retrospective definitive confirmation of the initially suspected involved drugs based on the clinical approach.

Poisoning is one of the most frequent causes of patient admission in hospital, either to the emergency department or the ICU. The central nervous system (CNS) is a major target of toxicants possibly resulting in the development of life-threatening symptoms including coma, seizures, movement disorders, and encephalopathy. The main exposures declared to the American Poison Centers in 2009 included analgesics (11.80%), cosmetics (7.75%), sedatives (5.84%), antidepressants (3.58%), cardiovascular drugs (3.32%), and pesticides (3.1%) [1]. In France, 19 out of the 20 pharmaceuticals involved in the overdoses declared to the Poison Centre of Paris were psychoactive [2].

Three reasons can explain the severity of a poisoning and thus its required admission in the ICU: (1) presentation of life-threatening symptoms, including coma, seizures, respiratory failure, arrhythmias, and shock; (2) necessity of close monitoring due to exposure to a significant amount of toxicant; (3) underlying conditions corresponding to a more severe vulnerability, in aged or newborn patients or with significant comorbidities. In 2006, the French Society of Intensive Care Medicine (SRLF) published guidelines for the management of severe poisonings in the ICU, including those resulting in severe encephalopathy and other neurological impairments [3].

The objective of this chapter is to review the major features and specificities of drug-related encephalopathy resulting in the admission of a poisoned patient to the ICU, trying to highlight how to assess the diagnosis and to present the various features and their resulting consequences for patient management.

Brain Disorders in Critical Illness, ed. Robert D. Stevens, Tarek Sharshar, and E. Wesley Ely. Published by Cambridge University Press. © Cambridge University Press 2013.

Table 33.1 Neurotransmitter systems and cellular receptors involved in the central nervous system effects of the most frequent toxicants.

Acetylcholine receptors	Organophosphate pesticides
Adrenergic receptors	Sympathomimetics, sympatholytics, ergot alkaloids, antipsychotic agents
Cannabinoid receptors	Marijuana, hashish
Dopamine receptors	Antipsychotic drugs, apomorphine
GABA receptors	Benzodiazepine, zopiclone, zolpidem, barbiturates, ethanol, baclofen
Glycine receptors	Strychnine
Histamine receptors	Antihistamines, tricyclic antidepressants
Membrane lipid	Anesthetic drugs
MAO receptors	MAO inhibitors
Muscarinic receptors	Curare
Nicotinic receptors	Nicotine, neuromuscular blocking drugs
NMDA receptors	Ethanol, ketamine
Norepinephrine reuptake	Cocaine, amphetamine, tricyclic antidepressants
Opioid receptors	Opium, heroin, morphine, codeine, methadone, buprenorphine, tramadol
Potassium channels	4-aminopyridine, quinidine, phencyclidine, toxins from scorpion
Purine/adenosine receptors	Caffeine, theophylline
Serotonin receptors	Atypical neuroleptics, buspirone, LSD, mescaline, khat and cathinones
Serotonin reuptake	Tricyclic antidepressants, selective serotonin reuptake inhibitors, venlafaxin
Sodium channels	Local anesthetics, tricyclic antidepressants, tetrodotoxin (puffer fish), ciguatoxins, aconitine

GABA, Gamma-aminobutyric acid; LSD, lysergic acid diethylamide; MAO, monoamine oxidase; NMDA, N-methyl-D-aspartate.

Mechanisms of toxicity

When CNS impairments are directly related to a functional interaction between the toxicant and its specific receptors on its targeted cells, then a dose–response relationship with a short latency period after exposure and a rapid improvement after cessation of the exposure characterize the occurrence of its effects. Several neurotransmitters and receptors on neurons in the CNS are involved to explain the observed features [4] (Table 33.1). Moreover, there is a relatively good parallel between the intensity of the presented signs and symptoms (which defines the toxicodynamic (TD) variables) and the toxicant amount present in the body, whose better hallmark is the blood concentrations (defining the toxicokinetic (TK) variables) (Figure 33.1). Rarely, non-functional interactions may occur leading to non-reversible CNS injuries and causing focal neurological deficits: they involve mechanisms of cell hypoxia and hypoperfusion, or represent the consequences of major systemic metabolic disturbances like hypoglycemia or acidosis. Recently, nitric oxide-mediated brain damage in

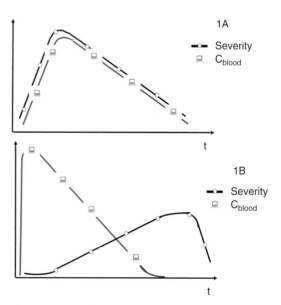

Figure 33.1 Classification of the psychoactive drugs according to the relationships between their central nervous system (CNS) effects and their blood concentrations: 1A, functional drugs with reversible CNS impairments after elimination from the body; 1B, injury-inducing drugs with potential non-reversible CNS impairments and possible sequelae despite their elimination from the body.

relation to peroxynitrite-induced oxidant stress has been identified as the pathway of toxicity resulting from carbon monoxide and paraquat poisonings. In these situations, there is no good TK/TD correlation between the intensity of symptoms and the corresponding blood concentrations of the involved toxicant (Figure 33.1).

Another important concern with toxicants is the necessity to cross the blood–brain barrier which protects neurons from the toxicant passive diffusion. Transport at the blood–brain barrier represents a major source of inter-individual variability and vulnerability. Several ATP-binding cassette (ABC) transporters such as P-glycoprotein (P-gp; ABCB1, MDR1), BCRP (ABCG2), and MRPs (ABCCs) expressed at the blood–brain barrier influence the brain pharmacokinetics of their substrates by restricting their uptake or enhancing their clearance from the brain into the blood, which has consequences for their CNS effects [5]. The effects of morphine, methadone, and loperamide on the CNS are modulated by P-gp. Recently, we demonstrated that P-gp plays a protective key role in buprenorphine-related respiratory effects, by allowing the efflux of its active and toxic metabolite, norbuprenorphine, at the blood–brain barrier, while P-gp inhibition may explain the occurrence of buprenorphine-associated respiratory depression [6]. In the upcoming years, investigating the role of these transporters will probably help to better understand the consequences of drug–drug interactions and the observed vulnerability in some of our patients, who develop severe neurological impairments in relation to moderate drug exposures.

Lithium intoxication represents a typical situation enhancing the role of the toxicant distribution into the brain in the occurrence and degree of severity of its resulting features. Lithium passage across the blood–brain barrier is slow, resulting in approximately a 24-h delay in the peak brain concentrations [7]. Moreover, lithium's slow distribution kinetics into and out of the brain explain the intensity of symptoms. Features of lithium toxicity are more severe in patients with chronic rather than acute poisoning, even though the plasma lithium concentration is usually lower. It is therefore essential that the pattern and duration of poisoning are taken into account in interpreting the plasma lithium concentration, as misinterpretation may result in delayed treatment and the risk of neurological damage or death, particularly in those suffering from chronic poisoning.

Three patterns of poisoning need to be distinguished, defining different TK/TD relationships.

1. Acute poisoning that occurs in previously untreated patients. Patients generally present mild symptoms, despite elevated plasma lithium concentrations. Consistently, it is possible to observe a patient with a plasma concentration of 8 mmol/l who did not develop any neurological impairment.

2. Acute-on-chronic (or acute-on-therapeutic) poisoning that occurs in previously treated patients who take an overdose. Patients can develop severe or life-threatening symptoms, usually with plasma lithium concentrations above 3–4 mmol/l.

3. Chronic poisoning that occurs in treated patients who develop progressive lithium accumulation due to renal dysfunction, underlying disease, low sodium intake, and drug–drug interactions (such as loop diuretics, angiotensin-converting enzyme inhibitors, or non-steroidal anti-inflammatory drugs); the elderly are particularly vulnerable to these conditions. Serum concentrations as low as 1.5 mmol/l may be associated with mild toxicity, whereas concentrations between 2.5 and 3.5 mmol/l may be associated with severe toxicity, and concentrations greater than 3.5 mmol/l may be life threatening.

Drug-induced neurological impairments

Alterations in consciousness result from drug-induced suppression of the activity of the reticular activating system, located in the upper brainstem, spread through the rostral pontine, the thalamus and the midbrain, and developing tight connections with the whole cerebral cortex. This interaction with the toxicant is either direct with the neurons from the reticular activating system or with the cerebral cortex.

Several degrees of toxicant-induced changes in mental status can be described. Usually, alterations in the level (i.e., the quantitative aspects from lethargy to coma) and in the content (i.e., the qualitative aspects including confusion, delirium, and agitation) of consciousness are distinguished. However, they are generally tightly associated in the drug-induced CNS effects. Lethargy corresponds to the inability of a patient to maintain a wakeful state without any verbal or manual stimulation. Stupor is the patient's arousability in response to a noxious stimulation. Delirium or acute cortical–subcortical neuronal encephalopathy is characterized by confusion, disorientation, and irritability that develops over a short period of time. Coma corresponds to the endpoint of consciousness impairment and represents one of the major presentations of poisoned patients to the ICU. The Glasgow Coma Scale (GCS), originally developed to assess severity in head trauma patients, is routinely used to describe the depth and time course of drug-induced coma and to take decisions regarding the poisoned patient's management including tracheal intubation.

Drug-induced encephalopathy may result in other neurological symptoms including seizures, abnormal movements, disturbances in the pyramidal tract, the brainstem, and the sensorial transmission. Various areas of the brain can be targeted by a toxicant, sometimes resulting from a specific interaction with one kind of neurotransmitter or receptor. Specific TD consequences are helpful for identifying the involved drug, if present among the multiple non-specific other signs of encephalopathy. Diagnosis is based on the recognition of such signs of high value of orientation based either on the general or the neurological physical examination of the poisoned patient, characterizing the clinical toxidrome-based approach of the poisoned patient.

General examination of a patient with a suspected drug-induced encephalopathy

The first step of diagnosis relies on the collection of features mandating consideration of a toxic exposure, including a history of drug overdose or abuse, a history of psychiatric illness, and prior suicide attempts. Although sometimes unreliable or incomplete, the history of exposure is essential, based on the information given by the patient (if he can answer the questions) and the family members, friends, witnesses, first-aid services, pharmacists, and treating physicians. Physical examination including neurological evaluation should be daily repeated and written in the patient's record.

General presentation

General physical examination with the measurement of vital signs is an essential step in the diagnosis of drug-induced neurological disturbances. Skin lesions including erythematous patches and blisters are much more frequently present in drug-induced coma than in cases from non-toxic causes. However, they have no specific value in differentiating among the different toxicants. Presence of skin needle tracks may suggest an intravenous abuse of opioids, cocaine, amphetamines, or insulin. Smelling a patient's breath or clothing may also be helpful to identify a toxicant with a characteristic odor: ethanol, ether, isopropylic alcohol (acetone odor), trichlorethylene or organophosphate pesticides (petroleum solvent), arsenic (garlic), cyanide (bitter almonds), camphor (mothballs), hydrogen sulfide (rotten eggs), and smoke inhalation (burning and fire). Skin color may suggest a possible orientation. Carbon monoxide is responsible for a reddish coloration of the skin. Jaundice could be attributable to the late presentation of a poisoning with hepatotoxins like acetaminophen or *Amanita* mushrooms. Flushed skin suggests anticholinergic drugs, serotonin syndrome, alcohol/disulfiram antabuse reaction, or scombroid fish poisoning (histamine release). A relatively well presentation despite an intense cyanosis not reversed with oxygen and blood sampling, with a chocolate brown color suggest the presence of methemoglobinemia in relation to amyl nitrite "poppers" inhalation or to the ingestion of dapsone, chlorate, and aniline derivates. A red coloration of the urine can be attributable to the ingestion of rifampicine, while a muddy brown color is suggestive of myoglobinuria (secondary to rhabdomyolysis), hemoglobinuria (secondary to intravascular hemolysis), or an associated massive methemoglobinemia. Hair loss can be related to an exposure to radiation or radioactive substances, a chemotherapy, colchicine, arsenic, or thallium. The association of peripheral neuropathy, gastroenteritis, and alopecia is specific of an exposure 2 weeks previously to arsenic or thallium [8]. The presence of associated cholera-like diarrhea is suggestive of colchicine poisoning.

Body temperature

Several toxicants are able to disturb central temperature. Hypothermia generally results from a deep coma even if occurring at home. In the case of severe associated vasodilation, thermal loss can occur by means of the skin. Fever may result from an excessive production of heat due to muscle rigidity (neuroleptic malignant syndrome), seizures, extreme agitation (antihistamines), or excessive vasoconstriction (cocaine). Other mechanisms are possible including oxidative dephosphorylation (aspirin and phenols), sweating inhibition (anticholinergic drugs), or direct injury (fire victim). Most frequently in a comatose patient, fever is attributed to the onset of an aspiration pneumonia that should be confirmed by pulmonary auscultation and chest X-rays.

Respiratory pattern

Respiratory failure may contribute to the onset of drug-induced encephalopathy. Bradypnea or apnea indicates that the patient has been exposed to a toxicant able to interact with the centers of ventilation control such as an opioid, a barbiturate, cyanide, or hydrogen sulfide. The ingestion of a benzodiazepine or any similar sedative molecule cannot be responsible for a decrease in respiratory frequency. Elevated respiratory rate in the presence of hypoxemia (cyanosis or decreased SpO_2) suggests aspiration bronchopneumonia, non-cardiogenic pulmonary edema, or inhalation of a pulmonary irritant such as chlorine. In the absence of decreased SpO_2, polypnea can be related to the use of psychostimulant drugs (such as cocaine or amphetamine) or associated metabolic acidosis (with Kussmaul breathing).

Circulation

Circulation may contribute to the onset of drug-induced encephalopathy. Measurement of blood pressure and heart rate should systematically be completed by an ECG. Association of hypotension and tachycardia is suggestive of circulatory failure and non-well tolerated ventricular or supraventricular arrhythmia. Association of hypotension and bradycardia is suggestive of conduction disturbances in relation to the ingestion of a beta-blocker (possible sinus bradycardia), calcium channel blocker (sino atrial or atrio-ventriuclar block), sodium channel blocker (membrane stabilizing effects and intraventricular block), or digitalis (sinus dysfunction and atrio-ventriuclar block). Deep hypoxemia (respiratory depression) or tissue hypoxia (cyanide intoxication) may also be responsible for bradycardia and hypotension, all resulting in the onset of encephalopathy. Association of tachycardia and hypertension suggests an alpha-sympathic stimulation in relation to an exposition to cocaine, amphetamine, phenylephedrine, or monoamine oxidase inhibitors. Association of hypertension and bradycardia suggests a massive vasoconstriction (sympathomimetic drugs, central alpha-2 agonists), but can also result from an acute complication due to a hypertensive crisis such as cerebral hemorrhage after cocaine use.

Neurological examination of a patient with suspected toxic coma or encephalopathy

General presentation

The toxic origin of a coma should be suspected in the absence of focal signs (unless hypoglycemia is involved) and meningeal irritation. However, exceptionally in single case reports, transient lateralizing signs have been described after overdoses with barbiturates [9] and phenytoin [10]. A rapid and easy orientation requires an evaluation of the spontaneous motility (calm versus agitated), the tone (hypo- versus hypertonia), the deep tendon reflexes (hypo- versus hyperreflexia), and the plantar reflexes (flexor or indifferent versus extensor).

A calm or sedated presentation suggests the ingestion of a sedative drug or tranquilizer, while an agitated presentation with tremor or seizures suggests the ingestion of a psychostimulant or hypoglycemic drug. A lethargic syndrome (defined by the association of hypotonia, hyporeflexia, and indifferent plantar responses) suggests the ingestion of hypnotics, tranquilizers or ethanol; a pyramidal syndrome (defined by the association of hypertonia, hyperreflexia, and extensor plantar responses) suggests the ingestion of antidepressants, first-generation antihistamines, or hypoglycemic substances; an extrapyramidal syndrome suggests the ingestion of antipsychotic drugs and especially substituted benzamides or butyrophenones. However, variants can exist: a coma following a massive ingestion of the recently banned meprobamate (Mépronizine® or Equanil®) from the French market is hypotonic; however, in less than 10% of the cases, it can be hypertonic.

Pupil abnormalities

Miotic pupils suggest exposure to an opioid-receptor agonist (morphine derivative) or an anticholinesterasic drug (organophosphate or carbamate insecticide). Pupils in mydriasis suggest the ingestion of a tricyclic antidepressant, a serotonin reuptake inhibitor, an antihistamine, a sympathomimetic compound, or cocaine. Pupil dilation may also be the first sign of visual impairment complicating intoxication with quinine or methanol [11]. Inequality of the pupil size as well as inequality to their reaction to light are seldom evidence of brainstem compression; however, in some rare cases, unequal pupils have been reported in poisonings while patients exhibiting this sign recovered uneventfully.

Disturbances in brainstem functions

Abnormalities in the posture or movements of the eyes can occur in acute poisonings with a large variety of psychotropic drugs as described under anesthesia. Ophthalmoplegia is possible when consciousness is minimally altered [12,13]. Vertical or horizontal strabismus has been observed in carbamazepine, phenytoin, and tricyclic antidepressant poisonings. Roving eye movements (generally reported as dysconjugated) as well as loss of the doll's eye and oculovestibular reflexes have been observed in benzodiazepine, barbiturate, ethanol, phenothaizine, and tricyclic antidepressant poisonings [14]. A recent case with diplopia and cranial neuropathies including ataxia was attributed to the subcutaneous injection of elemental mercury [15]. Signs of decerebration and decortication were also described. Apparent brain death with an isoelectric EEG can be observed following a massive intoxication with barbiturates, chloral, meprobamate, benzodiazepine, and baclofen [16]. Similarly, profound hypothermia resulting from drug-induced coma can mimic an apparent brain death. All these situations of extreme brain injuries should be interpreted with caution, as full uneventful recovery could be obtained, with the complete elimination of the toxicant. Any organ procurement should only be discussed after disclosing a possible massive psychotropic drug poisoning [17].

Sensory alterations

Visual impairment suggests a possible poisoning with quinine, ethambutol, cyclosporine, and methanol (which may cause irreversible blindness). Hearing impairment characterizes acute salicylate and quinine (cinchonism) intoxication. Anecdotal cases of temporary deafness following heroin injection, carbon monoxide poisoning, and non-steroidal drug overdoses have been reported.

Seizures

Seizures can be induced by several drugs (Table 33.2). Antidepressants, either tricyclic or serotonin reuptake inhibitors, are the most frequently involved in poisoned patients who are admitted to the ICU. In a festive context, drugs of abuse should be suspected including the classical substances such as cocaine and

Table 33.2 Toxicants frequently involved in the occurrence of seizures.

Pharmaceuticals
Tri- or tetracyclic antidepressants
Serotonin reuptake inhibitors
Monoamine oxidase inhibitors
Lithium
Phenothiazines
Antihistamines
Piperazine or non-piperazine anti-cough derivatives
Anticonvulsive drugs (carbamazepine, valproic acid)
Bupropion
Baclofen
Chloral
Hypoglycemic compounds
Isoniazid
Minaprine
Chloroquine
Xanthine derivatives e.g., theophylline
Salicylates (pediatrics)
Atropine (pediatrics)
Sedative or hypnotic withdrawal syndrome (benzodiazepines, ethanol, meprobamate, barbiturates)

Non-pharmaceutical compounds
Cocaine
Amphetamines
Carbon monoxide
Organophosphate insecticides
Anticholinesterasic carbamate pesticides
Chlorinated hydrocarbons
Anticholinergic plants (Datura)
Nicotine
Metaldehyde
Camphor and terpen derivatives (e.g., menthol)
Ethylene glycol
Fluorides and oxalates
Strychnine
Water intoxication in psychogenic polydipsia

amphetamines, and the emergent smart ones including mephedrone and other cathinones [18], the ketamine derivative methoxetamine [19], the bath salts, and legal highs (novel psychoactive substances) [20,21]. In patients on psychoactive treatments, chronic lithium overdose, phenothiazine, and serotonin syndrome are usually responsible for seizures. Finally, a withdrawal syndrome in relation to the brutal interruption of ethanol or any sedative hypnotics can result in the development of seizures, requiring the rapid reintroduction of the pharmaceuticals previously used in the long term.

Involuntary movements

Parkinsonism, tremor, chorea-ballismus, choreoathetosis, dystonia, myoclonus, tics, tardive dyskinesia (i.e., involuntary asymmetrical movements of the muscles), and akathisia (i.e., feeling of motor restlessness) can be induced by many drugs [22]. The most frequently implicated drugs in movement disorders are first-generation antipsychotics, calcium antagonists, orthopramides, substituted benzamides (e.g., metoclopramide, sulpiride, clebopride, domperidone), CNS stimulants, antidepressants, anticonvulsants, antiparkinsonian drugs, and lithium. Metoclopramide is also an increasingly recognized cause of tardive dyskinesia. Acute dystonic movements, torticollis (muscular spasms of neck), orolingual dyskinesias, and oculogyric crises are attributed, mainly in infants, to the ingestion of metoclopramide more often than to the other dopamine antagonists [23]. It is possible for a single drug to induce two or more types of movement disorders in the same intoxicated patient. The physician should be aware that movement disorders are not always reversible after drug withdrawal.

The main neurological toxidromes

A "toxidrome" or toxic syndrome includes symptoms, signs, laboratory test and electrocardiographic abnormalities suggestive when grouped in a clinical entity of its toxicological origin. A toxidrome is suggestive but not completely specific of the involvement of a class of toxicants in the observed features [3]. It is generally more sensitive than any other emergent analytical biomarker. Thus, diagnosis in clinical toxicology is based on the identification of toxidromes (Table 33.3). However, multi-drug poisonings or non-specific complications can modify clinical features when compared with the typical presentation (Figure 33.2). In a patient with drug-induced coma, encephalopathy, confusion, or agitation, the toxidrome-based diagnosis approach is requested not only to assess the adequate toxicological diagnosis but also to rule out any alternative non-toxicological diagnosis.

The lethargic syndrome

This syndrome consists of a calm, hypotonic, and hyporeflexic coma or sometimes a simple sedation. A consequent hypotension and respiratory depression can be observed. The most frequently involved drugs are the following: benzodiazepines, imidazopyridines (zolpidem, zopiclone), barbiturates, meprobamate, phenothiazines, phenytoin, sodium valproate, and ethanol. The titrated intravenous administration of flumazenil can

Table 33.3 The main toxidromes with central nervous system involvement.

Sedative hypnotic	Confusion, stupor, and coma Slurred speech Respiratory depression
Opioid	Coma Miosis Bradypnea Hypotension, bradycardia
Anticholinergic "hot as a hare, dry as a bone, red as a beet, mad as a hatter"	Mydriasis Dry skin, flushing Urinary retention Ileus Tachycardia, hypertension Coma, seizures, myoclonus
Cholinergic "SLUDGE"	Salivation Lacrimation Urination Diarrhea Gastrointestinal cramps Emesis Wheezing Diaphoresis Bronchorrhea Bradycardia Miosis
Adrenergic	Tachycardia Tremor Diaphoresis, dry mucus membranes Hypertension (alpha), hypotension (beta)
Serotonin	Flushing Diarrhea Diaphoresis Fever Trismus Hyperreflexia Tremor Myoclonus

be safely used as a pharmacodynamic test in such comatose patients after disclosing any past medical history of epilepsy, any possible co-ingestion of pro-epileptic drugs (especially antidepressants), any anticholinergic features, ECG abnormalities, or significant respiratory complications of coma (like aspiration pneumonia) [24]. The recommended regimen is an initial administration of 0.3 mg in 1 minute followed by additional doses of 0.1 mg each minute until a cumulative dose of 1–2 mg [3]. The absence of any response with 2 mg flumazenil rules out a possible intoxication with benzodiazepines or analogs. The adequate use of flumazenil including its strict administration to patients presenting

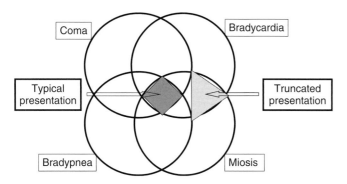

Figure 33.2 Toxidromes are defined for the typical presentations after exposition to one given toxicant. In real life, atypical aspects are much more frequent in relation to multidrug ingestions.

lethargic syndromes avoids complication and may indicate in certain situations against intubation of a benzodiazepine-poisoned patient [24].

The opioid syndrome

This syndrome is characteristic and includes: (i) impaired consciousness with calm, hypotonic, and hyporeflexic coma; (ii) bradypnea (defined as reduced respiratory rate < 12/minute); and (iii) bilateral constricted to pinpoint miosis [25]. Sinus bradycardia and hypotension are also frequently observed. If the patient is not deeply comatose, bradypnea is inducible with an acceleration of the respiratory rate when the patient is stimulated. This syndrome is related to an opioid overdose, although the identification of the exact molecule is impossible based only on the clinical presentation. Buprenorphine, an opioid used as maintenance therapy of heroin addicts, is responsible for coma and respiratory depression despite its ceiling respiratory effects: its resulting features are not significantly different from those of heroin and methadone regarding coma depth and respiratory depression intensity [26]. Buprenorphine overdoses are attributed to the injection of crushed pills or the association with benzodiazepines [27]. The titrated intravenous administration of naloxone represents a useful pharmacodynamic test. In cases of buprenorphine overdose, we did not observe a significant improvement in patients' GCS when using a 0.4–0.8 mg dose of naloxone [26], probably due to the very elevated affinity of buprenorphine to its receptor. For all other opioids, the absence of a complete awakening after naloxone administration suggests a possible co-intoxication with another psychotropic drug or the occurrence of severe anoxic brain injuries, especially if management was delayed.

The anticholinergic syndrome

This syndrome is suspected in the presence of (i) encephalopathy with confusion, hallucinations, delirium, myoclonic jerks, frequent seizures, and varying degree of coma; and (ii) atropinic signs including sinus tachycardia, bilateral mydriasis, dry skin, urinary retention, and decreased bowel sounds. Urinary retention generally represents an additional cause of agitation with encephalopathy. Coma is usually not profound, with pyramidal but no focal signs. Early-onset seizures (incidence: 6–11%) in relation to antidepressant overdose (one of the major drug-induced convulsions) are generalized, usually multiple (50%), and often of short duration (about 30–60 s but exceptionally > 24 h) [28]. Their occurrence is predictable by the enlargement of the QRS complex (> 0.120 s) and may result in a deterioration of the patient's hemodynamics [29]. Some antidepressants including dosulepine, amoxapine, and maprotiline are particularly responsible for seizures. Recognition of encephalopathy with anticholinergic syndrome suggests an exposition to one of the following toxicants: cyclic antidepressant, H1-antihistamines, anti-Parkinson's medications, antipsychotics with anticholinergic effects (piperazinated phenothiazines), and the *Solanaceae* family (Datura).

The cholinergic syndrome

The cholinergic syndrome results from poisoning with anticholinesterasic pesticides belonging either to the organophosphate or carbamate family. Organophosphates represent a large family of chemical compounds developed in the 1940s as chemical arms or pesticides. They are still widely used in agriculture and veterinary medicine and are responsible for frequent accidental or suicidal intoxications. They represent a major health problem all over the world with about 3 million severe intoxications and more than 220,000 deaths each year in the developing world [30]. By contrast, in developed countries, these intoxications have become rare as the less toxic pyrethroid insecticides have progressively taken over from the organophosphate compounds.

Cholinergic syndrome includes CNS impairment resulting in confusion, ataxia, and convulsive coma. It associates two distinct syndromes, the muscarinic and the nicotinic. Features due to the overstimulation of muscarinic acetylcholine receptors in the parasympathetic system are bradycardia, hypotension, miosis, lacrymation, blurred vision, ocular pain, bronchorrhea, bronchospasm (mimicking an acute pulmonary edema), gastrointestinal cramps, meteoric abdomen, vomiting, diarrhea, and urination. Features due to overstimulation of nicotinic acetylcholine receptors in the sympathetic system are tachycardia, mydriasis, hypertension, and sweating, as well as several biological abnormalities including hyperglycemia, hypokalemia, hypophosphoremia, and lactic acidosis, while those related to the overstimulation of the nicotinic receptors at the neuromuscular junction result in muscle weakness, paralysis, and fasciculation. All cholinergic features contribute to the development of acute respiratory failure that is responsible for the majority of cholinergic syndrome fatalities.

Typical organophosphate intoxication has three stages, i.e., early, intermediate, and late. The early stage includes the three previously described cholinergic syndromes, at varying degrees, depending on the organophosphate molecule, the time since exposure, and the route of penetration into the body. After ingestion, gastrointestinal signs are the first to develop. In contrast, following an inhalation, the ocular and CNS features are more rapid. Interestingly, following the sarin gas attack on the Tokyo subway in 1995, ocular and CNS symptoms were observed in almost all the victims [31]. In contrast, carbamate insecticide-induced cholinergic features do not include nicotinic syndrome and its duration usually does not exceed 24 h. Toxicity of petroleum solvent should be added to the insecticide-related cholinergic syndrome. It is responsible for diarrhea, consciousness impairment, and aspiration pneumonia, which accounts for an additional cause of hypoxemia.

In its typical form, diagnosis is easy based on the assessment of clinical features. In atypical forms, diagnosis may be difficult, requiring the measurement of plasma butyrylcholinesterase (or pseudo-cholinesterase) activity [30]. Although relatively sensitive and routinely available in the emergent setting, this laboratory test is not specific as a significant decrease in activity can be obtained in cases of pregnancy, anemia, or liver failure. Measurement of the erythrocyte acetylcholinesterase activity can be of a confirmatory value, but should be performed in a specialized laboratory.

Recognition of muscarinic signs in a patient presenting with an encephalopathy requires the intravenous administration of high-dose atropine (2–4 mg as initial bolus, followed by 2 mg each 5–10 minutes according to the feature severity). The endpoint is to maintain clear chest auscultation and reduce respiratory secretions. Mydriasis, agitation, and pyrexia should be rather considered as indicators of atropine toxicity.

The adrenergic syndrome

The adrenergic syndrome consists of: (i) neurovegetative signs including psychomotor agitation, bilateral mydriasis, sweating, tremor, and convulsions; (ii) cardiovascular signs including tachycardia, hypertension (for toxicants with alpha-stimulant activity) or hypotension (for toxicants with beta-2 stimulant activity); (iii) ECG abnormalities including sinus tachycardia, ventricular arrhythmia; (iv) metabolic signs including hyperglycemia, lactic acidosis, hypokalemia due to cellular transfer of potassium, hyperleucocytosis, and hypophosphoremia. This syndrome can correspond to poisoning with cocaine, amphetamines, lysergic acid diethylamide (LSD), ephedrine, or caffeine (alpha stimulant activity), as well as theophylline or salbutamol (beta-2 stimulant activity). Central nervous system complications are frequent in relation to cocaine overdose with myocardial infarction (coronary vasospasm), brain ischemic stroke (vasoconstriction of the brain vessels), or cerebral hemorrhage (hypertension). In a patient admitted with encephalopathy and hypertension in the emergency room, the identification of an associated adrenergic syndrome suggests cocaine overdose and should thus contraindicate beta-blockers that may increase the risk of coronary vasospasm [32]. Only beta-blockers with alpha-blocking properties such as labetolol should be used.

The serotonin syndrome

Clinical features of the serotonin syndrome include: (i) CNS impairment with agitation, confusion, hallucinations, myoclonus, tremor, pyramidal syndrome, seizures, and coma; (ii) neurovegetative signs with mydriasis, sweating, tachycardia, tachypnea, hyperthermia, hypotension, diarrhea, and respiratory arrest; (iii) biologic abnormalities including hyperglycemia, hyperleucocytosis, hypokalemia, hypocalcemia, disseminated intravascular coagulation, lactic acidosis, and rhabdomyolysis [33]. The criteria of diagnosis were defined by Sternbach in 1991 [34]. Diagnosis requires first to rule out any endocrine impairment, infectious disease, withdrawal syndrome, as well as any recent modification in an antipsychotic treatment. Differentiation with other toxicological syndromes may be difficult (Figure 33.3). Myoclonus are the most constant feature and should be searched first as indicated in the Hunter diagram (Figure 33.4), in order to increase the specificity of the clinical diagnosis [35].

Incidence of the serotonin syndrome is increasing but remains underestimated, due to the banality of the observed signs. However, features may be life-threatening and thus require an exact assessment. This syndrome may correspond either to an overdose or frequently to the side effects of a pro-serotonin treatment enhanced by drug–drug interactions. Features are attributed to the increase of serotonin activity in the CNS triggered by a serotonin reuptake inhibitor, a monoamine oxidase inhibitor, lithium, a tricyclic antidepressant, ecstasy, or L-tryptophan, for instance (Table 33.4). 5-HT$_{1A}$ and 5-HT$_2$ receptors are believed to be involved. The identification of serotonin syndrome in a patient presenting with an encephalopathy requires cessation of the involved pharmaceutical (in case of drug–drug interaction) and administration of optimal supportive care to avoid the occurrence of a malignant hyperthermia which may result in multiorgan failure and death. In severe cases, external cooling, mechanical ventilation, and muscle paralysis may be required. No antidote has been shown as efficient, based on a randomized control trial in the treatment of serotonin syndrome. The efficiency of cyproheptadine (12–32 mg/day by oral route) or dantrolene (mainly for ecstasy) has been suggested, but remains debated.

The neuroleptic malignant syndrome

This neuroleptic malignant syndrome is more often due to a side effect and rarely to an overdose with any neuroleptics. Diagnosis is suggested if the patient presents a body temperature > 38 °C, confusion, consciousness impairment, generalized hypertonia,

	Serotonin syndrome	Anticholinergic syndrome	Neuroleptic malignant syndrome	Malignant fever
Toxicant	Serotoninergic	Anticholinergic	Dopaminergic agonist	Inhaled anesthetics
Delay	<12h	<12h	1–3 days	30 min to 24 h
Vital signs	+++	+	+++	++++
Pupils	Mydriasis	Mydriasis	N	N
Mucosa	Salivation	Dryness	Salivation	N
Skin	Diaphoresis	Flushing	Diaphoresis	Mottled, diaphoresis
Gastrointestinal signs	↑	↓	N or ↓	↓
Tonus	↑, lower limb	↑, N	↑↑	Rigor mortis
Reflexes	Hyperreflexia, clonus	N	Bradyreflexia	Hyporeflexia
Consciousness	Coma, agitation	Delirium, agitation	Stupor, muteness, coma	Agitation

Figure 33.3 Differentiation of the serotonin syndrome with other toxicological syndromes.

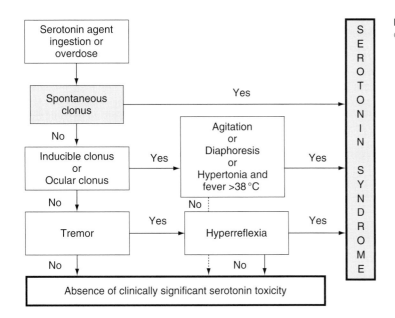

Figure 33.4 The Hunter diagram to aid the clinical diagnosis of the serotonin syndrome [35].

hyperreflexia, axial muscle rigidity, sweating, hemodynamic instability, and rhabdomyolysis. Fever may exceed 43 °C and become life-threatening. It occurs after a few hours to 7 days regarding the immediate-release antipsychotics and between 2–4 weeks for delayed-release antipsychotics. This syndrome should be distinguished from a serotonin syndrome-induced malignant hyperthermia (such as after ecstasy use) and from halogenated anesthetic-related malignant fever (Figure 33.3). Recognition of this syndrome requires an immediate massive fluid repletion and the administration of a specific treatment like dantrolene or bromocriptine.

Role of laboratory and radiological investigations

Routine laboratory tests

Management of poisoning mainly relies on a clinical approach and supportive treatments. Routine laboratory tests are more important than toxicological analysis. Metabolic disturbances should be systematically ruled out in a patient presenting with an encephalopathy (see Chapter 34, this volume), even if a toxic cause is suspected. These abnormalities can be sometimes induced by the drug itself: alteration in serum sodium in relation to lithium overdose, hypoxia and hypercapnia in relation to drug-induced coma with aspiration pneumonia or CNS depression, or hepatic

encephalopathy induced by acetaminophen. Investigating the amplitude of drug-induced impairment in a biological parameter is more useful for patient management than measuring the involved drug concentration. Finally, in the alcoholic encephalopathy patient, multiple issues have to be clarified based on laboratory tests, including withdrawal symptoms, delirium tremens, the Wernicke–Korsakoff syndrome, seizures, depression, polysubstance abuse, electrolyte disturbances, and liver diseases. Such complicated patients require a coordinated, multidisciplinary approach.

Cerebral imaging

Neuroimaging techniques, mainly magnetic resonance imaging, have improved the delineation of parenchyma drug-induced injuries even at the early stage of poisoning. Moreover they help in characterizing the mechanism of tissue impairment (vasogenic edema versus cytotoxic edema or hemorrhage). Toxic injuries are usually bilateral and symmetrical. Their exact location is assessed, either within the gray or white matter. Basal ganglia are preferentially involved due to a relative susceptibility to higher metabolic/energetic demands. However, injuries within the basal ganglia are not specific of any particular toxicant. Moreover, these areas are also preferentially affected by anoxic processes from non-toxic origin and by metabolic disorders, thus requiring an expert comparison between the medical history, the clinical features, and the imaging. Neuroimages after acute exposure to industrial products (methanol,

Table 33.4 The main pharmaceuticals and non-pharmaceutical drugs reported to have induced a serotonin syndrome.

Specific serotonin reuptake inhibitors: sertraline, fluoxetine, fluvoxamine, paroxetine, citalopram, escitalopram

Antidepressant drugs: trazodone, nefazodone, buspirone, clomipramine, venlafaxine

Monoamine oxidase inhibitors: phenelzine, moclobemide, clorgiline, isocarboxazid

Anticonvulsants: valproate

Analgesics: meperidine, fentanyl, tramadol, pentazocine

Antiemetic agents: ondansetron, granisetron, metoclopramide

Antimigraine drugs: sumatriptan

Bariatric medicatons: sibutramine

Antibiotics: linezolide, ritonavir

Over-the-counter cough and cold remedies: dextromethorphan

Drugs of abuse: amphetamines, ecstasy, LSD, foxy methoxy, Syrian rue

Dietary supplements and herbal products: tryptophan, *Hypericum perforatum* (St John's wort), Panax ginseng

Lithium

Bupropion

Typical association resulting in serotonin syndrome
- Phenelzine and mepiridine
- Tranylcypromine and imipramine
- Olanzapine and clomipramine
- Phenelzine and SSRI
- Paroxetine and buspirone
- Linezolide and citalopram, mepiridine
- Moclobemide and SSRI
- Tramadol, venlafaxine, and mirtazapine
- Fluconazole and citalopram
- Cyclosporin and escitalopram

LSD, lysergic acid diethylamide; SSRI, selective serotonin reuptake inhibitor.

ethylene glycol), environmental agents (cyanide, carbon monoxide), pharmaceuticals (insulin, valproic acid), and illicit substances (heroin, cocaine) were recently reviewed by Hantson and Duprez [36]. Different kinds of lesions lacking specificity for toxic injury were observed. Deep gray matter lesions with symmetrical distribution throughout basal ganglia were most often seen, although all the described findings have been also reported after anoxic-ischemic insults and metabolic disturbances. The emergent neuroimaging findings of alcohol-related CNS non-traumatic disorders were recently reviewed by Zuccoli *et al.* [37]. The three best-defined toxic leukoencephalopathies correspond to delayed posthypoxic leukoencephalopathy including delayed neurological sequelae after carbon monoxide poisoning, heroin inhalation leukoencephalopathy, and posterior reversible encephalopathy syndrome [38]. The final prognostic value of imaging in all these situations remains debatable. Quantitative or molecular imaging techniques such as magnetic resonance diffusion-weighted imaging or magnetic resonance spectroscopy will increase their predictive value in the coming years.

Electroencephalography

Electroencephalography findings in drug-induced encephalopathy are various and may help in assessing the mechanisms of toxicity. An EEG is essential to assess drug- or withdrawal-induced seizures, especially in cases of non-convulsive status epilepticus, as patients may be encephalopathic because of ongoing epileptic activity with minimal or no motor movements. An EEG may also be required to monitor an antiepileptic treatment in case of seizures. Drug-induced metabolic disturbances like hepatic or renal dysfunction, are often characterized by slowing of background rhythms and triphasic waves. Drug-induced hypoxia can produce a number of abnormal EEG patterns such as burst suppression, alpha coma, and spindle coma. In the case of drug-induced supratentorial injury, an EEG may show focal disturbances such as delta and theta activity, epileptiform abnormalities, and attenuation of faster frequencies. In contrast, in infratentorial lesions, the EEG may appear normal, particularly with a pontine lesion. Finally, an EEG is required to assess brain death, after the elimination of the involved psychoactive drug.

Toxicological analysis

Toxicological tests aim to identify and/or quantify the toxicant in order to confirm or rule out the diagnosis of drug-induced neurological disturbances, to evaluate the severity of poisoning, and to monitor the effectiveness of treatment. Whenever possible, assays to determine blood concentrations should be preferred to screening tests. Toxicological analysis is essential to obtain a definitive diagnosis of poisoning, mainly in cases of medico-legal issues and to understand a mechanism of drug–drug interaction (TK or TD) or individual variability (tolerance for example).

Indications for tracheal intubation in drug-induced coma

Intubation is not always necessary in the presence of cough, gag reflexes, and adequate spontaneous ventilation. However, if airway protection is compromised or clinical situation deteriorates, airway securing is recommended. The GCS is largely used to indicate intubation of poisoned patients, although its predictive value has been poorly assessed in the field of toxicology [39,40]. Usually, a cut-off value of GCS of less than 8 is used to intubate, as generally accepted for intubation after head injury [41]. Based on studies observing current practice, this criterion was found to be a useful guideline for intubation, although it should be used in conjunction with the clinical context [40]. Endotracheal intubation decreases but does not eliminate the risk of aspiration which was evaluated at about 10–15% in comatose poisoned patients [42,43]. However, it has clearly been demonstrated that the loss of airway reflexes and risk of aspiration cannot be reliably predicted using the GCS alone [42]. Protective cough reflexes have been shown to be present in patients with a GCS score less than or equal to 8 from a pharmacological cause [44]. Thus, for psychotropic drugs, the decision should not only take into account the degree of sedation but also the severity of encephalopathy, such as in antidepressant poisonings [3]. Agitation, seizures, muscle rigidity, trismus, and myoclonus, which are frequent features in drug-induced anticholinergic, serotoninergic, and adrenergic syndromes, represent facilitating conditions for aspiration in the course of poisonings. The expected time course of symptoms should also be considered, when treating patients poisoned with toxicants which may cause relatively rapid recovery such as ethanol or gamma-hydroxybutyrate [45,46]. Interestingly, the simple alert/verbal/painful/unresponsive (AVPU) responsiveness scale (alert, responsive to verbal stimulation, responsive to painful stimulation, and unresponsive), widely taught in advanced life support courses and used by paramedics in the out-of-hospital setting, was shown to provide a rapid method of assessing consciousness level in most poisoned patients, although difficulty was observed in assessing alcohol-intoxicated patients [47]. More recently, a clinical study suggested that it can be safe to observe poisoned patients in the emergency department without tracheal intubation despite a decreased consciousness, with a GCS of 8 or less [48].

Physically combative or violent or delirious poisoned patients can potentially become dangerous to themselves or to the staff. Rarely, they may need to be controlled through sedation and intubation, when aggressive chemical or physical restraints have proven ineffective, and further studies such as computed tomography of the brain are required to aid in diagnosis and care [49]. However, such action should be considered an extreme measure and not taken lightly or inappropriately used.

Decision to intubate is left to the clinical judgment of the treating physicians. Timing the intubation can be tricky as changes in mental status with subsequent loss of protective airway mechanisms, or hemodynamic status can occur suddenly in the acutely poisoned, but initially well-appearing patient, as in the case of a cyclic antidepressant overdose. The physician must, therefore, anticipate and estimate the possibility of such an occurrence to decide if and when to intubate. Based on the American and European position statements on gastrointestinal decontamination [50,51], it is no longer recommended to intubate a patient solely for the purposes of systematic decontamination. However, whether a gastrointestinal decontamination is judged beneficial for the patient, the procedure is contraindicated, unless the patient has an intact or protected airway. If antidotes (including naloxone and flumazenil) were first administered and continuously infused, close patient monitoring in the intensive or intermediate level care units is required in order to decide for any further delayed tracheal intubation if respiratory presentation or neurological status worsen [3].

Conclusion

Drug-induced encephalopathy is a frequent presentation by ICU patients, requiring rapid management as it may result in life-threatening conditions. Identification of the involved drugs is essential and based on a clinical approach using the toxidromes. Central nervous system features may involve several toxidromes including the lethargic, opioid, anticholinergic, cholinergic, adrenergic, and serotonin ones. Laboratory tests are mandatory to rule out any associated biological impairment. Neuroimaging and electroencephalograms may be helpful in certain situations to understand the mechanisms of CNS injuries. Toxicological analysis is necessary for a final definitive diagnosis, mainly when a medico-legal issue exists.

References

1. Bronstein AC, Spyker DA, Cantilena LR Jr, *et al*. 2009 Annual Report of the American Association of Poison Control Centers' National Poison Data System (NPDS): 27th Annual Report. *Clin Toxicol (Phila)* 2010;**48**:979–1178.

2. Villa A, Cochet A, Guyodo G. Les intoxications signalées aux centres antipoison français en 2006. *Rev Prat* 2008;**58**:825–31.

3. Mégarbane B, Donetti L, Blanc T, Chéron G, Jacobs F, panel of experts convened by the SRLF. ICU management of severe poisoning with medications or illicit substances. *Réanimation* 2006;**15**:343–53.

4. Ford M, Delanay KA, Ling L, Erickson T. *Clinical Toxicology*. Philadelphia, PA: WB Saunders; 2001, p. 135.

5. Tournier N, Declèves X, Saubaméa B, Scherrmann JM, Cisternino S. Opioid transport by ATP-binding cassette transporters at the blood–brain barrier: implications for neuropsychopharmacology. *Curr Pharm Des* 2011;**17**:2829–42.

6. Alhaddad H, Cisternino S, Declèves X, *et al*. Respiratory toxicity of buprenorphine results from the blockage of P-glycoprotein-mediated efflux of norbuprenorphine at the blood–brain barrier in mice. *Crit Care Med* 2012; **40**(12):3215–23.

7. El Balkhi S, Megarbane B, Poupon J, Baud FJ, Galliot-Guilley M. Lithium poisoning: is determination of the red blood cell lithium concentration useful? *Clin Toxicol (Phila)* 2009;**47**(1):8–13.

8. Hoffman RS. Thallium toxicity and the role of Prussian blue in therapy. *Toxicol Rev* 2003;**22**:29–40.

9. Carroll BJ. Barbiturate overdosage: presentation with focal neurological signs. *Med J Aust* 1969;**1**:1133–5.

10. Sandyk R. Transient hemiparesis – a rare complication of phenytoin toxicity. *Postgrad Med J* 1983;**59**:601–2.

11. Coulter CV, Farquhar SE, McSherry CM, Isbister GK, Duffull SB. Methanol and ethylene glycol acute poisonings – predictors of mortality. *Clin Toxicol (Phila)* 2011;**49**:900–6.

12. Spector RH, Davidoff RA, Schwartzman RJ. Phenytoin-induced ophthalmoplegia. *Neurology* 1976;**26**:1031–4.

13. Ng K, Silbert PL, Edis RH. Complete external ophthalmoplegia and asterixis with carbamazepine toxicity. *Aust N Z J Med* 1991;**21**:886–7.

14. Barret LG, Vincent FM, Arsac PL, Debru JL, Faure JR. Internuclear ophthalmoplegia in patients with toxic coma frequency, prognostic value, diagnostic significance. *J Toxicol Clin Toxicol* 1983;**20**:373–9.

15. Malkani R, Weinstein JM, Kumar N, Victor TA, Bernstein L. Ataxia and cranial neuropathies from subcutaneously injected elemental mercury. *Clin Toxicol (Phila)* 2011;**49**:334–6.

16. Sullivan R, Hodgman MJ, Kao L, Tormoehlen LM. Baclofen overdose mimicking brain death. *Clin Toxicol (Phila)* 2012;**50**:141–4.

17. Marrache F, Mégarbane B, Pirnay S, Rhaoui A, Thuong M. Difficulties in assessing brain death in a case of benzodiazepine poisoning with persistent cerebral blood flow. *Hum Exp Toxicol* 2004;**23**:503–5.

18. Wood DM, Davies S, Puchnarewicz M, Johnston A, Dargan PI. Acute toxicity associated with the recreational use of the ketamine derivative methoxetamine. *Eur J Clin Pharmacol* 2012;**68**(5):853–6.

19. Wood DM, Davies S, Greene SL, *et al*. Case series of individuals with analytically confirmed acute mephedrone toxicity. *Clin Toxicol (Phila)* 2010;**48**:924–7.

20. Gibbons S. 'Legal highs' – novel and emerging psychoactive drugs: a chemical overview for the toxicologist. *Clin Toxicol (Phila)* 2012;**50**:15–24.

21. Spiller HA, Ryan ML, Weston RG, Jansen J. Clinical experience with and analytical confirmation of "bath salts" and "legal highs" (synthetic cathinones) in the United States. *Clin Toxicol (Phila)* 2011;**49**:499–505.

22. Jiménez-Jiménez FJ, García-Ruiz PJ, Molina JA. Drug-induced movement disorders. *Drug Saf* 1997;**16**:180–204.

23. Pasricha PJ, Pehlivanov N, Sugumar A, Jankovic J. Drug insight: from disturbed motility to disordered movement – a review of the clinical benefits and medicolegal risks of metoclopramide. *Nat Clin Pract Gastroenterol Hepatol* 2006;**3**:138–48.

24. Gueye PN, Hoffman JR, Taboulet P, Vicaut E, Baud FJ. Empiric use of flumazenil in comatose patients: limited applicability of criteria to define low risk. *Ann Emerg Med* 1996;**27**:730–5.

25. Hoffman JR, Schriger DL, Luo JS. The empiric use of naloxone in patients with altered mental status: a reappraisal. *Ann Emerg Med* 1991;**20**:246–52.

26. Mégarbane B, Buisine A, Jacobs F, *et al*. Prospective comparative assessment of buprenorphine overdose with heroin and methadone: clinical characteristics and response to antidotal treatment. *J Subst Abuse Treat* 2010;**38**:403–7.

27. Kintz P. Deaths involving buprenorphine: a compendium of French cases. *Forensic Sci Int* 2001;**12**:65–9.

28. Taboulet P, Michard F, Muszynski J, Galliot-Guilley M, Bismuth C. Cardiovascular repercussions of seizures during cyclic antidepressant poisioning. *J Toxicol Clin Toxicol* 1995;**33**:205–11.

29. Boehnert MT, Lovejoy FH Jr. Value of the QRS duration versus the serum drug level in predicting seizures and ventricular arrhythmias after an acute overdose of tricyclic antidepressants. *N Engl J Med* 1985;**313**:474–9.

30. Eddleston M, Buckley NA, Eyer P, Dawson AH. Management of acute organophosphorus pesticide poisoning. *Lancet* 2008;**371**:597–607.

31. Nozaki H, Hori S, Shinozawa Y, *et al.* Relationship between pupil size and acetylcholinesterase activity in patients exposed to sarin vapor. *Intensive Care Med* 1997;**23**:1005–7.

32. Hoffman RS. Treatment of patients with cocaine-induced arrhythmias: bringing the bench to the bedside. *Br J Clin Pharmacol* 2010;**69**:448–57.

33. Boyer EW, Shannon M. The serotonin syndrome. *N Engl J Med* 2005;**352**:1112–20.

34. Sternbach H. The serotonin syndrome. *Am J Psychiatry* 1991;**148**:705–13.

35. Isbister GK, Buckley NA, Whyte IM. Serotonin toxicity: a practical approach to diagnosis and treatment. *Med J Aust* 2007;**187**:361–5.

36. Hantson P, Duprez T. The value of morphological neuroimaging after acute exposure to toxic substances. *Toxicol Rev* 2006;**25**:87–98.

37. Zuccoli G, Siddiqui N, Cravo I, *et al.* Neuroimaging findings in alcohol-related encephalopathies. *AJR Am J Roentgenol* 2010;**195**:1378–84.

38. Tormoehlen LM. Toxic leukoencephalopathies. *Neurol Clin* 2011;**29**:591–605.

39. Heard K, Bebarta VS. Reliability of the Glasgow Coma Scale for the emergency department evaluation of poisoned patients. *Hum Exp Toxicol* 2004;**23**:197–200.

40. Chan B, Gaudry P, Grattan-Smith TM, McNeil R. The use of Glasgow Coma Scale in poisoning. *J Emerg Med* 1993;**11**:579–82.

41. Gentleman D, Dearden M, Midgley S, Maclean D. Guidelines for resuscitation and transfer of patients with serious head injury. *Br Med J* 1993;**307**:547–52.

42. Marik PE. Aspiration pneumonitis and aspiration pneumonia. *N Engl J Med* 2001;**344**:665–71.

43. Adnet F, Baud F. Relation between Glasgow Coma Scale and aspiration pneumonia. *Lancet* 1996;**348**:123–4.

44. Moulton C, Pennycook AG. Relation between Glasgow Coma Score and cough reflex. *Lancet* 1994;**343**:1261–2.

45. Galicia M, Nogue S, Miró O. Liquid ecstasy intoxication: clinical features of 505 consecutive emergency department patients. *Emerg Med J* 2011;**28**:462–6.

46. Yost DA. Acute care for alcohol intoxication. Be prepared to consider clinical dilemmas. *Postgrad Med* 2002;**112**:14–6, 21–2, 25–6.

47. Kelly CA, Upex A, Bateman DN. Comparison of consciousness level assessment in the poisoned patient using the alert/verbal/painful/unresponsive scale and the Glasgow Coma Scale. *Ann Emerg Med* 2004;**44**:108–13.

48. Duncan R, Thakore S. Decreased Glasgow Coma Scale score does not mandate endotracheal intubation in the emergency department. *J Emerg Med* 2009;**37**:451–5.

49. Muakkassa FF, Marley RA, Workman MC, Salvator AE. Hospital outcomes and disposition of trauma patients who are intubated because of combativeness. *J Trauma* 2010;**68**:1305–9.

50. Vale JA. Position statement: gastric lavage. American Academy of Clinical Toxicology; European Association of Poisons Centres and Clinical Toxicologists. *J Toxicol Clin Toxicol* 1997;**35**:711–19.

51. Chyka PA, Seger D. Position statement: single-dose activated charcoal. American Academy of Clinical Toxicology; European Association of Poisons Centres and Clinical Toxicologists. *J Toxicol Clin Toxicol* 1997;**35**:721–41.

Chapter 34

Metabolic encephalopathies: inborn errors of metabolism causing encephalopathies in adults

Frederic Sedel

SUMMARY

Inborn errors of metabolism (IEM) are caused by deficiencies in enzymes or other proteins involved in cell metabolism. Numerous IEM are treatable and it is therefore important to make the diagnosis before irreversible neurological lesions occur. Inborn errors of metabolism can present at any age from infancy to late adulthood, in some instances with unexplained coma or encephalopathy. These late-onset acute presentations are often triggered by apparently non-specific external factors such as benign fever episodes, prolonged exercise, prolonged fasting, surgery, etc. (1) Disorders of energy metabolism and (2) intoxication syndromes such as hyperammonemias, hyperhomocysteinemias, porphyrias, aminoacidopathies, and organic acidurias are the two main categories of IEM presenting with acute encephalopathies or coma. In such situations, the most important metabolic investigations are blood lactate and ammonia, followed by plasma, aminoacids, homocysteine, urinary organic acids, porphyrins, and porphobilinogen. Interpretation of biochemical results and corresponding treatments require a specific expertise obtained in specific reference centers.

Introduction

Inborn errors of metabolism (IEM) represent a subgroup of genetic disorders characterized by dysfunction of an enzyme or other protein involved in cellular metabolism. With around 500 different diseases identified to date, IEM as an entity represent about one third of genetic diseases. In contrast with other genetic disorders, the diagnosis of which relies predominantly on specific molecular analysis, diagnosis of IEM can usually be accomplished by biochemical analysis of blood and urine samples, which can be rapidly obtained in specialized metabolic laboratories. Inborn errors of metabolism can affect many organs, including liver, kidney, heart, and muscle, but in most cases they involve the nervous system and can present as neurological or psychiatric disorders. The first clinical symptoms usually manifest in infancy or childhood, but in a proportion of cases they can appear in adolescence or adulthood [1]. Late-onset forms of IEM presenting initially in adulthood are often unrecognized, so their exact prevalence is unknown. Most often they have psychiatric or neurological manifestations, such as acute encephalopathy or coma, atypical psychosis or depression, peripheral neuropathy, cerebellar ataxia, spastic paraparesis, dementia, movement disorders, leukodystrophy, or epilepsy [1–5].

In this chapter, we will discuss late-onset acute encephalopathies caused by IEM. Nevertheless, one should bear in mind that advances in treatment have allowed patients diagnosed in childhood to live to advanced ages. These forms of early-onset IEM maintained with specific treatments or regimen are likely to decompensate in adulthood when a specific treatment or a specific diet is stopped. These late decompensations may be catastrophic and this raises the need for specialized units in the management of these patients after the pediatric age.

Classification of IEM

From a pathophysiological point of view, with few exceptions, two major types of metabolic diseases can lead to acute encephalopathies: intoxication diseases and disorders of energy metabolism. Diseases in each of these groups share common clinical and radiological features, a similar clinical course, as well as similar diagnostic and therapeutic principles.

Brain Disorders in Critical Illness, ed. Robert D. Stevens, Tarek Sharshar, and E. Wesley Ely. Published by Cambridge University Press. © Cambridge University Press 2013.

Intoxication disorders

Intoxication disorders are related to the endogenous accumulation of an offending metabolite upstream of an enzymatic block (Table 34.1). Most often, the deficient enzyme lies in the liver but the toxic metabolites will impair the nervous system. Intoxication diseases include acute intermittent porphyrias, urea cycle disorders, organic acidurias (glutaric aciduria type 1, methylmalonic aciduria, propionic, isovaleric, and deficits in multiple carboxylase) and amino acidopathies (non-ketotic hyperglycinemia, maple syrup urine disease, homocystinurias, tyrosinemia). In most of these diseases, acute decompensation may occur under certain predisposing circumstances, often a catabolic event (intercurrent infection, fever, surgery, prolonged fasting), unusual protein intake, use of certain medications (valproate in urea cycle disorders, porphyrinogenic drugs). Beside acute encephalopathies, intoxication diseases may be responsible for chronic neurological or psychiatric disorders (leukoencephalopathies, psychiatric disorders, spastic paraparesis, dementia, etc.). The principle of treatment is to reduce the accumulation of a toxic metabolite by dialysis (hyperammonemia), cleansing drugs (sodium benzoate and phenylacetate in disorders of the urea cycle), synthesis inhibitors (heme arginate in acute attacks of porphyria), specific diets (protein-restricted diet in urea cycle disorders, organic acidurias, and amino acidopathies), or cofactors (betaine, folate, vitamin B12 in homocysteine remethylation disorders). The diagnosis of these diseases is based, depending on the clinical situation, on a relatively small number of laboratory tests including the determination of ammonemia, amino acids chromatography in plasma, urinary organic acids, the determination of homocysteine and the search for urinary porphyrins and porphobilinogen.

Energy metabolism disorders

Energy metabolism disorders (Table 34.2) constitute a group of diseases characterized by defects in ATP production by the mitochondria, either by malfunction of the respiratory chain itself; by dysfunction of upstream pathways (pyruvate dehydrogenase, Krebs cycle, fatty acids β oxidation) or of synthesis, recycling, or transport of co-factors (thiamine, biotin, riboflavin, coenzyme Q10). These diseases are likely to decompensate acutely in certain circumstances (benign infections, prolonged fasting, drugs). Some neurological or myopathic syndromes are immediately suggestive of an energy metabolism disorder. This is the case for Leigh syndrome, an acute necrotizing encephalopathy involving basal ganglia. Lesions are visible on brain MRI as bilateral and symmetrical hyperintensities of the putamen, caudate nuclei, thalami, dentate nuclei, and brainstem (see Figures 34.1 and 34.2). Rhabdomyolysis triggered by exercise or fasting strongly suggests a fatty acid β oxidation defect. Pseudo-strokes are very suggestive of mitochondrial diseases such as the MELAS syndrome (Mitochondrial Encephalopathy Lactic Acidosis and Stroke-Like Episodes). Status epilepticus can be a presentation of certain mitochondrial disorders such as *POLG1* mutations. Some of the energy metabolism disorders can be treated effectively by cofactors. High doses of thiamine (vitamin B1) may be effective in pyruvate dehydrogenase deficiency or in Wernicke-like encephalopathy caused by mutations in SLC19A3, a gene encoding the THTR-2 thiamine transporter [6]. Biotin may be effective in biotinidase deficiency, holocarboxylase synthase deficiency and in "Biotin responsive basal ganglia disease," a Leigh syndrome caused by SLC19A3 mutations [7]. Riboflavin may be efficacious in electron transport flavoprotein (ETF) dehydrogenase deficiency, and in certain Leigh syndromes caused by complex I deficiency. CoQ10 may work in CoQ10 synthesis disorders as well as in some "CoQ10 responsive Leigh syndromes." A ketogenic diet may be beneficial in pyruvate dehydrogenase deficiency.

The diagnosis of energy metabolism disorders can be difficult, especially in the case of respiratory chain disorders requiring muscle biopsy, measurement of different enzymatic complexes as well as complex genetic analyses not obtainable in an emergency department. In emergency situations, the exploration of energy metabolism is mainly based on simple blood, urinary, and eventually cerebrospinal fluid (CSF) measures of lactate, pyruvate, amino acids, and organic acids. Plasma acylcarnitines are mandatory in cases of rhabdomyolysis caused by fatty acid β oxidation defects [8].

Circumstances of diagnosis: when to think to an IEM?

The functioning of all organs being dependent on cell metabolism, it can be anticipated that IEM can affect

Table 34.1 Inborn errors of metabolism causing encephalopathies in adults: intoxications.

Disease	Mode of inheritance/ age at onset	Major clinical and radiological signs (late-onset forms)	Major biological disturbances	Treatment	Screening tests (mandatory tests in bold)
UCD	X-linked (OTC deficiency), AR/any age	Metabolic crisis triggered by high protein intake or catabolism: nausea, vomiting, cephalalgia confusion, psychiatric troubles, ataxia, stroke-like episodes, epilepsy, coma. MRI: normal or cerebral edema or high signal of the cortex on T2-weighted sequences. Subacute paraplegia in arginase deficiency	High ammoniemia above 80–100 µM and high glutamine. Other abnormalities depend on the metabolic block	Protein restriction, sodium benzoate or phenylbutyrate, L-arginine, dialysis	**Ammoniemia**, AAC, urinary orotic acid
MTHFR deficiency	AR/any age	Psychiatric troubles, confusion, coma, paraplegia, thromboembolic events, polyneuropathy. MRI : leukoencephalopathy	Homocysteine > 100 µM, low methionine, low folates	Folinic acid, betaine, cobalamin	**Homocysteinemia**, AAC, blood folates
CblC	AR/any age	Psychiatric troubles, confusion, subacute spinal cord degeneration, peripheral neuropathy, optic atrophy, retinitis pigmentosa, thromboembolic events, macrocytosis. MRI: leukoencephalopathy, high signal of spinal pyramidal tracts and posterior columns	Homocysteine > 100 µM, low methionine high methylmalonic aciduria	Hydroxocobalamin, folic acid, bétaine	Homocysteinemia, AAC, OAC
NKH	AR/any age	Acute signs: paroxysmal movement disorders, confusion, supranuclear gaze palsy Chronic signs: mental retardation, behavioral problems	Hyperglycinemia, hyperglycinuria, CSF/blood glycine ratio > 0.04	Sodium benzoate, dextromethorphan, ketamine	AAC
MSUD	AR/any age	Episodes of nausea, vomiting, encephalopathy, coma triggered by high protein intake or circumstances of high protein catabolism	High levels of leucine, valine, isoleucine, 2-oxo and 2-iso organic acids. Ketosis	Low branched-chain amino acids diet	**AAC**, OAC
Triple H syndrome	AR/any age	Episodes of nausea, vomiting, triggered by high protein intake, spastic paraparesis, cerebellar ataxia, mild mental retardation	High ornithine, ammoniemia, homocitrulline, orotic acid	Protein restriction, ornithine, arginine, or citrulline	**Ammoniemia**, AAC, urinary orotic acid
Glutaric aciduria type 1	AR/any age	Cephalalgia, oro-facial dyskinesias, supranuclear ophtalmoparesis, epilepsy, cognitive disorders, macrocephaly. MRI : leukoencephalopathy	High urinary glutaric acid and 3OH glutaric acid	Carnitine (Levocarnyl)	**OAC**, acylcarnitines profile
Propionic aciduria	AR/any age	Chorea, dementia, mental retardation, acute episodes of nausea or lethargia	High urinary propionic acid, glycine, 3OH propionate and propionyl glycine	Low branched-chain amino acids diet	**OAC**, acylcarnitines
Acute porphyrias	AD/adult	Acute signs: digestive signs, acute peripheral neuropathy, psychiatric troubles, confusion, epilepsy, dysautonomia hyponatremia, dark urines Chronic signs: cutaneous signs (coproporphyria, porphyria variegata)	High urinary excretion of δ-aminolevulinate and porphobilinogen	Avoid triggering factors, glucose and heme perfusion	Urinary δ-amino-levulinate and porphobilinogen
CBS deficiency	AR/any age	Mental retardation, psychiatric troubles, epilepsy, strokes, dystonia, thromboembolic events, Marfan-like appearance, lens dislocation, myopia	Hyperhomocysteinemia > 100 µM, hypermethioninemia	Vitamin B6, protein restriction diet	Homocysteinemia, AAC

AAC, amino acids chromatography (plasma); AD, autosomal dominant; AR, autosomal recessive; CBS, cystathionine beta synthase; CblC, cystathionine beta synthase; MSUD, maple syrup urines diseases; MTHFR, methylene tetrahydrofolate reductase; NKH, non-ketotic hyperglycinemia; OAC, organic acid chromatography (urines); OTC, ornithine transcarbamylase deficiency; UCD, urea cycle disorders.

Table 34.2 Inborn errors of metabolism (IEM) causing metabolic encephalopathies in adults: defects of energy metabolism.

Disease	Mode of inheritance/ age at onset	Major clinical and radiological signs (late-onset forms)	Major biological disturbances	Treatment	Screening tests
Defects of energy metabolism					
Coenzyme Q10 deficiency	AR/any age	(A) Myopathic form: myoglobinuria, exercise intolerance, central nervous system disorders (B) Ataxic form: cerebellar ataxia, epilepsy, pyramidal signs, mental retardation (C) Leigh's syndrome	Low respiratory chain activity restored by coenzyme Q10. Low levels of coenzyme Q10 (muscle biopsy)	Coenzyme Q10	Muscular biopsy with measurement of coenzyme Q10
PDH deficiency	X-linked or AR/ any age	Acute signs: Episodes of ataxia, dystonia, limb weakness, encephalopathy, coma triggered by fever or exercise Chronic signs: Mental retardation, axonal polyneuropathy, optic atrophy, movement disorders (dystonia, chorea, parkinsonism). MRI: normal or putaminal necrosis	High lactate and pyruvate in blood and CSF with low lactate/pyruvate ratio. Low PDH activity on leukocytes or fibroblasts	Vitamin B1	Blood lactate and pyruvate (before and 1 hour after lunch), CSF lactate and pyruvate
Fatty acid ß-oxidation defects	AR/any age	Acute signs: encephalopathy, coma, rhabdomyolysis, cardiac arrhythmias, liver dysfunction Chronic signs: cardiomyopathy, proximal myopathy (axonal polyneuropathy in trifunctional protein deficiency)	Non-ketotic hypoglycemia, high urinary dicarboxylic acids, high blood acylcarnitines	Avoid prolonged exercise or fasting, medium chain triglycerides	Acylcarnitines profile (blood), OAC
Cerebral glucose transporter (GLUT-1) deficiency	AD (de novo mutations)/child	Epilepsy, movement disorders, confusion, lethargy, triggered by fasting (morning)	Ratio of CSF/blood glucose below 0.4 (normal > 0.6)	Ketogenic diet, avoid fasting	Blood and CSF glucose (measured at the same time)
Biotinidase deficiency	AR/child or adolescence	Bilateral optic atrophy, spastic paraparesis, cerebellar ataxia, motor neuropathy, deafness, alopecia, seborrheic dermatitis	High lactate, high urinary 3OH isovalerate, 3OH propionate, 3 methylcrotonyl glycine, low biotinidase activity (erythrocytes)	Biotin	Lactates, OAC, therapeutic trial with biotin, biotinidase activity (blood)
Biotin responsive basal ganglia disease	AR/child	Acute signs: encephalopathy, coma, epilepsy, rigidity Chronic signs: dystonia. MRI: bilateral lesions of basal ganglia (head of caudate nuclei and putamen)	SLC19A3 gene mutations	Biotin	Therapeutic trial with high doses of biotin

AD, autosomal dominant; AR, autosomal recessive; OAC, organic acid chromatography (urines); PDH, pyruvate dehydrogenase.

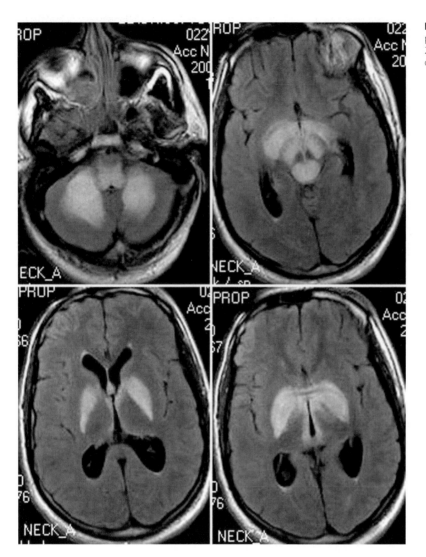

Figure 34.1 Leigh syndrome caused by pyruvate dehydrogenase deficiency in a 22-year-old male (F Sedel, unpublished observation).

all organs and cellular systems in all scenarios at any age and with all modes of transmission. But of course this does not mean that metabolic investigations are required in all patients! Two pitfalls await the clinician: to ignore some IEM amenable to life-saving treatments, or conversely, to conduct inappropriate unselected tests in clinical circumstances not suggestive of an IEM.

Inborn errors of metabolism involving the nervous system may present acutely as (1) "unexplained" encephalopathy or coma; (2) strokes or pseudo-strokes; (3) acute polyneuropathy mimicking a Guillain–Barré syndrome (mainly during attacks of acute intermittent porphyria); (4) acute or

subacute paraplegia, usually in the context of subacute combined degeneration of the spinal cord; (5) acute cerebellar ataxia (Table 34.3).

In all these situations, the following criteria are suggestive of an IEM, and each of them warrants specialized investigations.

The existence of a triggering factor

Metabolic encephalopathies are often triggered by an infectious event (often benign), situations of metabolic stress (surgery, intensive exercise), high protein intake or certain drugs. In clinical practice, there is a risk to misinterpret the trigger as the

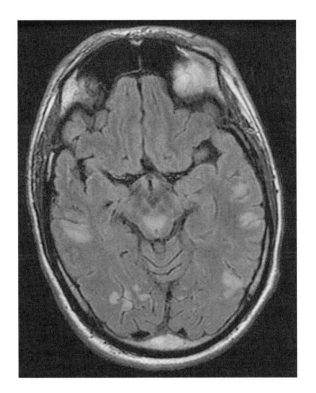
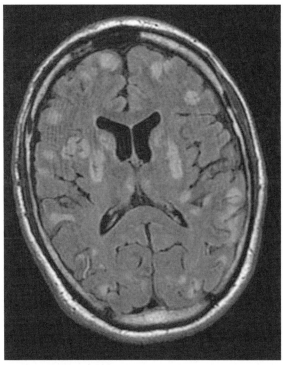
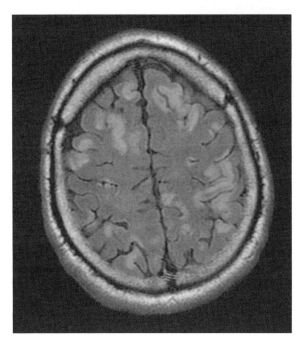

Figure 34.2 Leigh syndrome and diffuse encephalopathy in a 33-year-old male with SLC19A3 mutations. The patient recovered after treatment with very high dose of biotin and thiamine [7].

Table 34.3 Specialized metabolic investigations in acute situations.

Main clinical entries	Treatable metabolic diseases	Screening tests	First-line treatment*, **
Encephalopathy/ coma	UCD Homocysteine remethylation defects Porphyrias Organic acidurias Beta-oxidation defects Aminoacidopathies Biotin responsive basal ganglia disease Pyruvate dehydrogenase deficiency	Ammonemia Homocysteinemia Urinary porphyrins Urinary OAC Plasma acylcarnitines Plasma AAC Therapeutic trial with biotin Blood lactate, pyruvate	NH3 chelators***, stop protein intake, arginine Folinic acid, B12, betaine Heme arginate, high glucose infusion rate Carnitine, stop protein intake Carnitine, high glucose infusion rate Stop protein intake Very high doses of biotin Ketogenic diet
Strokes and pseudo-strokes	UCD Homocystinurias Respiratory chain disorders (MELAS) Alpha methyl acyl CoA racemase deficiency	Ammonemia Homocysteinemia Lactate/pyruvate Pristanic acid	 Arginine (to be evaluated) None
Acute polyneuropathy	Porphyrias Pyruvate dehydrogenase deficiency	Urinary porphyrins Blood lactate, pyruvate	
Acute/subacute paraplegia	Homocysteine remethylation defects Arginase deficiency Biotinidase deficiency Copper deficiency	Homocysteine Plasma AAC Therapeutic trial with biotin Copper, ceruloplasmin	 Stop protein intake, ammonia chelators Copper
Acute cerebellar ataxia	Pyruvate dehydrogenase deficiency UCD Respiratory chain disorders	Blood lactate, pyruvate Ammonemia Lactate/pyruvate	

AAC, amino acids chromatography; UCD, urea cycle disorders.
* For details, see Table 34.1. In all situations, mostly in UCD, homocystinurias, organic acidurias, and aminoacidopathies, it is important to stop protein catabolism.
** Sodium benzoate, sodium phenylbutyrate. In life-threatening situations, hemodialysis should be discussed.
*** D penicillamine, zinc, trientine.

sole cause of the disease. Indeed, during metabolic comas triggered by an infectious episode, a common raised diagnosis is "infectious encephalitis."

Brain MRI

The presence of bilateral lesions of the basal ganglia (Leigh syndrome, Figures 34.1 and 34.2) is pathognomonic for a disorder of energy metabolism and requires adequate investigations. Pseudo-strokes usually manifest as episodes of encephalopathy accompanied by cephalalgia, epilepsy, high signals of the cortex, and of the subcortical white matter with local edema (see below).

Family history

The existence of similar family history suggests the existence of a hereditary disease, however, given the usual recessive mode of inheritance of IEM, these diseases most often appear sporadically.

Personal history

The existence of similar episodes of decompensation from childhood is very important when they exist. The existence of a "childhood disease" followed for years in a specialized center, treated by diet or vitamin strongly suggests the existence of an underlying metabolic disease.

Diagnostic approach

Two main groups of IEM are responsible for encephalopathies in adults: intoxication syndromes and energy metabolism defects (Tables 34.1 and 34.2). In the first group MRI is usually normal or shows non-specific features [brain edema, generalized leukoencephalopathy, posterior reversible encephalopathy syndrome (PRES)], whereas in the second group MRI is almost always abnormal, showing bilateral lesions of basal ganglia (Leigh syndrome) or high signals of the cortex (stroke-like episodes). Thus, the diagnostic approach is mainly based on MRI.

In addition, some clinical signs suggest specific diagnoses. Encephalopathies in the context of urea cycle disorders, organic aciduria, and aminoacidopathies are usually associated with gastrointestinal symptoms such as nausea or vomiting. Porphyria crises are associated with abdominal pain, acute neuropathy, or hyponatremia. Homocysteine remethylation defects cause acute or subacute myelopathy and are often preceded by psychiatric symptoms lasting for months or years [9].

Fatty acid oxidation disorders usually cause muscular symptoms; however, patients with medium chain AcylCoA dehydrogenase (MCAD) deficiency may present with isolated encephalopathies starting in adolescence or adulthood with normal MRI.

Lastly, alpha-methyl-acyl-CoA racemase (AMACR) deficiency can cause a very severe relapsing encephalopathy [10]. Patients with this disease often have characteristic MRI findings including abnormal signals of thalami and brainstem, with cortical lesions mimicking infectious encephalitis or pseudo-strokes.

Some IEM cause ischemic strokes in adulthood. This is the case in Fabry disease and homocystinuria. In the former, strokes typically involve small arteries of the vertebrobasilar system, leading to acute deafness, vertigo, diplopia, and hemiplegia among others. In homocystinuria (cystathionine beta-synthase deficiency or homocysteine remethylation defects), thrombosis or dissection of large vessels (carotid arteries) is typically observed. Recently, ischemic brain lesions have also been reported in patients with Pompe disease. In addition, acute focal neurological signs mimicking strokes (pseudo-strokes) can be seen in patients with urea cycle disorders, Wilson's disease, mitochondriopathies, and AMACR deficiency. These pseudo-strokes differ from real strokes in that they do not correspond to usual arterial territories and are often associated with signs of encephalopathy, including cephalalgia, confusion, and epileptic seizures. A good way to distinguish pseudo-strokes from true ischemic strokes is diffusion imaging: the diffusion coefficient is typically normal or increased in the former and decreased in the latter. Another typical feature is that in pseudo-strokes, brain arteries imaging is normal despite extensive cortical signal abnormalities.

Metabolic testing: what to ask, what to expect?

In emergency situations the investigation protocol to identifying acute-onset metabolic diseases essentially comprises the simultaneous determination, in plasma and urine, of a set of metabolites that have to be carried out before any therapeutic intervention.

These investigations should include, in addition to standard biological investigations (electrolytes, urea, creatinine, etc.), arterial blood gas, analysis of blood ammonia, lactates, pyruvate, and urinary ketones.

The discovery of a metabolic acidosis with an anion gap is suggestive of organic acidurias or of lactic acidosis. A respiratory alkalosis is suggestive of hyperammonemia. Hyperlactacidemia and hypoglycemia without ketosis suggests a fatty acid β oxidation defect. Hyponatremia is observed in acute attacks or porphyria. However in many situations these first-line tests may be normal. Thus further investigations are needed. In the emergency, urine and plasma should be kept frozen for further specialized tests, such as the determination of homocysteine, plasma amino acids chromatography, urinary organic acids chromatography, the search for precursors of porphyrins, and plasma acylcarnitines profiles. These second-line investigations should be guided by the clinical context (see Table 34.3). Generally, it is recommended at this stage to contact a reference center for IEM since the interpretation of tests and the initiation of appropriate treatments require special expertise.

A few examples

Example 1. Hyperammonemia > 100 micromol/l is highly suggestive of a disorder of the urea cycle, but can also occur in cases of hepatic insufficiency, portosystemic shunts (sometimes with normal liver function), treatment with asparaginase, urinary tract infection by urease positive bacteria, and multiple myeloma [11,12]. Once hyperammonemia is found, plasma amino acids chromatography, the search for urinary orotic acid, and abdominal imaging are required. Glutamine is usually very high in urea cycle disorders whereas it remains normal or only slightly increased in other situations (shunt, myeloma, etc.). Low citrullinemia with high urine orotic acid strongly suggests ornithine transcarbamylase (OTC) deficiency, the most common urea cycle disorder in adulthood [3].

Example 2. Measurements of lactate and pyruvate are mandatory in case of Leigh syndrome to differentiate a mitochondrial respiratory chain disorder from pyruvate dehydrogenase deficiency. These measures should be repeated during the day (usually before and 1 hour after a meal, then a third time during the day). Increased pyruvate values (greater than 150–200 µmol/l) with a low lactate/pyruvate ratio around "10" suggests pyruvate dehydrogenase deficiency (or thiamine deficiency). This situation requires treatment with a high dose of thiamine (> 500 mg/day i.v.) and a ketogenic diet. In contrast, increased lactate with moderately high pyruvate (and thus with increased lactate/pyruvate ratio at 20 or greater) suggests a dysfunction of the respiratory chain or a sampling problem. Note that the interpretation of the lactate/pyruvate ratio has no diagnostic value in the absence of hyperlactacidemia. If there is a doubt concerning sampling, the existence of a hyper-alaninemia on amino-acids chromatography suggests a real pyruvate increase since excess pyruvate is trans-aminated into alanine in vivo.

Example 3. Hyperhomocysteinemia above 100 µmol/l together with hypomethioninemia suggests a disorder in the homocysteine remethylation pathway [9]. In this case, an increase of methylmalonic acid suggests B12 deficiency or a disorder of the B12 metabolism (such as CblC) while a normal methylmalonic acid suggests folate deficiency or MTHFR deficiency. In all cases, treatment is urgent and should combine parenteral vitamin B12 together with high doses of folic or folinic acid.

Example 4. In case of "biotin responsive basal ganglia disease" caused by SLC19A3 mutations, all laboratory tests are normal and only the positive response to a very high dose of biotine (5 to 10 mg/kg/day) and thiamine (500 mg/day) suggests the diagnosis [7].

Management

When a metabolic encephalopathy is suggested, therapeutic measures should be taken urgently based on first-line tests.

In any case, it is necessary to identify and treat a potential triggering factor (treatment of an infection, drug withdrawal, etc.).

Several practices are potentially harmful and must be avoided: (1) infusion of corticosteroids; (2) treatment with valproate; and (3) prolonged fasting (which would increase catabolism and worsen an energy metabolism defect).

In practice several situations do exist:

1. The suspicion of an intoxication disease (urea cycle disorder, aminoacidopathy, organic aciduria, porphyria) requires the cessation of protein intake and infusion of glucose solution to maintain an adequate caloric intake avoiding protein catabolism.

2. Treatment with folate and vitamin B12 intramuscularly (e.g., Lederfoline 25 mg three times a day) is required if a homocysteine remethylation disorder is suspected.

3. If an energy metabolism disorder is suspected e.g., brain imaging showing lesions of the basal ganglia suggestive of a Leigh syndrome, infusion of glucose is potentially harmful, especially in the case of pyruvate dehydrogenase deficiency. A ketogenic diet consisting mainly of fat (80% of calories) and proteins (15%) with low glucose (5%) should be introduced. In such situations, various cofactors of energy metabolism can be tested sequentially or in combination: thiamine (500 mg/day), biotin (10 mg/kg/day), riboflavin (60 mg/day) and/or coenzyme Q10 (Ubiten 10 mg/kg/day). However, CoQ10 can be harmful in the case of respiratory chain complex III deficiency (personal experience).

References

1. Sedel F. Inborn errors of metabolism in adults: a diagnostic approach to neurological and psychiatric presentations. In Saudubray J-M., Van den Berghe G, Walter JH, editors. *Inborn Metabolic Diseases.* 5th edn. Berlin: Springer-Verlag; 2012:55–74.

2. Lee PJ, Lachmann RH. Acute presentations of inherited metabolic disease in adulthood. *Clin Med* 2008;**8**(6):621–4.

3. Maillot F, Crenn P. Urea cycle disorders in adult patients. *Rev Neurol (Paris)* 2007;**163**(10):897–903.

4. Saudubray JM, Sedel F, Walter JH. Clinical approach to treatable inborn metabolic diseases: an introduction. *J Inher Metab Dis* 2006;**29**:261–74.

5. Sedel F, Lyon-Caen O, Saudubray JM. Therapy insight: inborn errors of metabolism in adult neurology – a clinical approach focused on treatable diseases. *Nat Clin Pract Neurol* 2007;**3**:279–90.

6. Kono S, Miyajima H, Yoshida K, *et al.* Mutations in a thiamine-transporter gene and Wernicke's-like encephalopathy. *N Engl J Med* 2009;**360**:1792–4.

7. Debs R, Depienne C, Rastetter A, *et al.* Biotin-Responsive Basal Ganglia Disease (BBGD) in Europeans with novel SLC19A3 mutations. *Arch Neurol* 2010;**67**(1):126–30.

8. Berardo A, DiMauro S, Hirano M. A diagnostic algorithm for metabolic myopathies. *Curr Neurol Neurosci Rep* 2010;**10**:118–26.

9. Michot JM, Sedel F, Giraudier S, Smiejan JM, Papo T. Psychosis, paraplegia and coma revealing

methylenetetrahydrofolate reductase deficiency in a 56 year-old woman. *J Neurol Neurosurg Psychiatry* 2008;**79**(8):963–4.

10. Kapina V, Sedel F, Truffert A, *et al*. Relapsing rhabdomyolysis due to peroxisomal α-methylacyl-CoA racemase deficiency. *Neurology* 2010;**75**(14):1300–2.

11. Weiss N, Levi C, Hussenet C, *et al*. A urinary cause of coma. *J Neurol* 2011;**258**(5):941–3.

12. Bénet B, Alexandra JF, Andrieu V, *et al*. Multiple myeloma presenting as hyperammonemic encephalopathy. *J Am Geriatr Soc* 2010;**58**(8): 1620–2.

Chapter 35

Encephalopathy associated with alcohol or drug withdrawal

Felix Kork and Claudia D. Spies

SUMMARY

Alcohol consumption causes numerous health problems, hospitalizations, and deaths. Despite increasing research activity in prevention, therapy, and detoxification, the absolute numbers of alcohol-related health damage have not changed over the last decade. Illicit drug use also causes health damage, depending on the substance used. Additionally, alcohol use disorder (AUD) and smoking are common comorbidities. Discontinuation of those substances leads to withdrawal symptoms, depending on the substance, the amount, and period of time of prior intake. Withdrawal syndromes can potentially be life threatening and are often seen in critical care medicine. Diagnosing, prevention, and treatment possibilities are presented within this chapter.

Diagnosing withdrawal syndromes in ICU patients can be difficult because of the complexity of possible differential diagnoses. Cognitive disorders and productive-psychotic symptoms such as hallucinations are difficult to recognize in intubated patients. Furthermore, before the diagnosis of a withdrawal syndrome can be established in ICU patients, common complications must be excluded.

Most of the treatment options in withdrawal syndromes can also be used to prevent those. Hence, the transition from prophylaxis to treatment can be continuous. Specific treatment should be symptom-oriented, regarding type and dosage adaptation to the severity of the symptoms. Specific treatment options depend on the substance of withdrawal.

Introduction

In 2010, 51.8% of Americans above 12 used alcohol, 27.3% tobacco products, and 8.9% illicit substances (www.samha.gov). The World Health Organization (www.who.int) identifies alcohol as the world's third largest risk factor for disease burden. In the USA, it is the largest risk factor, and in Europe it is the second largest risk factor. Its consumption affects the health of the consumer but also the health of others. Estimates suggest per capita pure ethanol consumption in the USA of 9.44 liters per year. In 2010 in the USA, approximately 46.7 million (15% of the population) engaged in binge drinking (five or more drinks on at least one occasion in the previous month) and approximately 15.6 million (5% of the population) were heavy drinkers (drinking five or more drinks per occasion on 5 or more days in the previous 30 days; www.cdc.gov). These numbers have only slightly varied during the past 5–10 years. Worldwide, alcohol consumption causes approximately 2.5 million deaths and an assumed 79,000 in the USA. The Centers for Disease Control and Prevention (CDC) report about 1.6 million hospitalizations and 4 million emergency room visits for alcohol-related conditions per year, costing billions [1].

The risk of being admitted to a hospital due to chronic alcohol misuse increases with the amount consumed daily. Chronic alcohol misuse is more common in surgical patients (e.g., up to 43% in otorhinolaryngological departments) than in psychiatric (30%) or neurological (19%) patients [2]. Alcohol influences many organ systems and promotes carcinogenesis. More than 50% of patients with carcinomas of the gastrointestinal tract are chronic alcoholics [3]. Patients who were injured while under the influence of alcohol occupy almost half of all trauma beds [4]. In addition to the life-threatening complications of alcohol withdrawal syndrome (AWS), the rate of morbidity and mortality due to infections, cardiopulmonary insufficiency, or bleeding disorders is 2–4 times greater in chronic alcoholics [5].

Brain Disorders in Critical Illness, ed. Robert D. Stevens, Tarek Sharshar, and E. Wesley Ely. Published by Cambridge University Press. © Cambridge University Press 2013.

In the perioperative setting, alcohol dependency has been linked to severe complications, all reasons qualifying for intensive care unit (ICU) admission: increased postoperative pneumonia and other infections as well as sepsis, adult respiratory distress syndrome (ARDS), cardiovascular complications, secondary hemorrhage, and other surgical complication as well as AWS [6]. All of these complications affect patients' outcomes after surgery, trauma, or critical illness [7].

Alcohol withdrawal syndrome occurs in approximately 25% of intensive care patients. It may be the reason for the admission or it may occur during the ICU stay as result of the withdrawal and may lead to a life-threatening state. More importantly, its mortality is significantly dependent on whether AWS is treated or not: AWS untreated results in mortality of 15% that can be reduced to mortality of 2% when treated [5].

Illicit drug use can cause a variety of diseases and predispositions depending on the substance used. Polydrug use is frequently observed and especially AUD and smoking are relevant comorbidities in most clinical cases [8]. Equally, the withdrawal syndrome highly depends on the substance(s) used. Drug withdrawal syndromes present diverse clinical appearances. Although the intensivist is most commonly confronted with acute life-threatening intoxications, drug withdrawal can – depending on the substrate withdrawn – also impose as such. For most drug withdrawal syndromes, there is no evidence-based specific therapy, and craving remains the major symptom. Acute states of arousal can be treated symptom-oriented with benzodiazepines or alpha agonists, yet lacking sufficient evidence against or for it. Therefore, only specifics on certain substances will be presented.

Pathophysiology

Effects of alcohol on cellular level

The effects of ethanol on neuronal systems are complex [9]: the pharmacological effects of ethanol are non-selective but very specific. Due to its mainly hydrophilic and also lipophilic functional groups, ethanol is well soluble in water and poorly soluble in lipids. This characteristic is responsible for its possible effects on membrane organization, the function of membrane-bound enzymes, enzymes and proteins involved in signal transduction, ion channels, receptor-coupled ionophores, carrier proteins, and gene expression. Additionally, ethanol affects discrete sites on particular proteins that are relevant for its function and consequently for cell and system functioning.

Effects of chronic ethanol exposure on NMDA receptors

One criterion for dependence is the development of tolerance to the substance, a kind of learning process. N-methyl-D-aspartate (NMDA) receptors are of relevance in neuro-adaptational processes such as learning and memory and in phenomena such as conditioning and associative learning. Supposedly, the development of tolerance to substances is also facilitated via NMDA receptors. The blockade of NMDA receptor antagonists has been shown to prevent tolerance to substances such as morphine, benzodiazepines, and also ethanol. In this manner, dizocilpine and ketamine are able to prevent the development of tolerance to alcohol-induced ataxia, hypothermia, and hypnotic effects. These effects seem to be redeemable as well when the antagonists are administered after ethanol consumption.

Effects of chronic ethanol exposure on GABA receptors

Gamma-aminobutyric acid (GABA) is an inhibitory neurotransmitter in the brain and the data on $GABA_A$ receptors on response to ethanol are inconclusive. A number of studies reported a potentiation of $GABA_A$ receptor response by ethanol, while other studies could not confirm this effect. Interestingly, $GABA_A$ receptors vary in response to ethanol in different regions of the brain. Chronic ethanol exposure differentially modifies the expression of $GABA_A$ receptor subunits e.g., in the cerebral cortex and hippocampus. The mechanism of this difference is not well understood. Current theories favor ethanol-induced changes in $GABA_A$ receptor function to be caused by a change in subunit stoichiometry of the receptor by chronic alcohol exposure [10].

Alcohol withdrawal

Chronic alcohol exposure exerts numerous pharmacological effects by means of interactions with various neurotransmitters and neuromodulators. During chronic ethanol administration, compensatory changes can result in an up-regulation of glutamatergic transmission. This is mainly caused by an up-regulation of NMDA receptors and a decreased

GABA$_A$ receptor function and leads to equilibrium in the presence of ethanol but results in withdrawal hyperactivity in the absence of ethanol [11].

The most widely accepted mechanism of adaptation to chronic ethanol exposure is up-regulation of the cyclic adenosine monophosphate (cAMP) pathway. Whereas acute ethanol exposure stimulates the cAMP pathway in many neurons in the brain, chronic exposure is inhibiting, therefore leading to a compensatory up-regulation of the cAMP pathway in certain brain regions. Upon removal of the drug, the up-regulated cAMP pathway can overshoot and contribute to features of withdrawal. Up-regulation of the cAMP pathway interferes with glutamatergic, GABAergic, dopaminergic, serotonergic, and opioidergic actions of the neurons [12].

Because of the various neurotransmitter systems affected, it is not surprising to find a complex pathophysiology of AWS [9]. On the one hand, there is an increased activity of excitatory mechanisms; on the other hand, there is a decreased function of inhibitory systems. Withdrawal also seems to interact with the hypothalamic-pituitary-adrenal axis. An increase in corticotropin-releasing factor and a decrease in ß-endorphin has been reported after alcohol withdrawal, which has been suggested to predispose patients to relapse to alcohol misuse. Kindling phenomena are reported after repeated withdrawal, i.e., there is evidence for sensitization so that repeated withdrawals become progressively more severe. However, treatment of withdrawal may retard this sensitization process. Despite long-term abstinence, selective changes such as loss of serotonergic or GABAergic neurotransmission may persist [5].

Diagnosis

World Health Organization Taxonomy: F10.3 and F10.4

The *International Statistical Classification of Diseases and Related Health Problems* (ICD–10) requires encoding withdrawal states in Chapter V (F), mental and behavioral disorders (http://apps.who.int/classifications/apps/icd/). The subsection F1, mental and behavioral disorders due to substance use is subdivided by the causative substances (0–9 representing the substance, e.g., 0 = alcohol). The last digit of the code represents the actual disorder that is caused and is similar for all substances, e.g., 3 represents 'withdrawal state' and 4

'withdrawal state with delirium'. Specific symptoms are only provided for delirium tremens, yet lacking definite criteria for the diagnosis.

Diagnostic and Statistical Manual of Mental Disorders classification: 291.0 and 291.81

The more accurate taxonomy and diagnostic tool for mental disorders, the *Diagnostic and Statistical Manual of Mental Disorders*, Fourth Edition (DSM–IV), provides the user explicitly with criteria that have to be fulfilled completely to diagnose alcohol withdrawal and alcohol withdrawal delirium. Contrary to the ICD–10 classification, the DSM–IV rather subsumes by symptoms than categories of disease: whereas "alcohol withdrawal" is categorized under *Substance-related Disorders*, "alcohol withdrawal delirium" is categorized under *Delirium, Dementia, and Amnestic and Other Cognitive Disorders* [13]. Unlike the ICD–10, the DSM–IV only provides diagnoses of withdrawal and withdrawal delirium for (a) alcohol (with possible delirium), (b) amphetamines, (c) cocaine, (d) nicotine, (e) opioids, (f) sedatives, hypnotics and anxiolytics (with possible delirium), or other (with possible delirium).

Detection

The Alcohol Use Disorder Identification Test (AUDIT) presents a well-established screening tool for the detection of AUD [14] and can be enhanced by laboratory testing [7]. The AUDIT is a 10-item questionnaire that is more suited for differentiation of AUD severity ranging from risky use to dependence. Ten questions sum up to a score between 0 and 40 points. The test is positive when more than 8 points are counted. The AUDIT has been criticized for its length, yet an advantage of the AUDIT is its validation for use by a proxy. This can be helpful to objectify AUD in ICU patients who may be incapable of answering questions due to their severity of illness and consequent use of sedatives or the need of mechanical ventilation [15].

Standard laboratory parameters for detecting AUD are mean corpuscular volume (MCV), gamma-glutamyl transpeptidase (GGT), and carbohydrate-deficient transferrin (CDT). Yet, sensitivity and specificity differ depending on the population tested and none of the markers is sufficiently sensitive [16–19]. These biomarkers should be tested as early as possible after hospitalization since they are altered by hemorrhage or volume substitution. Still, no biomarker is capable of discriminating alcohol dependency from AUD. High blood alcohol concentrations indicate tolerance, which is linked to dependence. Ethylglucuronide or other ethanol metabolites may be useful to monitor abstinence because detection is possible for a longer period in blood or urine [7].

Whereas heavy users or dependent patients of all substances are often easily detected – especially when intoxicated or consumption has become the primary aim – illicit substance use is poorly reported and detected [8]. Severity of withdrawal commonly depends on the amount of regular consumption before cessation.

Severity evaluation

The ICD–10 and DSM–IV–TR both describe the symptoms of AWS as heterogeneous. The severity of the alcohol withdrawal can be assessed using the Clinical Institute Withdrawal Assessment of Alcohol Scale, revised (CIWA-Ar). The CIWA-Ar is a 10-item scale including (1) nausea and vomiting, (2) tremor, (3) paroxysmal sweats, (4) anxiety, (5) agitation, (6) tactile disturbances, (7) auditory disturbances, (8) visual disturbances, (9) headaches, and (10) orientation and clouding of sensorium. Medication should be titrated until the CIWA-Ar score is ≤ 10 points. The CIWA-Ar is standard in monitoring symptom-triggered therapy in the general hospital setting but not evaluated for the ICU setting. It can be used by nursing staff but requires the patient to be conscious. Another less commonly used scale for assessing the severity of AWS is that developed by Cushman [20,21]. It contains (1) heart rate, (2) systolic blood pressure, (3) respiratory frequency, (4) tremor, (5) sweating, (6) agitation, and (7) sensoric disorders. Withdrawal from opiates can be monitored using the "Objective Opiate Withdrawal Scale" (OOWS) and the "Subjective Opiate Withdrawal Scale" (SOWS). The Delirium Detection Score (DDS) is evaluated to monitor delirium and treatment success on the ICU and may be an alternative [22].

Differential diagnosis: I WATCH DEATH

Diagnosing AWS in ICU patients is difficult in many cases for the complexity of possible differential diagnoses. Additionally, cognitive disorders and productive-psychotic symptoms such as hallucinations are difficult to recognize in intubated patients. Before the diagnosis of withdrawal syndromes can be established in an ICU patient, common ICU complications, such as bleeding, metabolic, or electrolyte disorders, infection, hypoxia, pain, or focal neurological signs must be excluded. The acronym "I WATCH DEATH" (standing for: Infections, Withdrawal, Acute metabolic, Trauma, Central nervous system pathology, Hypoxia, Deficiencies, Endocrinopathies, Acute vascular events, Toxins/drugs, Heavy metals) can render assistance. The complex differential diagnosis and the symptoms being rather common in ICU patients, adequate therapy is in danger of being delayed and the patient's condition may deteriorate [5]. Since each of the differential diagnoses requires a specific therapy, differentiation is of utmost importance. Consequences are equally severe either in delaying AWS therapy for unnecessary diagnostics in the search for somatic causes or in misconceiving a somatic disorder for an AWS. Unfortunately, there is no failsafe way to a correct diagnosis. Taking exact anamneses, third-party anamneses, conducting thorough physical examinations, systematically eliminating possible differential diagnoses as well as closely monitoring the patient for improvement or deterioration can emphasize or annihilate existing suspicions of the cause for the patients' condition.

Prevention of withdrawal, delirium, and sequelae

Prediction of alcohol withdrawal syndrome

Delay of delirium therapy worsens patient outcome by increasing morbidity and mortality. Early treatment could be facilitated if prediction of AWS was simple. It would also prevent patients from deteriorating when AWS transits into delirium tremens. One of the strongest predictors for the development of AWS is either a personal or family history of AWS or delirium tremens. The literature suggests that African American patients develop less severe AWS than other hospital admissions. Both these factors indicate a possible genetic predisposition to develop AWS. Biochemical and other clinical measurements such as aminotransferases, magnesium, erythrocyte parameters, histopathological cirrhosis, are of doubtful prediction quality. A few small studies have shown homocysteine levels to be helpful in the prediction of seizures and admission ethanol levels ≥ 150 mg/dl to be a rather good predictor in at-risk patients for severity of AWS [23].

Preoperative preventive measures

Length of stay in the ICU and other postoperative complications are increased in AUD patients and can be decreased, when prophylaxis is applied in patients having AUD and drinking more than 60 g ethanol daily [5,24,25]. In these patients, postoperative AWS can be reduced from 50% to 25% if preventive measures are taken [5,24]. Hence, prevention needs to start before elective surgery and preoperative abstinence or even detoxification could be an option for patients with scheduled surgery. Furthermore, alcohol-induced pathophysiological alterations and dysfunctions are potentially reversible and 3–8 weeks abstinence before surgery will significantly reduce the incidence of several serious postoperative complications, such as wound and cardiopulmonary complications as well as infections [26]. Brief interventions, non-confronting short conversations based on FRAMES criteria (Feedback, Responsibility, Advice, Menu of Options, Empathy), have been shown to decrease alcohol consumption and result in reduction of withdrawal and delirium [27].

A randomized controlled trial has shown that benzodiazepines, alpha-2 agonists, and neuroleptics as well as ethanol were equally efficient in pharmacological prophylaxis of AWS in ICU patients [28]. Additionally, patients with AWS show an augmented stress response to surgical trauma, induced by the hypothalamic-pituitary-adrenal (HPA) axis. Perioperative treatment, e.g., with low-dose morphine or if consented by the patient 0.5 g ethanol per day, has been shown to block this response and decrease postoperative pneumonia rate and ICU length of stay [29].

General preventive measures

Patients with severe AUD often suffer from dehydration in the form of intravascular volume depletion and have a high prevalence of various electrolyte abnormalities such as hypokalemia, hypomagnesemia, and hypophosphatemia. Additionally, they often suffer from malnutrition and therefore metabolic acidosis. Compensation of these disorders should be striven for and facilitated promptly since they may worsen the clinical situation and lead to the development of further complications, such as cardiac arrhythmias [15,23].

Wernicke's encephalopathy and Korsakoff's psychosis

Alcohol abuse is a possible cause of vitamin B1 (thiamine) deficiency. It can lead to Wernicke's encephalopathy or Korsakoff's psychosis. Wernicke's encephalopathy is usually characterized by oculomotor abnormalities, cerebellar dysfunctions and an altered mental state, Korsakoff's psychosis by confabulation, disorientation, and retrograde as well as anterograde amnesia and both can present jointly as Wernicke–Korsakoff syndrome. Critically ill patients with a history of AUD are at increased risk to develop either or both of these disorders and should be treated parenterally over several days with 200 mg of thiamine [7,15].

Delirium

There exist several non-pharmacologic preventive measures for delirium of any cause. The patients' circadian rhythm should be maintained (prevention of sleep deprivation, mobilization during the day) and (re)orientation should be supported by providing visual and hearing aids and time of day as early as possible [27] (see also Chapter 24, this volume).

Treatment of withdrawal syndromes

Treatment of alcohol withdrawal syndrome

Alcohol withdrawal syndrome should be treated early in order to avoid deterioration of symptoms and to reduce the ICU length of stay. Delirium management in ICU patients should be protocol-based with continuous re-evaluation [30] for sedation and pain management. Unfortunately, there are no evidence-based guidelines for the treatment of AWS in the ICU setting. Evidence-based guidelines for treatment in non-ICU settings recommend sedative or hypnotic agents that are capable of reducing duration of AWS and mortality. While psychiatric patients usually receive monotherapy, more than half of ICU patients require a combination of medications. The most frequently used drug category for the treatment of AWS is benzodiazepines because of their comparatively high safety margin and the most extensive data. Most of the drugs used to treat AWS can also be used to prevent AWS. Hence, the transition from prophylaxis to treatment can be continuous.

Benzodiazepines

Benzodiazepines have been shown to effectively reduce withdrawal severity, incidence of delirium and seizures with a greater margin of safety and lower abuse potential when compared with other therapies. The rationale of the use of benzodiazepine is to modulate CNS hyperactivity due to the alcohol withdrawal by interacting with GABA receptors.

Administration of benzodiazepines should be symptom-triggered (see scores above) rather than on a fixed schedule since symptom-triggered therapy results in lower incidence of pneumonia, a decrease of ventilation time and hospital length of stay [30]. There is little evidence that supports favoring one benzodiazepine over another. A Cochrane database review including systematic reviews on the efficacy and safety of pharmacological interventions for the treatment of AWS found that (1) benzodiazepines performed better for seizures than other treatments (moderate evidence); (2) benzodiazepines performed better than antipsychotics for seizures compared with other treatment options (high level of evidence); and that (3) between benzodiazepines, chlordiazepoxide performed best [31]. Thus, benzodiazepines show a protective benefit against alcohol withdrawal symptoms, in particular seizures, when compared with placebo and a potentially protective benefit for many outcomes when compared with antipsychotic drugs. The review included inpatients and outpatients and therefore applicability for the ICU setting may be doubted. Moreover, the favored substance chlordiazepoxide can only be administered orally and its use in ICU patients is frequently not possible. Yet, in several ICU studies, benzodiazepines have been shown to be beneficial against AWS, especially seizures, and should be used to treat agitation, anxiety, and seizures, preferably with long-acting substances [25,30–32].

Alpha agonists

Clonidine or dexmedetomidine can be used to decrease central sympathetic activity and plasma catecholamine levels resulting in attenuation of autonomic signs, such as tachycardia and tremor. Yet, they do not have any effect on the occurrence of AWS or seizures. A systematic review found clonidine and dexmedetomidine may provide additional benefit as adjunctive treatment to benzodiazepines in treating AWS [33].

Neuroleptics

Neuroleptics are commonly and successfully used in ICU patients, mostly in combination with sedatives. There is evidence that neuroleptic monotherapy in AWS results in adverse outcome. Neuroleptics furthermore have a proconvulsive effect and low therapeutic index. They can cause QT prolongation and neuroleptic malignant syndrome.

Anticonvulsants

Despite the widespread use of anticonvulsants, their exact role for the treatment of alcohol withdrawal has not yet been adequately assessed. They sometimes are used to prevent seizures. It is unknown whether different anticonvulsants and different forms of administration may have the same merits.

Gamma-hydroxybutyric acid

Gamma-hydroxybutyric acid (GHBA) is also an effective treatment option for AWS. In surgical ICU patients, it has been shown to reduce autonomic nervous system symptoms, but cannot successfully treat hallucinations [5]. Evidence for the application on the ICU is very limited. Withdrawal from chronic GHBA consumption can also cause withdrawal. There are also case reports describing severe delirium after cessation of GHBA in dependent patients.

Ethanol

Although oral or intravenous ethanol administration has been used to treat alcohol withdrawal delirium in a few uncontrolled trials, it is not recommended because of its inconsistent pharmacokinetic profile, its narrow therapeutic index, and the potential adverse effects [34].

Baclofen

Lately baclofen has been revived for the treatment of AWS, although a recent Cochrane Database review found the evidence of recommending baclofen for AWS to be insufficient [35].

Treatment of opioid withdrawal

Substitution

The opioid-dependent patient requires substitution in order to prevent withdrawal, unless detoxification was planned. Substitution can be conducted by either Polamidone or buprenorphine and should be done upon consultation with a specialist. The substitution can be considered as baseline opioid maintenance, should be extended with opioids as required, and can be monitored using the "Objective Opiate Withdrawal Scale" (OOWS) and the "Subjective Opiate Withdrawal Scale" (SOWS). Besides patient testimony, monitoring for clinical signs of over- and underdosing is necessary. Additionally, patients require laxatives and are at risk of hyperhidrosis.

Antagonization

Administration of antagonists induces a severe withdrawal syndrome in opioid-dependent patients and causes – even under general anesthesia – a heavy cardiovascular stimulation and often life-threatening hypokalemia. Antagonists should therefore only be administered in severe intoxication, titrated to return of spontaneous respiration, since overdone antagonization endangers patients with organ dysfunction.

Detoxification programs

Besides substitution treatment and later detoxification of the substitution, possibilities are limited to "cold turkey." Both methods are feared by opioid-dependent patients and both are associated with high drop-out rates. Especially abortive weaning from Polamidone is common, due to the long substance half-life.

Treatment of cocaine withdrawal

The main symptoms of cocaine withdrawal are fatigue, depressed mood, and a strong craving that can already be observed after the first intake's effect fades. Agitation, psychomotor activation, and restlessness are seldom the main symptoms of cocaine withdrawal. Cocaine withdrawal commonly does not result in delirium and poses no acute life-threatening state. In heavy users withdrawal can lead to major depression and suicide. Often, patients try to soothe their withdrawal and (over-)compensate with intake of alcohol or benzodiazepines. There are pharmacotherapeutic treatment options for cocaine addiction that relieve withdrawal symptoms, evaluated for outpatient detoxification programs.

Treatment of amphetamine withdrawal

The DSM–IV–TR criteria of amphetamine withdrawal include dysphoric mood and two or more symptoms of the following: fatigue, vivid or unpleasant dreams, insomnia or hypersomnia, increased appetite, and psychomotor agitation or retardation that occur following discontinuation of the drug. Most patients experience amphetamine withdrawal as clinically severe and report suicide thoughts and attempts. Typically, withdrawal symptoms start within 24 hours after the last use and begin most likely with increased sleep, appetite, and depressive mood ("crash"). Symptoms can be measured using the Amphetamine Withdrawal

Questionnaire or the Amphetamine Selective Severity Assessment [36,37]. Most of the symptoms disappear in a week or less, while some symptoms, may continue for weeks or months.

References

1. Epidemiology, AALS. *Health Disparities and Inequalities Report – United States.* 2011. http://www.cdc.gov/mmwr/pdf/other/su6001.pdf. (Accessed December 12, 2011)

2. Vokes EE, Weichselbaum RR, Lippman SM, *et al.* Head and neck cancer. *N Engl J Med* 1993;**328**:184–94.

3. Seitz HK, Maurer B, Stickel F. Alcohol consumption and cancer of the gastrointestinal tract. *Dig Dis* 2005;**23**:297–303.

4. Gentilello LM, Donovan DM, Dunn CW, *et al.* Alcohol interventions in trauma centers. Current practice and future directions. *JAMA* 1995;**274**:1043–8.

5. Spies CD, Rommelspacher H. Alcohol withdrawal in the surgical patient: prevention and treatment. *Anesth Analg* 1999;**88**:946–54.

6. Schiemann A, Hadzidiakos D, Spies C. Managing ICU delirium. *Curr Opin Crit Care* 2011;**17**:131–40.

7. Kork F, Neumann T, Spies C. Perioperative management of patients with alcohol, tobacco and drug dependency. *Curr Opin Anaesthesiol* 2010;**23**:384–90.

8. Kleinwächter R, Kork F, Weiss-Gerlach E, *et al.* Improving the detection of illicit substance use in preoperative anesthesiological assessment. *Minerva Anestesiol* 2010;**76**:29–37.

9. Fadda F, Rossetti ZL. Chronic ethanol consumption: from neuroadaptation to neurodegeneration. *Prog Neurobiol* 1998;**56**:385–431.

10. Lingford-Hughes A, Nutt D. Neurobiology of addiction and implications for treatment. *Br J Psychiatry* 2003;**182**:97–100.

11. Hughes JR. Alcohol withdrawal seizures. *Epilepsy Behav* 2009;**15**:92–7.

12. Pandey SC. The gene transcription factor cyclic AMP-responsive element binding protein: role in positive and negative affective states of alcohol addiction. *Pharmacol Ther* 2004;**104**:47–58.

13. American Psychiatric Association. *Diagnostic and Statistical Manual of Mental Disorders, Fourth edition, Text Revision* (DSM–IV–TR). Washington, DC: American Psychiatric Association; 2000.

14. National Institute for Health and Clinical Excellence. *Alcohol-use Disorders: Preventing the Development of Hazardous and Harmful Drinking.* 2010. www.nice.org.uk/guidance/PH24. (Accessed November 4, 2011)

15. Moss M, Burnham EL. Alcohol abuse in the critically ill patient. *Lancet* 2006;**368**:2231–42.

16. Eggers V, Tio J, Neumann T, *et al.* Blood alcohol concentration for monitoring ethanol treatment to prevent alcohol withdrawal in the intensive care unit. *Intensive Care Med* 2002;**28**:1475–82.

17. Kip MJ, Spies CD, Neumann T, *et al.* The usefulness of direct ethanol metabolites in assessing alcohol intake in nonintoxicated male patients in an emergency room setting. *Alcohol Clin Exp Res* 2008;**32**:1284–91.

18. Miller PM, Spies C, Neumann T, *et al.* Alcohol biomarker screening in medical and surgical settings. *Alcohol Clin Exp Res* 2006;**30**:185–93.

19. Neumann T, Spies C. Use of biomarkers for alcohol use disorders in clinical practice. *Addiction* 2003;**98** (Suppl):281–91.

20. Cushman P, Forbes R, Lerner W, *et al.* Alcohol withdrawal syndromes: clinical management with lofexidine. *Alcohol Clin Exp Res* 1985;**9**:103–8.

21. Cushman P. Clonidine and alcohol withdrawal. *Adv Alcohol Subst Abuse* 1987;**7**:17–28.

22. Luetz A, Heymann A, Radtke FM, *et al.* Different assessment tools for intensive care unit delirium: which score to use? *Crit Care Med* 2010;**38**:409–18.

23. Sarff M, Gold JA. Alcohol withdrawal syndromes in the intensive care unit. *Crit Care Med* 2010;**38**:S494–501.

24. Spies CD, Nordmann A, Brummer G, *et al.* Intensive care unit stay is prolonged in chronic alcoholic men following tumor resection of the upper digestive tract. *Acta Anaesthesiol Scand* 1996;**40**:649–56.

25. Spies CD, Dubisz N, Neumann T, *et al.* Therapy of alcohol withdrawal syndrome in intensive care unit patients following trauma: results of a prospective, randomized trial. *Crit Care Med* 1996;**24**:414–22.

26. Tønnesen H, Nielsen PR, Lauritzen JB, *et al.* Smoking and alcohol intervention before surgery: evidence for best practice. *Br J Anaesth* 2009;**102**:297–306.

27. Paupers M, Schiemann A, Spies CD. Alcohol withdrawal and delirium in the intensive care unit. *Neth J Crit Care* 2012;**16**(3):84–92.

28. Spies CD, Dubisz N, Funk W, *et al.* Prophylaxis of alcohol withdrawal syndrome in alcohol-dependent patients admitted to the intensive care unit after tumour resection. *Br J Anaesth* 1995;**75**:734–9.

29. Spies C, Eggers V, Szabo G, *et al.* Intervention at the level of the neuroendocrine-immune axis and postoperative pneumonia rate in long-term alcoholics. *Am J Respir Crit Care Med* 2006;**174**:408–14.

30. Spies CD, Otter HE, Hüske B, *et al.* Alcohol withdrawal severity is decreased by symptom-orientated adjusted bolus therapy in the ICU. *Intensive Care Med* 2003;**29**:2230–8.

31. Amato L, Minozzi S, Davoli M. Efficacy and safety of pharmacological interventions for the treatment of the alcohol withdrawal syndrome. *Cochrane Database Syst Rev* 2011;CD008537.

32. Amato L, Minozzi S, Vecchi S, *et al.* Benzodiazepines for alcohol withdrawal. *Cochrane Database Syst Rev* 2010;CD005063.

33. Muzyk AJ, Fowler JA, Norwood DK, *et al.* Role of α2-agonists in the treatment of acute alcohol withdrawal. *Ann Pharmacother* 2011;**45**:649–57.

34. Mayo-Smith MF, Beecher LH, Fischer TL, *et al.* Management of alcohol withdrawal delirium. An evidence-based practice guideline. *Arch Intern Med* 2004;**164**:1405–12.

35. Liu J, Wang L. Baclofen for alcohol withdrawal. *Cochrane Database Syst Rev* 2011;CD008502.

36. Shoptaw SJ, Kao U, Heinzerling K, *et al.* Treatment for amphetamine withdrawal. *Cochrane Database Syst Rev* 2009;CD003021.

37. Srisurapanont M, Jarusuraisin N, Jittiwutikan J. Amphetamine withdrawal: I. Reliability, validity and factor structure of a measure. *Aust N Z J Psychiatry* 1999;**33**:89–93.

Chapter 36

Posterior reversible encephalopathy syndrome (PRES): the essential elements

Walter S. Bartynski and Hebah M. Hefzy

SUMMARY

Posterior reversible encephalopathy syndrome (PRES) is a syndrome which has non-specific clinical features coupled with a unique and usually specific appearance on computed tomography (CT) or magnetic resonance (MR) imaging. Posterior reversible encephalopathy syndrome most commonly occurs in the setting of pregnancy (preeclampsia/eclampsia), allogeneic or solid organ transplantation, autoimmune disease, infection/sepsis/shock, or following cancer chemotherapy, conditions which have or can have significant immune system challenges including T-cell and endothelial activation. Clinically, patients present with altered mentation, headache, vision disturbance, and/or generalized seizures. Evidence of systemic inflammatory response and multiple organ dysfunction syndrome are often observed (thrombocytopenia, renal, hepatic, and/or pulmonary dysfunction). Treatment of PRES includes withdrawal or management of the offending trigger and management of evolving critical clinical events including seizure activity, hypertension, and organ hypoperfusion. In most instances the clinical neurotoxicity and imaging features disappear without sequelae, hence the term "reversible."

Introduction

Posterior reversible encephalopathy syndrome (PRES) is a condition characterized by non-specific clinical presentation coupled with unique findings on CT or MR imaging studies [1]. Posterior reversible encephalopathy syndrome was originally described in association with pregnancy (eclampsia), following solid organ or hematopoietic transplantation, and in patients with significant hypertension [1] who had abnormalities primarily identified in the posterior portions of the cerebral hemispheres [2]. Pathogenesis is believed to reflect an immunological mechanism [3].

Basic clinical and imaging features seen in PRES

Clinically, patients usually present with headache, vision disturbance, and altered mentation (30%) or seizures (70%). Cortical blindness has been seen in severe cases of PRES, and has always resolved with resolution of brain edema. Blood pressure is elevated in approximately 50% of patients with mild hypertension in 10–15% and normal blood pressure in approximately 30–35%. At presentation, blood pressure is normal in 25–30% of patients with mild BP elevation in 15% (MAP: 106–115 mmHg) [4]. Moderate–severe hypertension (MAP: 120–140 mmHg) at presentation is seen in ~50% of patients and is rarely noted to be above MAP 150 mmHg [3,4]. Blood pressure lability is common, in particular in unstable patients such as those after stem cell transplant. A focal neurological deficit is occasionally present and occasionally psychiatric or spinal cord symptoms may occur. Posterior reversible encephalopathy syndrome most commonly occurs in the setting of transplantation (solid organ transplant or stem cell transplant; cyclosporine or tacrolimus toxicity), pregnancy (preeclampsia/eclampsia), infection/sepsis/shock, autoimmune disease, or post-cancer chemotherapy. The syndrome has been reported in the setting of other unique immune conditions including medical-renal diseases, thrombotic thrombocytopenic purpura, and hemolytic-uremic syndrome.

Basic imaging features

The hallmark on CT or MR imaging studies is a characteristic pattern of brain vasogenic edema,

---

Brain Disorders in Critical Illness, ed. Robert D. Stevens, Tarek Sharshar, and E. Wesley Ely. Published by Cambridge University Press. © Cambridge University Press 2013.

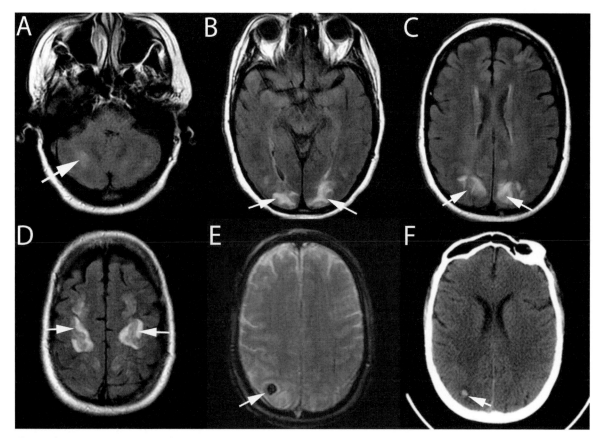

Figure 36.1 Patient is a 52-year-old female with Crohn's disease and suspected vasculitis with headache, altered mentation then seizure. Baseline blood pressure fluctuated between120/88 to 158/110 mmHg with toxicity blood pressures ranging between 160/90 to 200/80 mmHg. (A–D) Axial MR imaging (FLAIR) demonstrates PRES vasogenic edema in the cerebellar hemispheres (A: large arrow), occipital lobes, parietal lobes, and superior frontal sulcus bilaterally (smaller arrows). (E) Axial gradient image demonstrates a minute hemorrhage in the right parietal region (arrow). (F) Axial CT image in the same region demonstrates the small hemorrhage in the right parietal region (arrow).

typically present in the watershed zones (Figure 36.1). Brain edema is most commonly present in the occipital and parietal lobes (95%, hence "posterior") but other portions of the brain develop vasogenic edema including the frontal lobes (60–70%, in particular the superior frontal sulcus), inferior temporal-occipital junctions (40%), and cerebellar hemisphere watershed (30%). The splenium of the corpus callosum is involved in approximately 10% of patients (watershed between posterior peri-callosal and callosal-marginal branches). The brainstem as well as basal ganglia and deep white matter can be involved in 5–10% of patients. The exact location of initial edema development has not been established but appears to be related to the gray–white junction.

Three primary patterns of vasogenic edema are typically seen with near equal frequency (~25%) including: (1) holo-hemispheric, (2) superior frontal sulcal, and (3) dominant posterior (parietal/occipital lobes) [5]. In approximately 25% of patients the imaging pattern demonstrates either partial expression of the typical PRES patterns or marked asymmetric expression of the typical patterns. The primary PRES patterns reflect the locations of the watershed areas of the brain. The most extreme watershed is at the junction of the anterior cerebral artery (ACA), middle cerebral artery (MCA), and posterior cerebral artery (PCA) branches, which primarily resides in the parietal and occipital lobes. The holo-hemispheric pattern most clearly demonstrates the junctional character of the location of the vasogenic edema with a location that reflects the junction between medial brain branches (ACA and PCA) and lateral hemispheric branches (MCA). The superior frontal sulcal pattern is in many ways a diminutive form of the holo-hemispheric pattern with partial involvement but not complete frontal extension of edema along the superior frontal sulcus. In most respects the PRES pattern reflects the watershed zones of the brain and mimics the pattern of watershed infarction [6]. These patterns appear to be independent of either the clinical setting (i.e., eclampsia vs. organ transplant) or the blood pressure at presentation.

With partial expression of the PRES pattern, the neurotoxicity may still be easy to diagnose if enough elements of the vasogenic edema locations are identified. As less brain involvement is present, the diagnosis of PRES may be challenging. In characteristic clinical settings such as pregnancy or transplantation, subtle amounts of vasogenic edema in typical locations will commonly be recognized as PRES (eclampsia, cyclosporine/tacrolimus toxicity) but in other circumstances (i.e., infection) subtle amounts of edema might not be recognized as PRES. Isolated or predominant brainstem or cerebellar involvement can occur and is difficult to recognize as PRES. Severe cerebellar edema has rarely been reported with the development of hydrocephalus or cerebellar herniation. Occasionally the edema is wholly or primarily uni-hemispheric suggesting infiltrative tumor and while very rare, the term tumifactive PRES has been suggested.

The mechanism behind PRES

The mechanism behind PRES is as yet unproven. Two prevailing theories are: (1) brain hypoperfusion with secondary ischemia leading to the development of vasogenic edema and (2) severe hypertension with loss of autoregulatory protection and subsequent vasogenic edema. The hypoperfusion or ischemic theory is more substantially supported by observations in most PRES patients [3].

Hypoperfusion and PRES

Insight into the mechanism behind PRES can be gained by observing the broad clinical picture in which PRES presents. First, PRES typically occurs in patients who have a profound immune-system challenge, such as pregnancy, infection/sepsis/shock, transplantation (solid organ, allogeneic stem cell), autoimmune disease (i.e. Lupus), and patients who have had cancer chemotherapy [3,4]. These conditions have in common an immunological trigger such as the placenta, transplanted organ/cells, immune response to infection, auto-immune disease, or potential immune response to oncogenetic protein. Evidence of endothelial injury is often present with platelet

consumption and schistocyte formation. Systemic inflammatory response syndrome (SIRS) and multiple organ dysfunction syndrome (MODS) may occur due to platelet consumption, hypoperfusion (liver, kidney), and pulmonary dysfunction. Endothelin production occurs in many of these conditions likely due to endothelial cell activation, leading to blood pressure instability and hypertension. In conditions such as infection/sepsis/shock, a systemic inflammatory response might be observed with resultant T-cell trafficking. Understanding the multiple physiological responses present in these patients can help explain the clinical presentations in PRES.

Problems surrounding the hypertension/hyperperfusion theory

The hypertensive theory suggests that with significant elevation of blood pressure, the upper limits of brain autoregulation (the blood pressure-responsive brain vessel vasoconstriction/vasodilation mechanism responsible for maintaining stable cerebral blood flow) are exceeded, resulting in endothelial disruption and vasogenic edema. This 'forced hyper-perfusion' is a very different concept from simple loss of autoregulatory tone with passive hyperperfusion, often called luxury perfusion. Several critical flaws are present in the hypertension/hyperperfusion theory and, to date, this model has not been convincingly demonstrated in PRES. The upper limit of brain autoregulation is relatively high (MAP: 150–160 mmHg) and few patients with PRES develop blood pressure levels this high. Secondly, the upper limit of autoregulation is increased in the setting of both chronic hypertension and sympathetic system activation [7,8].

Initial reports of PRES focused on accompanying hypertension and therefore the term "hypertensive encephalopathy" was commonly applied. The initial imaging report suggesting hyperperfusion associated with PRES vasogenic edema had only two patients studied with SPECT brain perfusion imaging, one with mixed brain perfusion demonstrated, and the second with a complex perfusion pattern somewhat distant from the location of the vasogenic edema [9]. A second, frequently cited article may represent a selective population (absence of normotensive patients) using only blood pressure averaging to garner proof of a hypertensive mechanism [10]. Additional observations suggested that sympathetic stimulation occurred in the setting of PRES and that inadequate sympathetic neural innervation of "posterior" brain vasculature reduced autoregulation control but as mentioned above, the limits of autoregulation are increased in the setting of sympathetic stimulation [8].

Histology in PRES

Few histopathological studies are available in the acute phase of PRES. Vasogenic edema is noted, typical of the edema noted on CT or MR imaging. Endothelial activation has been observed (plump activated endothelial cells) with evidence of T-cell trafficking at the microvascular or capillary level (CD4 or CD8 T-cells adherent to the endothelial surface, progressing through the endothelium and present surrounding vessels) [11,12]. In addition, increased vascular endothelial growth factor (VEGF) and cellular VEGF expression have been identified suggesting a hypoxemic micro-cellular environment. These findings point to hypoperfusion with resultant hypoxemia as an important mechanism in PRES.

Advanced imaging features in PRES and associated clinical conditions

Stippled enhancement can be observed in PRES but is not common. Extensive parenchymal enhancement or gyral enhancement is not usually observed. Some degree of blood–brain barrier permeability change can be recognized in some patients with contrast crossing to the extracellular space, but enhancement is infrequent.

Several vascular changes have been identified in PRES. Reduced cerebral blood flow can be seen on late arterial, capillary and early venous phases at catheter angiography. With MR angiography, evidence of vasculopathy, vasoconstriction, and distal vessel "pruning" can be observed with either reduced distal vessel flow or vessel constriction and luminal irregularity, best recognized as the vessels normalize after the PRES toxicity process subsides (Figure 36.2) [1,13]. This vasculopathy, vasoconstriction, and reduced distal flow (pruning) will be seen to reverse if follow-up MRA is obtained (Figure 36.2D, F). At catheter angiography a similar vasculopathy can occasionally be observed with evidence of vasoconstriction, luminal irregularity and string of bead appearance, similar to what is described in vasculitis. This might represent large vessel overlap with the microvascular process. Vessel irregularity has occasionally been observed in

the extracranial carotid or vertebral arteries, mimicking the appearance of dissection or fibromuscular disease. Similar to reduced cerebral blood flow noted during the capillary phase of a catheter angiogram, reduced perfusion has been noted on SPECT nuclear medicine scans as well as at MR perfusion imaging [1,13].

Evidence of restricted diffusion and infarction are known to occur in PRES. Minute areas of infarction can be seen as well as areas of infarction in the watershed zone. The exact incidence of stroke and restricted diffusion in PRES is somewhat difficult to confirm since many lesions appear small on the diffusion-weighted sequence and are challenging to confirm on the ADC map. It is likely that restricted diffusion and ischemic stroke occur in approximately 10–15% of patients.

Hemorrhage occurs in 15–20% of patient with PRES (Figure 36.1D, E) [4]. Hemorrhage can be present as minute foci of blood, frank hematoma, or as sulcal-subarachnoid hemorrhage. Mass effect can occur in the presence of significant hematoma. Patients with PRES and hemorrhage are often more significantly neurologically impaired with more severe altered mentation, seizures, and even coma. The frequency of hemorrhage is essentially the same among the clinical conditions that develop PRES. The frequency of hemorrhage also is essentially the same whether the presenting blood pressure is normal or severe hypertension is present.

Preeclampsia and eclampsia

The classic, most natural, and extensively studied condition in which PRES develops is preeclampsia and eclampsia [1,3]. Preeclampsia occurs in approximately 5% of pregnancies with eclampsia currently occurring in 1/3000 (historically 1/700). Blood pressure elevation, systemic vasoconstriction, and blood pressure instability develop (hence initial description as hypertensive disorder of pregnancy), the causes of which are complex. Thrombocytopenia, red blood cell fragmentation (schistocytes), and increased lactate dehydrogenase levels are observed suggesting endothelial injury with altered renal function (endothelial activation/alteration), liver function (HELLP syndrome), hypomagnesemia, systemic edema, and occasionally pulmonary edema. Systemic VEGF is elevated. With altered mentation or seizure, eclampsia is defined. With delivery of the fetus and placenta, the condition reverses.

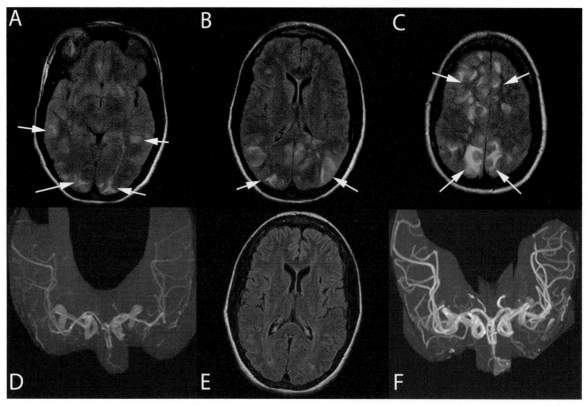

Figure 36.2 Patient is a 22-year-old female with sickle cell disease, membranous glomerulonephritis with new pneumonia (*Streptococcus viridans*), and acute renal failure who presents with a seizure. Blood pressure on admission was 210/110 mmHg. (A–C) Axial MR imaging (FLAIR) at toxicity demonstrates patchy vasogenic edema in the occipital poles, inferior temporal-occipital junctions, parietal region, and frontal lobes bilaterally consistent with PRES. (D) 3D Time of Flight MRA image axial projection at toxicity demonstrates small, irregular cerebral vessels and reduced overall flow signal in the anterior circulation (ACA, MCA), in particular the middle cerebral arteries bilaterally, consistent with vasoconstriction, vasculopathy, and cerebral hypoperfusion. (E) Axial MR image (FLAIR) after symptom resolution demonstrates resolution of the PRES vasogenic edema. (F) Repeat 3D Time of Flight MRA image axial projection after symptom resolution now demonstrates marked improvement in the size, uniformity, and flow characteristics of the anterior cerebral vessels consistent with reversal of vasoconstriction and hypoperfusion.

Infection, sepsis, or shock

At the opposite extreme, PRES is often seen in the setting of infection, sepsis, or shock, conditions known to develop MODS or SIRS [1,3]. Severe bacterial infection is the most common association, but PRES has now also been noted following viral infection including childhood and adult influenza and in association with malaria [14]. Evidence of vasculopathy can be identified by MRA in particular if follow-up studies are obtained. Blood pressure may be normal at presentation or hypertension may be present and, similar to solid organ transplant, the quantity of brain edema is greater when the patient is normotensive and less when severe hypertension is present. Postviral infection and postimmunization PRES has also been described.

The trigger for PRES in the setting of infection, sepsis, or shock has not as yet been defined. Given the uniform characteristics of the clinical and imaging presentation of PRES among the high-risk groups, it would be expected that the mechanism is similar among the groups as well. With immune challenge present in these conditions, T-cell activation, vascular activation, and T-cell trafficking are most likely central to the process. In the setting of bacterial or viral infections, antigen-presenting cells typically display partially fragmented protein components of the offending organism to either CD4 or CD8 T-cells [15]. In the setting of severe infection, sepsis, or the septic response, more extensive T-cell activation occurs with development of a systemic inflammatory response, T-cell trafficking, and resultant reduced organ blood flow with the development of MODS [16–19]. Coagulation may also be affected including thrombocytopenia [19]. It is likely that a "unique" protein-antigenic combination is being presented to the patient's T-cells in this setting leading to the exaggerated T-cell response with excessive up-regulation and subsequent cytokine expression (TNFα and IL-1) [17]. This process most likely proceeds to endothelial up-regulation including cell surface trafficking molecules, vasoactive molecules [endothelin, nitric oxide (NO)] and platelet adhesion (thromboxane release) resulting in non-specific T-cell trafficking (central to systemic inflammatory response) and vascular instability [16,17,20–29].

In PRES, the features of vascular instability can be seen with observable reversible cerebral vasoconstriction (when follow-up MRA is obtained) and labile blood pressure with a subset of patients becoming moderately hypertensive (endothelin, NO, thromboxane). Non-specific T-cell trafficking might be the pathophysiology behind vessel pruning seen on MRA in infection, contributing to brain hypoperfusion. This combination might be the brain's reflection of organ hypoperfusion, central to the MODS process. Systemic hypertension might even worsen brain hypoperfusion through cerebral autoregulatory vasoconstriction. If sufficient hypoxemia develops, VEGF would become up-regulated by the endothelium and brain parenchyma resulting in altered endothelial permeability and cerebral edema [30–34]. T-cell trafficking and cellular/endothelial VEGF up-regulation have been demonstrated in selected case reports of PRES and reversible encephalopathy when acute-phase histology has been obtained [11,12].

If brain hypoperfusion is central to the PRES process, then blood pressure management becomes complex. When hypertension accompanies PRES, the effects of blood pressure reduction could be deleterious. Careful management of blood pressure when the patient is hypertensive is essential.

Stem cell transplantation

Posterior reversible encephalopathy syndrome is frequently identified following stem cell or allogeneic bone marrow transplantation (allo-BMT) [1,3]. Initially referred to as "cyclosporin toxicity" the development of PRES is likely complex in these patients. Infection and graft-vs.-host disease is commonly encountered and PRES is likely related to the immune process as affected by the immune-suppressive drugs.

Posterior reversible encephalopathy syndrome is typically seen in the first 3 months following allo-BMT with an incidence of approximately 7–8% likely depending upon the intensity of the conditioning regimen (myelo-ablative vs. non-myelo-ablative) and underlying hematopoietic malignancy or condition.

Solid organ transplant

Posterior reversible encephalopathy syndrome is less frequent after solid organ transplant as compared with allo-BMT. Often referred to as "tacrolimus toxicity" the incidence is approximately 0.5% among most solid organ transplants but some significant differences exist [35]. Evidence of bacterial or viral infection (e.g., cytomegalovirus) and organ rejection are commonly noted. Posterior reversible encephalopathy syndrome after liver transplant usually occurs early (months after transplant) with blood pressure near normal but amount of brain edema substantial. In contrast, PRES after kidney transplants tends to be a late event (years after transplant), blood pressure tends to be high (MAP: 130–140mmHg) but amount of brain edema much less.

Immune-triggered and auto-immune disease

Posterior reversible encephalopathy syndrome has been reported in a variety of auto-immune conditions [1]. Most commonly seen in systemic lupus erythematosus, PRES has also occurred in patients with scleroderma, Wegener's, and polyarteritis nodosa. These are conditions with complex immune activation events including T-cell dysfunction and autoantibody production. Other immune-related conditions in which PRES has been observed include medical-renal diseases. Guillain-Barré syndrome, neuromyelitis optica, allergy, and post-transfusion.

Post-cancer chemotherapy

Another setting in which PRES is observed is following chemotherapy. The cause is not established but T-cell activation from oncogene-produced proteins is a consideration [3].

Vasoconstrictive states

Posterior reversible encephalopathy syndrome is occasionally observed in the setting of metabolic change or drugs that might induce severe vasoconstriction [1].

Early reports related hypomagnesemia to PRES and more recently hypercalcemia-related PRES has been noted (Mg^{2+} is a competitive inhibitor of Ca^{2+}). Drugs such as Ephedra, phenylpropanolamine, and caffeine have been implicated in PRES as has licorice over-ingestion. These may be inducing cerebral as well as systemic vasoconstriction.

Multiple organ dysfunction syndrome (MODS) and systemic inflammatory response syndrome (SIRS)

Features and signatures of MODS can be recognized in many patients with PRES with acute change in associated parameters including: thrombocytopenia, creatinine, bilirubin, pulmonary function (ARDS) and neurological function [3]. Organ dysfunction in MOD is related to hypoperfusion and vasculopathy has been noted in other organs in patients with PRES. Episodes of MODS are common in infection or sepsis, are part of the typical presentation in patients with preeclampsia/eclampsia (thrombocytopenia, renal dysfunction, hepatic dysfunction, i.e., HEELP) and are frequently seen in patients after solid organ or stem cell transplants (veno-occlusive disease of the liver [VOD]; bone marrow transplant thrombotic microangiopathy [BMT-TM]).

Recurrent PRES

Posterior reversible encephalopathy syndrome can recur with an incidence of approximately 3% [1]. Recurrent PRES is likely due to re-exposure of the underlying clinical condition triggering multisystem dysfunction such as infection or transplant rejection.

Clinical management

Treatment of PRES should be initiated early to reduce the risk of permanent neurological damage. If not recognized and treated quickly, PRES can result in cerebral infarction and hemorrhage. Management is often achieved through a multidisciplinary approach centering on reversal of underlying triggers and controlling early neurological symptoms. Neurological manifestations of PRES can be as mild as headaches, or as severe as status epilepticus. As there have not been clinical trials, treatment of PRES and its manifestations has been guided by pathophysiological reasoning and expert opinion [36].

General treatment considerations

Given the preponderance of reduced circulating intravascular volume in patients with PRES, generous hydration with intravenous fluids is recommended. Coagulopathies should be corrected to decrease the likelihood of a hemorrhagic complication. Electrolyte disturbances should be corrected as hypomagnesemia and/or hypercalcemia can worsen PRES [36].

Managing underlying PRES triggers

When PRES is caused by calcineurin inhibitor therapy (CNI) in the context of solid organ transplantation (typically cyclosporine or tacrolimus), successful recovery is frequently seen with cessation of these medications [37,38]. In circumstances where complete cessation of CNI therapy is contraindicated, such as with lung transplantation, switching to the alternative CNI is the accepted therapeutic approach [37]. It is important to note that serum drug trough levels of CNI have poor correlation with the occurrence of PRES, and that even severe cases of neurotoxicity are reversible with discontinuation of the offending drug [39].

In the setting of infection, sepsis, shock, and/or multi-organ dysfunction, fluid management and continuous invasive blood pressure monitoring is advised [40]. When patients are extremely hypertensive, nitrates (such as nitroglycerin and nitroprusside) should be avoided, as this class of antihypertensives can worsen cerebral edema and/or neurotoxicity [41]. A reduction of no more than 20% of the MAP is suggested, and intravenous labetalol and/or calcium channel blockers have frequently been employed as the first-line agents [36].

When PRES is found in pregnant women with eclampsia, urgent delivery of the baby almost always leads to a complete recovery. Prior to delivery, all patients should receive a bolus of magnesium sulfate 5 g i.v. followed by a continuous infusion of 1 g/h. Nimodipine as treatment of hypertension in eclamptic patients has been hypothesized to be neuroprotective through its prevention of vasospasm [36].

Posterior reversible encephalopathy syndrome has been described in isolated case reports in the context of intravenous immunoglobulin (IvIg) use. In most of these reports, there is another known PRES trigger present at the same time, such as chemotherapy [42] or active systemic autoimmune disease [43]. In fact, PRES has been shown to resolve following treatment of the underlying trigger with IvIg [44,45]. Therefore, if the underlying PRES trigger warrants treatment with IvIg, it can be used; however, IvIg is not a treatment for PRES per se.

Managing neurological complications of PRES

Often, the only neurological symptom noted in patients with PRES is an alteration in mental status. Altered mental status may represent non-convulsive status epilepticus; for this reason, it is essential to evaluate with EEG. Previous series have found that renal failure and history of epilepsy are risk factors for developing status epilepticus in PRES, but in any patient with PRES who has a delayed recovery in their mental status, or a witnessed clinical seizure, electro-encephalographic (EEG) monitoring should be considered to look for episodes of subclinical seizures [46]. First-line antiepileptic drugs are benzodiazepines, fos-phenytoin, and/or valproic acid. In patients found to be in status epilepticus on EEG, continuous EEG monitoring until the patient is seizure free is mandatory. Most patients are kept on short-term antiepileptic medications (ranging from 1 week to 4 months) after their seizures, unless they are known to have underlying chronic epilepsy, and typically have a very good prognosis without recurrent seizures [46].

Hemorrhage has been seen to occur with PRES, regardless of blood pressure at the time of hemorrhage. In patients with hemorrhage, it has been the standard to aggressively lower blood pressure with i.v. medications, with systolic blood pressure goal < 160 mmHg. Thrombocytopenia and coagulopathies predispose to hemorrhage, and transfusion of platelets and/or fresh frozen plasma in patients with hemorrhage until platelet and coagulation values normalize is necessary [47]. These laboratory values should be monitored closely in all patients with PRES so as to avoid hemorrhage when possible.

Clinical outcome after PRES

Outcome after PRES depends on several factors. Most of the conditions that develop PRES are complex biologically, making targeting of the specific trigger difficult to define and therefore control. In eclampsia, delivery with placenta removal is technically curative. With the development of moderate or severe hypertension, onset of the PRES may be clear. In patients who develop PRES in the setting of transplantation or infection, in particular if normotensive or only mildly hypertensive, onset of the toxic state may be difficult to pinpoint. In addition, complicated PRES, with development of either stroke or hemorrhage, will undoubtedly affect neurological outcome. In the setting of selected clinical states (autoimmune disease, preeclampsia/eclampsia, transplantation) it may be difficult to separate the specific effects of PRES from the course of the underlying condition.

Clinical resolution likely parallels imaging resolution. Most patients clinically improve in days or 1–2 weeks after the onset of PRES [36,48,49]. In patients with eclampsia, postpartum neurological complications such as coma can develop but most deficits are transient [50–52]. Permanent deficits have been described including the development of epilepsy [36,53,54] as well as permanent neurological deficits [36,55–57].

Imaging resolution of PRES likely depends on the amount of vasogenic that has developed. Edema typically resolves completely over the course of 1–2 weeks [48,58]. This larger series experience parallels observations in the majority of the small series and case reports. In the setting of hemorrhage or stroke with restricted diffusion, damage will likely persist and residual neurological deficit remain [54,57–59].

Conclusion

Posterior reversible encephalopathy syndrome is generally observed in conditions with significant immune system challenge. Clinical presentation and classic imaging features generally secure the diagnosis. Blood pressure elevation and instability are commonly observed but the role of hypertension is as yet not established. Management of PRES is aimed at withdrawing offending agents and treating seizures when present. No guidelines exist regarding treatment of hypertension, but the consensus has been to carefully lower blood pressure when it is severely elevated.

References

1. Bartynski WS. Posterior reversible encephalopathy syndrome, part 1: fundamental imaging and clinical features. *AJNR Am J Neuroradiol* 2008;**29**(6):1036–42.

2. Hinchey J, Chaves C, Appignani B, *et al*. A reversible posterior leukoencephalopathy syndrome. *New Engl J Med* 1996;**334**(8):494–500.

3. Bartynski WS. Posterior reversible encephalopathy syndrome, part 2: controversies surrounding pathophysiology of vasogenic edema. *AJNR Am J Neuroradiol* 2008;**29**(6):1043–9.

4. Hefzy HM, Bartynski WS, Boardman JF, Lacomis D. Hemorrhage in posterior reversible encephalopathy syndrome: imaging and clinical features. *AJNR Am J Neuroradiol* 2009;**30**(7):1371–9.

5. Bartynski WS, Boardman JF. Distinct imaging patterns and lesion distribution in posterior reversible encephalopathy syndrome. *AJNR Am J Neuroradiol* 2007;**28**(7):1320–7.

6. Bartynski WS, Grabb BC, Zeigler Z, Lin L, Andrews DF. Watershed imaging features and clinical vascular injury in cyclosporin A neurotoxicity. *J Comp Assist Tomog* 1997;**21**(6):872–80.

7. Ferrer I, Kaste M, Kalimo H. Vascular diseases. In Love S, Louis DN, Ellison DW, editors. *Greenfield's Neuropathology*. 8th edn. London: Hodder Arnold; 2008:121–240.

8. Barrett KE, Barman SM, Boitano S, Brooks HL, editors. Circulation through special beds. In *Ganong's Review of Medical Physiology*. 23rd edn. New York, NY: McGraw Hill; 2010:569–85.

9. Schwartz RB, Jones KM, Kalina P, et al. Hypertensive encephalopathy: findings on CT, MR imaging, and SPECT imaging in 14 cases. *AJR Am J Roentgenol* 1992;**159**(2):379–83.

10. Schwartz RB, Bravo SM, Klufas RA, et al. Cyclosporine neurotoxicity and its relationship to hypertensive encephalopathy: CT and MR findings in 16 cases. *AJR Am J Roentgenol* 1995;**165**(3):627–31.

11. Horbinski C, Bartynski WS, Carson-Walter E, et al. Reversible encephalopathy after cardiac transplantation: histologic evidence of endothelial activation, T-cell specific trafficking, and vascular endothelial growth factor expression. *AJNR Am J Neuroradiol* 2009;**30**(3):588–90.

12. Kofler J, Bartynski WS, Reynolds TQ, et al. Posterior reversible encephalopathy syndrome (PRES) with immune system activation, VEGF up-regulation, and cerebral amyloid angiopathy. *J Comp Assist Tomogr* 2011;**35**(1):39–42.

13. Bartynski WS, Boardman JF. Catheter angiography, MR angiography, and MR perfusion in posterior reversible encephalopathy syndrome. *AJNR Am J Neuroradiol* 2008;**29**(3):447–55.

14. Bartynski WS, Upadhyaya AR, Boardman JF. Posterior reversible encephalopathy syndrome and cerebral vasculopathy associated with influenza A infection: report of a case and review of the literature. *J Comp Assist Tomogr* 2009; **33**(6):917–22.

15. Abbas AK, Lichtman AH, editors. Activation of T lymphocytes. In *Cellular and Molecular Immunology*. 5th edn. Philadelphia, PA: Elsevier Saunders; 2005:163–88.

16. Munford RS. Sepsis, severe sepsis and septic shock. In Mandell GL, Bennett JE, Dolin R, editors. *Principles and Practice of Infectious Disease*. Philadelphia, PA: Elsevier; 2005:906–26.

17. Cohen J. The immunopathogenesis of sepsis. *Nature* 2002;**420**(6917):885–91.

18. Varon J, Marik PE. Multiple organ dysfunction syndrome. In Irwin RS, Rippe JM, editors. *Irwin and Rippe's Intensive Care Medicine*. 5th edn. Philadelphia, PA: Lippincott-Williams, Wilkins; 2003:1834–8.

19. Vincent JL, Moreno R, Takala J, et al. The SOFA (Sepsis-related Organ Failure Assessment) score to describe organ dysfunction/failure. On behalf of the Working Group on Sepsis-Related Problems of the European Society of Intensive Care Medicine. *Intensive Care Med* 1996;**22**(7):707–10.

20. Parent C, Eichacker PQ. Neutrophil and endothelial cell interactions in sepsis. The role of adhesion molecules. *Infectious Dis Clin North Am* 1999;**13**(2):427–47.

21. Symeonides S, Balk RA. Nitric oxide in the pathogenesis of sepsis. *Infectious Dis Clin North Am* 1999;**13**(2):449–63, x.

22. McCuskey RS, Urbaschek R, Urbaschek B. The microcirculation during endotoxemia. *Cardiovascular Res* 1996;**32**(4):752–63.

23. Wanecek M, Weitzberg E, Rudehill A, Oldner A. The endothelin system in septic and endotoxin shock. *Eur J Pharmacol* 2000;**407**(1–2):1–15.

24. Weitzberg E, Lundberg JM, Rudehill A. Elevated plasma levels of endothelin in patients with sepsis syndrome. *Circulatory Shock* 1991;**33**(4):222–7.

25. Pittet JF, Morel DR, Hemsen A, et al. Elevated plasma endothelin-1 concentrations are associated with the severity of illness in patients with sepsis. *Annals Surg* 1991;**213**(3):261–4.

26. Marsden PA, Brenner BM. Transcriptional regulation of the endothelin-1 gene by TNF-alpha. *Am J Physiol* 1992;**262**(4 Pt 1):C854–61.

27. Mantovani A, Bussolino F, Dejana E. Cytokine regulation of endothelial cell function. *FASEB J* 1992;**6**(8):2591–9.

28. Maemura K, Kurihara H, Morita T, Oh-hashi Y, Yazaki Y. Production of endothelin-1 in vascular endothelial cells is regulated by factors associated with vascular injury. *Gerontology* 1992;**38**(Suppl 1):29–35.

29. Sugiura M, Inagami T, Kon V. Endotoxin stimulates endothelin-release in vivo and in vitro as determined by

radioimmunoassay. *Biochem Biophys Res Comms* 1989;**161**(3):1220–7.

30. Kevil CG, Payne DK, Mire E, Alexander JS. Vascular permeability factor/vascular endothelial cell growth factor-mediated permeability occurs through disorganization of endothelial junctional proteins. *J Biological Chem* 1998;**273**(24):15099–103.

31. Levy AP, Levy NS, Wegner S, Goldberg MA. Transcriptional regulation of the rat vascular endothelial growth factor gene by hypoxia. *J Biological Chem* 1995;**270**(22):13333–40.

32. Shweiki D, Itin A, Soffer D, Keshet E. Vascular endothelial growth factor induced by hypoxia may mediate hypoxia-initiated angiogenesis. *Nature* 1992;**359**(6398):843–5.

33. Schoch HJ, Fischer S, Marti HH. Hypoxia-induced vascular endothelial growth factor expression causes vascular leakage in the brain. *Brain* 2002;**125**(Pt 11):2549–57.

34. Xu L, Fukumura D, Jain RK. Acidic extracellular pH induces vascular endothelial growth factor (VEGF) in human glioblastoma cells via ERK1/2 MAPK signaling pathway: mechanism of low pH-induced VEGF. *J Biological Chem* 2002;**277**(13):11368–74.

35. Bartynski WS, Tan HP, Boardman JF, Shapiro R, Marsh JW. Posterior reversible encephalopathy syndrome after solid organ transplantation. *AJNR Am J Neuroradiol* 2008;**29**(5):924–30.

36. Servillo G, Bifulco F, De Robertis E, *et al.* Posterior reversible encephalopathy syndrome in intensive care medicine. *Intensive Care Med* 2007;**33**(2):230–6.

37. Tsang BK, Kermeen FD, Hopkins PM, Chambers DC. Reversible posterior leukoencephalopathy syndrome: diagnosis and management in the setting of lung transplantation. *Internal Med J* 2010;**40**(10):716–20.

38. de Oliveira RA, Fechine LM, Neto FC, *et al.* Posterior reversible encephalopathy syndrome (PRES) induced by cyclosporine use in a patient with collapsing focal glomeruloesclerosis. *Int Urol Nephrol* 2008;**40**(4):1095–8.

39. Wijdicks EF. Neurotoxicity of immunosuppressive drugs. *Liver Transpl* 2001;**7**(11):937–42.

40. Fearnley RA, Lines SW, Lewington AJ, Bodenham AR. Influenza A-induced rhabdomyolysis and acute kidney injury complicated by posterior reversible encephalopathy syndrome. *Anaesthesia* 2011;**66**(8):738–42.

41. Finsterer J, Schlager T, Kopsa W, Wild E. Nitroglycerin-aggravated pre-eclamptic posterior reversible encephalopathy syndrome (PRES). *Neurology* 2003;**61**(5):715–16.

42. Delanghe JR. How to estimate GFR in children. *Nephrol Dialysis Transplant* 2009;**24**(3):714–16.

43. Gratton D, Szapary P, Goyal K, *et al.* Reversible posterior leukoencephalopathy syndrome in a patient treated with ustekinumab: case report and review of the literature. *Arch Dermatol* 2011;**147**(10):1197–202.

44. Elahi A, Kelkar P, St Louis EK. Posterior reversible encephalopathy syndrome as the initial manifestation of Guillain-Barré syndrome. *Neurocritical Care* 2004;**1**(4):465–8.

45. Abraham A, Ziv S, Drory VE. Posterior reversible encephalopathy syndrome resulting from Guillain-Barré-like syndrome secondary to West Nile virus infection. *J Clin Neuromuscul Dis* 2011;**12**(3):113–17.

46. Kozak OS, Wijdicks EF, Manno EM, Miley JT, Rabinstein AA. Status epilepticus as initial manifestation of posterior reversible encephalopathy syndrome. *Neurology* 2007;**69**(9):894–7.

47. Aranas RM, Prabhakaran S, Lee VH. Posterior reversible encephalopathy syndrome associated with hemorrhage. *Neurocritical Care* 2009;**10**(3):306–12.

48. Shah-Khan FM, Pinedo D, Shah P. Reversible posterior leukoencephalopathy syndrome and anti-neoplastic agents: a review. *Oncol Rev* 2007;**1**:152–61.

49. Lee VH, Wijdicks EF, Manno EM, Rabinstein AA. Clinical spectrum of reversible posterior leukoencephalopathy syndrome. *Archiv Neurol* 2008;**65**(2):205–10.

50. Sibai BM. Eclampsia. VI. Maternal-perinatal outcome in 254 consecutive cases. *Am J Obstet Gynecol* 1990;**163**(3):1049–54; discussion 54–5.

51. Striano P, Striano S, Tortora F, *et al.* Clinical spectrum and critical care management of posterior reversible encephalopathy syndrome. *Med Sci Monit* 2005;**11**(11):CR549–53.

52. Baizabal-Carvallo JF, Barragan-Campos HM, Padilla-Aranda HJ, *et al.* Posterior reversible encephalopathy syndrome as a complication of acute lupus activity. *Clin Neurol Neurosurg* 2009;**111**(4):359–63.

53. Parasole R, Petruzziello F, Menna G, *et al.* Central nervous system complications during treatment of acute lymphoblastic leukemia in a single pediatric institution. *Leukemia Lymphoma* 2010;**51**(6):1063–71.

54. Morris EB, Laningham FH, Sandlund JT, Khan RB. Posterior reversible encephalopathy syndrome in children with cancer. *Pediatr Blood Cancer* 2007;**48**(2):152–9.

55. Pirker A, Kramer L, Voller B, *et al.* Type of edema in posterior reversible encephalopathy syndrome depends on serum albumin levels: an MR imaging study in 28 patients. *AJNR Am J Neuroradiol* 2011;**32**(3):527–31.

371

56. Burrus TM, Wijdicks EF, Rabinstein AA. Brain lesions are most often reversible in acute thrombotic thrombocytopenic purpura. *Neurology* 2009;**73**(1):66–70.

57. Stott VL, Hurrell MA, Anderson TJ. Reversible posterior leukoencephalopathy syndrome: a misnomer reviewed. *Intern Med J* 2005;**35**(2):83–90.

58. Donmez FY, Basaran C, Kayahan Ulu EM, Yildirim M, Coskun M. MRI features of posterior reversible encephalopathy syndrome in 33 patients. *J Neuroimaging* 2010;**20**(1):22–8.

59. Pande AR, Ando K, Ishikura R, *et al.* Clinicoradiological factors influencing the reversibility of posterior reversible encephalopathy syndrome: a multicenter study. *Radiation Med* 2006;**24**(10):659–68.

Hypoxic-ischemic encephalopathy

Fabio Silvio Taccone and Alain Cariou

SUMMARY

Hypoxic-ischemic encephalopathy (HIE) is a condition in which the entire brain is almost completely deprived of its oxygen supply because of inadequate blood flow or oxygenation. Brain damage that is observed following resuscitation from cardiac arrest is considered to be the most representative pattern of HIE.

Although complex, the pathophysiology of HIE is well understood. Cerebral ischemia triggers a complex cascade of pathways that will result in the peroxidation of lipids with cell membrane layers, protein oxidation, and DNA fragmentation, all contributing to brain cell death. Following this initial insult, brain injury continues even after restoration of cerebral perfusion and oxygenation, in a process known as "reperfusion injury." Particularly, the accumulation of reactive oxygen species and the early depletion of antioxidant reserves, such as glutathione, will lead to an oxidative stress that will promote damage to membrane, cytoskeletal proteins, and nucleic acids, thereby causing diffuse neuronal necrosis. Finally, even after the restoration of adequate blood supply and cellular energy stores, there can be a global hypoperfusion state that may further lead to secondary brain injury and aggravate neurological impairment after initial ischemia.

Initial clinical manifestations of HIE include: disorders of consciousness, movement disorders, seizures, and myoclonus status epilepticus (MSE). Autonomic impairment, such as respiratory abnormalities, temperature, heart rate, and blood pressure variability may also be observed. In survivors, mid- and long-term symptoms include memory and cognitive impairment, late-onset seizures, and cerebral palsy. Disorders of consciousness range from mild confusion and delirium to coma. Most severe patients will evolve towards a severely cognitively disabling and fully dependent state as a consequence of HIE. Some of them will remain in a minimally conscious or vegetative state, but very few will awake in a neurologically intact state.

At the early stage, a rigorous clinical evaluation that includes an exhaustive neurological examination remains the cornerstone of the prognostication process. In addition, various methods can be used to refine the neurological prognosis of comatose cardiac arrest victims, including mainly electrophysiological tests and marginally neuroimaging techniques and biochemical markers.

Regarding treatments, the existence of further cerebral damage during the reperfusion phase has encouraged intense research on the benefit of treatments aimed at limiting the neurological consequences of the post-cardiac arrest syndrome. Currently, induced hypothermia is the only treatment that is demonstrated to be associated with an increase in the rate of neurologically preserved patients after cardiac arrest. Despite numerous attempts, no drug has clearly demonstrated an ability to reduce the consequences of cerebral anoxo-ischemia after CA. In the future, new pharmacological and non-pharmacological treatments might contribute to further improve the prognosis of these patients.

Introduction

Hypoxic-ischemic encephalopathy (HIE) is a condition in which the entire brain is almost completely deprived of its oxygen supply, for at least a few minutes, because of inadequate blood flow or oxygenation [1]. Although the definition of HIE generally refers to brain injury occurring after adult cardiac arrest (CA) or asphyxia in newborn infants, other pathological conditions may potentially cause HIE, such as severe respiratory or cardiovascular failure,

Brain Disorders in Critical Illness, ed. Robert D. Stevens, Tarek Sharshar, and E. Wesley Ely. Published by Cambridge University Press. © Cambridge University Press 2013.

with prolonged hypoxia or hypotension, carbon monoxide or cyanide poisoning, open heart surgery, drowning, strangulation, and high altitudes. Also, severe hypoglycemia and protracted generalized epilepsy could result in a form of "hypoxic" injury, because the brain has no energy stores and is dependent on a continuous glucose supply that could be impaired in the case of low blood glucose levels or critical increase in neurons' needs, such as in seizures [1]. The mechanisms of injury are different in these patient populations, as is the prognosis for neurological recovery. During an isolated hypoxic event, cerebral blood flow (CBF) is maintained, glucose and other nutrients are still supplied to the brain, toxic metabolites are normally removed and cerebral glutamate levels, a marker of local excitotoxicity, are only moderately increased, these conditions being all severely altered in the case of CA [19]. Thus, isolated hypoxic events are generally associated with a better chance for survival than those with cerebral perfusion collapse. Considering that numerous investigations on HIE are related to CA, the present chapter will mainly focus on characteristics of brain injury following this condition.

Epidemiology

Sudden CA, defined as the abrupt loss of cardiac activity and concomitant fall in systemic blood flow, is one of the leading causes of death worldwide. In the USA, nearly 200,000 people suffer from out-of-hospital cardiac arrest (OHCA) and less than 10% of those will survive after cardiopulmonary resuscitation (CPR) and hospital stay [2]. Cardiac arrest occurring in the hospital (IHCA) is also associated with poor survival rates and functional outcome in these patients can be further aggravated by concomitant or pre-existing pathological conditions [3].

The occurrence of HIE after CA recently has been integrated in the so-called "post-resuscitation syndrome," which is characterized by post-arrest brain injury and myocardial dysfunction associated with a systemic inflammatory response following the ischemia/reperfusion process [4], that may potentially contribute to enhance HIE. Although HIE is considered as responsible for more than two-thirds of deaths among CA patients [5], a complex interplay remains between these pathological phenomena that eventually determine clinical presentation and overall outcome.

The economic impact of CA survivors is enormous, because intensive care and monitoring are required for several days, as well as organ support therapy and diagnostic tests to evaluate the severity of HIE and assess prognosis [1]. As such, clinical research has focused on a better comprehension of the mechanisms responsible for severe HIE as well as the development of several neuroprotective strategies to improve outcome in these patients.

Pathophysiology

Cerebral ischemia triggers a complex cascade of pathways [6] that will eventually induce extensive brain injury. As neurons are particularly vulnerable to ischemia because of high metabolic demand, the depletion of adenosine triphosphate (ATP) cellular stores will lead to the Na^+/K^+ ATPase pump failure and membrane depolarization, with accumulation of Ca^{2+} through extracellular influx and intracellular stores within the cytosol [7]. Elevated extracellular levels of glutamate may enhance these events by a further increase of intracellular Ca^{2+} levels; concomitantly, other transmitters that modulate the deleterious effects of glutamatergic activity, such as glycine and gamma-aminobutyric acid (GABA) are decreased [8]. Deregulation of intracellular Ca^{2+} homeostasis activates multiple second messengers and enzymes, which amplifies the detrimental effects of ischemia and interferes with the mitochondrial oxidative phosphorylation [9]. The final result of these reactions is the peroxidation of lipids with cell membrane layers, protein oxidation, and DNA fragmentation, all contributing to brain cell death [1].

Brain injury continues even after restoration of cerebral perfusion and oxygenation, in a process known as "reperfusion injury." Particularly, the accumulation of reactive oxygen species and the early depletion of antioxidant reserves, such as glutathione, will lead to an oxidative stress that will promote damage to membrane, cytoskeletal proteins, and nucleic acids, thereby causing diffuse neuronal necrosis [10]. Oxidative stress reduces the availability of nitric oxide (NO) in endothelial cells, which exacerbates vasoconstriction and capillary clot formation in the ischemic territory. Post-ischemic inflammation also enhances neuronal damage after ischemia and reperfusion injury and is characterized by an activation of coagulation and endothelial cells, an altered permeability of the blood–brain barrier, and the endothelial expression of adhesion molecules that promote the infiltration of leukocytes in ischemic brain areas and lead to production of IL-1β, TNFα, IL-6, and other cytokines [11]. Although post-ischemic inflammation is a self-limiting process, the pathophysiological cascade of cerebral ischemia may activate apoptosis or trigger a chronic inflammatory response involving microglia, which becomes a vicious cycle leading to a slow progressive neurodegeneration [12]. These injurious mechanisms are modulated by brain temperature: local hyperthermia activates glutamate receptors activity on neurons, increases intracellular calcium levels, and enhances the production of free radicals. Also, brain temperature can modify the tissue oxygen demand and contribute to limit the tolerance of brain cells to the anoxic insult [13].

Finally, even after the restoration of adequate blood supply and cellular energy stores, there can be a global hypoperfusion state, called the "no reflow phenomenon," which results from the combination of increased blood viscosity, microvascular alterations, and altered cerebral flow regulation [14]. This hypoperfusion, potentially associated with other secondary injury, such as alterations in blood glucose concentrations, low carbon dioxide levels, seizures, and hyperthermia, may further lead to secondary brain injury and aggravate neurological impairment after initial ischemia.

Clinical manifestations: short term and long term

Clinical manifestations after cerebral ischemia depend on the different susceptibilities of brain regions to anoxia, which results in heterogeneous neurological signs and symptoms. Large projection neurons of the cerebral cortex, the reticulus nucleus of the thalamus, the amygdala, the cerebellum, and hippocampus are the most vulnerable areas [15]. The subcortical areas, such as brainstem, thalamus, and hypothalamus, are more resistant to the injury than the cortex [16]. These differences could be related either to the poor circulation (i.e., watershed areas or CBF-impaired autoregulation), to the higher energy requirement and glutamate release of brain cells or to the lower expression of some proteins, such as heat-shock proteins, which confer a relative tolerance to ischemia, in these vulnerable brain regions [1].

The clinical evaluation of HIE patients is challenging, especially in the case of CA. Indeed, most of the clinical observations in such patients concerned those who were not treated with therapeutic hypothermia [17], and the use of this intervention, requiring sedative and neuromuscular blocking agents, may

significantly change the spectrum and time course of neurological abnormalities following global ischemia. Thus, a complete neurological evaluation should be undertaken after the exclusion of confounding factors, which include also the use of illicit drugs, cerebral hypoperfusion, non-convulsive seizures, electrolyte abnormalities, and metabolic derangements.

Neurological dysfunction in HIE predominantly includes disorders of consciousness, which range from mild confusion (difficulty concentrating, poor judgment, or euphoria) and delirium to coma [1]. The degree of neurological impairment will depend on the injury on subcortical and brainstem functions, which promote and maintain the arousal, or on the cortex, which is important for awareness. During coma status, patients do not respond to any external stimuli; this condition may be irreversible or evolve towards the minimally conscious state (MCS), the vegetative state (VS), or brain death. Clinically, VS could present periodic episodes of arousal in absence of consciousness and response to external stimuli while MCS shows intermittent behavioral evidence of consciousness, suggesting awareness. These severe conditions represent the leading cause of mortality and disability in such patients.

Hypoxic-ischemic encephalopathy also includes other manifestations of neurological dysfunction, such as seizures and MSE. The occurrence of seizures after CA was largely variable in clinical observational studies and is probably related to extensive lesions in cortical and subcortical brain areas. While some reported a 30–40% incidence of epileptic events, others observed a much lower rate [18]. Myoclonus status epilepticus is a prolonged epileptic condition in which the patient is affected by nearly continuous, spontaneous, and repeated myoclonic jerks in the face, arms, limbs, and trunk that are mainly asymmetrical and asynchronous. This condition clearly affects most of the brain cortex, especially the cortex and the pyramidal tract. Other forms of movement disorders include post-anoxic myoclonus, which is often triggered by an external stimulus and gradually resolves over time, akinetic-rigid syndrome, and dystonia [1], which are probably secondary to ischemic injury in the basal ganglia, these latter two occurring after several weeks from the initial ischemic insult. Cerebellar Purkinje cells injury may account for movement disorders and ataxia that are often seen during HIE. Patients with carbon monoxide poisoning have a preferential injury to the basal ganglia, while a primary myelinolytic process in the subcortical areas has been observed in patients undergoing a prolonged period of hypoxia [19].

The presence of autonomic impairment, such as respiratory abnormalities, temperature, heart rate, and blood pressure variability may be observed and is called the "sympathetic storm." Long-term symptoms include the impairment of memory functioning, which is related to the injury of pyramidal neurons in the hippocampus, cognitive impairment, late-onset seizures, and cerebral palsy.

Prognosis

Among acute illnesses, HIE due to cardiac arrest represents a particular challenge since the decision to forgo or to stop initial life-sustaining therapies will have immediate and major effects on survival. Unfortunately, most studies focusing on prognostication are potentially influenced by the occurrence of a so-called "self-fulfilling prophecy." This results from the improper use of variables evaluated for the prediction of poor prognosis that are concomitantly considered to withdraw supportive care in comatose CA patients. This bias may affect the predictive values of such variables in predicting outcome since it remains sometimes difficult to determine whether mortality is or is not influenced by decisions to withdraw or withhold care based on a self-perceived poor neurological prognosis.

In the immediate post-cardiac arrest period, no clinical signs or investigations can accurately predict the patient's outcome, especially when sedation is used in conjunction with hypothermia. Accurate prognostication can only occur after 72 hours have elapsed from all confounding factors that may alter neurological assessment. During this "waiting period," half of these patients will subsequently suffer from a post-resuscitation disease, which could include a severe shock leading by itself to death in the absence of adapted organ supports. In our opinion, this shock should be treated without limitation during the very first hours and days in order to reach the time window that permits an adequate neurological evaluation.

In patients without HIE, awakening generally takes place within 3–4 days after return of spontaneous circulation (ROSC). By contrast, cerebral damage should always be suspected in patients who fail to do so. Regrettably these patients will often evolve towards a severely cognitively disabling and fully dependent state as a consequence of HIE. Some of them will remain in a minimally conscious or vegetative state, but very few will awake in a neurologically intact state. The simultaneous presence of poor neurological examination and negative indicators beyond the "waiting period" can be incorporated into the prognosis assessment, and may enable the family and the ICU team to reach a consensus on prognosis and management.

Importantly, in the most severe patients, brain death will occur in about 10% in the following days after cardiac arrest, because of cerebral damages due to initial cerebral anoxia [20]. In these patients, life support will be stopped, in conjunction with an organ donation process in most cases.

Can we predict outcome?

It is generally estimated that not more than 20–30% of patients hospitalized in the intensive care unit (ICU) after a cardiac arrest will survive the first days. This figure needs re-evaluation taking into account comorbidity, duration of initial CPR, and also by considering additional arguments. However, even if circumstances surrounding initial resuscitation (anoxia time, duration of CPR, cause of cardiac arrest) are strongly related to outcome, none of these variables can undoubtedly discriminate accurately between patients with poor and those with favorable outcome [21]. Thus these elements should be incorporated in the analysis but decisions to withdraw life-sustaining therapies cannot be solely based on these elements.

A rigorous clinical evaluation that includes an exhaustive neurological examination remains the cornerstone of the prognostication process [18,22,23]. However this process cannot be performed in the first few hours since there are no specific clinical signs that can predict outcome in this early stage. After the first 72 hours, the value of the clinical examination becomes much more acceptable. At that time, the absence of motor response to pain remains the most demonstrated clinical predictor of poor prognosis. Several additional clinical findings accurately predict poor outcome, such as MSE within the first 24 hours, absence of pupillary responses within days 1–3 after resuscitation, absence of corneal reflexes within days 1–3 after CPR, and absent or extensor motor responses after 3 days. Conversely, single seizures and sporadic focal myoclonus do not accurately predict poor outcome. In the same way, although permanent status epilepticus is associated with a mortality approaching 100%, exceptions to this dismal outcome have been reported.

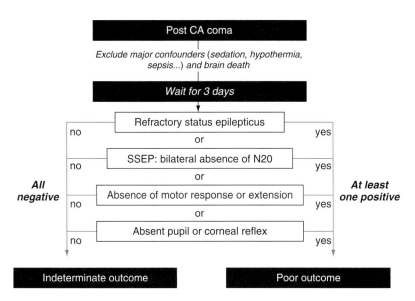

Figure 37.1 Prognosis assessment. CA, cardiac arrest; SSEP, somatosensory evoked potential.

In addition to physical examination, various methods can be used to refine the neurological prognosis of comatose cardiac arrest victims, including mainly electrophysiological tests, neuroimaging techniques, and biochemical markers. Electrophysiological tests consist of electroencephalograms (EEG) and evoked/event-related potential studies. Routine EEG are not supported by the results of the published reviews, but should be used if ongoing seizure activity is suspected to confirm it [24]. Seizures are very common in the course of HIE (10–40%). However they can be clinically unapparent and can also be confounded with other abnormal movements. Even if the benefit to treat seizures remains to be demonstrated, EEG is important to confirm and/or to detect them. In this way, continuous EEG (cEEG), which is now routinely available with minimal equipment, could help with early detection of malignant aspects [25]. Generalized suppression pattern, burst-suppression pattern with generalized epileptiform activity, or generalized periodic complexes on a flat background are strongly but not invariably associated with poor outcome. Burst suppression or generalized epileptiform discharges on EEG predict poor outcomes but with insufficient prognostic accuracy. By contrast with EEG, systematic reviews of outcome prediction in comatose post-cardiac arrest patients have concluded that somatosensory evoked potentials (SSEPs) are helpful for predicting bad outcome. The assessment of poor prognosis can be guided by the bilateral absence of cortical SSEPs (N20 response) within 2–3 days. After

that time or later, bilateral absence of the N20 component of the SSEPs with median nerve stimulation accurately predicts the lack of future awakening [24]. Conversely, the presence of the N20 response is not helpful in predicting outcome as many patients who fail to recover could have preserved N20 responses (Figure 37.1).

Post-cardiac arrest HIE is associated with the blood release of various biochemical markers, and their peak plasma level is thought to be correlated with the amount of neuronal definitive death. A large peak of serum neuron-specific enolase (NSE) and/or S100 protein (S100) concentration is a highly specific but only moderately sensitive marker for a poor neurological outcome after cardiopulmonary resuscitation. The search for a simple, reliable, and readily available biological test remains an exciting challenge but clinical decisions with potentially irreversible consequences should never rely on a single marker and can only be made in the context of all available prognostic information [26].

Even if it can obviously help to detect cerebral causes of cardiac arrest, the use of routine neuroimaging techniques is debatable. There are no trials indicating that systematic CT-scan imaging adds to clinical assessment unless stroke, bleeding, or trauma is suspected on the basis of history or clinical examination [27]. Ongoing clinical studies on functional magnetic resonance imaging (fMRI) will probably provide information regarding the additional value of this test in this setting.

Neuroprotective treatments

The existence of further cerebral damage during the reperfusion phase has encouraged intensive research on the benefit of treatments aimed at limiting the neurological consequences of the post-cardiac arrest syndrome.

Unfortunately, most of the accomplished efforts have not resulted in significant therapeutic advances in the field of HIE, except for the implementation of induced hypothermia at the acute phase. In the past, numerous experimental data demonstrated that mild hypothermia (32–34 °C) can exert neuroprotective effects through multiple mechanisms of action: decrease of cerebral metabolism, reduction of apoptosis and mitochondrial dysfunction, slowing of the cerebral excitatory cascade, decrease of local inflammatory response, reduction of free oxygen radicals production, and decrease of vascular and membrane permeability. Two landmark clinical studies concomitantly published in 2002 confirmed these convergent experimental data [28,29]. In both trials, the implementation of mild hypothermia achieved a survival rate without major sequel in around 40–50% of a highly "selected" population (cardiac arrest with an initial rhythm of ventricular fibrillation in front of a bystander). In both trials, hypothermia was achieved by external cooling methods (blanket, ice packs), associated with routine use of neuromuscular paralysis. At the targeted levels of hypothermia (32–34 °C), theoretical adverse effects (arrhythmias, coagulopathy, infection) were very rare. A trend toward greater frequency of bleeding and infectious events was observed in cooled patients, but was greatly outweighed by the neurological and survival benefit. The publication of these two studies was decisive and led to a rapid change in international recommendations on the management of patients surviving after CA. It is now strongly recommended to routinely use moderate hypothermia (32–34 °C) for 12–24 hours in any comatose adult successfully resuscitated after OHCA caused by ventricular fibrillation/tachycardia [30]. In patients presenting an initial non-shockable rhythm, the level of evidence is weaker and some recent data suggest a lack of neurological benefit [31]. Considering that the risk–benefit ratio is sufficiently favorable, it is reasonable to discuss the indication for treatment on a case-by-case basis. Finally, no single cooling method has been shown to be superior in terms of clinical outcome.

Despite numerous attempts, no drug has clearly demonstrated its ability in the early or late phase of resuscitation to reduce the consequences of cerebral anoxo-ischemia after CA, despite encouraging animal data and early administration after ROSC. Similarly, the different sedative agents have not proven their efficiency. Thus, apart from special situations (therapeutic hypothermia for instance), there is no argument for recommending the routine use of pharmacological agents in CA survivors. Currently, several molecules with cytoprotective effects during ischemia–reperfusion phenomena (antioxidants, cyclosporine, and erythropoietin) are clinically investigated [32,33].

Prevention of secondary cerebral damages

Achieving and maintaining a perfect homeostasis (particularly in terms of metabolism) are the major goals of post-cardiac arrest management. Hypoxemia should be avoided by setting the oxygen fraction of inspired gas to maintain arterial oxygen saturation above 92% and 96%, so as to maintain a sufficient oxygen transport to peripheral tissues. It is not necessary to set a target of "supraphysiological" PaO_2. Even if debatable, hyperoxia should probably be avoided [34]. The level of $PaCO_2$, which is completely controlled by the ventilatory settings in this sedated and sometimes paralyzed patient, is exposed to significant variations. Hypocapnia, meanwhile, should be avoided because it causes a reduction of cerebral blood flow. In animal models of CA, ROSC is accompanied by a brief and transient cerebral hyperemia, followed by a secondary and more prolonged decline in cerebral blood flow. In a canine model of CA using therapeutic hypothermia, hyperventilation appeared to worsen the neurological outcome [35]. In addition, hyperventilation may be responsible for increased intracranial pressure by increasing positive end-expiratory pressure. Conversely, hypercapnia, leading to cerebrovascular vasodilation and increased intracranial pressure, should also be proscribed. Overall, despite the absence of clinical studies specifically addressing the ventilatory settings, it seems logical to maintain a $PaCO_2$ within normal limits [29]. For this, it is necessary to monitor the quality of ventilation using, whenever possible, measurement of expiratory tidal CO_2 and regular monitoring of arterial blood gases, especially during cooling and warming phases which significantly alter production of CO_2.

The correction of electrolyte disturbances is crucial and special attention should be given to those that may participate in the recurrence of CA or worsening of organ dysfunction. Regarding glycemia, converging data underline that blood glucose variability more seriously impairs the outcome of critically ill patients, rather than the mean level of glycemia. This observation has recently been confirmed in cardiac arrest survivors [36], so attention should probably be paid to avoid such large glycemia fluctuations.

Mid- and long-term outcome of survivors

Beyond recurrence of cardiac arrest, quality of life and the possibility of regaining social activity in patients who are sometimes young and active are often poorly taken into consideration. Of the 681 patients studied after discharge from hospital for a period of 6 months, 69% of them were considered to have a good neurological recovery at discharge [37]. For 70% of patients followed, the neurological status remained stable, or even improved in 12% of cases; only 1% of the patients exhibited a decrease in neurological performance. In this cohort, the 6-month mortality of 17% was mainly due to cardiovascular causes. To go further, a precise evaluation of the quality of life was performed 3 years after resuscitation from ventricular fibrillation, using the standardized questionnaire SF-36, which explores both physical and mental aspects [38]. Results were quite similar to those observed in a matched population, except for a lower sense of vitality. Hypoxic insult may nevertheless result in a number of disorders considered as minor, but having a strong impact on quality of life, such as memory problems. They may be even more frequent in younger patients than in older subjects. Overall, health status of these patients is considered as satisfactory.

Conclusion

Recent improvements in the understanding of HIE pathophysiology have undoubtedly enhanced the management of this syndrome. In these patients, the primary objective of care remains to minimize neurological sequelae in future survivors. By influencing the vital and functional prognosis of patients, cerebral protection is now an essential part of the management of HIE. Currently, it relies mainly on therapeutic hypothermia. In the future, new pharmacological and non-pharmacological treatments might contribute to further improve the prognosis of these patients.

References

1. Xiong W, Hoesch RE, Geocadin RG. Post-cardiac arrest encephalopathy. *Semin Neurol* 2011;**31**:216–25.

2. Thom T, Haase N, Rosamond W, *et al*. Heart disease and stroke statistics – 2006 update. *Circulation* 2006;**113**:85–151.

3. Levy PD, Ye H, Compton S, *et al*. Factors associated with neurologically intact survival for patients with acute heart failure and in-hospital cardiac arrest. *Circ Heart Fail* 2009;**2**:572–81.

4. Adrie C, Laurent I, Monchi M, *et al*. Postresuscitation disease after cardiac arrest: a sepsis-like syndrome? *Curr Opin Crit Care* 2004;**10**:208–12.

5. Laver S, Farrow C, Turner D, Nolan J. Mode of death after admission to an intensive care unit following cardiac arrest. *Intensive Care Med* 2004;**30**:2126–8.

6. Illievich UM, Zornow MH, Choi KT, Scheller MS, Strnat MA. Effects of hypothermia metabolic suppression on hippocampal glutamate concentrations after transient global cerebral ischemia. *Anesth Analg* 1994;**78**:905–11.

7. Wagner SR, IV, Lanier WL. Metabolism of glucose, glycogen, and high-energy phosphates during complete cerebral ischemia. A comparison of normoglycemic, chronically hyperglycemic diabetic and acutely hyperglycemic rats. *Anesthesiology* 1994;**81**:1516–26.

8. Globus MY, Ginsberg MD, Busto R. Excitotoxic index – a biochemical marker of selective vulnerability. *Neurosci Lett* 1991;**127**:39–42.

9. Traystman RJ, Kirsch JR, Koehler RC. Oxygen radical mechanisms of brain injury following ischemia and reperfusion. *J Appl Physiol* 1991;**71**:1185–95.

10. Martin LJ, Brambrink AM, Price AC, *et al*. Neuronal death in newborn striatum after hypoxia-ischemia is necrosis and evolves with oxidative stress. *Neurobiol Dis* 2000;**7**:169–91.

11. Iadecola C, Anrather J. The immunology of stroke: from mechanisms to translation. *Nat Med* 2011;**17**:796–808.

12. Tu YF, Tsai YS, Wang LW, *et al*. Overweight worsens apoptosis, neuroinflammation and blood–brain barrier damage after hypoxic ischemia in neonatal brain through JNK hyperactivation. *J Neuroinflammation* 2011;**8**:40.

13. Chio CC, Kuo JR, Hsiao SH, Chang CP, Lin MT. Effect of brain cooling on brain ischemia and damage markers after fluid percussion brain injury in rats. *Shock* 2007;**28**:284–90.

14. Ames A, III, Wright RL, Kowada M, Thurston JM, Maino G. Cerebral ischemia. the no-reflow phenomenon. *Am J Pathol* 1968;**52**:437–53.

15. Wijdicks EF, Campeau NG, Miller GM. MR imaging in comatose survivors of cardiac resuscitation. *AJNR Am J Neuroradiol* 2001;**22**:1561–65.

16. Fujioka M, Okuchi K, Sakaki T, *et al.* Specific changes in human brain following reperfusion after cardiac arrest. *Stroke* 1994;**25**:2091–5.

17. Levy DE, Caronna JJ, Singer BH, *et al.* Predicting outcome from hypoxic-ischemic coma. *JAMA* 1985;**253**:1420–6.

18. Oddo M, Rossetti AO. Predicting neurological outcome after cardiac arrest. *Curr Opin Crit Care* 2011;**17**:254–9.

19. Greer DM. Mechanisms of injury in hypoxic-ischemic encephalopathy: implications to therapy. *Semin Neurol* 2006;**26**:373–9.

20. Adrie C, Haouache H, Saleh M, *et al.* An underrecognized source of organ donors: patients with brain death after successfully resuscitated cardiac arrest. *Intensive Care Med* 2008;**34**:132–7.

21. Adrie C, Cariou A, Mourvillier B, *et al.* Predicting survival with good neurological recovery at hospital admission after successful resuscitation of out-of-hospital cardiac arrest: the OHCA score. *Eur Heart J* 2006;**27**:2840–5.

22. Fugate JE, Rabinstein AA, Claassen DO, White RD, Wijdicks EF. The FOUR score predicts outcome in patients after cardiac arrest. *Neurocrit Care* 2010;**13**:205–10.

23. Booth CM, Boone RH, Tomlinson G, Detsky AS. Is this patient dead, vegetative, or severely neurologically impaired? Assessing outcome for comatose survivors of cardiac arrest. *JAMA* 2004;**291**:870–9.

24. Zandbergen EG, Hijdra A, Koelman JH, *et al.* Prediction of poor outcome within the first 3 days of postanoxic coma. *Neurology* 2006;**66**:62–8.

25. Rossetti AO, Urbano LA, Delodder F, Kaplan PW, Oddo M. Prognostic value of continuous EEG monitoring during therapeutic hypothermia after cardiac arrest. *Crit Care* 2010;**14**:R173.

26. Tiainen M, Roine RO, Pettila V, Takkunen O. Serum neuron-specific enolase and S-100B protein in cardiac arrest patients treated with hypothermia. *Stroke* 2003;**34**:2881–6.

27. Weiss N, Galanaud D, Carpentier A, Naccache L, Puybasset L. Clinical review: prognostic value of magnetic resonance imaging in acute brain injury and coma. *Crit Care* 2007;**11**:230.

28. Bernard SA, Gray TW, Buist MD, *et al.* Treatment of comatose survivors of out-of-hospital cardiac arrest with induced hypothermia. *N Engl J Med* 2002;**346**:557–63.

29. HACA Study Group. Mild therapeutic hypothermia to improve the neurologic outcome after cardiac arrest. *N Engl J Med* 2002;**346**:549–56.

30. Neumar RW, Nolan JP, Adrie C, *et al.* Post-cardiac arrest syndrome: epidemiology, pathophysiology, treatment, and prognostication. A consensus statement from the International Liaison Committee on Resuscitation (American Heart Association, Australian and New Zealand Council on Resuscitation, European Resuscitation Council, Heart and Stroke Foundation of Canada, InterAmerican Heart Foundation, Resuscitation Council of Asia, and the Resuscitation Council of Southern Africa); the American Heart Association Emergency Cardiovascular Care Committee; the Council on Cardiovascular Surgery and Anesthesia; the Council on Cardiopulmonary, Perioperative, and Critical Care; the Council on Clinical Cardiology; and the Stroke Council. *Circulation* 2008;**118**:2452–83.

31. Dumas F, Grimaldi D, Zuber B, *et al.* Is hypothermia after cardiac arrest effective in both shockable and nonshockable patients? Insights from a large registry. *Circulation* 2011;**123**:877–86.

32. Cariou A, Claessens YE, Pene F, *et al.* Early high-dose erythropoietin therapy and hypothermia after out-of-hospital cardiac arrest. a matched control study. *Resuscitation* 2008;**76**:397–404.

33. Piot C, Croisille P, Staat P, *et al.* Effect of cyclosporine on reperfusion injury in acute myocardial infarction. *N Engl J Med* 2008;**359**:473–81.

34. Kilgannon JH, Jones AE, Shapiro NI, *et al.* Association between arterial hyperoxia following resuscitation from cardiac arrest and in-hospital mortality. *JAMA* 2010;**303**:2165–71.

35. Safar P, Xiao F, Radovsky A, *et al.* Improved cerebral resuscitation from cardiac arrest in dogs with mild hypothermia plus blood flow promotion. *Stroke* 1996;**27**:105–13.

36. Cueni-Villoz N, Devigili A, Delodder F, *et al.* Increased blood glucose variability during therapeutic hypothermia and outcome after cardiac arrest. *Crit Care Med* 2011;**39**(10):2225–31.

37. Arrich J, Zeiner A, Sterz F, *et al.* Factors associated with a change in functional outcome between one month and six months after cardiac arrest. a retrospective cohort study. *Resuscitation* 2009;**80**:876–80.

38. Bunch TJ, White RD, Gersh BJ, *et al.* Long-term outcomes of out-of-hospital cardiac arrest after successful early defibrillation. *N Engl J Med* 2003;**348**:2626–33.

Sepsis-associated encephalopathy

Romain Sonneville, C. Rauturier, F. Verdonk, F. Chretien, and Tarek Sharshar

SUMMARY

Sepsis is often characterized by an early and acute encephalopathy, which is associated with increased morbidity and mortality. Its pathophysiology is highly complex, resulting from both inflammatory and non-inflammatory processes, including microglial activation, production of pro-inflammatory cytokines in brain parenchyma, blood–brain barrier dysfunction, altered neurotransmission, and oxidative stress. The diagnosis of brain dysfunction relies essentially on neurological examination and neurological tests, such as electroencephalography (EEG) and neuroimaging. Factors that can aggravate or prolong brain dysfunction have to be screened and treated systematically. These notably include circulatory failure, metabolic disturbances, sedative overdoses, medications, withdrawal syndromes, and Wernicke's encephalopathy. A brain MRI should be considered in case of persistent brain dysfunction after control of sepsis and exclusion of major confounding factors. Recent MRI studies suggest that septic shock can be associated with acute cerebrovascular lesions and white matter abnormalities. Currently, the treatment of sepsis-associated encephalopathy (SAE) mainly consists of controlling sepsis and supportive measures, including management of organ failure(s), and prevention of all aggravating factors. Modulation of microglial activation, prevention of blood–brain barrier alterations, and use of antioxidants represent relevant therapeutic targets that may impact significantly on neurological outcomes. In the future, investigations in patients with sepsis should be undertaken to reduce the duration of brain dysfunction and to study the impact of this reduction on important health outcomes, including functional and cognitive status in survivors.

Introduction

Sepsis is often characterized by an acute brain dysfunction ranging from confusion to coma, which is associated with increased mortality [1,2]. This encephalopathy is characterized by inattention, disorganized thinking, and fluctuating mental status changes, and therefore, matches with current criteria for delirium. Among the myriad of conditions that can induce acute brain dysfunction in critically ill patients, sepsis, in the form of sepsis-associated encephalopathy, represents the most frequent and severe cause [3,4]. Several nomenclatures have been proposed to describe the encephalopathy in sepsis [5]. For this chapter, we will refer to it as SAE, about which we will draw on references that use both the terms encephalopathy and delirium. Diagnosing encephalopathy in a patient with sepsis implies a systematic diagnostic approach of all potential factors, additionally to sepsis, that can contribute to brain dysfunction. The aim of this chapter is to describe the pathophysiology of SAE and to propose a diagnostic approach to a critically ill patient with encephalopathy in the context of sepsis.

Pathophysiology

Brain signaling and microglial activation

The encephalopathy in sepsis is considered a diffuse cerebral dysfunction as a consequence of the systemic inflammatory response to an infection, with no direct central nervous system (CNS) infection. The response to stress is physiologically triggered by an activating signal that is mediated by three pathways (Figure 38.1). The first one is the vagus nerve, which can detect visceral inflammation through its axonal cytokine receptors: inflammatory products produced in damaged tissues activate afferent signals that are

Brain Disorders in Critical Illness, ed. Robert D. Stevens, Tarek Sharshar, and E. Wesley Ely. Published by Cambridge University Press. © Cambridge University Press 2013.

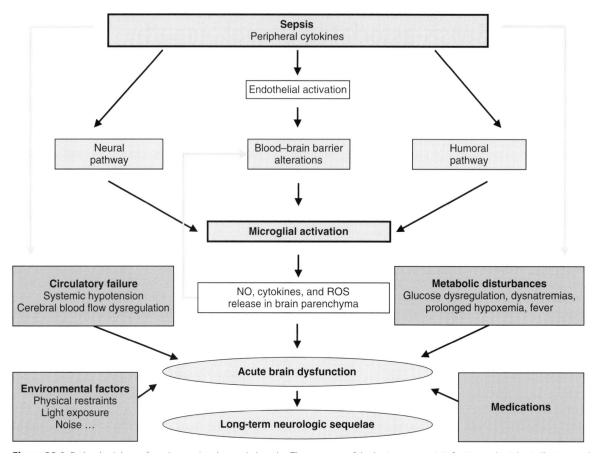

Figure 38.1 Pathophysiology of sepsis-associated encephalopathy. The response of the brain to systemic infection is physiologically triggered by an activating signal that is mediated by three pathways. (1) The neural pathway that requires activation of primary afferent nerves, such as the vagal or the trigeminal nerves, by involving peripherally produced pathogen-associated molecular patterns (PAMPs) and cytokines. (2) The humoral pathway involves circulating cytokines. They reach the brain at the level of the choroid plexus and the circumventricular organs that lie outside the blood–brain barrier. (3) The blood–brain barrier alterations induced by the activation of cerebral endothelial cells results in the release of various mediators into the brain. This activation is due to the production, at the early phase of sepsis, of nitric oxide synthase-derived nitric oxide. All these pathways instigate the activation of microglial cells, which are the resident immune cells of the brain. When activated, microglial cells may negatively affect the brain by the production of nitric oxide, cytokines, and reactive oxygen species that lead to cell death within vulnerable areas of the brain. This production is, in itself, responsible for an increase of the blood–brain barrier alterations, and thus causes a vicious circle increasing brain dysfunction and injury. These mechanisms are compounded by common metabolic disturbances that occur in septic patients (such as prolonged hyperglycemia, severe hypoxemia), hemodynamic failure, use of medications, and iatrogenic and environmental factors. Sepsis-related brain dysfunction may be associated with neurological sequelae in survivors, including functional and cognitive decline, probably by neurodegenerative mechanisms.

relayed to the nucleus *tractus solitarius* in the brainstem. Subsequent activation of vagus efferent activity inhibits cytokine synthesis in damaged tissues through a cholinergic anti-inflammatory pathway (the inflammatory reflex) [6]. The vagus nerve is also connected to other autonomic nuclei, notably the hypothalamic paraventricular nucleus that controls adrenal axis and vasopressin secretion [7]. The second pathway involves the circumventricular organs (CVOs), which are located near neuroendocrine and autonomic nuclei. Circumventricular organs are deprived of a

blood–brain barrier, and express components of innate and adaptive immune systems. Once visceral or systemic inflammation is detected by the first or the second pathway, the activating signal will spread to behavioral, neuroendocrine, and autonomic centers. Sepsis enhances the transcription of several pro- and anti-inflammatory cytokines and chemokines in the brain, including tumor necrosis factor alpha (TNFα), interleukin-1 beta (IL-1β), transforming growth factor beta (TGF-β), and monocyte chemoattractant protein 1 (MCP1) [8]. These mediators will affect microglial cells, astrocytes, and neurons, inducing brain dysfunction. Microglial activation may represent one of the earliest changes observed in sepsis-associated encephalopathy and prolonged microglial activation may negatively affect other brain cells during sepsis [9]. Early microglial activation in sepsis was evidenced in mice models within 4 hours following LPS injection, as assessed by the increased pro-inflammatory cytokine IL-1β level in microglia [10]. Using positron emission tomography (PET) imaging in non-human primates, another study demonstrated microglia activation only 1 h after LPS-induced systemic inflammation [11]. There is also increasing evidence that an excess of pro-inflammatory mediators released in the CNS at the onset of sepsis will lead to cell death within vulnerable areas of the brain [12–14]. Finally, blood–brain barrier alterations induced by the activation of cerebral endothelial cells represent a third pathway by which different mediators may reach the brain.

Endothelial activation and blood–brain barrier dysfunction

Endothelial cells play a major role in sepsis-associated brain inflammation. Sepsis induces their activation, which results in blood–brain barrier dysfunction and release of various mediators into the brain. Experimental data indicate that during early sepsis, eNOS-derived nitric oxide (NO) exhibits pro-inflammatory characteristics and contributes to the activation and dysfunction of cerebrovascular endothelial cells [15]. The activated endothelium relays the inflammatory response into the brain by releasing pro-inflammatory cytokines and NO that are able to interact with surrounding brain cells. The other consequences of endothelial activation may include impairment of metabolic supply (oxygen, glucose, and other nutrients), microcirculatory dysfunction, which might compromise cerebral perfusion, and blood–brain barrier alterations. Experimental data suggest that endotoxemia leads to inflammation in the brain, with alteration in blood–brain barrier, up-regulation of aquaporin 4 (AQP4) and associated edema, neutrophil infiltration, astrocytosis, as well as apoptotic cellular death, all of which appear to be mediated by TNFα signaling through TNFR1 [16]. Alterations of the blood–brain barrier have also been evidenced in patients with septic shock, with help of brain magnetic resonance imaging [17]. Blood–brain barrier breakdown can be localized in the cortex around the Virchow–Robin spaces or have a more diffuse pattern in the whole white matter. It can also predominate in posterior lobes, being consistent with a posterior reversible encephalopathy syndrome [18]. Blood–brain barrier alterations might also facilitate the passage of potential neurotoxic factors.

Alteration of neurotransmission

Significant neurotransmitter alterations have been described during experimental sepsis, including cholinergic, brain beta-adrenergic, gamma-aminobutyric acid, and serotoninergic release [19]. These phenomena predominate in cortex and in hippocampus, and may be mediated by NO, cytokines, and prostaglandins [20]. Neurotransmitter synthesis is also altered by ammonium and tyrosine, tryptophan and phenylalanine, whose plasma levels are increased secondary to liver dysfunction and muscle proteolysis [21]. Their neurotoxic effect might be potentiated by the decrease in branched-chain amino acids. Deficit in cholinergic function and imbalance between dopaminergic and cholinergic pathways have been postulated as a major mechanism of delirium [22,23]. It has been also hypothesized that reduced cholinergic inhibition of microglia is involved in delirium [9]. However, administration of rivastigmine, an agent that increases extracellular acetylcholine activity and may restore cholinergic control of microglia, did not decrease duration of delirium and might have been linked to increased mortality of critically ill patients with delirium [24]. Data from critically ill patients also suggest that use of GABA agonists, such as benzodiazepines, is associated with an increased risk of brain dysfunction [25]. Noradrenergic neurotransmission might be also particularly involved in SAE as dexmedetomidine, an agonist of alpha-2 adrenoceptors which are highly expressed in the locus coeruleus, is associated with less brain dysfunction and better outcomes in septic patients when compared with midazolam [26,27].

Microcirculatory dysfunction and coagulopathy

Endothelial activation alters vascular tone and induces both microcirculatory dysfunction and coagulopathy, which will in turn favor ischemic and/or hemorrhagic lesions [28]. It has to be noted that ischemia is consistently observed in brain areas susceptible to low cerebral flow [28,29]. Furthermore, it has been recently shown that SAE is more likely associated with disturbed autoregulation than with altered cerebral blood flow or tissue oxygenation [30]. One major unanswered issue is whether targeting higher systemic blood pressures will result in improved cerebral perfusion and oxygenation, given the presence of a microcirculatory dysfunction. Finally, neuropathological examination of non-survivors of septic shock reveals hemorrhages in about 10% of cases, which were always associated with clotting disorders [31].

Oxidative stress, mitochondrial dysfunction, and apoptosis

Experimental data suggest that oxidative damage, assessed by the thiobarbituric acid reactive species and the protein carbonyl assays, occurred early (after 6 h) in the course of sepsis [32]. Moreover, the combined use of antioxidants (N-acetyl-cysteine and deferoxamine) attenuated oxidative damage in hippocampus 6 h after sepsis induction [33]. Mitochondrial-mediated apoptosis has been evidenced in experimental sepsis and might be related to a decrease of intracellular anti-apoptotic (Bcl-2) and an increase of pro-apoptotic (Bax) factors [12]. In patients who had died from septic shock, neuronal and microglial apoptosis have been detected in autonomic and neuroendocrine nuclei as well as in amygdala, and the magnitude of apoptosis correlated with expression of endothelial iNOS [29]. Additionally to NO, other pro-apoptotic factors have been incriminated, such as glutamate, TNFα, and hyperglycemia [34].

Diagnosis
Clinical examination

Detection of acute brain dysfunction in the intensive care unit (ICU) is based on repeated daily neurological examination (Table 38.1). Sepsis-associated encephalopathy is characterized by acute changes in mental status, cognition, alteration of sleep–wake cycle, disorientation, impaired attention, and/or disorganized thinking. Sometimes exaggerated motor activity with agitation, and/or hallucinations can be observed and agitation and somnolence can occur alternatively. Other but less frequent motor symptoms include paratonic rigidity, asterixis, tremor, and multifocal myoclonus. Physicians have at their disposal validated clinical instruments for detecting brain dysfunction in critically ill patients, including the Confusion Assessment Method for the ICU (CAM–ICU) which has been shown to be highly reliable in the detection of ICU delirium in mechanically ventilated patients [35], and the Intensive Care Delirium Screening Checklist (ICDSC) [36]. For awareness, Glasgow Coma Scale is commonly used; for monitoring of arousal and sedation, the Richmond Agitation–Sedation Scale (RASS) or the Assessment to Intensive Care Environment (ATICE) can be used [37]. Once brain dysfunction is identified, an exhaustive neurological examination assessing neck stiffness, motor responses, muscular strength, plantar and deep tendon reflexes, and cranial nerves is mandatory. The main limitation of clinical detection is sedation, as sedatives alter awareness and cognition, even after their

Table 38.1 Neurological approach in sedated patients.

Domain	Phenotype	Interrupt sedation?	Additional tests
Spontaneous motor activity	Agitated	Careful	If no obvious explanation*
Awareness/awakeness	Comatose	Yes	If persistent* #
Cognition	Delirious	Yes	If persistent*
Motor and brainstem responses	1. Modification not explained by sedation 2. Focal signs 3. Myoclonus	1. Yes 2. Not necessary 3. No	1. If persistent* 2. Necessary (MRI) 3. Necessary (EEG, MRI...)

Four domains have to be evaluated when performing clinical examination in sedated patients: (1) spontaneous motor activity, (2) awareness, (3) cognition, and (4) motor and brainstem responses. Depending on the phenotype, a "sedation stop" test can be performed. Additional tests have then to be discussed in case of persistent neurological abnormality.
* Biological, neuroradiological, and electrophysiological complementary investigations have to be discussed.
# Use of antagonist of benzodiazepines and/or opioids have to be discussed.

Table 38.2 Brain magnetic resonance imaging (MRI) findings in sepsis.

Brain MRI findings	References
Acute changes	
Cytotoxic edema (hippocampus, cortex)	[17,66]
Ischemic lesions	
Vasogenic edema	[17,66]
Posterior reversible encephalopathy syndrome (PRES)	[18,67]
Chronic changes observed in survivors	
White matter disruption	[68]
Brain atrophy (Frontal cortex, hippocampus)	[69]

Table 38.3 Electroencephalographic (EEG) patterns in sepsis.

Electroencephalographic findings	Association with adverse outcome	References
Normal EEG	0	[47]
Theta (mild generalized slowing)	+	[47]
Delta (severe slowing)	+	[47]
Triphasic waves	++	[47]
Periodic epileptiform discharges	++	[39]
Electrographic seizures	++	[39]
Generalized suppression or burst-suppression	+++	[40,47]

discontinuation. It was recently suggested that brainstem reflexes may be maintained and retain short-term prognostic value even in patients receiving sedative infusions [38]. The occurrence of sudden fluctuations in mental status or inattention unexplained by modification of sedative infusion rate, occurrence of focal neurological sign, seizure, and neck stiffness should prompt the physician to consider neuroimaging, EEG, and/or lumbar puncture.

Other investigations

First of all, a direct CNS infection (e.g., meningitis, brain abscess) should be ruled out. Other factors that can contribute to brain dysfunction include iatrogenic and environmental factors, metabolic disturbances, or drugs toxicity. In the presence of focal neurological signs, brain imaging is indicated. Following seizure(s), neuroimaging and an EEG will be required, with an emphasis on excluding non-convulsive status epilepticus. Main MRI and electroencephalographic findings observed in sepsis are described in Tables 38.2 and 38.3, respectively. It has been recently shown that sepsis can be associated with electrographic seizures or periodic epileptiform discharge [39]. Other EEG abnormalities include increased theta rhythms, triphasic waves and, less often but more pejorative, burst suppression [40]. Assessments of plasma levels of brain injury biomarkers, such as neuron-specific enolase and S100-β protein, have been proposed for detecting brain dysfunction in sedated septic patients [41,42].

Although neuroimaging is clearly indicated in the presence of focal neurological deficits, it should also be considered when no cause for encephalopathy has been identified. Brain MRI has a higher sensitivity than computed tomography (CT) for detecting acute CNS disorders such as recent ischemic or hemorrhagic stroke, white matter disorders, or brain abscess. However, before transporting the critically ill patient, risks and benefits of brain MRI studies should be carefully balanced. In addition to the importance of etiological diagnosis, assessment of the nature and extent of brain damage may also influence the patient's treatment. For example, evidence for brain hemorrhage should lead to discontinuation of any drug with an anticoagulant activity.

In the absence of focal sign(s) or when neuroimaging is normal, physicians should carefully screen all potential metabolic or toxic causes of confusion that can be easily treated. Standard laboratory tests should be performed for detecting common metabolic disturbances that can impair consciousness (such as hypoglycemia, hypercalcemia, hypo- or hypernatremia). Encephalopathy in critically ill patients can result from various causes, which can be entwined, masked, or worsened by a septic process. Sepsis can be the triggering and/or aggravating factor of hepatic or uremic encephalopathy. A careful screening of the drug chart should be systematically performed in order to identify potential neurotoxic substances that could be then discontinued (or tapered according to their plasma levels or to the liver and/or renal function). Additional to sedative and analgesics, many classes of drugs currently administered in critically ill patients can induce acute brain dysfunction, notably a number

Table 38.4 Medications associated with brain dysfunction in the intensive care unit.

Agent	Mechanism of action
Benzodiazepines (long- and short-acting)	Sedation Neuronal inhibition by membrane hyperpolarization (GABA-agonist)
Opioids	Anticholinergic toxicity CNS sedation Urinary retention, fecal impaction
Antibiotics Penicillins, cephalosporins, carbapenems Quinolones	Inhibition of $GABA_A$ receptors
Antiarrhythmics Flecaine, Amiodarone Digoxin	Strong anticholinergic effects Sodium channel blockage Unknown
Beta-blockers	Not yet described Association with delirium
Diuretics	Dehydration and electrolyte disturbances
Steroids	Anticholinergic toxicity Increase of catecholamine activity GABA-agonist Altered serotonin activity
Inhaled anesthetics	Beta-amyloid protein generation Cytotoxicity of beta-amyloid potentiating Apoptosis inducing
Ketamine	NMDA-antagonism
Histamine-2 blocking agents Cimetidine	Anticholinergic toxicity
Non-steroidal anti-inflammatory drugs	Blood–brain barrier dysfunction
Anticholinergics Oxybutinin, bladder antispasmodics	Anticholinergic toxicity
Anticonvulsants Phenobarbital, phenytoin	CNS sedation
Antiparkinsonian agents L-Dopa, dopamine agonists, amantadine	Dopaminergic toxicity
Antidepressants (amitryptiline, imipramine, doxepin)	Anticholinergic toxicity

CNS, central nervous system; GABA, gamma-aminobutyric acid; NMDA, N-methyl-D-aspartate.

of antibiotics, steroids, and cardiac drugs (Table 38.4). It must be emphasized that encephalopathy is often multifactorial. Finally, reappearance or persistence of encephalopathy may indicate that sepsis is not controlled.

Differential diagnosis and other specific causes of encephalopathy

As aforementioned, a brain infection must always be suspected and relevance of brain imaging and lumbar puncture always addressed in a septic patient with any central neurological symptoms. Critically ill patients

are also susceptible to drug overdose but also drug withdrawal, notably of benzodiazepines and opioids. The chronological link and the neurological improvement after their re-administration are arguments for a withdrawal syndrome. Tobacco dependency is a risk factor for delirium in critically ill patients that may be prevented by use of a nicotine patch in chronic smokers admitted to the ICU [43]. Alcohol withdrawal-related delirium is often evoked in an alcoholic patient who develops an encephalopathy. This represents a potentially fatal complication that occurs in only 5% of hospitalized alcohol-dependent patients and usually within 48–72 hours of the last drink. The predominance of psychomotor agitation, hallucinosis, and autonomic signs (hyperpyrexia, tachycardia, hypertension, and diaphoresis) are suggestive of the diagnosis. In malnourished or alcoholic patients, Wernicke's encephalopathy must always be evoked and treated with intravenous thiamine, especially if there is evidence of ophthalmoplegia or ataxia [44]. Thiamine deficiency can be aggravated by infusion of glucose. In a patient with unexplained neurological symptoms (focal neurological sign or confusion) and bloodstream infection, an infective endocarditis should be systematically ruled out [45]. Finally, air embolism is an iatrogenic cause of sudden coma, agitation, seizure, or focal neurological signs, and for which hyperbaric oxygen is recommended.

Outcomes

Eidelman *et al.* showed in a landmark study that about one third of patients with sepsis had a Glasgow Coma Scale score less than 12, and that alteration of alertness and consciousness was an independent prognostic factor, increasing mortality rate up to 63% when Glasgow Coma Scale score was less than 8 [1]. More recent studies have shown that in addition to being highly prevalent in the ICU, delirium is an independent risk factor for 3-fold increase in mortality, with elderly patients being at an increased risk [4]. The number of days of ICU delirium was associated with higher 1-year mortality after adjustment for relevant covariates in an older ICU population [46]. Mortality also increases with severity of electrophysiological abnormalities, ranging from 0 when EEG is interpreted as normal to 67% when it shows burst suppressions [39,47]. Electrographic seizures and periodic discharges are also associated with increased mortality [17,39]. The prognosis value of MRI findings remains to be assessed [17]. The impact of brain dysfunction during sepsis on secondary outcomes is not known but is certainly close to that reported for delirium in critically ill patients. It is clearly established that delirium in critically ill patients is associated with a prolonged length of stay in the ICU and hospital, a longer duration of mechanical ventilation, and extra costs. It has been established that sepsis is associated with cognitive decline in elderly patients, as it has been reported in critically ill patients who developed delirium in the ICU and in survivors from acute respiratory distress syndrome [48–50]. As aforementioned, it can be related to an Alzheimer-type degenerating process involving prolonged microglial activation and

vascular-type process related to diffuse ischemic damage. This hypothesis is supported by data showing that elevated levels of beta-amyloid in ICU patients with delirium are correlated with long-term cognitive impairment [51]. Insults of the hippocampus, which is liable to inflammatory and ischemic damage, are certainly a determinant of neuropsychological sequelae in survivors of critical illness. Indeed, it has been reported that critically ill patients, including septic patients, are at risk to develop depression, anxiety, and posttraumatic stress syndrome [52]. However, the relationships between dementia and delirium are complex, as pre-existing cognitive impairment is a major risk factor of delirium and as delirium can aggravate or induce cognitive disorders [53]. While advances in clinical care provided to septic patients have greatly improved outcomes, several studies now indicate that sepsis survivors suffer from residual deficits in cognitive function and physical performance that represent a downward and lasting trajectory change in their lives [54,55].

Therapeutic perspectives

There is no specific treatment for SAE, hence management should focus on control of infection source and on supportive measures such as management of organ failure(s), prevention of metabolic disturbances, and avoidance of neurotoxic drugs. Preventive strategies to reduce occurrence and duration of brain dysfunction should be applied for every patient admitted to the ICU. Symptomatic treatment of delirium and agitation does not differ from that proposed in critically ill patients and has been described elsewhere [56]. Adjunctive therapies of septic shock may protect the blood–brain barrier or reduce endothelial activation but their effect has not been established. For instance, activated protein C in septic shock patients with impaired consciousness significantly reduced plasma levels of S100-β protein [57]. Steroids have been shown to reduce posttraumatic stress syndrome [58] and prevention of prolonged hyperglycemia may also be neuroprotective [59].

Various therapeutic interventions have been experimentally tested. Inhibition of iNOS reduces neuronal apoptosis in septic animals but does not improve the state of consciousness and may even aggravate ischemic injuries of the brain [60]. Another study showed that sepsis-induced cognitive impairment at 2 months was prevented in iNOS knockout mice [14]. Interestingly, cognitive impairment was associated with activation of glial cells and not neuronal death. Experimental studies show a protective effect on the blood–brain barrier with the use of magnesium [61,62], riluzole [62], hyperbaric oxygenotherapy [63], calcium channel blockers, steroids, or anti-cytokine antibodies [64]. Intravenous immunoglobulins, administered prior to cecal ligation and perforation, preserve blood–brain barrier integrity [65]. Regarding oxidative stress, antioxidant treatment with N-acetyl-cysteine and deferoxamine prevents cognitive impairment in septic mice [33].

Conclusion

Brain dysfunction is frequent in sepsis but too often neglected, despite its dramatic impact on outcomes. Its pathophysiology is highly complex, resulting from both inflammatory and non-inflammatory processes that affect all types of brain cells. The diagnosis of encephalopathy relies essentially on neurological examination and selected additional tests, including EEG and neuroimaging. Brain dysfunction during sepsis is frequently linked with other factors that have to be screened systematically, including withdrawal syndrome, drugs overdose, and severe metabolic disturbances. Currently, the treatment of sepsis-associated encephalopathy mainly consists of controlling sepsis and supportive measures, including management of organ failure(s), prevention of metabolic disturbances, and avoidance of sedatives and neurotoxic drugs.

References

1. Eidelman LA, Putterman D, Putterman C, Sprung CL. The spectrum of septic encephalopathy. Definitions, etiologies, and mortalities. *JAMA* 1996;**275**:470–3.

2. Sprung CL, Peduzzi PN, Shatney CH, *et al.* Impact of encephalopathy on mortality in the sepsis syndrome. The Veterans Administration Systemic Sepsis Cooperative Study Group. *Crit Care Med* 1990;**18**:801–6.

3. Bleck TP, Smith MC, Pierre-Louis SJ, *et al.* Neurologic complications of critical medical illnesses. *Crit Care Med* 1993;**21**:98–103.

4. Ely EW, Shintani A, Truman B, *et al.* Delirium as a predictor of mortality in mechanically ventilated patients in the intensive care unit. *JAMA* 2004;**291**:1753–62.

5. Morandi A, Pandharipande P, Trabucchi M, *et al.* Understanding international differences in terminology for delirium and other types of acute brain dysfunction

in critically ill patients. *Intensive Care Med* 2008;**34**:1907–15.

6. Tracey KJ. The inflammatory reflex. *Nature* 2002;**420**:853–9.

7. Sharshar T, Annane D. Endocrine effects of vasopressin in critically ill patients. *Best Pract Res Clin Anesthesiol* 2008;**22**:265–73.

8. Semmler A, Hermann S, Mormann F, *et al.* Sepsis causes neuroinflammation and concomitant decrease of cerebral metabolism. *J Neuroinflamm* 2008;**5**:38.

9. van Gool WA, van de Beek D, Eikelenboom P. Systemic infection and delirium: when cytokines and acetylcholine collide. *Lancet* 2010;**375**:773–5.

10. Henry CJ, Huang Y, Wynne AM, Godbout JP. Peripheral lipopolysaccharide (LPS) challenge promotes microglial hyperactivity in aged mice that is associated with exaggerated induction of both pro-inflammatory IL-1beta and anti-inflammatory IL-10 cytokines. *Brain, Behav Immun* 2009;**23**:309–17.

11. Hannestad J, Gallezot JD, Schafbauer T, *et al.* Endotoxin-induced systemic inflammation activates microglia: [^{11}C]PBR28 positron emission tomography in nonhuman primates. *NeuroImage* 2012;**63** (1):232–9.

12. Semmler A, Okulla T, Sastre M, Dumitrescu-Ozimek L, Heneka MT. Systemic inflammation induces apoptosis with variable vulnerability of different brain regions. *J Chem Neuroanatomy* 2005;**30**:144–57.

13. Semmler A, Frisch C, Debeir T, *et al.* Long-term cognitive impairment, neuronal loss and reduced cortical cholinergic innervation after recovery from sepsis in a rodent model. *Exp Neurol* 2007;**204**:733–40.

14. Weberpals M, Hermes M, Hermann S, *et al.* NOS2 gene deficiency protects from sepsis-induced long-term cognitive deficits. *J Neuroscience* 2009;**29**:14177–84.

15. Handa O, Stephen J, Cepinskas G. Role of endothelial nitric oxide synthase-derived nitric oxide in activation and dysfunction of cerebrovascular endothelial cells during early onsets of sepsis. *Am J Physiol Heart Circ Physiol* 2008;**295**:H1712–19.

16. Alexander JJ, Jacob A, Cunningham P, Hensley L, Quigg RJ. TNF is a key mediator of septic encephalopathy acting through its receptor, TNF receptor-1. *Neurochemistry Int* 2008;**52**:447–56.

17. Sharshar T, Carlier R, Bernard F, *et al.* Brain lesions in septic shock: a magnetic resonance imaging study. *Intensive Care Med* 2007;**33**:798–806.

18. Fugate JE, Claassen DO, Cloft HJ, *et al.* Posterior reversible encephalopathy syndrome: associated clinical and radiologic findings. *Mayo Clin Proc* 2010;**85**:427–32.

19. Kadoi Y, Saito S. An alteration in the gamma-aminobutyric acid receptor system in experimentally induced septic shock in rats. *Crit Care Med* 1996;**24**:298–305.

20. Pavlov VA, Ochani M, Gallowitsch-Puerta M, *et al.* Central muscarinic cholinergic regulation of the systemic inflammatory response during endotoxemia. *Proc Natl Acad Sci USA* 2006;**103**:5219–23.

21. Basler T, Meier-Hellmann A, Bredle D, Reinhart K. Amino acid imbalance early in septic encephalopathy. *Intensive Care Med* 2002;**28**:293–8.

22. Hshieh TT, Fong TG, Marcantonio ER, Inouye SK. Cholinergic deficiency hypothesis in delirium: a synthesis of current evidence. *J Gerontol A Biol Sci Med Sci* 2008;**63**:764–72.

23. Field RH, Gossen A, Cunningham C. Prior pathology in the basal forebrain cholinergic system predisposes to inflammation-induced working memory deficits: reconciling inflammatory and cholinergic hypotheses of delirium. *J Neurosci* 2012;**32**:6288–94.

24. van Eijk MM, Roes KC, Honing ML, *et al.* Effect of rivastigmine as an adjunct to usual care with haloperidol on duration of delirium and mortality in critically ill patients: a multicentre, double-blind, placebo-controlled randomised trial. *Lancet* 2010;**376**:1829–37.

25. Pandharipande P, Shintani A, Peterson J, *et al.* Lorazepam is an independent risk factor for transitioning to delirium in intensive care unit patients. *Anesthesiology* 2006;**104**:21–6.

26. Pandharipande P, Sanders RD, Girard TD, *et al.* Effect of dexmedetomidine versus lorazepam on outcome in patients with sepsis: an a priori-designed analysis of the MENDS randomized controlled trial. *Crit Care* 2010;**14**:R38.

27. Pandharipande PP, Pun BT, Herr DL, *et al.* Effect of sedation with dexmedetomidine vs lorazepam on acute brain dysfunction in mechanically ventilated patients: the MENDS randomized controlled trial. *JAMA* 2007;**298**:2644–53.

28. Sharshar T, Annane D, de la Grandmaison GL, *et al.* The neuropathology of septic shock. *Brain Pathol* 2004;**14**:21–33.

29. Sharshar T, Gray F, Lorin de la Grandmaison G, *et al.* Apoptosis of neurons in cardiovascular autonomic centres triggered by inducible nitric oxide synthase after death from septic shock. *Lancet* 2003;**362**:1799–805.

30. Pfister D, Siegemund M, Dell-Kuster S, *et al.* Cerebral perfusion in sepsis-associated delirium. *Crit Care* 2008;**12**:R63.

31. Sharshar T, Annane D, de la Grandmaison GL, *et al.* The neuropathology of septic shock. *Brain Pathol* 2004;**14**:21–33.

32. Barichello T, Fortunato JJ, Vitali AM, *et al.* Oxidative variables in the rat brain after sepsis induced by cecal ligation and perforation. *Crit Care Med* 2006;**34**:886–9.

33. Barichello T, Machado RA, Constantino L, *et al.* Antioxidant treatment prevented late memory impairment in an animal model of sepsis. *Crit Care Med* 2007;**35**:2186–90.

34. Polito A, Brouland JP, Porcher R, *et al.* Hyperglycaemia and apoptosis of microglial cells in human septic shock. *Crit Care* 2011;**15**:R131.

35. Ely EW, Inouye SK, Bernard GR, *et al.* Delirium in mechanically ventilated patients: validity and reliability of the confusion assessment method for the intensive care unit (CAM-ICU). *JAMA* 2001;**286**:2703–10.

36. Bergeron N, Dubois MJ, Dumont M, *et al.* Intensive care delirium screening checklist: evaluation of a new screening tool. *Intensive Care Med* 2001;**27**:859–64.

37. De Jonghe B, Bastuji-Garin S, Fangio P, *et al.* Sedation algorithm in critically ill patients without acute brain injury. *Crit Care Med* 2005;**33**:120–7.

38. Sharshar T, Porcher R, Siami S, *et al.* Brainstem responses can predict death and delirium in sedated patients in intensive care unit. *Crit Care Med* 2011;**39**:1960–7.

39. Oddo M, Carrera E, Claassen J, Mayer SA, Hirsch LJ. Continuous electroencephalography in the medical intensive care unit. *Crit Care Med* 2009;**37**:2051–6.

40. Watson PL, Shintani AK, Tyson R, *et al.* Presence of electroencephalogram burst suppression in sedated, critically ill patients is associated with increased mortality. *Crit Care Med* 2008;**36**:3171–7.

41. Piazza O, Russo E, Cotena S, Esposito G, Tufano R. Elevated S100B levels do not correlate with the severity of encephalopathy during sepsis. *Br J Anaesth* 2007;**99**:518–21.

42. Nguyen DN, Spapen H, Su F, *et al.* Elevated serum levels of S-100beta protein and neuron-specific enolase are associated with brain injury in patients with severe sepsis and septic shock. *Crit Care Med* 2006;**34**:1967–74.

43. Lucidarme O, Seguin A, Daubin C, *et al.* Nicotine withdrawal and agitation in ventilated critically ill patients. *Crit Care* 2010;**14**:R58.

44. Sechi G, Serra A. Wernicke's encephalopathy: new clinical settings and recent advances in diagnosis and management. *Lancet Neurol* 2007;**6**:442–55.

45. Sonneville R, Mirabel M, Hajage D, *et al.* Neurologic complications and outcomes of infective endocarditis in critically ill patients: the ENDOcardite en REAnimation prospective multicenter study. *Crit Care Med* 2011;**39**:1474–81.

46. Pisani MA, Kong SY, Kasl SV, *et al.* Days of delirium are associated with 1-year mortality in an older intensive care unit population. *Am J Respir Crit Care Med* 2009;**180**:1092–7.

47. Young GB, Bolton CF, Archibald YM, Austin TW, Wells GA. The electroencephalogram in sepsis-associated encephalopathy. *J Clin Neurophysiol* 1992;**9**:145–52.

48. Hopkins RO, Herridge MS. Quality of life, emotional abnormalities, and cognitive dysfunction in survivors of acute lung injury/acute respiratory distress syndrome. *Clin Chest Med* 2006;**27**:679–89.

49. Hopkins RO, Jackson JC. Assessing neurocognitive outcomes after critical illness: are delirium and long-term cognitive impairments related? *Curr Opin Crit Care* 2006;**12**:388–94.

50. Hopkins RO, Jackson JC. Short- and long-term cognitive outcomes in intensive care unit survivors. *Clin Chest Med* 2009;**30**:143–53, ix.

51. van den Boogaard M, Kox M, Quinn KL, *et al.* Biomarkers associated with delirium in critically ill patients and their relation with long-term subjective cognitive dysfunction; indications for different pathways governing delirium in inflamed and noninflamed patients. *Crit Care* 2011;**15**:R297.

52. Boer KR, van Ruler O, van Emmerik AA, *et al.* Factors associated with posttraumatic stress symptoms in a prospective cohort of patients after abdominal sepsis: a nomogram. *Intensive Care Med* 2008;**34**:664–74.

53. Iwashyna TJ, Ely EW, Smith DM, Langa KM. Long-term cognitive impairment and functional disability among survivors of severe sepsis. *JAMA* 2010;**304**:1787–94.

54. Girard TD, Jackson JC, Pandharipande PP, *et al.* Delirium as a predictor of long-term cognitive impairment in survivors of critical illness. *Crit Care Med* 2010;**38**:1513–20.

55. Iwashyna TJ, Cooke CR, Wunsch H, Kahn JM. Population burden of long-term survivorship after severe sepsis in older Americans. *J Am Geriatr Soc* 2012;**60**:1070–7.

56. Girard TD, Pandharipande PP, Ely EW. Delirium in the intensive care unit. *Crit Care* 2008;**12**(Suppl 3):S3.

57. Spapen H, Nguyen DN, Troubleyn J, Huyghens L, Schiettecatte J. Drotrecogin alfa (activated) may attenuate severe sepsis-associated encephalopathy in clinical septic shock. *Crit Care* 2010;**14**:R54.

58. Schelling G, Roozendaal B, Krauseneck T, *et al.* Efficacy of hydrocortisone in preventing posttraumatic stress disorder following critical illness and major surgery. *Ann N Y Acad Sci* 2006;**1071**:46–53.

59. Sonneville R, den Hertog HM, Guiza F, *et al.* Impact of hyperglycemia on neuropathological alterations during critical illness. *J Clin Endocrinol Metab* 2012;**97**:2113–23.

60. Kadoi Y, Goto F. Selective inducible nitric oxide inhibition can restore hemodynamics, but does not improve neurological dysfunction in experimentally-induced septic shock in rats. *Anesth Analg* 2004;**99**:212–20.

61. Esen F, Erdem T, Aktan D, *et al.* Effect of magnesium sulfate administration on blood-brain barrier in a rat model of intraperitoneal sepsis: a randomized controlled experimental study. *Crit Care* 2005;**9**:R18–23.

62. Toklu HZ, Uysal MK, Kabasakal L, *et al.* The effects of riluzole on neurological, brain biochemical, and histological changes in early and late term of sepsis in rats. *J Surg Res* 2009;**152**:238–48.

63. Avtan SM, Kaya M, Orhan N, *et al.* The effects of hyperbaric oxygen therapy on blood-brain barrier permeability in septic rats. *Brain Res* 2011;**1412**:63–72.

64. Wratten ML. Therapeutic approaches to reduce systemic inflammation in septic-associated neurologic complications. *Eur J Anaesthesiol Suppl* 2008;**42**:1–7.

65. Esen F, Senturk E, Ozcan PE, *et al.* Intravenous immunoglobulins prevent the breakdown of the blood–brain barrier in experimentally induced sepsis. *Crit Care Med* 2012;**40**:1214–20.

66. Bozza FA, Garteiser P, Oliveira MF, *et al.* Sepsis-associated encephalopathy: a magnetic resonance imaging and spectroscopy study. *J Cereb Blood Flow Metab* 2010;**30**:440–8.

67. Bartynski WS, Boardman JF, Zeigler ZR, Shadduck RK, Lister J. Posterior reversible encephalopathy syndrome in infection, sepsis, and shock. *AJNR Am J Neuroradiol* 2006;**27**:2179–90.

68. Morandi A, Rogers BP, Gunther ML, *et al.* The relationship between delirium duration, white matter integrity, and cognitive impairment in intensive care unit survivors as determined by diffusion tensor imaging: the VISIONS prospective cohort magnetic resonance imaging study. *Crit Care Med* 2012;**40**:2182–9.

69. Gunther ML, Morandi A, Krauskopf E, *et al.*; VISIONS Investigation, VISualizing ICU SurvivOrs Neuroradiological Sequelae. The association between brain volumes, delirium duration, and cognitive outcomes in intensive care unit survivors: the VISIONS cohort magnetic resonance imaging study. *Crit Care Med* 2012;**40**(7):2022–32.

Chapter 39

Seizures and status epilepticus in critical illness

Brandon Foreman and Jan Claassen

SUMMARY

Seizures are frequently encountered in the medical, surgical, or neurological intensive care unit (ICU). They typically are seen in patients with either systemic illness or direct injury to the brain: sepsis, post-cardiac arrest, ischemic or hemorrhagic stroke, or traumatic brain injury (TBI). Evidence suggests seizures, particularly status epilepticus, may contribute independently to the severity of critical illness. A high index of suspicion in conjunction with continuous electroencephalographic monitoring (cEEG) is essential for the diagnosis of seizures in the critically ill, as the majority of seizures and status epilepticus in this population are non-convulsive. Continuous EEG findings such as periodic discharges or stimulus-induced rhythmic, periodic, or ictal discharges are potentially associated with the development of seizures or with worse outcomes, and in some cases, may represent ongoing seizures. However, interpretation of these patterns is controversial. The treatment of convulsive status epilepticus should be aggressive and occur within the shortest possible time, and may necessitate the use of anesthetics or, if super-refractory, additional pharmacological and non-pharmacological interventions. Typically, treatment of non-convulsive status epilepticus should be the same as convulsive status epilepticus, but in certain circumstances may require a more nuanced approach, particularly when ambiguous cEEG patterns are involved. In certain scenarios, preventing seizures may be appropriate, although there is little consensus. In general, the timely diagnosis and appropriate treatment of seizures and status epilepticus may have the potential to create better outcomes.

Overview of the clinical problem

Seizures and status epilepticus (SE) are common in neurological, surgical, and medical ICUs. In the neurological ICU (NICU), up to one in three patients develop seizures, similar to the proportion among hospitalized patients with altered mental status undergoing cEEG. In patients without known acute brain injury admitted to a medical intensive care unit (MICU), 8–10% overall have seizures. In specific medical conditions such as liver failure or transplant, this may be up to one third of patients. It has been increasingly recognized that patients with direct brain injury and patients with systemic illness alike may develop seizures in the course of their care.

Brain injury acts to disrupt and irritate pre-existing neuronal networks and may cause seizures or SE, particularly in the NICU population. In patients with acute ischemic stroke (AIS), 2–5% will develop seizures within 24 hours [1]. Intracerebral hemorrhage (ICH) carries twice this risk [2], particularly in the setting of lobar or enlarging hemorrhage, and may result in seizures in up to one third of patients [3], most occurring within the first day. Subarachnoid hemorrhage (SAH) and TBI may precipitate seizures in around 20%. Central nervous system (CNS) infection is often presumptive, but seizures and SE may occur in up to half and, in cases of herpes simplex (HSV) infection, as many as 90% [4]. After cardiac arrest, when the brain has experienced hypoxic-ischemic injury, the incidence of seizures is around 10% in patients treated with hypothermia and up to 36% in older series [5,6].

Seizures and SE are not only observed during critical illness; evidence also suggests that they may contribute to its severity. Several studies have found

Brain Disorders in Critical Illness, ed. Robert D. Stevens, Tarek Sharshar, and E. Wesley Ely. Published by Cambridge University Press. © Cambridge University Press 2013.

Table 39.1 Synergistic effect of seizures and status epilepticus on acute brain injury.

Acute brain injury	Synergistic effect	Source
TBI	Increased intracranial pressure; increased lactate/pyruvate ratio, glutamate, glycerol on microdialysis; long-term hippocampal atrophy	[9–11]
SAH	Increased mortality	[12,13]
ICH	Increased midline shift, expansion of hemorrhage volume	[3,10]
AIS	Increased mortality (up to 3x with status epilepticus)	[14–16]

AIS, acute ischemic stroke; ICH, intracerebral hemorrhage; SAH, subarachnoid hemorrhage; TBI, traumatic brain injury.

that in-hospital mortality after SE is higher; in fact, the onset of SE while a patient is hospitalized is associated with poor outcome [7]. In the MICU, seizures recorded during cEEG in patients without coincident brain injury have been associated with worse outcome, even when other variables were accounted for, such as age, physical exam, and associated organ dysfunction [8]. Seizures and SE act synergistically with brain injury (see Table 39.1). Depending on the underlying injury, this may be the result of increased energy demands either affecting an area of vascular compromise or resulting in increased perfusion in the setting of reduced brain compliance, or a combination of the two. These data suggest that seizures and SE lead to collateral damage in the context of critical illness, particularly when there is already direct injury to the brain.

Definitions and diagnosis

Organ systems have varying degrees of complexity, but typically one primary function that is vulnerable to failure in response to critical illness. While organs such as the heart or the kidney may develop mechanical failure, encephalopathy or global dysfunction of the brain may be seen in the setting of hypoxia, metabolic disarray, or focal destructive lesions. Normal brain function is associated with characteristic electrical activity, while critical illness may lead to electrical failure (i.e., diffuse background attenuation or slowing) or seizures.

Seizures are classically defined by their clinical appearance. A loss of awareness defines a complex

versus a simple seizure. Motor movements, including tonic stiffening and clonic jerking movements, are identified with convulsive seizures (see Figure 39.1). If these occur in one area of the body, the seizures have partial (or focal) onset, in contrast to generalized seizures that may begin as focal prior to spread of the seizure to other regions in the brain.

Typically, seizures last no longer than 2 minutes [9], but as seizures last more than 5 minutes, or as shorter seizures recur over the span of 5 minutes or more without full recovery of the patient in between, they are termed SE. The pathophysiology of this transition has not been fully clarified, but involves a variety of complex interactions at the cellular, synaptic, neurovascular, and network levels [10,11]. Initially, excitatory impulses overwhelm the ability of a set of firing neurons to generate appropriate hyperpolarizing ionic gradients and to respond to inhibitory neurotransmitters. During this initial failure of inhibition, receptor composition alters quickly, and some inhibitory receptors (such as $GABA_A$) are desensitized. With time, these abnormal depolarizations are able to propagate unchecked, in part via gap junctions, as the synaptic receptor balance shifts toward excess excitation. In some cases, subcortical networks may be unable to prevent the generalization of this cascade of repetitive, synchronized neuronal firing. As SE progresses, inhibitory receptors and glial signaling become paradoxically excitatory as secondary blood–brain barrier breakdown and inflammation perpetuate the ongoing SE. Early in this process, there is increased cerebral metabolism, which results in increased oxygen demand and compensatory cerebral blood flow. At this point it is unclear if this mechanism remains intact and what role it may play in the observation that both seizures and SE during acute brain injury may lead to further brain injury. Ultimately, the exhaustion of available energy may be implicated in the subsequent necrosis and apoptosis of cortical neurons.

Generalized convulsive SE is always a medical emergency with serious morbidity and mortality [12,13]. However, many seizures do not have prominent motor manifestations, termed non-convulsive seizures (NCSz). In the critically ill, these represent the majority of all seizures (up to 92%) [14]. Continuous EEG is crucial to the diagnosis of NCSz (see Table 39.2 and Figure 39.2). When these electrographic patterns are seen in the setting of prolonged mental status changes (for 5 minutes or more), are accompanied by subtle or no motor symptoms, and

Table 39.2 Criteria for the diagnosis of non-convulsive seizures.

Any pattern lasting > 10 seconds fulfilling one of the following:

Primary Criteria:
(1) Repetitive generalized or focal spikes, sharp-waves, spike-and-wave or sharp-and-slow-wave complexes at 3/s or more.
(2) Repetitive generalized or focal spikes, sharp-waves, spike-and-wave or sharp-and-slow-wave complexes at < 3/s plus secondary criterion.
(3) Sequential rhythmic, periodic, or quasi-periodic waveforms at 1/s or more and unequivocal evolution in frequency (gradually increasing or decreasing by at least 1/s, e.g., from 2 to 3/s), morphology, or location (gradual spread into or out of a region involving at least two electrodes). Evolution in amplitude alone is not sufficient. Change in sharpness without other change in morphology is not adequate to satisfy evolution in morphology.

Secondary Criterion:
Significant improvement in clinical state or appearance of previously absent normal electroencephalography (EEG) patterns (such as a posterior dominant rhythm) temporally coupled to acute administration of a rapidly acting antiepileptic drug. Resolution of the "epileptiform" discharges leaving diffuse slowing without clinical improvement and without appearance of previously absent normal EEG patterns would not satisfy the secondary criterion.

Reproduced with permission from Chong and Hirsch, 2005 [23].

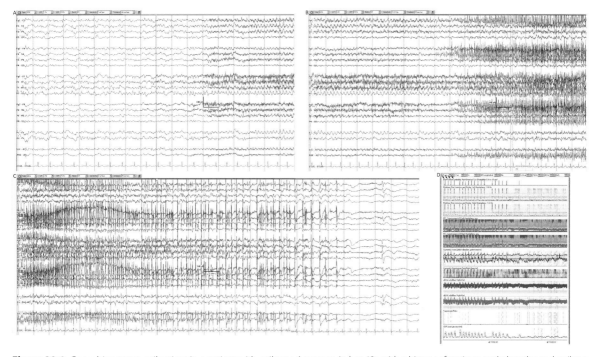

Figure 39.1 Convulsive status epilepticus in a patient with epilepsy. A woman in her 40s with a history of static encephalopathy and epilepsy who presented with hyponatremia and subtherapeutic anticonvulsant levels. Continuous electroencephalography (cEEG) demonstrated left temporal 1–2 Hz quasi-periodic sharp waves (not clearly seen here) with (A) gradual evolution to 4–5Hz sharply contoured ictal theta. (B, C) Seizures lasted 50–80 seconds and manifest as behavioral arrest followed by tonic right arm movement, leftward head deviation, and rightward eye deviation. (D) On quantitative EEG, there was a clear cyclic component with seizures occurring at regular intervals every 5–20 minutes. From the top to the bottom, rows on this quantitative EEG montage include: seizure probability, rhythmic run detection on left and right, color spectrogram on left and right, relative and absolute asymmetry indices, asymmetry spectrogram, amplitude integrated EEG on left and right, suppression ratio, and alpha/delta ratio on left and right. Four typical seizures on the quantitative montage are indicated by arrows. This figure is presented in color in the color plate section.

occur continuously or repetitively, they may be considered non-convulsive status epilepticus (NCSE) [15]; this definition varies in the literature. How the pathophysiology of NCSE differs from generalized convulsive SE is not clear. In the critically ill or comatose, NCSE alone is clearly associated with significant mortality, although much of the available data comes from indirect observation. For instance, there is

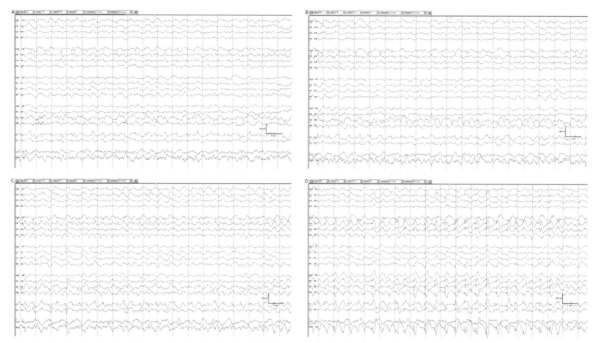

Figure 39.2 Non-convulsive status epilepticus in a critically ill patient with acute brain injury. A woman in her 30s six days postpartum who developed a decrease in her level of arousal. Emergency computed tomography (CT) demonstrated right frontal hemispheric intracerebral hemorrhage with intraventricular extension. Surgical evacuation was performed successfully, but her mental status did not improve. Continuous electroencephalography (cEEG) demonstrated diffuse delta frequency slowing and attenuation, more pronounced over the right side. (A) During the recording, subtle superimposed sharply contoured theta developed over the right hemisphere, best seen over the frontal region. (B, C) This theta rhythm continued to develop and organize into a clear 5–6 Hz ictal rhythm and (D) finally ended in 2 Hz spike-wave discharges with spread into adjacent areas. There was no clinical correlate. Her mental status improved after the seizures were controlled.

increased mortality when associated age and etiology are controlled [16]. In addition, both delays to diagnosis and duration of NCSE lead to increased mortality [17].

The most common clinical manifestation of NCSz in the critically ill is coma without focal neurological abnormalities [18]. Additional signs that might suggest the diagnosis include: waxing and waning mental status, repetitive blinking, nystagmus, or eye deviation. The subtlety of these symptoms often leads to a delay in diagnosis or misdiagnosis in the ICU. Some retrospective case series suggest that non-convulsive seizures may be missed for up to 24 hours in the NICU [17], 48 hours in the MICU, and 72 hours in the surgical ICU setting (SICU) [19]. Standard EEG, typically 20–60 minutes, will miss half of these NCSz. A full 48 hours of cEEG is necessary to detect seizures in comatose patients to a sensitivity of about 90% [14]. In the ICU, there must be a very high index of suspicion for NCSz and NCSE in any patient with impaired mental status or coma [20].

Once a diagnosis of seizures or SE has been made, it is crucial to establish its underlying cause. Between 50–70% of SE cases in population-based studies result from an acute symptomatic cause: either a new brain injury or systemic illness. In the critically ill, more than 80% are the result of an acute symptomatic cause [21]. In addition to routine serologies (e.g., metabolic panel, blood count, and liver function panel), a non-contrast computed tomography (CT) study of the head is warranted for almost all cases. If there is any concern for meningoencephalitis or CT-negative subarachnoid hemorrhage, a lumbar puncture is essential. Depending on the clinical scenario, other considerations include an evaluation for viral infections (i.e., Arbovirus or Enterovirus) and inflammatory, neoplastic, or autoimmune conditions.

An ictal–interictal continuum

In the ICU, many comatose patients undergoing cEEG exhibit patterns that appear potentially ictal, but do not fulfill strict criteria for NCSz (Table 39.2). These include periodic epileptiform discharges (PEDs), stimulus-induced rhythmic, periodic, or ictal discharges (SIRPIDs), and cyclic patterns. While there

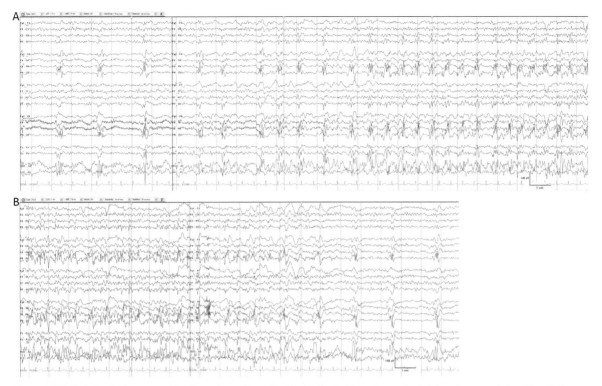

Figure 39.3 Periodic discharges evolving into seizures in a critically ill patient with no known brain injury. A woman in her 40s with liver dysfunction and sepsis. She had done well after a course of antibiotics and was transferred out of the intensive care unit (ICU) initially, but developed deterioration of her mental status over 24 hours with partial seizures on continuous encephalography (cEEG). (A) Her EEG demonstrated 0.5 Hz right hemispheric periodic lateralized epileptiform discharges (PLEDs). These gradually involved faster, sharply contoured activity (PLEDs Plus) before evolving into frank non-convulsive seizures with 2 Hz sharp waves superimposed on rhythmic theta frequencies without significant spread. (B) These abruptly ended as the more simply configured PLEDs returned.

is significant debate over whether these discharges constitute NCSz or merely some epiphenomenon of underlying brain injury, clinically there is often overlap between these conditions. This phenomenon has been labeled by some as the ictal–interictal continuum reflecting a dynamic link between neuronal injury and the metabolic derangements associated with critical illness [22]. While some patterns are clearly harmful, such as status epilepticus, and others are not, such as triphasic waves, much more uncertainty exists when talking about patterns on the ictal–interictal continuum [23].

The hallmarks of PEDs are repetitive and morphologically stereotyped discharges occurring at frequencies less than 3 Hz (at which point they fulfill criteria for NCSz, according to many experts [23]). Periodic epileptiform discharges may occur focally (periodic lateralized epileptiform discharges [PLEDs], or if multifocal, bilateral independent periodic epileptiform discharges [BIPLEDs]) or generally (generalized periodic epileptiform discharges [GPEDs]). In reality,

these discharges often fluctuate with regard to morphology and display additional features such as superimposed rhythmic slowing or very fast, low amplitude, sharp activity, termed PEDs Plus (see Figure 39.3) [24]. Periodic epileptiform discharges most often reflect acute systemic or CNS pathology, although they may rarely occur chronically [25]. While controversy exists as to where on the ictal–interictal continuum PEDs lie, they at the very least confer an increased risk for developing seizures, particularly when they are considered PED Plus (see Table 39.3). In some cases, PEDs clearly represent an ictal rhythm as suggested by positron emission tomography (PET) studies showing concordant focal hypermetabolism [26] or by the presence of clinically time-locked motor movements [23]. Similar to NCSE, a variety of negative symptoms have been described in ictal PEDs [27], and although controversial, the presence of PEDs appears to independently correlate with worse outcomes in conditions such as sepsis [8], ICH [3], and SAH [28]. Both GPEDs and BIPLEDs have been associated with

Table 39.3 Ictal–interictal continuum: associations with seizures and mortality.

	Hospital-based prevalence	% with seizures	Mortality*	Sources
PLEDs	13–22%	49–90%	27–52%	[21,22,34–36]
PEDs Plus	17–60% of LPDs	74–100%	Unknown	[32,34]
GPEDs	4.5–9.4%	26.5% (NCSz) 21.5% (NCSE) 29.4–46% (any)	41–64%	[37–39]
BIPLEDs	1–5%	35–78%	52–61%	[34,40]
SIRPIDs	9–22%	52%	Unknown	[13,41]
Total	16–23%	29–59%	27%	[8,22]

BIPLEDs, bilateral independent periodic lateralized epileptiform discharges; GPEDs, generalized periodic epileptiform discharges; PLEDs, periodic lateralized epileptiform discharges; PED, periodic epileptiform discharges; SIRPIDs, stimulus-induced rhythmic, periodic, or ictal discharges.
* Mortality is largely dependent on underlying etiology in the majority of the literature, although there are independent associations with PDs in sepsis (in combination with seizures [8]), ICH [3], SAH [13], and cardiac arrest [42].

poor outcomes in the context of cardiac arrest [29], yet GPEDs do not associate with outcome when age, etiology, and neurological exam are controlled [30] and several reviews have observed that the mortality associated with PEDs results largely from the underlying disease process.

The interaction of subcortical arousal pathways may interact with neuronal injury and metabolic dysfunction to produce a variety of disordered patterns including SIRPIDS [31]. These carry the features of PLEDs, GPEDs, BIPLEDs, or NCSz, but consistently and stereotypically occur after stimulation. Seen after acute brain injury, they may reflect a dysregulation of thalamocortical projections exacerbated by intact arousal pathways. They may be associated with SE when focal or ictal in appearance, but further study is needed to determine whether these have any impact clinically or if they should be treated as more typical spontaneous seizure activity. Cyclic arousal patterns may also occur in the critically ill in which periods of high-amplitude slowing alternate with 2–3 seconds of lower amplitude faster frequencies without discrete discharges. These are rare (0.2%) but probably underreported. Unlike in patients with SIRPIDS, the EEG is typically reactive in these patients and survival outcomes were greater than 90% in one small series [32]. These patterns may reflect recovering sleep, and in fact the absence of sleep architecture in comatose SAH patients is an independent predictor of poor outcome [28]. Interestingly, NCSE in the critically ill may also occur in a cyclic pattern in which brief but clearly ictal events occur approximately every 5–10 minutes [33]. These may be related to endogenous inhibitory

mechanisms that become overwhelmed in a repetitive pattern as opposed to cycling arousal, but should be kept in mind whenever periodic or cyclic patterns are encountered on EEG.

Treatment

Patients who demonstrate convulsive SE should be treated aggressively and within the shortest amount of time possible. Data are robust that these events create significant morbidity and mortality that increase with time spent in SE. Emergent initial therapy should start with administration of a benzodiazepine and many recommend intravenous (i.v.) lorazepam (4 mg over 2 minutes) based on randomized controlled trials (RCT) of first-line agents [12,34]. This should be given immediately in conjunction with strict attention to the patient's airway, breathing, and circulation. Each of these may be affected by SE alone or in combination with the medications used to treat it, although it should be pointed out that prehospital administration of lorazepam actually decreased the need for intubation in one RCT when compared with placebo. The administration of 10 mg intramuscular midazolam appears to be a safe and effective alternative to i.v. lorazepam for prehospital SE [35].

Urgent control therapy, formerly referred to as second-line agents, may be chosen based on patient characteristics. Fosphenytoin, a diphosphate sodium ester of phenytoin, may be loaded quickly (20 mg/kg i.v. at up to 150 ml/min) and avoids some of the hypotension, cardiac arrhythmia, and respiratory depression associated with phenytoin. However, it remains hepatically cleared and exhibits zero-order kinetics and significant drug–drug interactions due to protein binding and cytochrome P450 induction. An alternative that may have similar efficacy is valproate, which may also be loaded quickly (20–40 mg/kg i.v. over 10 min) with no substantial cardiopulmonary effects, making it perhaps more ideal in patients who are elderly, who already exhibit cardiovascular compromise, or who have do-not-intubate directives. Valproate is also hepatically cleared, inhibits the P450 system, and may be associated with pancreatitis, hyperammonemia, thrombocytopenia, or other qualitative platelet defects. Consider avoiding valproate in patients with liver failure, a bleeding diathesis, or diffuse intravascular coagulopathy. Levetiracetam may emerge as an alternative but so far experience is limited.

It is important to note that up to a third of patients with convulsive SE will go on to have NCSz or NCSE after cessation of clinical movements. A cEEG should be considered urgently if a patient treated "successfully" for SE does not improve within 20 minutes or return to baseline within 60 minutes. The persistence of both non-convulsive and convulsive SE despite emergent and urgent therapeutic interventions, referred to as refractory status epilepticus (RSE), should prompt aggressive seizure control intervention, usually involving the use of continuous i.v. anesthetic agents, such as midazolam or propofol. For these patients, cEEG is crucial to guide the use of these medications. If cEEG is unavailable, these patients should be transferred to a center with appropriate capabilities.

Midazolam should be loaded with 0.2 mg/kg boluses every 5 minutes, followed by titration of infusion rates by 0.2mg/kg/hour until seizures stop, to a maximum maintenance dose of up to 2.9 mg/kg/hour. This rate is up to 10 times higher than conventional dosing, but early evidence suggests that while causing higher rates of hypotension [36] higher-dose midazolam therapy may be associated with better seizure control. If administered in an ICU setting, severe hypotension due to high-dose midazolam is not associated with worse outcome and overall outcome is better for patients treated with high- vs. lower-dose midazolam for RSE [36,37]. Propofol is used similarly, with 1–2 mg/kg boluses every 5 minutes and infusion rates up to 5 mg/kg/hour. Long-term use of higher infusion rates are contraindicated due to the risk of the propofol infusion syndrome, a potentially deadly combination of hypertriglyceridemia and acidosis, and prolonged use of propofol in refractory SE may be associated with higher morbidity and mortality [38]. However, if SE has not been controlled within 30–60 minutes even by aggressive bolusing, pentobarbital titrated to seizure control or burst-suppression should be initiated. Ultimately, whether midazolam, propofol, or pentobarbital are used as initial therapy for RSE [39], mortality rates are essentially the same and the agent that controls the seizures is the agent of choice, as illustrated in a recent randomized controlled trial of propofol vs. pentobarbital for refractory SE [40]. Stopped early due to lack of patient enrollment, and therefore underpowered, this study also demonstrated the difficulty in conducting quality evidence-based research on this heterogeneous and relatively rare condition.

Occasionally, SE may continue despite the use of anesthetics, termed "malignant" or "super-refractory" SE. In addition to stopping the seizures, further treatment strategies for super-refractory SE also focus on neuroprotection and addressing possible underlying etiologies. Of course, there is little reason to exclude neuroprotection and the treatment of underlying etiologies in the early stages of SE. There are likely few, if any, differences pathophysiologically between refractory and super-refractory SE. However, in the absence of any clear evidence-based data, alternative options are largely supported by case series or case reports alone [41], and are therefore used once more traditional therapies aimed at stopping the seizures fail. These options are summarized in Table 39.4.

How long to continue care remains a matter of significant debate, both medically and ethically [42]. The prolonged use of anesthetics, cEEG, and non-evidence-based therapies for weeks or even months costs significant money and time, requires the expertise of entire healthcare teams, takes a tremendous toll on the family of the patient, and provides no guarantee of success. In many regions, these resources may be denied others as a result. On the other hand, there is a paucity of data regarding both the treatment and the prognosis of RSE patients to guide clinicians, in contrast to conditions that have been relatively well studied, such as cardiac arrest and TBI. In situations wherein resources are available, it is clear that some patients with super-refractory status lasting many months may survive with good outcome [43,44].

The treatment of patients in the ICU with changes in mental status or coma found to be in NCSE differs

397

Table 39.4 Alternative treatment for refractory seizures and status epilepticus.

Treatment	Mechanism	Considerations
Ketamine (c.i.v.)	NMDA antagonism	Possible neuroprotectant Sympathetomimetic side-effect profile (in contrast to phenobarbital, propofol, and midazolam)
Inhaled anesthetics (isoflurane, desflurane)	Non-specific blockade of neuronal conduction	Logistically difficult in standard intensive care unit Long-term use may lead to reversible neurotoxicity Frequent seizure recurrence
Lidocaine (i.v., c.i.v.)	Sodium channel conduction blockade	Non-sedating Frequent recurrence requires c.i.v. May cause hypotension or cardiac arrhythmia
Magnesium (i.v.)	Saturation of NMDA receptors, restoring tonic blockade	Few side effects (peripheral neuromuscular blockade at high serum concentrations) May be uniquely effective in certain etiologies (i.e., mitochondrial cytopathies or acute intermittent porphyria)
Ketogenic diet (PO)	Shifts metabolic substrate from glucose to ketones, suppressing seizures; anti-inflammatory	Easy to administer, particularly with secured enteral access May cause hypoglycemia or acidosis; cannot be combined with propofol or carbonic anhydrase inhibitors
Hypothermia	Decrease in metabolic demand; independent antiepileptic effects	Possible neuroprotectant Restores blood–brain barrier and decreases inflammation associated with ongoing SE Associated with medical complications (coagulopathy, immunosuppression, cardiac arrhythmias)
Immunotherapy (steroids, ACTH, IvIg, or plasma exchange)	Immunomodulation and suppression of inflammatory response	Restores blood–brain barrier and decreases inflammation associated with ongoing SE May treat unrecognized underlying etiologies (i.e., autoimmune or paraneoplastic) Infectious or medical complications (hyperglycemia, volume overload)
Electroconvulsive therapy	Increases endogenous anticonvulsant signaling pathways and prolongs refractory period	Requires weaning anesthetic agents and possibly other anticonvulsants Must be performed daily for 3–8 days by experienced physician
Surgery (e.g., resection, subpial transections, vagal nerve stimulation, or deep brain stimulation)	Removal of seizure onset zone or modulation of neural networks	Resective surgery only for clear focal seizure onset zone, requiring corroborative data (i.e., PET or SPECT) Invasive; may require surgeons with particular expertise in epilepsy surgery

ACTH, adrenocorticotropic hormone; c.i.v., continuous intravenous infusion; i.v., intravenous, IvIg, intravenous immunoglobulin; NMDA, N-methyl-D-aspartate; PET, positron emission tomography; PO, per os; SPECT, single photon emission computed tomography.

from the treatment of convulsive SE described above. Randomized controlled studies comparing different treatment approaches for patients with SE have excluded or were underpowered to study different treatment approaches for patients with NCSE. For most patients, in whom the airway is protected and there is no cardiovascular compromise, the use of traditional agents (fosphenytoin, valproate) followed quickly by anesthetic continuous i.v. medications is appropriate as in convulsive SE. However, particularly for patients with waxing and waning mental status who have yet to be intubated and for patients with do-not-intubate orders, alternative non-anesthetic medications may be used. Valproate does not appear to cause cardiovascular or respiratory dysfunction, and based on data demonstrating efficacy to control convulsive SE many practitioners also use valproate for NCSE. Levetiracetam is a well-tolerated medication that is available in i.v. form. There are no cardiovascular effects, and it is cleared renally with no significant protein binding. Particularly in the elderly or critically ill, levetiracetam may also be an attractive option. Lacosamide is a newer agent with similar tolerability, although there may be potential PR interval prolongation on electrocardiogram. Lacosamide may exhibit some protein binding. Data are limited for both levetiracetam and lacosamide in terms of efficacy, and these should be used in combination with other, more traditional agents for most patients.

Ictal–interictal continuum patterns pose a particularly difficult treatment scenario – do the patterns represent SE and therefore warrant more aggressive treatment? In the appropriate clinical scenario, corroborative evidence for either the ictal nature of the EEG pattern or its potential for neuronal injury may be employed to guide treatment aggressiveness. First, response to an antiepileptic medication (AED) may be used to assess whether or not there is clinical improvement. The caveat is that patients with electrographic SE after termination of convulsive SE [12] and patients with concurrent critical illness [19] may have, at best, only minimal and transient clinical response. Ictal and non-ictal EEG patterns alike may resolve with treatment, further confusing the picture. In these cases, imaging may demonstrate ongoing damage implicating the ictal nature of an EEG pattern: restricted diffusion on MRI, increased areas of regional blood flow on CT perfusion or SPECT, or areas of hypermetabolism on PET. Occasionally, serum markers such as

neuron-specific enolase (NSE) may be used, but remain useful only if there is clear correlation to the onset of the ictal–interictal pattern; there are no studies that have determined the ictal nature of EEG patterns based on NSE. Intracortical data such as tissue oxygenation, lactate/pyruvate ratio, glutamate, or glycerol have been looked at in NCSz, but not systematically studied with regard to determining the ictal nature of the ictal–interictal continuum [45]. If available data are concordant, suspected NCSE should be treated as such, but the risks and benefits of more aggressive treatment should be considered on a case-by-case basis. It is important to realize that none of these approaches allow the physician to gain certainty that the patient would benefit from more or less aggressive measures.

In some scenarios, seizure prophylaxis may have a role (see Table 39.5). In patients with TBI, phenytoin has been shown in a randomized controlled trial (RCT) to reduce early posttraumatic seizures up to 7 days with only mild short-term cognitive effects [46]. Valproate has similar efficacy but may cause higher mortality [47]. More recently levetiracetam appears to be as effective with improved 3- and 6-month outcomes compared with phenytoin [48]. In general, prophylaxis does not prevent late (> 1 week) seizures, and should not be continued past the initial posttraumatic period. In patients with SAH, prophylactic anticonvulsants have received Class IIb, Level of Evidence B recommendations during the immediate posthemorrhagic period. However, there are no RCTs to guide treatment and therefore the issue is highly controversial. Patients treated with AEDs (mostly phenytoin or phenobarbital) may have worse functional and cognitive outcomes at 3 months, more

Table 39.5 Summary of recommendations for prophylactic antiepileptic medication in select acute brain injury. Choice of antiepileptic medication should be left to the physician, as evidence at this time does not appear to favor one medication over another. Traditionally many physicians used phenytoin but increasingly other anticonvulsants such as levetiracetam are being used.

Condition	Rate of acute seizures	At risk	Duration*
TBI	5–20%	Moderate to severe TBI	7 days
SAH	10–20%	Hunt–Hess IV–V or thick cisternal blood	3–7 days
ICH	10–30%	Lobar hemorrhage, poor mental status, mass effect	7 days
AIS	2–5%	Large, cortical infarcts	None
Cardiac arrest	10–30%	Poor neurological exam	None

AIS, acute ischemic stroke; ICH, intracerebral hemorrhage; SAH, subarachnoid hemorrhage; TBI, traumatic brain injury.
*Based on expert opinion. Except in TBI, there are few data to support routine prophylaxis in acute brain injury.

symptomatic vasospasm, and more stroke but these data are very controversial as well [49,50]. A shorter, 3-day course of phenytoin has been successful in mitigating acute side effects and treating early seizures [51] but 3-day courses of levetiracetam may lead to increased in-hospital seizures requiring longer treatment duration [52]. Guidelines recommend against the general routine long-term use of anticonvulsants but admit that these may be considered for patients with risk factors such as prior seizure, parenchymal hematoma, infarct, or middle cerebral artery aneurysms [53]. Practically, prophylaxis may be argued for prior to treatment of an aneurysm (almost always less than 72 hours) and in patients at higher risk of seizures (for instance, poor Hunt–Hess grade or those with thick cisternal blood) [54]. Seizure prophylaxis is not recommended in recent guidelines for patients with acute ischemic stroke [55] or intracerebral hemorrhage (ICH) [56]. There is some evidence suggesting that the use of phenytoin in patients with ICH is associated with worse outcomes [57], but there are few existing data to guide clinicians otherwise. Only one small RCT exists which compared 1 month of valproate to placebo; early seizures were prevented and the NIH stroke scale was improved at 1 year [58], but again late seizures were not affected. Because there are patients who may be vulnerable to mass effect as a result of the effects of a seizure [3,59], some favor prophylaxis in high-risk ICH patients, such as those with lobar hemorrhage or impending herniation [54]. After AIS, both phenytoin and phenobarbital have been shown to delay motor improvement [1], and whereas levetiracetam shows promise in both seizure prevention and neuroprotection, performing an RCT has proven to be difficult [60]. Data regarding seizure prophylaxis for patients who have undergone cardiac arrest are limited to expert opinion, and there is no consensus; most would likely not give prophylaxis but perform cEEG and treat seizures if they are diagnosed.

Conclusion

Seizures occur frequently in the medical, surgical, or neurological ICU as a result of both systemic illness and direct injury to the brain. The underlying etiology may be quite varied including sepsis, post-cardiac arrest, stroke, or trauma. In addition, there is increasing evidence to suggest that seizures may affect the natural course of critical illness, increasing mortality or causing collateral brain injury. Seizures in the critically ill are commonly

non-convulsive, necessitating cEEG monitoring for detection. Associated phenomena, including PEDs and SIRPIDs, have been associated with seizures, worse outcomes, and may represent ictal phenomena in certain cases. The early recognition and treatment of these conditions is challenging but may have the potential to create better outcomes.

References

1. Camilo O, Goldstein LB. Seizures and epilepsy after ischemic stroke. *Stroke* 2004;**35**(7):1769–75.

2. Bladin CF, Alexandrov AV, Bellavance A, *et al.* Seizures after stroke: a prospective multicenter study. *Arch Neurology* 2000;**57**(11):1617–22.

3. Claassen J, Jette N, Chum F, *et al.* Electrographic seizures and periodic discharges after intracerebral hemorrhage. *Neurology* 2007;**69**(13):1356–65.

4. Glaser CA, Gilliam S, Honarmand S, *et al.* Refractory status epilepticus in suspect encephalitis. *Neurocrit Care* 2008;**9**(1):74–82.

5. Krumholz A, Stern BJ, Weiss HD. Outcome from coma after cardiopulmonary resuscitation: relation to seizures and myoclonus. *Neurology* 1988;**38**(3):401–5.

6. Rittenberger JC, Popescu A, Brenner RP, *et al.* Frequency and timing of nonconvulsive status epilepticus in comatose post-cardiac arrest subjects treated with hypothermia. *Neurocritical Care* 2012;**16**(1):114–22.

7. Vignatelli L, Rinaldi R, Baldin E, *et al.* Impact of treatment on the short-term prognosis of status epilepticus in two population-based cohorts. *J Neurol* 2008;**255**(2):197–204.

8. Oddo M, Carrera E, Claassen J, *et al.* Continuous electroencephalography in the medical intensive care unit. *Crit Care Med* 2009;**37**(6):2051–6.

9. Theodore WH, Porter RJ, Albert P, *et al.* The secondarily generalized tonic-clonic seizure: a videotape analysis. *Neurology* 1994;**44**(8):1403–7.

10. Chen JW, Wasterlain CG. Status epilepticus: pathophysiology and management in adults. *Lancet Neurol* 2006;**5**(3):246–56.

11. Lado FA, Moshe SL. How do seizures stop? *Epilepsia* 2008;**49**(10):1651–64.

12. Treiman DM, Meyers PD, Walton NY, *et al.* A comparison of four treatments for generalized convulsive status epilepticus. Veterans Affairs Status Epilepticus Cooperative Study Group. *N Engl J Med* 1998;**339**(12):792–8.

13. Delanty N, French JA, Labar DR, *et al.* Status epilepticus arising de novo in hospitalized patients: an analysis of 41 patients. *Seizure* 2001;**10**(2):116–19.

14. Claassen J, Mayer SA, Kowalski RG, et al. Detection of electrographic seizures with continuous EEG monitoring in critically ill patients. *Neurology* 2004;**62**(10):1743–8.

15. Walker M, Cross H, Smith S, et al. Nonconvulsive status epilepticus: Epilepsy Research Foundation Workshop Reports. *Epileptic Disord* 2005;**7**(3):253–96.

16. DeLorenzo RJ, Waterhouse EJ, Towne AR, et al. Persistent nonconvulsive status epilepticus after the control of convulsive status epilepticus. *Epilepsia* 1998;**39**(8):833–40.

17. Young GB, Jordan KG, Doig GS. An assessment of nonconvulsive seizures in the intensive care unit using continuous EEG monitoring: an investigation of variables associated with mortality. *Neurology* 1996;**47**(1):83–9.

18. Jordan KG. Nonconvulsive status epilepticus in acute brain injury. *J Clin Neurophysiol* 1999;**16**(4):332–40; discussion 53.

19. Drislane FW, Lopez MR, Blum AS, et al. Detection and treatment of refractory status epilepticus in the intensive care unit. *J Clin Neurophysiol* 2008;**25**(4):181–6.

20. Jordan KG, Hirsch LJ. In nonconvulsive status epilepticus (NCSE), treat to burst-suppression: pro and con. *Epilepsia* 2006;**47**(Suppl 1):41–5.

21. Foreman B, Hirsch LJ. Epilepsy emergencies: diagnosis and management. *Neurol Clin* 2012;**30**(1):11–41.

22. Pohlmann-Eden B, Hoch DB, Cochius JI, et al. Periodic lateralized epileptiform discharges – a critical review. *J Clin Neurophysiol* 1996;**13**(6):519–30.

23. Chong DJ, Hirsch LJ. Which EEG patterns warrant treatment in the critically ill? Reviewing the evidence for treatment of periodic epileptiform discharges and related patterns. *J Clin Neurophysiol* 2005;**22**(2):79–91.

24. Reiher J, Rivest J, Grand'Maison F, et al. Periodic lateralized epileptiform discharges with transitional rhythmic discharges: association with seizures. *Electroencephalogr Clin Neurophysiol* 1991;**78**(1):12–17.

25. Orta DSJ, Chiappa KH, Quiroz AZ, et al. Prognostic implications of periodic epileptiform discharges. *Arch Neurology* 2009;**66**:985–91.

26. Handforth A, Cheng JT, Mandelkern MA, et al. Markedly increased mesiotemporal lobe metabolism in a case with PLEDs: further evidence that PLEDs are a manifestation of partial status epilepticus. *Epilepsia* 1994;**35**(4):876–81.

27. Hughes JR. Periodic lateralized epileptiform discharges: do they represent an ictal pattern requiring treatment? *Epilepsy Behavior* 2010;**18**(3):162–5.

28. Claassen J, Hirsch LJ, Frontera JA, et al. Prognostic significance of continuous EEG monitoring in patients with poor-grade subarachnoid hemorrhage. *Neurocrit Care* 2006;**4**(2):103–12.

29. San-Juan OD, Chiappa KH, Costello DJ, et al. Periodic epileptiform discharges in hypoxic encephalopathy: BiPLEDs and GPEDs as a poor prognosis for survival. *Seizure* 2009;**18**(5):365–8.

30. Foreman B, Claassen J, Hirsch LJ. *A Controlled Study of 202 Patients with Generalized Periodic Discharges (GPDs): Relationship to Seizures and Outcome*. [Poster]. New Orleans, LA: American Clinical Neurophysiology Society; 2011.

31. Hirsch LJ, Claassen J, Mayer SA, et al. Stimulus-induced rhythmic, periodic, or ictal discharges (SIRPIDs): a common EEG phenomenon in the critically ill. *Epilepsia* 2004;**45**(2):109–23.

32. Kassab MY, Farooq MU, Diaz-Arrastia R, et al. The clinical significance of EEG cyclic alternating pattern during coma. *J Clin Neurophysiol* 2007;**24**(6):425–8.

33. Friedman DE, Schevon C, Emerson RG, et al. Cyclic electrographic seizures in critically ill patients. *Epilepsia* 2008;**49**(2):281–7.

34. Alldredge BK, Gelb AM, Isaacs SM, et al. A comparison of lorazepam, diazepam, and placebo for the treatment of out-of-hospital status epilepticus. *N Engl J Med* 2001;**345**(9):631–7.

35. Silbergleit R, Durkalski V, Lowenstein D, et al. Intramuscular versus intravenous therapy for prehospital status epilepticus. *N Engl J Med* 2012;**366**(7):591–600.

36. Lesch C, Lantigua H, Fernandez A, et al. Safety of high dose midazolam infusions for refractory status epilepticus (Poster). *Neurocrit Care* 2011;**15**:S147.

37. Fernandez A, Lesch C, Lantigua H, et al. Treatment of refractory status epilepticus with low vs. high dose midazolam infusions (Poster). *Neurocrit Care* 2011;**15**:S139.

38. Iyer VN, Hoel R, Rabinstein AA. Propofol infusion syndrome in patients with refractory status epilepticus: an 11-year clinical experience. *Crit Care Med* 2009;**37**(12):3024–30.

39. Claassen J, Hirsch LJ, Emerson RG, et al. Treatment of refractory status epilepticus with pentobarbital, propofol, or midazolam: a systematic review. *Epilepsia* 2002;**43**(2):146–53.

40. Rossetti AO, Milligan TA, Vulliemoz S, et al. A randomized trial for the treatment of refractory status epilepticus. *Neurocrit Care* 2011;**14**(1):4–10.

41. Shorvon S, Ferlisi M. The treatment of super-refractory status epilepticus: a critical review of available

therapies and a clinical treatment protocol. *Brain* 2011;**134**(10):2802–18.

42. Crippen D, Burrows D, Stocchetti N, *et al.* Ethics roundtable: 'Open-ended ICU care: can we afford it?'. *Crit Care* 2010;**14**(3):222.

43. Cooper AD, Britton JW, Rabinstein AA. Functional and cognitive outcome in prolonged refractory status epilepticus. *Arch Neurol* 2009;**66**(12):1505–9.

44. Bausell R, Svoronos A, Lennihan L, *et al.* Recovery after severe refractory status epilepticus and 4 months of coma. *Neurology* 2011;**77**(15):1494–5.

45. Claassen J, Perotte A, Albers D, *et al.* Electrographic seizures after subarachnoid hemorrhage lead to derangement of brain homeostasis in humans (Poster). *Neurocrit Care* 2011;**15**:S10.

46. Temkin NR, Dikmen SS, Wilensky AJ, *et al.* A randomized, double-blind study of phenytoin for the prevention of post-traumatic seizures. *N Engl J Med* 1990;**323**(8):497–502.

47. Bratton SL, Chestnut RM, Ghajar J, *et al.* Guidelines for the management of severe traumatic brain injury. XIII. Antiseizure prophylaxis. *J Neurotrauma* 2007;**24** (Suppl 1):S83–6.

48. Szaflarski JP, Sangha KS, Lindsell CJ, *et al.* Prospective, randomized, single-blinded comparative trial of intravenous levetiracetam versus phenytoin for seizure prophylaxis. *Neurocritical Care* 2010;**12**(2):165–72.

49. Rosengart AJ, Huo JD, Tolentino J, *et al.* Outcome in patients with subarachnoid hemorrhage treated with antiepileptic drugs. *J Neurosurgery* 2007;**107**(2):253–60.

50. Naidech AM, Kreiter KT, Janjua N, *et al.* Phenytoin exposure is associated with functional and cognitive disability after subarachnoid hemorrhage. *Stroke* 2005;**36**(3):583–7.

51. Chumnanvej S, Dunn IF, Kim DH. Three-day phenytoin prophylaxis is adequate after subarachnoid hemorrhage. *Neurosurgery* 2007;**60**(1):99–102; discussion –3.

52. Murphy-Human T, Welch E, Zipfel G, *et al.* Comparison of short-duration levetiracetam with extended-course phenytoin for seizure prophylaxis after subarachnoid hemorrhage. *World Neurosurg* 2011;**75**(2):269–74.

53. Bederson JB, Connolly ES, Jr., Batjer HH, *et al.* Guidelines for the management of aneurysmal subarachnoid hemorrhage: a statement for healthcare professionals from a special writing group of the Stroke Council, American Heart Association. *Stroke* 2009;**40**(3):994–1025.

54. Gilmore E, Choi HA, Hirsch LJ, *et al.* Seizures and CNS hemorrhage: spontaneous intracerebral and aneurysmal subarachnoid hemorrhage. *Neurologist* 2010;**16**(3):165–75.

55. Adams HP, Jr., del Zoppo G, Alberts MJ, *et al.* Guidelines for the early management of adults with ischemic stroke: a guideline from the American Heart Association/American Stroke Association Stroke Council, Clinical Cardiology Council, Cardiovascular Radiology and Intervention Council, and the Atherosclerotic Peripheral Vascular Disease and Quality of Care Outcomes in Research Interdisciplinary Working Groups: the American Academy of Neurology affirms the value of this guideline as an educational tool for neurologists. *Stroke* 2007;**38**(5):1655–711.

56. Morgenstern LB, Hemphill JC III, Anderson C, *et al.* Guidelines for the management of spontaneous intracerebral hemorrhage: a guideline for healthcare professionals from the American Heart Association/American Stroke Association. *Stroke* 2010;**41**(9):2108–29.

57. Naidech AM, Garg RK, Liebling S, *et al.* Anticonvulsant use and outcomes after intracerebral hemorrhage. *Stroke* 2009;**40**(12):3810–15.

58. Gilad R, Boaz M, Dabby R, *et al.* Are post intracerebral hemorrhage seizures prevented by anti-epileptic treatment? *Epilepsy Res* 2011;**95**(3):227–31.

59. Vespa PM, O'Phelan K, Shah M, *et al.* Acute seizures after intracerebral hemorrhage: a factor in progressive midline shift and outcome. *Neurology* 2003;**60**(9):1441–6.

60. van Tuijl JH, van Raak EP, de Krom MC, *et al.* Early treatment after stroke for the prevention of late epileptic seizures: a report on the problems performing a randomised placebo-controlled double-blind trial aimed at anti-epileptogenesis. *Seizure* 2011;**20**(4):285–91.

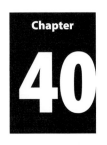

Chapter

40

Encephalopathy and coma in acute and chronic liver failure

Julia Wendon and Jennifer Ryan

SUMMARY

Brain failure, hepatic encephalopathy (HE) in association with liver failure is a common occurrence and may on occasions be difficult to separate from the delirium of critical illness and septic encephalopathy. Encephalopathy is graded from stages 1 to 4 with grades 3 and 4 (Glasgow Coma Scale of 9 and less) often requiring intubation to prevent aspiration and facilitate optimal care. In acute liver failure, and rarely in chronic liver failure, the syndrome is complicated by clinically important cerebral edema. The etiology of HE is multifactorial with inflammation and ammonia being the prime agents accountable for its progression and development.

Management is usually supportive with etiological factors being sought and treated as appropriate. Arterial ammonia may assist in risk stratification. Rate of onset and failure to be able to control brain osmolytes increases risk of cebebral edema in hyperacute and acute liver failure. Other risk factors for brain edema are young age, vasopressor need, hyponatraemia, renal failure, acute and hyperacute etiology, and arterial ammonia greater than 150 µmol/L.

Treatment is largely supportive and patients can be difficult to manage safely in a ward environment where administration of sedative agents may result in decreased conscious level, aspiration, and chest sepsis. Patients who require intubation will need use of appropriate sedative and analgesic agents. Drugs such as L-ornithine, L-arginine to decrease arterial ammonia have not been found to be beneficial in a controlled trial of patients with acute liver failure; similarly agents such as rifaxamin have not been investigated in this setting. Fluids and antimicrobials may be required and gastrointestinal (GI) function addressed to avoid ileus and promote transit of GI contents. Temperature and serum sodium should be controlled, ammonia monitored and manipulated as appropriate and screening for brain swelling utilizing middle cerebral artery Doppler may be useful. The role of intracranial pressure (ICP) monitoring remains controversial with no studies showing a mortality benefit. Treatment for surges in ICP may be with bolus mannitol or hypertonic saline. The incidence of cerebral edema and raised ICP appears to be decreasing steadily in the USA and Europe.

Introduction

The neurological features seen in patients with liver disease were eloquently described by Adams and Foley, asterixis, or flapping tremor being a characteristic feature of patients with hepatic encephalopathy [1]. The neurological manifestations of liver disease encountered in intensive care are numerous and dependent on the type of patient and etiology of liver disease. It is important to consider the patient with acute liver failure (ALF), acute-on-chronic liver failure (AoCLF) and those developing acute liver dysfunction in association with critical illness as clearly separate entities, albeit with common metabolic precipitants of brain failure. The latter group are likely to be increasingly encountered due to the rapidly growing cohort of patients with both undiagnosed alcohol-related and non-alcoholic fatty liver disease. These patients have "stiff," but often not cirrhotic livers highly susceptible to oxidative stress and commonly present with elevated bilirubin, portal hypertension, hyperammonemia, and in some cases an altered level of consciousness. Another cohort that deserves mention are those who undergo extended liver resections, especially in the context of previous chemotherapy which may render them at risk of fatty liver. This cohort of patients may develop ascites

Brain Disorders in Critical Illness, ed. Robert D. Stevens, Tarek Sharshar, and E. Wesley Ely. Published by Cambridge University Press. © Cambridge University Press 2013.

and portal hypertension alongside jaundice, often resultant upon a portal venous inflow that is excessive to the volume of the residual liver.

In this chapter, we will concentrate on HE within the critical care environment and will describe therapeutic modalities, focusing on the ALF and AoCLF patients.

Definitions

Hepatic encephalopathy describes the spectrum of neuropsychiatric abnormalities seen in patients with liver dysfunction, after exclusion of other known brain disease [2].

An understanding of the prognostic importance of the development of encephalopathy following liver injury led O'Grady and colleagues to classify ALF into three categories depending on the time between the onset of jaundice and encephalopathy [3]: (1) *Hyperacute liver failure* has a jaundice to encephalopathy time of within 7 days and a higher incidence of cardiovascular failure, severe coagulopathy, and intracranial hypertension. It is generally associated with a good survival rate without emergency liver transplantation. (2) *Acute liver failure* has a jaundice to encephalopathy time of between 8 and 28 days. Patients have moderate degrees of coagulopathy, jaundice, and intracranial hypertension with generally less favorable outcomes without liver transplantation. (3) *Subacute liver failure* has more of an indolent cause and frequently results from non-acetaminophen drug-induced liver injury and seronegative liver injury. A jaundice to encephalopathy time of 5–12 weeks is commonplace, with low levels of encephalopathy and increased levels of bilirubin.

Acute-on-chronic liver failure encompasses patients with cirrhosis in whom a precipitating factor such as infection or gastrointestinal bleeding results in an acute pathophysiological deterioration with progressive organ dysfunction. The acute episode is typically characterized by cardiovascular failure (hyperdynamic), renal dysfunction, and HE [4]. A proportion of these patients will be referred to intensive care and decision to admit will depend on the patient's background and precipitating factors; it is not possible to devise definitive rules regarding admission of this cohort and it is key that considered decisions are made on a case-by-case basis.

Table 40.1 summarizes the subgroups of patients with liver disease and neurological sequelae that may be encountered in the intensive care unit (ICU) [4].

The heterogeneous nature of the presentation of HE led to the development of consensus terminology (Table 40.2) [2]. The West Haven Criteria is perhaps the best-known scoring system, with the severity of HE being graded from 0 to 4 (Table 40.3) [5].

Table 40.1 The subgroups of patients with liver disease and neurological sequelae that may be encountered in the intensive care unit (ICU) [4].

The critically ill patient with cirrhosis; pre-existing cirrhosis with one or more of the following:
Major variceal hemorrhage requiring airway management Severe hepatic encephalopathy (grade 3/4) Acute renal dysfunction requiring renal replacement therapy Hypotension (requiring fluids and vasopressors) Intra-abdominal hypertension with end-organ dysfunction Metabolic acidosis
Acute liver dysfunction in association with critical illness; encompasses the following three groups:
Septic cholestasis "Small for size" syndrome post-liver resection (ascites, portal hypertension, cholestasis +/− hepatic encephalopathy) Liver trauma
Acute liver failure; acute liver dysfunction (with no pre-existing liver disease) in association with any of the following:
Coagulopathy Hepatic encephalopathy Metabolic acidosis Renal dysfunction Cardiovascular failure Respiratory failure

Table 40.2 Clinical presentation of hepatic encephalopathy [2].

Encephalopathy	Definition
Acute	Acute liver dysfunction
Recurrent or episodic	Episodes of mental alteration in a patient with cirrhosis
Persistent	Neurological deficit that persists despite the reversal of liver injury such as following transplantation or the removal of a precipitating factor
Minimal (previously known as subclinical)	No evidence of overt encephalopathy but subtle cognitive deficits may be detected with a neuropsychological function test battery

Table 40.3 Clinical scoring of hepatic encephalopathy.

Grade using West Haven Criteria [5]	Clinical features	Glasgow Coma Scale Score [22]
0	No abnormality apparent on clinical examination	15
1	Short-term memory loss, difficulty in concentrating, and reverse of sleep wake cycle	15
2	Lethargy, apathy, drowsiness, flapping tremor (asterixis), disorientation, confusion, inappropriate behavior	12–15 (Verbal response or obeying command typically impaired)
3	Stuporose but easily rousable, marked confusion, incoherent speech	6–12
4	Coma, unresponsive	3–6 (May respond to painful stimuli)

Pathogenesis

In normal health, the ammonia generated by the body is delivered to the liver through the portal vein (level of up to 300 μmol/L) with production of urea via the urea cycle. A small amount is also excreted through the kidney and used by the skeletal muscle producing glutamine. When individuals develop either significant liver dysfunction and/or increased portosystemic shunting there is increased delivery of ammonia to the systemic circulation and hence the brain. There is risk of development of encephalopathy.

Severe liver dysfunction results in impaired urea synthesis resulting in buildup of glutamine, from ammonia and glutamate. Increased ammonia is delivered and taken across the blood–brain barrier (passive and transport through cation channels) where it can result in cytotoxic cerebral edema. The cerebral metabolic rate and uptake of ammonia is increased in acute liver failure. Ammonia may result in altered neurotransmission directly and indirectly, specifically N-methyl-D-aspartate (NMDA) and gamma-aminobutyric acid (GABA) receptors have been shown to be modulated, as have serotoninergic and dopaminergic transmission. Overstimulation of NMDA receptors through release of glutamate results in neuronal modulation, degeneration, and eventually apoptosis. The glutamate–NO pathway is also linked to inflammatory changes.

Once ammonia crosses the blood–brain barrier glutamine synthesis found predominantly in astrocytes results in amidation of glutamate to glutamine utilizing ammonia. There is slowing of oxidative metabolism and substrate depletion of TCA cycle with depletion of energy-rich phosphate compounds and lactate buildup.

There is evidence of astrocyte swelling in acute liver failure and this is associated with increased glutamine. The "Trojan horse" hypothesis recognizes that glutamine may release ammonia when taken up into the mitochondria, with release of oxidative and nitrosative stress by release of free radicals and mitochondrial permeability transition (MPT), an apoptotic pathway that results in loss of inner membrane potential and cessation of adenosine triphosphate (ATP) synthesis. Aquaporins (AQP4 particularly) have been shown to be up-regulated in astrocytes in the presence of increased ammonia levels, with ex vivo increase in astrocyte cell volume.

Cerebral blood flow is also increased in ALF and AoCLF, possibly as a result of systemic and potentially central inflammation. This results in increased delivery of ammonia to the brain and also has the potential to exacerbate cell swelling through hydrostatic factors and the increased blood volume has the potential to exacerbate elevations in ICP if the pressure–volume relationship is situated on the steep part of the curve.

In ALF, astrocytes can swell rapidly and this has the potential to result in cytotoxic brain edema [6]. Cerebral hyperemia is also critical to the development of intracranial hypertension (ICH) in ALF [7].

Patients with cirrhosis appear to be more resilient to the development of cerebral edema that can be seen in acute liver failure. This is probably due to relatively decreased brain volume in cirrhosis as compared with younger people with ALF. In addition in cirrhosis, astrocytes appear to have decreased amounts of myo-inositol probably in response to chronic increases in glutamine – thus the cells become resistant to cell swelling and acute osmotic changes.

Clinically significant brain swelling and increased intracranial pressure (ICP) are effectively only seen in acute liver failure. Bernal and colleagues have shown that the incidence of ICH in ALF has fallen over the past three decades. Data from 3,300 patients showed that approximately 65% of the patients presenting between 1984 and 1988 developed ICH but this had reduced to 20% during 2004 and 2008 [8]. This probably represents a trend towards earlier referral to tertiary care and advances in intensive and neurocritical care. Ammonia is now well established as an independent risk factor for the development of HE and ICH in ALF; arterial ammonia concentrations of >150 mmol/L predicted a greater likelihood of raised ICP [9]. Recent work by Bernal *et al* showed an incidence of raised ICP of 20–25% overall with the incidence being seen almost entirely in those with acute and hyperacute etiologies. Younger age (tighter skull), requirement for vasopressors, and renal replacement therapy are all additional independent risk factors for the development of ICH [10].

It is also now well recognized that infection and/or the resulting systemic inflammatory response are important factors contributing to worsening brain edema and ICH in ALF [11,12].

The causes of "brain failure" in acute-on-chronic liver failure are diverse; sepsis, alcohol withdrawal, drugs, intracranial hemorrhage, Wernicke's, new-onset portal vein thrombosis/hepatocellular carcinoma, and electrolyte disturbance all need to be considered. Again the inflammatory response is thought to be of key importance in modulating the pathophysiological effects of ammonia on the brain. In patients with cirrhosis the existence of hyponatraemia is a major risk factor in the development of overt hepatic encephalopathy, the underlying pathogenesis thought to be a second osmotic hit to astrocytes [13]. Only in rare circumstances is clinically significant brain swelling seen; however this should be considered especially in patients post TIPS shunt without prior exposure to hyperammonemia [14]. Cerebral imaging may be required in certain circumstances and may help to define etiology when there is concern.

Clinical features

The onset of encephalopathy in ALF can be rapid and it is not uncommon for the patient to be fully alert and lucid initially, subsequently lapsing into coma within a few hours, often with an interim period of extreme agitation which can render management difficult. For that reason, patients with early grades of encephalopathy and acute/hyperacute etiologies should be assessed for safety of transfer to a tertiary centre; early intubation and ventilation is often the safest strategy in case of acute deterioration of consciousness. The onset of encephalopathy in ALF may not be as clearly delineated as that in cirrhosis. Experience over 35 years at King's Liver Intensive Care Unit in over 3,000 ALF patients is that the onset of aggressive behavior, hyperreflexia, and ankle clonus are indicative of risk of progression from grade 3–4 coma and subsequent development of brain edema [15]. Seizures have been reported in up to a third of patients with ALF and may be associated with elevated arterial ammonia concentrations [16]. It may be necessary to undertake electroencephalography (EEG) confirmation given the difficulties in clinical diagnosis of seizures at the bedside in the ICU. There is no role for routine cerebral CT imaging to detect brain edema, however if there are pupillary abnormalities or localizing neurological signs then this should be performed to look for intracranial bleed or cerebral herniation.

Intracranial pressure monitoring is used infrequently in current practice but is still considered in those who develop grade 3–4 coma with the following features: fulfill King's criteria for poor prognosis, acute/hyperacute liver failure, pupillary abnormalities, seizures, fever, tachycardia, ammonia >150 μmol/L, hyponatremia, vasopressor therapy, jugular venous oxygen saturations suggestive of very low or very high cerebral blood flow, age < 40 [16]. Measurement of the velocity of blood flow in the middle cerebral arteries by transcranial Doppler ultrasonography may be helpful, with characteristic changes seen with rising intracranial pressure. Clearly the non-invasive nature is advantageous, however it is not sensitive to mild or moderate intracranial pressure changes. Monitoring of the reverse jugular vein oxygen saturation is frequently used in our institution and provides useful information on cerebral metabolism and oxygenation.

The critically ill patient with cirrhosis may present with a range of neurological symptoms from subtle confusion to deep coma. The differentials as alluded to earlier are numerous and in this scenario computed tomography (CT) imaging may be more frequently employed to exclude intracranial events, particularly in the context of thrombocytopenia and coagulopathy.

A normal ammonia does not exclude the presence of HE (particularly in cirrhosis); clinical observations do not always show a correlation between arterial ammonia concentration and grade of HE. Sepsis is a common precipitant and patients may not come to the attention of the intensive care team until they have developed grade 3–4 coma and associated sepsis-related organ dysfunction, and the myriad of symptoms that accompanies this.

Management

Early identification of the patient with ALF and referral to centers experienced in ALF management with transplant facilities are essential. Strategies employed in patients with established ALF and HE aim to maintain freedom from infection, reduce inflammation, use adequate sedation, and correct hypo-osmolality (Figure 40.1).

Early volume expansion, usually with a combination of crystalloid and colloid, should be undertaken. Hypertonic saline is used to maintain sodium between 145 and 150 mmol/L; in a study of 30 patients randomized to either standard care or standard care with hypertonic saline to maintain sodium levels between 145 and 150 mmol/L, ICP decreased significantly relative to baseline in the treatment group and the incidence of ICH (defined as a sustained increase in ICP to a level of 25 mmHg or greater) was significantly higher in the control group [17]. The underlying mechanism relates to maintenance of the osmotic pressure gradient across the blood–brain barrier thereby reducing brain water and lowering ICP. Bolus mannitol (20%) is also effective in decreasing surges in ICP.

Ventilation is altered to ensure arterial CO_2 is maintained between 4 and 4.5 kPa; hyperventilation is not beneficial but may be used acutely to decrease surges in ICP by decreasing cerebral blood flow [18]. Cerebral blood flow may also be decreased by use of intravenous indomethacin in patients with resistant intracranial hypertension and evidence of elevated ICP unresponsive to standard interventions.

Propofol, which induces hypometabolic vasoconstriction within the brain and reduces the risk of seizures, is the sedative of choice; fentanyl is usually used in addition. Moderate hypothermia or avoidance of fever has several beneficial effects on ICP related to reduced cerebral uptake of ammonia, cerebral blood flow, and mediators of inflammation. Induction of hypothermia (32 °C) has been shown to be efficacious in patients with uncontrolled ICH who await emergency liver transplantation [19].

Prophylactic use of phenytoin has not been shown to be beneficial in preventing cerebral edema, seizures, or need for mechanical ventilation, and does not improve survival [20]. The largest randomized controlled trial in ALF examined the use of L-ornithine-L-aspartate (LOLA): 201 ALF patients were randomized to receive either placebo or LOLA infusions; reduced ammonia levels/increased survival were not seen in the treatment group [21]. Hemofiltration is used to aid with removal of ammonia and is effectively the best strategy to reduce ammonia levels.

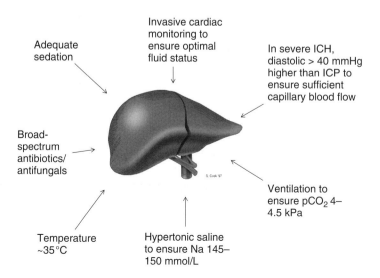

Figure 40.1 Management of acute liver failure. ICH, intracranial hypertension; ICP, intracranial pressure.

Adequate sedation

Invasive cardiac monitoring to ensure optimal fluid status

In severe ICH, diastolic > 40 mmHg higher than ICP to ensure sufficient capillary blood flow

Broad-spectrum antibiotics/ antifungals

Ventilation to ensure pCO$_2$ 4– 4.5 kPa

Temperature ~35°C

Hypertonic saline to ensure Na 145– 150 mmol/L

Broad-spectrum antibiotics and antifungals are used empirically in this group in order to try and prevent sepsis and worsening of encephalopathy. Survival has been transformed by emergency liver transplantation, which is now part of routine care for those who meet criteria indicative of a poor prognosis without contraindication.

There is no convincing evidence in ALF that liver support systems have benefit.

In acute-on-chronic liver failure management is centered around supportive measures whilst the precipitant is identified and treated. In this group where grade 3/4 HE has developed early management of the airway is key. Sepsis/inflammation is a frequent precipitant; again the early use of broad-spectrum antibiotics is recommended, these should then be rationalized at 48 hours depending on isolation from cultures.

Inflammation and infection

As alluded to throughout this chapter, there is a growing awareness of the synergistic role of inflammation, infection, and ammonia in the development of HE. The identification of biomarkers and the modulation of the immune system to develop novel treatment strategies in ALF are busy research areas. It is foreseeable that immunomodulatory therapies may become increasingly utilized, and with the development of further techniques to determine who may or may not benefit without liver transplantation, the number of patients managed 'medically' may increase over the next few decades.

Conclusion

Early identification of the ALF patient who has much in common with the patient with septic shock allows prompt resuscitation, referral to centers experienced in the management of acute liver failure, and goal-directed treatment as outlined above. Raised ICP and cerebral herniation has historically been the most feared complication of ALF; however this has reduced dramatically in frequency and patients are now more likely to succumb to sepsis and demise with multi-organ failure. Treatment strategies are aimed at reducing this risk to allow time for liver regeneration or emergency transplantation to take place. Cirrhotic patients who develop HE will be encountered much more frequently than the patient with ALF and this group may benefit from support in the ICU, particularly when there is a

reversible feature that has triggered the development of coma. Therapy in this cohort is again supportive and aimed at reducing the associated inflammation and worsening of infection. Modulation of the immune system is likely to be the focus of future treatment modalities and may change the number of patients requiring liver transplantation and life-long immunosuppression.

References

1. Adams R, Foley J. The neurological changes in the more common types of liver disease. *Trans Am Neurol Assoc* 1949;**74**:217–19.

2. Ferenci P, Lockwood A, Mullen K, *et al.* Hepatic encephalopathy – definition, nomenclature, diagnosis and quantification: final report of the working party at the 11th World Congresses of Gastroenterology, Vienna, 1998. *Hepatology* 2002;**35**:716–21.

3. O'Grady JG, Schalm SW, Williams R. Acute liver failure: redefining the syndromes. *Lancet* 1993;**342**:273–5.

4. Shawcross D, Wendon J. Acute-on-chronic liver failure in cirrhosis: defining and managing organ dysfunction. *Yearbook Intensive Care Emergency Med* 2009;**2009**:658–71.

5. Conn H, Lieberthal M. *The Hepatic Coma Syndromes and Lactulose.* Baltimore: Williams and Wilkins; 1979.

6. Kato M, Hughes R, Keays R, Williams R. Electron microscopic study of brain capillaries in cerebral oedema from fulminant hepatic failure. *Hepatology* 1992;**15**:1060–6.

7. Larsen FS, Adel HB, Pott F, *et al.* Dissociated cerebral vasoparalysis in acute liver failure. A hypothesis of gradual cerebral hyperaemia. *J Hepatol* 1996;**25**(2):145–51.

8. Bernal W, Hyyrylainen A, Gera A, *et al.* Evolution of natural history and treatment strategies in acute liver failure: lessons from a 35 year experience in 3300 patients. [Abstract]. *Hepatology* 2010;**52**(Suppl. 4).

9. Clemmesen J, Larsen F, Kondrup J, Hansen B, Ott P. Cerebral herniation in patients with acute liver failure is correlated with arterial ammonia concentration. *Hepatology* 1999;**29**:648–53.

10. Bernal W, Hall C, Karvellas C, *et al.* Arterial ammonia and clinical risk factors for encephalopathy and intracranial hypertension in acute liver failure. *Hepatology* 2007;**46**(6):1844–52.

11. Rolando N, Wade J, Davalos M, *et al.* The systemic inflammatory response syndrome in acute liver failure. *Hepatology* 2000;**32**:734–9.

12. Vaquero J, Polson J, Chung C, *et al.* Infection and the progression of hepatic encephalopathy in acute liver failure. *Gastroenterology* 2003;**125**(3):755–64.

13. Guevara M, Baccaro ME, Torre A, *et al.* Hyponatremia is a risk factor of hepatic encephalopathy in patients with cirrhosis: a prospective study with time-dependent analysis. *Am J Gastroenterology* 2009;**104**(6):1382–9.

14. Jalan R, Newby DE, Damink SW, *et al.* Acute changes in cerebral blood flow and metabolism during portosystemic shunting. *Liver Transpl* 2001;**7**:274–8.

15. Shawcross DL, Wendon JA. The neurological manifestations of acute liver failure. *Neurochem Int* 2011;**60**:662–71.

16. Ellis AJ, Wendon JA, Williams R. Subclinical seizure activity and prophylactic phenytoin infusion in acute liver failure: a controlled clinical trial. *Hepatology* 2000;**32**(3):536–41.

17. Murphy N, Auzinger G, Bernal W, Wendon J. The effect of hypertonic sodium chloride on intracranial pressure in patients with acute liver failure. *Hepatology* 2004;**39**:464–70.

18. Larsen F, Adel Hansen B, Pott F, *et al.* Dissociated cerebral vasospasm in acute liver failure. A hypothesis of gradual cerebral hyperaemia. *J Hepatol* 1996;**25**:145–51.

19. Jalan R, Olde Damink SW, Deutz NE, Hayes PC, Lee A. Moderate hypothermia in patients with acute liver failure and uncontrolled intracranial hypertension. *Gastroenterology* 2004;**127**(5):1338–46.

20. Bhatia V, Batra Y, Acharya SK. Prophylactic phenytoin does not improve cerebral edema or survival in acute liver failure – a controlled clinical trial. *J Hepatology* 2004;**41**(1):89–96.

21. Acharya SK, Bhatia V, Sreenivas V, Khanal S, Panda SK. Efficacy of L-ornithine-L-aspartate in acute liver failure: a double-blind, randomized, placebo-controlled study. *Gastroenterology* 2009;**136**(7):2159–68.

22. Teasdale G, Jennett B. Assessment of coma and impaired consciousness. A practical scale. *Lancet* 1974;**2**:81.

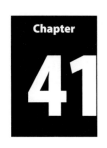

Chapter 41

Neurological complications of cardiac surgery: stroke, encephalopathy, and cognitive decline

Rebecca F. Gottesman, Maura A. Grega, Guy M. McKhann, and Ola A. Selnes

SUMMARY

Cardiac surgical procedures continue to be associated with postoperative neurological complications in a subset of patients, despite technological advances in surgical technique. This is primarily because individuals who are referred for cardiac surgery often have pre-existing risk factors that increase their risk of these complications. These risk factors include vascular risk factors as well as sometimes subclinical cerebrovascular disease. An increasing number of individuals undergoing cardiac surgery have old strokes, both clinical and radiographic, intra- and extracranial atherosclerosis, and leukoaraiosis. Thus, their risks for a postoperative neurological complication are increased. Specifically, individuals continue to experience stroke, delirium, and cognitive decline postoperatively, and rates of some of these complications – particularly stroke – are even more frequent in individuals having combined cardiac surgical procedures. In addition, with the increasing use of MRI diffusion-weighted imaging (DWI), individuals are found to have subclinical infarcts, which may be associated with subtle changes in cognition, or even global encephalopathy or delirium. Potential mechanisms of neurological injury after cardiac surgery are discussed, including embolization (both macro- and micro-), hypoperfusion, and inflammation. Data on the role of off-pump (as compared to on-pump) coronary artery bypass grafting surgery is discussed, particularly with regards to postoperative stroke and cognitive impairment, with no clear benefit from the use of off-pump surgery. Finally, the data on the short- and long-term cognitive outcomes of individuals undergoing cardiac surgery are discussed, including the controversy over the development of Alzheimer's disease in association with cardiopulmonary bypass.

Introduction

Individuals undergoing cardiac surgical procedures remain at risk for neurological injury, despite many improvements in surgical technique over the past decade. Neurological injury can take the form of stroke, encephalopathy or delirium, or postoperative cognitive decline. In addition, as MRI techniques have improved and allowed for detection of more subtle brain injury, subclinical brain infarction has been identified as another potential complication of cardiac surgery.

Specific patient-related factors appear to be most important in determining an individual's risk for neurological injury postoperatively. Medical comorbidities dictate likelihood of experiencing most neurological complications of cardiac surgery, and patients undergoing cardiac surgery in this era have more medical comorbidities, are older, and therefore are at higher risk for these neurological complications. In addition, many of the strategies implemented in cardiac surgery with the goal of improving neurological outcomes have not recognized this goal.

Surgery types

On-pump coronary artery bypass grafting

The use of the cardiopulmonary bypass pump (CPB) has made coronary revascularization surgery possible for the past several decades. However, numerous postoperative complications have been linked to the use of this technology. Possible mechanisms of neurological injury associated with the use of CPB include macro- and microemboli, hypoperfusion, hyperthermia, and a systemic inflammatory response, with an embolic etiology often considered as the primary mechanism

Brain Disorders in Critical Illness, ed. Robert D. Stevens, Tarek Sharshar, and E. Wesley Ely. Published by Cambridge University Press. © Cambridge University Press 2013.

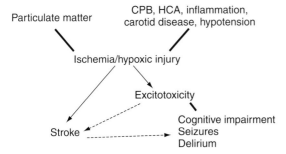

Figure 41.1 Potential mechanisms of neurological injury associated with cardiopulmonary bypass (CPB). HCA, hypothermic circulatory arrest.

(Figure 41.1). These emboli may take many forms – atheroemboli, surgical debris, fat or air emboli. Histopathological data show "small capillary arteriolar dilations," or SCADs, made of lipid, on autopsies of patients who have undergone cardiac surgery. These SCADs are thought to be due to suctioned cardiotomy blood that is returned to the bypass circuit, with some reduction in stroke with the use of a cell-saver device that filters blood before it is returned to the circulation [1]. Stroke still, however, remains a clinical problem, suggesting that additional mechanisms also contribute. Larger macroemboli originate both from the aorta and the heart, and some centers use epiaortic ultrasound to screen the extent of aortic disease. Knowledge of aortic plaque distribution can assist in decisions about aortic cross-clamp placement and might actually decrease rate of stroke when used in this intraoperative decision making [2,3].

It is likely that other factors, such as hypoperfusion and inflammation, play a role in the development of neurological complications in conjunction with embolic disease [4]. Thus, the focus should not be only on reduction of embolic injury, given evidence that hypoperfusion (in the form of relative [5] or absolute [6] reductions in blood pressure, or anemia [7]) is also associated with adverse postoperative outcomes, including stroke.

Off-pump coronary artery bypass grafting

Off-pump coronary artery bypass grafting (CABG) surgery is one particular approach that had the goal of reducing postoperative stroke, primarily because it was felt to reduce intraoperative emboli and other problems by eliminating the use of the bypass pump. Unfortunately, randomized studies have failed to show any difference in stroke rates for off-pump CABG vs. on-pump CABG [8], in either low-risk [9] or high-risk

[10] patients, providing further support that embolization may not be the only mechanism by which neurological injury occurs post-CABG. In addition, stroke is one type of postoperative neurological complication. At our institution, over 13 years of collecting data, neurological injury as a category (including delirium, coma, slowness to awaken from anesthesia) was more common among individuals undergoing off-pump CABG than among those undergoing on-pump CABG.

Combined surgeries

Cardiac surgery procedures can vary greatly, and the frequency of neurological complications varies depending on the type of surgery. An isolated CABG surgery has a lower rate of stroke (around 3%), for instance, than does CABG combined with valve replacement (around 6%) or carotid endarterectomy (CEA). In a German study, the stroke rates almost doubled when a single valve replacement was added to CABG, and if multiple valves were being replaced doubled again, to nearly 7% [11]. Repeat CABG surgery also increases stroke risk [2]. Carotid endarterectomy, combined with on-pump CABG, has been associated with higher stroke risk in some studies [12], although others have not found this result [13], and still others have noted lower rates of complications when CEA is combined with off-pump CABG [14]. Because of these variations between different procedure types, the incidence of neurological complications needs to be considered in the context of the surgical type.

Neurological complications

Stroke

Postoperative stroke is one of the most easily identified complications of CABG surgery. It occurred in 1.6% of isolated CABG patients in one single-institution study [2], with higher estimates reported elsewhere for combined surgical procedures. Post-CABG stroke may present like a typical clinical stroke, but, because these strokes are often multifocal, may present with less easily localizable or more diffuse signs and symptoms. In addition, other factors such as pain medication use or superimposed delirium may cloud neurological assessment in the early postoperative period. Strokes after CABG surgery are often split into "early" (within the first few days postoperatively) or "delayed" strokes; risk factors differ for these stroke types, with earlier strokes often associated with the amount of time on the CPB machine, aortic arch disease, and history of stroke. Later strokes are associated with atrial fibrillation and reduced cardiac output [15]. Other established risk factors for stroke include older age, female sex [16], and anemia and transfusion (independently) [7].

Individuals who experience stroke after CABG may also have other preoperative atherosclerosis; this may be subclinical, but is a strong predictor of stroke risk. In the past, most evaluations have been restricted to the extracranial carotid vasculature, as a measure of possible subclinical atherosclerosis burden: asymptomatic carotid stenosis, however, has not been clearly associated with postoperative stroke [17]. Cerebral atherosclerosis, measured on preoperative magnetic resonance angiography, however, does predict postoperative stroke (OR 1.35 for presence of intra- and extracranial cerebral atherosclerosis) [18]. Infarcts on preoperative brain MRI or leukoaraiosis [19] (Figure 41.2) have also been associated with an increasing risk of postoperative stroke rates: 1.4% in individuals with normal preoperative brain MRIs; 5.6% in those with small infarcts; and 8.4% in individuals with multiple infarctions on preoperative

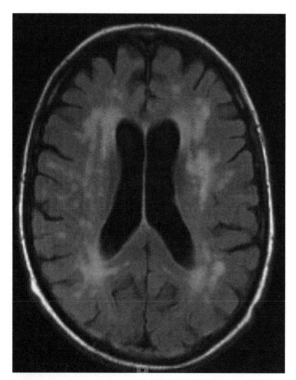

Figure 41.2 Fluid attenuated inversion recovery (FLAIR) MRI sequence demonstrating significant leukoaraiosis (white matter hyperintensities) in patients undergoing CABG surgery, suggesting significant premorbid cerebrovascular disease.

brain MRIs [20]. In addition, preoperative cognitive performance, which may be a marker of cerebrovascular disease in this population, also indicates increased risk of postoperative radiographic stroke [21]. As our ability to evaluate subclinical disease improves, it is increasingly likely that we will know more about an individual's subclinical atherosclerosis status before surgery occurs. The remaining question is whether selecting individuals for surgery on the basis of absence of this subclinical disease is practical or whether it actually improves outcomes.

Subclinical stroke

Stroke has traditionally been defined, in studies of post-CABG neurological complications, by clinical signs and symptoms. However, just as preclinical subclinical cerebrovascular disease is likely to impact postoperative outcomes, imaging studies of otherwise asymptomatic patients post-CABG have found that many of them do not have normal postoperative brain MRIs. Changes on diffusion-weighted imaging (DWI) MRI consistent with acute infarcts are not uncommon after CABG (Figure 41.3) and incidence of new DWI-positive lesions goes up for patients having combined surgical procedures.

When individuals undergoing cardiac surgical procedures are imaged with MRI postoperatively, over 40% of CABG patients [22] have been found to have new DWI-positive lesions, with estimates increasing with more complex surgical procedures. Postoperative cognitive performance may be completely normal [23] despite these infarct-like lesions. Although new subclinical ischemic lesions are most common postoperatively, one report of patients after valve replacement surgery has shown that some individuals postoperatively have new gradient echo-positive lesions, consistent with hemorrhage [24], despite the relatively low frequency of clinically apparent hemorrhagic strokes in this population.

With the increasing identification of subclinical disease, it is possible that many neurological symptoms not felt to have an anatomic correlate might actually be associated with subclinical ischemia on brain MRI. This includes delirium or encephalopathy, which might, in some cases, be related to subclinical infarcts. This area requires further investigation.

Delirium/encephalopathy

Delirium is a common postoperative complication in elderly patients after major cardiac and non-cardiac surgery. The reported incidence of delirium depends

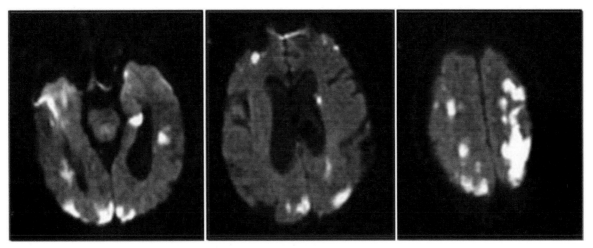

Figure 41.3 Diffusion-weighted imaging (DWI) MRI demonstrating acute infarcts in a post-CABG patient, in the absence of any focal neurological deficits, but with delirium and global encephalopathy.

on patient selection criteria and methodology used to identify delirium. It occurs in 10–60% of elderly patients after non-cardiac surgery [25], and from 3–43% in younger versus older patients after cardiac surgery [26,27]. One retrospective study found a higher rate of delirium after on-pump (11.9%) than after off-pump coronary artery bypass (OPCAB) surgery (5.1%), but the OPCAB patients were younger and had less severe cardiac disease [28]. There are no randomized trials comparing rates of delirium after on-pump versus OPCAB surgery, and it is therefore not known whether use of cardiopulmonary bypass by itself is associated with an increased risk of delirium. The range of potential causes and clinical manifestations of delirium makes analysis of delirium as an outcome, or as a predictor of other outcomes, difficult. Patient-related risk factors for delirium after cardiac surgery are similar to those for stroke, and include history of cerebrovascular disease, peripheral vascular disease, and atrial fibrillation [28]. Although delirium typically resolves before patients are discharged, it has nonetheless been associated with several serious outcomes after surgery, such as prolonged mechanical ventilation, longer ICU and hospital stays, and even increased mortality [29,30].

Future directions for delirium prevention

Despite recognition of risk factors for postoperative delirium [31], few strategies have emerged to reduce or prevent this complication. In a small, randomized study, postoperative sedation with dexmedetomidine reduced the duration but not the incidence of postoperative delirium [32]. Attempts to prevent postoperative delirium have focused on the role of sedative and analgesic agents as well as depth and type of anesthesia [33]. Further progress in understanding the pathophysiology of delirium might be obtained from brain-imaging studies that can quantify the degree of pre-existing cerebrovascular disease [34], but to date, no studies have examined brain imaging in patients with postoperative delirium.

Cognitive decline

Postoperative cognitive decline, as measured by neuropsychological testing, is the most commonly reported type of adverse neurological outcome associated with cardiac surgery. Prior studies estimated that more than 40% of patients undergoing CABG suffered some type of short-term cognitive deficits [35]. It was widely believed that microemboli, hypoperfusion, or the systemic inflammatory response associated with the use of extracorporeal CPB were directly responsible for the cognitive changes. In an attempt to reduce such postoperative cognitive deficits, techniques for coronary artery revascularization without the use of CPB were developed. Although results from initial studies suggested that the frequency of adverse postoperative neurological events were reduced in patients undergoing so-called off-pump surgery, later randomized controlled trials did not confirm these early findings (Table 41.1).

Table 41.1 Randomized trials comparing cognitive outcomes after on-pump and off-pump surgery.

Study	Year	Sample characteristics	Sample size	Follow-up interval	Proportion with decline		p-value
					On-pump	Off-pump	
[8]	2009	VA medical centers	2203	1 year	n/a	n/a	a
[43]	2007	Single center	201	Discharge	62%	52%	ns
				6 months	47%	44%	ns
[44]	2007	Single center	212	Discharge	n/a	n/a	b
				6 weeks	n/a	n/a	c
				6 months	n/a	n/a	c
[45]	2006	Single center	70	1 week	57%	58%	ns
				1 month	30%	12%	ns
				6 months	19%	15%	ns
[46]	2006	Single center	168	6 weeks	n/a	n/a	d
				6 months	n/a	n/a	e
[47]	2006	Single center	107	2 months	n/a	n/a	f
				6 months	n/a	n/a	g
[48, 49]	2006	High-risk patients	120	3 months	24%	20%	ns
	2008			1 year	19%	9%	ns
[50]	2005	Single center	120	3 months	23%	20%	ns
				1 year	23%	24%	ns
[51]	2003	Single center	60	2 weeks	15%	16%	ns
				1 year	15%	19%	ns
[52, 53]	2002	Low-risk patients	281	3 months	29%	21%	ns
		Single center		1 year	34%	31%	ns
	2007			5 years	35%	33%	ns

n/a, data not given as percentage; ns, not statistically significant.
[a] No difference between on- and off-pump in change in global z-score from baseline to follow-up.
[b] Higher global composite cognitive score (0.25 SD) in the off-pump group (p = 0.01).
[c] No significant difference in global composite score between on- and off-pump groups.
[d] Off-pump performed significantly better in 3/15 tests (p = < 0.001).
[e] Off-pump group performed significantly better in 2/15 tests (p < 0.001).
[f] No difference in incidence of cognitive impairment.
[g] Lower incidence of cognitive impairment in off-pump group for 1 test (word fluency).

More recent studies exploring cognitive outcomes after CABG have been methodologically more rigorous, and have incorporated one or more control groups, including patients with coronary artery disease (CAD) but no surgery, as well as improved statistical methods for estimating postoperative cognitive decline. The results of these studies have shown that while postoperative cognitive decline does still occur in some patients, the frequency is significantly lower than what was reported in earlier, uncontrolled studies. Nonetheless, despite many advances in the field of cardiac surgery, there is still considerable variability in surgical procedures among institutions. Some of these procedural differences, such as degree of hypothermia, rate of rewarming, use of pulsatile flow and cardiotomy suction, may be relevant to how well the brain is protected during surgery, and contribute to significant variability among institutions in actual rates of adverse cognitive outcomes.

Late cognitive decline

Although it is now generally accepted that for most patients, postoperative cognitive changes after cardiac surgery are generally relatively mild and transient in nature, these short-term cognitive changes may reflect subclinical injury, which may be a risk factor for future, or delayed, cognitive decline.

Newman and colleagues studied a group of 261 patients before surgery and followed them prospectively up to 5 years after CABG surgery [36]. At the

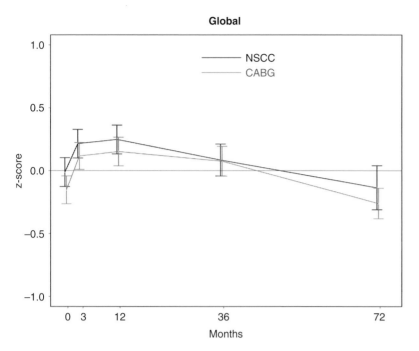

Figure 41.4 Composite longitudinal change in global cognitive z-score for individuals with coronary artery disease who underwent CABG surgery compared with the non-surgical cardiac controls (NSCC, who also had coronary artery disease). The lines and their trajectories do not differ statistically. Adapted from [37].

time of discharge, the incidence of cognitive decline was 53%, falling to 24% at 6 months. At 5 years, however, an alarming 42% of these patients were reported to have lower scores than their baseline performance on a composite measure of cognition. Predictors of long-term cognitive decline included older age, fewer years of education, higher baseline score, and cognitive decline at the time of discharge. The latter led to concerns that although early postoperative changes appeared to be transient, they might nonetheless be a risk factor for the development of future cognitive decline.

Because the Newman study did not include any control or comparison groups, it could not be determined if the late cognitive decline was related to the use of CPB or other factors. Selnes and colleagues followed 152 CABG patients and 92 non-surgical controls for 6 years. Although mild late cognitive decline was observed for both groups, no statistically significant differences were seen between the surgical and non-surgical groups in the degree of decline at 72 months after baseline testing (Figure 41.4) [37]. It was concluded therefore, that although late cognitive decline does occur, it is not specific to the use of CPB.

In summary, there is thus evidence that late cognitive decline may occur in some patients after CABG, but a specific link with the use of CPB has not been established. Alternative explanations for the late cognitive decline might include normal aging, progression of underlying cerebrovascular disease, or the development of Alzheimer's disease (AD).

Several studies have attempted to determine if patients who undergo CABG with CPB are at increased risk of developing AD years after the procedure [38,39]. In a retrospective study of Veterans Affairs patients, Lee and colleagues compared the incidence of dementia up to 5 years after conventional CABG (n = 5,216) with that after percutaneous coronary intervention (PCI) (n = 3,954). A total of 78 patients (1.5%) were diagnosed as having AD in the CABG group, compared with 41 (1.0%) in the PCI group, leading to an adjusted 1.71-fold greater risk of developing AD for the patients in the CABG group versus those in the PCI group [39].

There are several factors that should be considered in the interpretation of these results, however. First, in the absence of neuroimaging data, it is unclear whether these patients (1) had this condition pre-existing prior to surgery or (2) had actual AD as opposed to either a mixed AD/vascular dementia syndrome or a predominantly vascular dementia. Second, the overall 5-year incidence rate of AD reported for both study groups is several-fold lower than the 13% incidence previously reported in community cohorts with a history of cerebrovascular disease [40]. Therefore, it could be hypothesized that the low rate of AD in the VA study is because cardiac revascularization procedures may actually have protective effects against the progression of cerebrovascular disease and dementia. Since this was an uncontrolled study, this hypothesis could not be tested. A recent observational study from Canada did compare dementia outcomes for patients with surgical revascularization (CABG and PCI) versus medical therapy alone, and concluded that coronary revascularization procedures may be associated with lower incidence rates of future dementia than standard medical therapy [41].

There is also evidence from neuropathological and cognitive studies that a subset of patients with CAD of sufficient severity to require CABG may have pre-existing mild or preclinical AD [42]. These patients would be expected to have a progressive cognitive decline after their surgery. The prevalence of pre-existing cognitive impairment or AD in patients with less severe forms of CAD, as in those who can be treated with PCI, is not currently known.

Conclusion

In summary, neurological complications remain a problem after cardiac surgery, with higher rates associated with combined procedures or more extensive surgeries. In addition, the use of more sensitive screening instruments, particularly with the use of diffusion-weighted imaging MRI, is likely to lead to higher estimates of postoperative stroke, and possibly a better understanding of the etiologies of non-specific postoperative changes such as delirium and cognitive decline. Most cognitive change, if present, normalizes soon after surgery, and it is likely that any long-term decline or dementia previously attributed to CPB is actually due to the underlying vascular disease that led to the need for CABG surgery in the first place. Further studies in this field are needed to evaluate the interplay of causative factors in the development of neurological complications, with more of an emphasis on patient-based management, taking each individual's risk factors and previous history into account when planning surgical management.

References

1. Carrier M, Denault A, Lavoie J, Perrault LP. Randomized controlled trial of pericardial blood processing with a cell-saving device on neurologic markers in elderly patients undergoing coronary artery bypass graft surgery. *Ann Thorac Surg* 2006;**82**:51–6.

2. Tarakji KG, Sabik JF, III, Bhudia SK, Batizy LH, Blackstone EH. Temporal onset, risk factors and outcomes associated with stroke after coronary artery bypass grafting. *JAMA* 2011;**305**:381–90.

3. Nakamura Y, Kawachi K, Imagawa H, *et al.* The prevalence and severity of cerebrovascular disease in patients undergoing cardiovascular surgery. *Ann Thorac Cardiovasc Surg* 2004;**10**:81–4.

4. Caplan LR, Hennerici M. Impaired clearance of emboli (washout) is an important link between hypoperfusion, embolism, and ischemic stroke. *Arch Neurol* 1998;**55**:1475–82.

5. Gottesman RF, Sherman PM, Grega MA, *et al.* Watershed strokes after cardiac surgery: diagnosis, etiology, and outcome. *Stroke* 2006;**37**:2306–11.

6. Gold JP, Charlson ME, Williams-Russo P, *et al.* Improvements of outcomes after coronary artery bypass: a randomized trial comparing intraoperative high versus low mean arterial pressure. *J Thorac Cardiovasc Surg* 1995;**110**:1302–14.

7. Bahrainwala ZS, Grega MA, Hogue CW, *et al.* Intraoperative hemoglobin levels and transfusion independently predict stroke after cardiac operations. *Ann Thorac Surg* 2011;**91**:1113–18.

8. Shroyer AL, Grover FL, Hattler B, *et al.* On-pump versus off-pump coronary-artery bypass surgery. *N Engl J Med* 2009;**361**:1827–37.

9. Nathoe HM, van Dijk D, Jansen EWL, *et al.* A comparison of on-pump and off-pump coronary bypass surgery in low-risk patients. *N Engl J Med* 2003;**348**:394–402.

10. Moller CH, Perko MJ, Lund JT, *et al.* No major differences in 30-day outcomes in high-risk patients randomized to off-pump versus on-pump coronary bypass surgery: the Best Bypass Surgery trial. *Circulation* 2010;**121**:498–504.

11. Boeken U, Litmathe J, Feindt P, Gams E. Neurological complications after cardiac surgery: risk factors and correlation to the surgical procedure. *Thorac Cardiovasc Surg* 2005;**53**:33–6.

12. Cywinski JB, Koch CG, Krajewski LP, *et al.* Increased risk associated with combined carotid endarterectomy and coronary artery bypass graft surgery: a propensity-matched comparison with isolated coronary artery bypass graft surgery. *J Cardiothorac Vasc Anesth* 2006;**20**:796–802.

13. Dick AM, Brothers T, Robison JG, *et al.* Combined carotid endarterectomy and coronary artery bypass

grafting versus coronary artery bypass grafting alone: a retrospective review of outcomes at our institution. *Vasc Endovasc Surg* 2011;**45**:130–4.

14. Chiti E, Troisi N, Marek J, *et al.* Combined carotid and cardiac surgery: improving the results. *Ann Vasc Surg* 2010;**24**:794–800.

15. Hogue CW, Murphy SF, Schechtman KB, Davila-Roman VG. Risk factors for early or delayed stroke after cardiac surgery. *Circulation* 1999;**100**:642–7.

16. Hogue CW, Barzilai B, Pieper KS, *et al.* Sex differences in neurological outcomes and mortality after cardiac surgery. *Circulation* 2001;**103**:2133–7.

17. Naylor AR, Bown MJ. Stroke after cardiac surgery and its association with asymptomatic carotid disease: an updated systematic review and meta-analysis. *Eur J Vasc Endovasc Surg* 2011;**41**:607–24.

18. Lee EJ, Choi KH, Ryu JS, *et al.* Stroke risk after coronary artery bypass graft surgery and extent of cerebral artery atherosclerosis. *J Am Coll Cardiol* 2011;**57**:1811–18.

19. Andrell P, Jensen C, Norrsell H, *et al.* White matter disease in magnetic resonance imaging predicts cerebral complications after coronary artery bypass grafting. *Ann Thorac Surg* 2005;**79**:74–9.

20. Goto T, Baba T, Honma K, *et al.* Magnetic resonance imaging findings and postoperative neurologic dysfunction in elderly patients undergoing coronary artery bypass grafting. *Ann Thorac Surg* 2001;**72**:137–42.

21. Maekawa K, Goto T, Baba T, *et al.* Impaired cognition preceding cardiac surgery is related to cerebral ischemic lesions. *J Anesthesia* 2011;**25**:330–6.

22. Barber PA, Hach S, Tippett LJ, *et al.* Cerebral ischemic lesions on diffusion-weighted imaging are associated with neurocognitive decline after cardiac surgery. *Stroke* 2008;**39**(5):1427–33.

23. Cook DJ, Huston T, III, Brown RD, Zehr KJ, Sundt TM, III. Postcardiac surgical cognitive impairment in the aged using diffusion-weighted magnetic resonance imaging. *Ann Thorac Surg* 2007;**83**:1389–95.

24. Jeon SB, Lee JW, Kim SJ, *et al.* New cerebral lesions on t2*-weighted gradient-echo imaging after cardiac valve surgery. *Cerebrovasc Dis* 2010;**30**:194–9.

25. Parikh SS, Chung F. Postoperative delirium in the elderly. *Anesth Analg* 1995;**80**:1223–32.

26. Norkiene I, Ringaitiene D, Misiuriene I, *et al.* Incidence and precipitating factors of delirium after coronary artery bypass grafting. *Scand Cardiovasc J* 2007;**41**:180–5.

27. Rudolph JL, Inouye SK, Jones RN, *et al.* An independent predictor of functional decline after cardiac surgery. *J Am Geriatr Soc* 2010;**58**: 643–9.

28. Bucerius J, Gummert JF, Borger MA, *et al.* Predictors of delirium after cardiac surgery delirium: effect of beating-heart (off-pump) surgery. *J Thorac Cardiovasc Surg* 2004;**127**:57–64.

29. Kazmierski J, Kowman M, Banach M, *et al.* Incidence and predictors of delirium after cardiac surgery: results from the IPDACS study. *J Psychosom Res* 2010;**69**:179–85.

30. Gottesman RF, Grega MA, Bailey MM, *et al.* Delirium after coronary artery bypass graft surgery and late mortality. *Ann Neurol* 2010;**67**:338–44.

31. Afonso A, Scurlock C, Reich D, *et al.* Predictive model for postoperative delirium in cardiac surgical patients. *Seminars Cardiothoracic Vascular Anesthesia* 2010;**14**:212–17.

32. Shehabi Y, Grant P, Wolfenden H, *et al.* Prevalence of delirum with dexmedetomidine compared with morphine based therapy after cardiac surgery: a randomized controlled trial (dexmedetomidine compared to morphine-dexcom study). *Anesthesiology* 2009;**111**:1075–84.

33. Sieber FE. Postoperative delirium in the elderly surgical patient. *Anesthesiol Clin* 2009;**27**:451–64.

34. Shioiri A, Kurumaji A, Takeuchi T, *et al.* White matter abnormalities as a risk factor for postoperative delirium revealed by diffusion tensor imaging. *Am J Geriatr Psychiatry* 2010;**18**:743–53.

35. Hogue CW, Jr., Palin CA, Arrowsmith JE. Cardiopulmonary bypass management and neurologic outcomes: an evidence-based appraisal of current practices. *Anesth Analg* 2006;**103**:21–37.

36. Newman MF, Kirchner JL, Phillips-Bute B, *et al.* Longitudinal assessment of neurocognitive function after coronary-artery bypass surgery. *N Engl J Med* 2001;**344**:395–402.

37. Selnes OA, Grega MA, Bailey MM, *et al.* Do management strategies for coronary artery disease influence 6-year cognitive outcomes? *Ann Thorac Surg* 2009;**88**:445–54.

38. Knopman DS, Peterson RC, Cha RH, Edland SD, Rocca WA. Coronary artery bypass grafting is not a risk factor for dementia or Alzheimer's disease. *Neurology* 2005;**65**:986–90.

39. Lee TA, Wolozin B, Weiss KB, Bednar MM. Assessment of the emergence of Alzheimer's disease following coronary artery bypass graft surgery or percutaneous transluminal coronary angioplasty. *J Alzheimer's Dis* 2005;**7**:319–24.

40. Fitzpatrick AL, Kuller LH, Ives DG, *et al.* Incidence and prevalence of dementia in the Cardiovascular Health Study. *J Am Geriatr Soc* 2004;**52**:195–204.

41. Mutch WA, Fransoo RR, Campbell BI, *et al.* Dementia and depression with ischemic heart disease: a

population-based longitudinal study comparing interventional approaches to medical management. *PLoS ONE* 2011;**6**:e17457.

42. Emmrich P, Hahn J, Ogunlade V, *et al.* Neuropathological findings after cardiac surgery – retrospective study over 6 years. *Z Kardiol* 2003;**92**:925–37.

43. Hernandez F, Jr., Brown JR, Likosky DS, *et al.* Neurocognitive outcomes of off-pump versus on-pump coronary artery bypass: a prospective randomized controlled trial. *Ann Thorac Surg* 2007;**84**:1897–903.

44. Motallebzadeh R, Bland JM, Markus HS, Kaski JC, Jahangiri M. Neurocognitive function and cerebral emboli: randomized study of on-pump versus off-pump coronary artery bypass surgery. *Ann Thorac Surg* 2007;**83**(2):475–82.

45. Vedin J, Nyman H, Ericcson A, Hylander S, Vaage J. Cognitive function after on or off pump coronary artery bypass grafting. *Eur J Cardiothorac Surg* 2006;**30**(2):305–10.

46. Al-Ruzzeh S, George S, Bustami M, *et al.* Effect of off-pump coronary artery bypass surgery on clinical, angiographic, neurocognitive, and quality of life outcomes: randomised controlled trial. *Br Med J.* 2006;**332**:1365

47. Ernest CS, Worcester MU, Tatoulis J, *et al.* Neurocognitive outcomes in off-pump versus on-pump bypass surgery: a randomized controlled trial. *Ann Thorac Surg* 2006;**81**:2105–14.

48. Jensen BO, Hughes P, Rasmussen LS, Pederson PU, Steinbruchel DA. Cognitive outcomes in elderly high-risk patients after off-pump versus conventional coronary artery bypass grafting: a randomized trial. *Circulation* 2006;**113**:2790–5.

49. Jensen BO, Rasmussen LS, Steinbruchel DA. Cognitive outcomes in elderly high-risk patients 1 year after off-pump versus on-pump coronary artery bypass grafting. A randomized trial. *Eur J Cardiothorac Surg* 2008;**34**:1016–21.

50. Lund C, Sundet K, Tennoe B, *et al.* Cerebral ischemic injury and cognitive impairment after off-pump and on-pump coronary artery bypass grafting surgery. *Ann Thorac Surg* 2005;**80**:2126–31.

51. Lee JD, Lee SJ, Tsushima WT, *et al.* Benefits of off-pump bypass on neurologic and clinical morbidity: a prospective randomized trial. *Ann Thorac Surg* 2003;**76**:18–25.

52. van Dijk D, Jansen EW, Hijman R, *et al.* Cognitive outcome after off-pump and on-pump coronary artery bypass graft surgery: a randomized trial. *JAMA* 2002;**287**:1405–12.

53. van Dijk D, Spoor M, Hijman R, *et al.* Cognitive and cardiac outcomes 5 years after off-pump vs on-pump coronary artery bypass graft surgery. *JAMA* 2007;**297**:701–8

Glossary

ABCDE bundle: An evidence-based concept for the management of mechanically ventilated, critically ill patients that stands for Awakening and Breathing Coordination, attention to the Choice of Sedation, Delirium monitoring, and Early mobility and exercise.

Adrenal insufficiency: Inappropriate synthesis, delivery, or response to cortisol resulting in a syndrome of muscle weakness, electrolyte imbalance, and circulatory shock, as well as unchecked systemic inflammation. In the critically ill, this is better termed as "critical illness-related corticosteroid insufficiency."

Adverse drug reactions (ADR): Harm associated with the use of pharmacological agents at a normal dosage during normal use. ADRs may occur following a single dose or prolonged administration of a drug or result from the combination of two or more drugs.

Allostasis: Capacity of an organism to maintain biological stability through changes caused by stressors which mobilize the hypothalamic-pituitary-adrenal axis, the autonomic nervous system, cardiovascular and immune systems.

Amino acid neurotransmitters: Non-peptide neurotransmitters derived from amino acid metabolism. These are classified as excitatory (glutamate, aspartate, cysteine, homocysteine) and inhibitory (gamma-amino butyric acid, glycine, beta-alanine, and taurine).

Anticholinergic syndrome: Syndrome precipitated by antagonists of the muscarinic acetylcholine receptors, including encephalopathy, tachycardia, pupillary dilation, dry skin, urinary retention, and decreased bowel sounds.

Atypical antipsychotic: Second-generation antipsychotics, including olanzapine, risperidone, quetiapine, ziprasidone; decreased D_2 receptor binding affinity, relatively more activity at other receptors (serotonin, muscarinic, alpha-adrenergic, histaminergic); overall associated with fewer extrapyramidal symptoms relative to haloperidol, but similar risk for QTc prolongation and torsades de pointes.

Autonomic dysfunction: Deviation from the normal function of the autonomic nervous system, which may be observed in a range of neurological disorders, but also in sepsis and multi-organ dysfunction.

Burst-suppression: EEG pattern characterized by alternating periods of generalized electrical suppression and generalized bursts of high voltage, chaotic, often epileptiform activity. It may be induced by anesthetic agents or global cortical injury.

Cecal ligation and puncture (CLP): Well-established animal model for polymicrobial sepsis. It involves ligation and subsequent puncture of the caecum, generating local and systemic inflammatory responses.

Cerebral pressure autoregulation: The physiological regulatory mechanism that maintains a relatively constant CBF over a wide range of mean arterial pressures (c. 60–160 mmHg) or cerebral perfusion pressures (c. 50–150 mmHg). It can be regarded as the brain's second defense mechanism against hypo- and hyperperfusion, superimposed on the baroreceptor reflex.

Cholinergic deficiency hypothesis: States that impairments in the cholinergic system are central in eliciting signs and symptoms during delirium, through its effects on attention combined with the disinhibitory effects on microglia, sustaining a neuroinflammatory reaction in the brain.

Cholinesterase inhibitors: Medications that inhibit cholinesterase, an enzyme responsible for the breakdown of acetylcholine in the synapse. Used to treat dementia in the elderly; not recommended for treatment of ICU delirium.

Cognitive impairment: Abnormal and clinically significant deficits in cognitive function that affect executive function, learning, memory, attention, concentration, intelligence, or other cognitive functions.

Cognitive rehabilitation: Interventions that seek to restore lost or degraded cognitive functions, or compensatory strategies that allow individuals to "work around" their cognitive impairments.

Cognitive reserve: Moderates the association between brain pathology and expression; individuals with higher reserve are better able to cope with brain pathology than those with lower reserve.

Coma: Severe impairment in arousal and in awareness. A comatose patient is eye-closed and does not awake under stimulation.

Consciousness: A cognitive state enabling subjective reports (conscious contents), which can be related either to the self (self-consciousness or self-awareness) or to the environment (perceptual consciousness). Being in a conscious state requires a minimal level of arousal, but this necessary condition is not sufficient (e.g., vegetative states or complex epileptic seizures). From a clinical perspective, consciousness is defined by the presence of reproducible intentional behaviors.

Critical illness-associated hyperglycemia: Increased glucose synthesis, resulting from an up-regulation of stress hormones combined with a cytokine-mediated insulin resistance.

Cytokines: Inflammatory-signaling peptides that activate immune cells towards proliferation or differentiation. They serve as communication signals between immune and non-immune cells, generally require *de novo* synthesis, and mostly act in a paracrine manner at very low concentrations.

Delirium: A neuropsychiatric syndrome characterized by an acute onset of impaired attention, associated with altered level of consciousness, disorganized thinking, and a fluctuating course, generally associated with an underlying medical or physiological disturbance or exposure to psychoactive medications. Signs may include agitation, perceptual disturbances, altered sleep–wake cycle, increased or decreased psychomotor activity, and memory impairment.

Delirium tremens: Severe delirium associated with alcohol withdrawal syndrome.

Dementia: Cognitive deficits including primarily, but not exclusively, impaired memory along with disturbance in at least one additional cognitive domain; severity impacts functional ability, with a typical pattern of progression.

Electron paramagnetic resonance: A technique for studying materials with unpaired electrons.

Endoplasmic reticulum stress: Damage to endoplasmic reticulum lipids and proteins and loss of calcium stores causes accumulation of newly synthesized unfolded proteins, which impairs translation of new proteins.

Endothelial activation: Process by which endothelial cells produce and express adhesion molecules, including E-selectin, P-selectin, ICAM, and VCAM, which attract and adhere to immune cells. This can lead to passage of immune cells through the capillary-venous endothelial surface and into the perivascular space.

Endothelin: Peptide synthesized primarily in the endothelium, which is among the most potent vasoconstrictors known.

Energy metabolism disorders: Enzymatic defects in metabolic pathways leading to ATP production. Since neurons and glial cells use glucose as a principal source of energy, the energy metabolism disorders causing encephalopathies tend to be on the mitochondrial part of the glucose metabolism pathway (pyruvate oxidation, Krebs cycle, and oxidative phosphorylation).

Executive function: A set of cognitive abilities, mediated largely by frontal brain regions, that are responsible for the successful execution of complex, goal-directed activities such as decision making, planning, organization, developing strategies, working memory, and managing time.

Extrapyramidal symptoms: Spectrum of movement disorders associated with dopamine receptor blockade.

Most common side effect of antipsychotics, especially haloperidol; symptoms include involuntary movements, restlessness, uncontrollable speech, dystonia, or inability to initiate movement.

False neurotransmitter hypothesis: Theory attributing encephalopathy to the action of small molecules which act as neurotransmitters disrupting normal synaptic function.

Flow-metabolism coupling: The brain's (regional) adaptation of blood flow to changing metabolic requirements or function.

Heart rate variability (HRV): Variability in the beating pattern of the heart, often quantified from ECG data. HRV is clinically important as it has been shown to correlate with some disease states, and observable changes in HRV can arise before there are significant changes in other physiological signals.

Hepatic encephalopathy: The spectrum of neuropsychiatric abnormalities seen in patients with liver dysfunction, after exclusion of other known brain disease. Ammonia is the main pathophysiological factor.

Human endotoxemia: A model of systemic inflammation consisting of the treatment of healthy human subjects with small doses of endotoxin (lipopolysaccharides, LPS). LPS binds to Toll-like receptor 4 (TLR4) leading to the production of inflammatory mediators. This provides a controlled experimental model of TLR4 agonist-induced systemic inflammation, which is a component of the early sepsis response.

Hyperacute liver failure: Distinguished on time from jaundice to encephalopathy (7 days or less). Hyperacute liver failure may present with encephalopathy prior to onset of clinical jaundice and has the greatest severity of coagulopathy, severity of encephalopathy, and increased intracranial hypertension as compared with acute and subacute forms of the disease. It is associated with a greater chance of spontaneous recovery without need for liver transplantation compared with acute disease presentation.

Hyperammonemia: Ammonia is mainly delivered to the liver through the portal vein, and urea is produced via the urea cycle. In significant liver dysfunction and/or increased portosystemic shunting, there is increased delivery of ammonia to the brain. Ammonia crosses the blood–brain barrier and is used by astrocytes to transform glutamate into glutamine. Astrocyte metabolic dysfunction, apoptosis, and swelling are the main consequences that will contribute to alteration of GABA, glutaminergic, dopaminergic, and serotoninergic neurotransmission.

Hypoxic-ischemic encephalopathy (HIE): Neurological disorder provoked by a sudden and global decrease in brain oxygen supply, most commonly seen after cardiac arrest, refractory circulatory shock, and severe hypoxemia.

I WATCH DEATH: Mnemonic for the differential diagnosis of delirium: Infections, Withdrawal, Acute metabolic, Trauma, Central nervous system pathology,

Hypoxia, Deficiencies, Endocrinopathies, Acute vascular events, Toxins/drugs, Heavy metals.

Ictal–interictal continuum: The dynamic link between damaged neurons and the abnormal systemic and cerebral metabolism associated with critical illness, as manifest on EEG by patterns such as periodic discharges or rhythmic delta activity.

Immune-to-brain communication pathways: Enable the transmission of information from the peripheral immune system to the brain. However, the neural pathway involving the sensory nerves innervating the site of infection plays a predominant role in the induction of sickness behavior.

Indoleamine 2,3 dioxygenase: A ubiquitous enzyme that metabolizes tryptophan along the kynurenine pathway. Activation of this enzyme is normally responsible for some aspects of immunotolerance. However, activation during inflammation also acts as a molecular switch that favors the transition from sickness behavior to depression.

Induced hypothermia: Treatment that aims to cool patients in order to protect tissues (particularly brain) from ischemia–reperfusion injuries.

Instrumental activities of daily living (IADL): Complex skills needed to successfully live independently (e.g., managing finances). Standardized assessments of IADLs are commonly used as a measurement of the functional status of a person.

Intensive Care Delirium Screening Checklist (ICDSC): A delirium assessment tool that utilizes eight diagnostic features to evaluate brain function.

Intensive Care Unit-Acquired Weakness (ICUAW): Clinically detectable, generalized neuromuscular weakness in critically ill patients. This is caused by a myopathy, polyneuropathy, or neuromyopathy acquired in the setting of an underlying critical illness (e.g., sepsis, multiple organ failure).

ISPOR Principles of Good Practice: Outline of a structured translation and cultural adaptation process established by the International Society for PharmacoEconomics and Outcomes Research.

Leigh syndrome: A characteristic acute necrotizing encephalopathy involving the deep grey matter. It is exclusively observed in energy metabolism disorders that can be inherited or acquired.

Lipopolysaccharide (LPS): A key component of the cell wall of Gram-negative bacteria, which activates Toll-like receptor 4 and is used to mimic sepsis in experimental settings.

Long-term potentiation (LTP): A stimulus-induced increase in the efficiency of synaptic transmission sustained above the baseline response for hours or longer.

Luxury perfusion: Following events such as stroke or brain infarction, the intrinsic mechanism of autoregulation can fail, with loss of vascular tone, leading to passive excess blood flow passing through a brain region, which is also termed "hyperperfusion."

Major depression (MD): A disturbance of mood characterized by depressed mood, diminished self-attitude, anhedonia, and at least three of the following: inability to fall asleep or excessive sleep, impaired concentration, diminished energy, decreased or increased appetite, psychomotor retardation or agitation, and suicidal ideation. Symptoms are present for at least 2 weeks. MD is characterized by changes in central monoamine levels, elevated GC release, and alterations in the HPA feedback mechanisms.

Metabolic encephalopathy: A potentially reversible alteration of cognitive processes or consciousness in response to systemic toxins, such as byproducts of metabolism, pharmacological agents, or systemic illness. It frequently produces characteristic patterns of diffuse, rhythmic EEG slowing.

Microglia: Resident macrophages of the brain and spinal cord that are exquisitely sensitive to changes in brain homeostasis and rapidly change their morphology and antigen expression to insult or injury, acting as the first and main form of active immune defense in the central nervous system.

Microglial priming: Activation of microglial cells by features of chronic neurodegeneration, so they produce exaggerated responses to subsequent stimulation with lipopolysaccharide. The partially activated state is referred to as primed.

MicroPET: Positron emission tomography images obtained in living systems by recording high-energy gamma-rays emitted from within the subject.

Minimally conscious state: Patients with unequivocal but inconsistent behaviors indicating conscious arousal.

Monoamine transmitters: Dopamine, noradrenaline, and serotonin (5-hydroxytryptamin).

Muscarinic syndrome: Drug-induced cholinergic excess presenting as altered mental status, bradycardia, hypotension, pupillary constriction, tearing, bronchorrhoea, bronchospasm, gastrointestinal cramps, vomiting, diarrhea, and urination.

Necroptosis: A caspase-independent, extrinsic cell death pathway, in which ligand binding to a tumor necrosis factor superfamily receptor leads to formation of a complex of receptor interacting protein-1 and receptor interacting protein-3, through the kinase activity of receptor interacting protein-1, and in which the cell morphology resembles necrosis.

Neural compensation: The adoption of new neural networks, due to injury or pathology, interrupting pathways normally in use for a given task.

Neural reserve: Brain networks or cognitive paradigms that are efficient and flexible, making them adaptable and less prone to disruption. This is an important coping mechanism that brain-injured individuals utilize when faced with task demands.

Neuroimmunomodulation: Mechanisms by which local and systemic immune processes act upon the brain, and how the brain modulates the susceptibility and course of inflammatory, infectious, neoplastic, and autoimmune diseases.

Neuromodulation: How neurotransmission, neuronal networks, and neuronal properties may be affected.

Neuroprotection: Aims to prevent cell loss by interrupting the biochemical cascade leading to neuronal damage, until homeostatic mechanisms are able to provide the balance necessary to maintain neuronal integrity.

Non-convulsive seizures and status epilepticus: Seizures that do not exhibit clinically apparent signs or symptoms. While the most common sign is non-focal coma, others include nystagmus or eye deviation. These are most common in the critically ill, and require an electroencephalogram (EEG) for diagnosis.

Opioid syndrome: Association of sedation, bradypnea, and pinpoint miosis.

Ornithine transcarbamylase (OTC) deficiency: The most frequent urea cycle disorder. The gene coding for OTC lies on the X chromosome. Hemizygote men are usually affected more severely than heterozygote females. Adult forms of the disease are usually observed in heterozygotes, but late-onset presentations have been described in hemizygotes as well.

Parthanatos: A caspase-independent cell death pathway, in which oxidative damage to DNA leads to overactivation of poly(ADP-ribose) polymerase, translocation of apoptosis-inducing factor from the mitochondria to the nucleus, and initiation of large-scale DNA fragmentation.

Penumbra: An ischemic region that has the potential to be salvaged if reperfusion is instituted.

Pharmacogenomics: Studies the influence of genetic variation on drug response in patients by correlating gene expression or single-nucleotide polymorphisms with a drug's efficacy or toxicity.

Pharmacokinetics: Evaluation of the mechanisms of absorption, distribution, metabolism, and excretion of administered drugs.

Phasic alertness: Increased capacity to rapidly respond to an external target, induced by a warning stimulus presented before the target.

Post-resuscitation syndrome: Clinical and biological abnormalities observed after cardiac arrest, resulting from ubiquitous tissue ischemia–reperfusion and associated with a systemic inflammatory response.

Posttraumatic stress disorder (PTSD): An anxiety disorder occurring after experiencing a traumatic stressor that is either actually or perceived to be life-threatening. PTSD is characterized by intrusive recollections of the event, symptoms of hyperarousal, and avoidant behavior related to the traumatic event. Symptoms are present for at least 1 month.

RASS or Richmond Agitation–Sedation Scale: A scale ranging from −5 to +4 (negative numbers indicate sedation, positive numbers indicate agitation, 0 indicates alert and calm) used to assess the level of arousal in ICU patients, that can detect variations in the level of consciousness over time or in response to changes in sedative and analgesic drug use.

Riker Sedation–Agitation Scale: An arousal scale ranging from 1 to 7 used to assess level of sedation or agitation, scored by degree of stimulation required to obtain arousal (level 1–3) or the most severe degree of patient's agitation (level 5–7), with 4 indicating a calm patient.

Seizures: Paroxysmal neurological events resulting from abnormal, excessive, or hypersynchronous activity of neuronal networks. They present clinically with a wide variety of transient signs or symptoms, may be focal or generalized, and typically last no more than 2–3 minutes.

Selective attention: Mechanisms determining more extensive processing of some inputs than others.

Sepsis: Infection associated with a systemic inflammatory response.

Serotonin syndrome: Features attributed to a pro-serotonin drug and including myoclonus, encephalopathy, pupillary dilation, sweating, tachycardia, hyperthermia, hypotension, diarrhea, and characteristic biological abnormalities, in the absence of any withdrawal syndrome or recent modification in an antipsychotic treatment.

Sickness behavior: Profound behavioral alterations, induced by innate immune stimulation, that develop during an infection. Responses include reduced motor activity, suppressed appetite, reduced motivation, and altered sleep–wake cycle. By conserving energy and reducing the probability of spreading the infection, sickness behavior contributes to adaptation. These altered behavioral patterns can act as a significant confound in assessing cognitive function.

Somatosensory evoked potentials (SSEPs): Electrophysiological signals recorded along the spinothalamic tract from the peripheral nervous system through the spinal cord, brainstem, thalamus, and cortex, in response to electrical stimulation.

Spatial cueing: A response time paradigm to study spatial attention by presenting visual targets preceded by cues.

Spatial neglect: A neurological condition resulting from dysfunction of fronto-parietal networks in the non-dominant hemisphere, causing unawareness of events occurring on the left.

Spontaneous recovery: The time period (weeks to months) after brain injury in which there is some restitution of lost function due to neuronal structural changes, such as neurogenesis, neuroplasticity, and neural reorganization.

Status epilepticus (SE): A single, unremitting seizure lasting more than 5 minutes, or recurring seizures without an interictal return to the baseline clinical state. When SE does not respond to medications, it is termed "refractory." If SE returns after anesthetic medications have been used, it is termed "malignant" or "super-refractory."

Subsyndromal delirium (SSD): A syndrome that does not include all key features of delirium. Patients with SSD have a significantly worse outcome compared with patients without any delirium symptoms.

Sympatho-adrenal response: The synergistic cross-talk between the noradrenergic system and the hypothalamic-pituitary-adrenal axis to mount an appropriate response to stress.

Systemic inflammatory response syndrome (SIRS): The host response to a severe insult of infectious or non-infectious origin, mediated by pro-inflammatory signaling cascades. Defined according to criteria of fever (or hypothermia), tachycardia, tachypnea, leukocytosis (or leukopenia). Lies on a spectrum that includes sepsis, severe sepsis, septic shock, and refractory septic shock.

Toxidrome or toxic syndrome: Cluster of symptoms, signs, laboratory test results, and electrocardiographic abnormalities associated with drug or poison intoxication.

Triphasic waves: Bilaterally synchronous bursts of complexes with an initial negative deflection, followed by a positive deflection, then another negative deflection, with a characteristic frontal predominance and anterior-posterior lag. These are commonly seen in metabolic encephalopathies.

Vascular endothelial growth factor (VEGF): A protein up-regulated in the setting of tissue hypoxemia. Effects include angiogenesis and altered endothelial permeability, with the development of vasogenic edema.

Vegetative state: This is seen in patients in whom phenotypes of arousal are preserved (e.g., eyes open), even if still abnormal (no clear architecture of sleep–wake cycles), but without any awareness of self or environment.

Index

Number or Greek letter prefixes are filed as if spelt out.
Locators in **bold** refer to tables.